The "Golden Beads"

A Compilation From Leading Materia Medicas

OF

Kent, Boericke, Clarke, Blackwood and Allen

Dr. A.K.C. KUNJ

B. Jain Publishers (P) Ltd.
New Delhi

Note

Any information given in this book is not intended to be taken as a replacement for medical advice. Any person with a condition requiring medical attention should consult a qualified practitioner or therapist.

Price:

First Edition : 1997
Reprint edition 1998, 2002

Published by :
Kuldeep Jain
For
B. Jain Publishers (P.) Ltd.
1921, Street No. 10, Chuna Mandi,
Paharganj, New Delhi 110 055 (INDIA)
Phones: 3670430; 3670572; 3683200; 3683300
FAX 011-3610471 & 3683400
Email: bjain@vsnl.com

Printed in India by:
Unisons Techno Financial Consultants (P) Ltd.
522, FIE, Patpar Ganj, Delhi - 110 092

BOOK CODE : BK-5203

Preface

I took nearly 10 years to complete this book compiling from Materia Medicas of M/s William Boericke, John Henry Clarke, A.L. Blackwood, J.T. Kent, H.C. Allen (Key Notes) and so many other leading ones. The following abbreviations are used in the text, for showing the respective authors.

1. Boericke	for William Boericke
2. JHC	for John Henry Clarke
3. Blackwood	for A.L. Blackwood
4. Kent	for J.T. Kent
5. HCA	for H.C. Allen

Here I could reflect my 35 years of experience in Homoeo System of medicine, and my understanding after going through hundreds of books and literature available on this system.

I did not venture to write a separate Repertory for this Compilation, because I feel that one can use any one of the Repertories available with the materia medica of the above mentioned authors. Moreover in my opinion that a Homoeopath should know the disease totally, i.e., Mental, Physical, General and Particular - thereafter he should try to find out drugs available in the Materia Medica - matching for those conditions of the disease.

Repertory is helpful to some extent for narrowing down the group of drugs for the selection, but without mastering the Materia Medica, selecting the drug will always lead to wrong prescription.

After going through this compilation, I hope that one may develop the inquisity to know more from the quoted Original Books of the Authors, and enhance their knowledge on this subject.

The philosophy of Homoeopathy i.e. Similia Similibus Curentur and its application is known to all of us, who practise this system. But in the next chapter, I tried to explain it further in my Article 'A thought for all of us' in which one can comprehend vividly.

I hope that this book is going to be very useful for the students of Homoeopathy and the practising doctors of this science.

I submit this book at the feet of Dr. Samuel Hahnemann, founder and teacher of this science.

New Delhi-5
Dated. 1.9.1996

Dr. A.K.C. KUNJ

A THOUGHT FOR ALL OF US

All of us Homoeopaths know that the Homoeo system of medicine is very effective in curing diseases. How these drugs are effective in the curing process has been explained in many ways. The theory is that when a drug is potentised, i.e., when the material quantity of the drug is reduced by diluting it in a suitable medium, the power of that substance is increased for the purpose of healing. All explanations that we hear in this regard are not fully convincing and lack 'something' which can satisfy an enquiring intellect. Hence within the contraints of this article, I am endeavouring to explain this phenomenon in a different way from what I have learnt and gathered through the works and teachings of the great masters of this science.

In order to simplify my concept of this science, I have divided the interpretation into two main headings:

1. Disease

2. Drugs

Disease:

What is meant by the word 'Disease'? It is a way of expressing that one is not 'at ease', and that the harmonious functioning of the body organs is disturbed. In such a condition, we observe that the body has deviated from its normal functioning behaviour. This disturbance is manifested in the body, subjectively and objectively, by bringing out certain 'Symptoms'. Though at this point of time one feels disturbed, it is to be understood that there is a purpose behind these 'Symptoms' creating uneasiness. The manifestation of 'Symptoms' only goes to show that the body is struggling to bring back the 'balanced' level of the body's normal functioning. It is therefore, to be understood, that these 'Disease Symptoms' are actually, necessary Factors at that 'Point of time', thereby enabling the body to re-establish its normalcy.

At the same time, however, it should be known, that at the onset of a disease all the Symptoms required to overcome that condition do not develop immediately or manifest in the body. This takes its own course, time and sequence, depending upon the existing 'Dynamic strength' of the body.

A body having sufficient dynamic strength, thereby being able to develop all the required symptoms immediately, will not go into a condition of disease at all. The disease condition can be felt, only when the body cannot bring out all the required symptoms immediately-in other words, some of the required symptoms at that point of time are still to surface.

The period of struggle by the body to bring out these "required lacking symptoms" is the period of that disease. As soon as these "required lacking symptoms" are brought out, the harmony of the body is re-established and it becomes disease free.

A disease free state can be achieved either by the body's own dynamic strength, or by the application of such medicine which assists in bringing out these "Required Lacking

Symptoms". It is known that these symptoms are a reaction of the body organs and its complex system, manifested inwardly or outwardly either to accommodate or repel a certain thing unsuitable to it at that point of time.

Drugs

Regarding the Micro quantity dose of drugs and its Homoeopathic application, it was clearly defined by Dr. Hahnemann, the founder of Homoeopathy, that when a certain drug, in a large material dose, is administered to a healthy body, it will vitiate the normal functioning of the body and bring out a group of 'Disease like Symptoms'. He had also said that the drug when administered in a Micro Quantity dose will also bring out the same group of symptoms, but with a lesser intensity, since there will be a 'Struggle in the body' to accommodate or discard the foreign substance within it. If in case, all the required symptoms are not produced by the body then the body's "Struggle" will continue in a progressive way, bringing out more and more symptoms within the limits of the Body's dynamic strength and this process will continue until all the required symptoms are produced, or else it will collapse in the process.

It is therefore, for the physician to identify a Drug which has symptom similar in character to the symptoms manifested by the disease condition of the body. This selection can be done with the help of a "Materia medica". In a Materia medica the symptoms available in a drug may exceed in number than the symptoms manifested in the body with the disease. These extra available symptoms of the selected drug are the real curing factors for that Natural disease for which the Drug has been selected.

In a natural disease the body is in a state of 'Struggle' in trying to develop the 'Extra Symptoms' which are the "CURING FACTORS". Strangely enough the law of Nature is that when a group of 'Characteristic Symptoms' is found in a Natural disease there are Drugs also existing, which can produce a similar group of characteristic symptoms, PLUS some extra symptoms of its own. Generally, it is found that these extra symptoms available in a selected Drug are the "REQUIRED LACKING SYMPTOMS" for the dearth of which the body is in a state of struggle at that point of time of the Natural disease. Hence, as described earlier, in case the body is incapable of bringing out these "Required lacking symptoms" using its own dynamic strength, the administering of a similar symptom producing drug with its "Extra Symptoms", will assist in the process of healing of that natural disease.

This phenomenon is illustrated as follows:

Let the number of Symptoms produced by a body, using its own dynamic strength at a point of time to combat a certain disease force, thus endeavouring to re-establish its functional normalcy.	(A+B+C)
Let the total number of symptoms required by the body to combat the above said disease force in order to regain its functional normalcy.	(A+B+C+D+E+F)

Hence the number of "REQUIRED LACKING SYMPTOMS" for the above said disease condition.	(A+B+C+D+E+F)minus(A+B+C)=(D+E+F)
The total number of symptoms produced by a healthy body after administration of a selected drug having some similar characteristics of the above said disease found in a Materia Medica. (Symptoms of the selected drug alone)	(A+B+C+D+E+F+G+H)
Therefore the total symptoms produced by the body with the above said disease condition after administering the above said 'similar symptom' producing Drug.	(A+B+C)+(A+B+C+D+E+F+G+H) =(2A+2B+2C+D+E+F+G+H)
Hence the "Residual symptoms" after body acquires the "Required Lacking Symptoms" from the administered Drug.	(2A+2B+2C+D+E+F+G+H) minus(A+B+C+D+E+F)=(A+B+C+G+H)

The above illustration shows that the 'Extra Symptom' (D+E+F) of the Drug have been utilised by the body to activate its Dynamic strength in order to cure the existing disease condition. At the same time, the Un-utilised Residual Symptoms i.e. (A+B+C+G+H), are the unwanted Factors in this applications, thus creating a negligible disturbance in the body. The duration and the intensity of this will be too short to be felt, as the administered Drug is in a 'Micro' quantity. The more the Micro quantity of the Drug, the lesser is the residual drug reaction.

When the dynamic strength of a body is sufficient enough to produce most of the required symptoms, a more diluted, similar symptom producing Drug (High Potency-in Homoeo terms) only will be required to create the necessary reaction to combat the disease force. On the other hand, when the dynamic strength of the patient is feeble and low or genetically something is lacking in the body constitution, the Required Symptoms developed to combat disease will naturally be lesser; this results in the disease becoming chronic in nature. In such a situation, a less diluted (Low Potency) similar symptom producing drug is administered as a supportive agent to the body systems.

The drug symptoms produced by a Micro-dose, are very mild in intensity, exciting the nervous system by its mere contact or proximity (nearness). For example, a foul smell or sight can elicit vomiting, or in the field of emanation of certain substances, skin allergies, bronchial disturbances etc., are caused. Hence, it is interesting to note that the material quantity of a Drug does not have much relevance in Homoeo Therapy.

From the above theorization one can find more vivid explanations for the following questions:

Q.1 Why are Homoeo Medicines harmless as compared to allopathic medicines, even when administered on a non-similimum selection by a Novice?

A. The symptoms produced by the Drug are very mild in intensity, even though the required 'Lacking Symptoms' are not available in it.

Q.2 Why is the solvent used in potentization process also not in a Potentised form? Would it not act as a potentised Drug when administered with a selected Drug?

A.2 The selected Drug gets diluted in the potentisation process but the Solvent Material used is an inert substance and in its own symptoms, the 'Required Lacking Symptoms' may not be present, and stay inactive when administered with selected Drug in it.

Q.3 How are curative results found to be achieved by combining a number of Drugs together in Mother Tincture form or in low potencies and administered as a mixture?

A.3 As long as the 'Required Lacking Symptoms' are there in the combination, the curative power will be in it. However, the 'Unwanted Symptoms' produced by the surplus Drugs, will disturb the body adversely.

Q.4 It has been found that in several diseases, two, three or more potentised Drugs are used simultaneously for effecting a cure?

A.4 The 'Required Lacking Symptoms' will be provided by those Drugs combinedly thus a Cure is achieved.

In this way, it is now possible to rationally find answers to questions, which was, so far, not possible.

I urge my colleagues and other readers, to read this Write-up. I shall be happy to receive their comments.

Dr. A.K.C.Kunj
Homoeopath

Elakkat Villa
Near Karuna Temple
P.O. Kumaranellore
Trichur Dist (Kerala State)
Pin - 680590

INDEX

S. No. Name Of Medicine *Page No*

Preface iii
1 Abies canadensis 1
2 Abies nigra 1
3 Abrotanum 1
4 Absinthium 2
5 Acalypha indica 3
6 Acetanilidum 3
7 Acetic acid 3
8 Aconitum nap 4
9 Aconitinum 6
10 Actea spicata 6
11 Adonis vernalis 7
12 Adrenalin 7
13 Aesculus hippocastanum 9
14 Aethiops mercurialis 10
15 Aethusa cynapium 10
16 Agaricus muscarius 11
17 Agave americana 13
18 Agnus cactus 13
19 Agraphis nutans 14
20 Ailanthus glandulosa 14
21 Aletris farinosa 15
22 Alfalfa 16
23 Allium cepa 17
24 Allium sativum 17
25 Alnus rubra 18
26 Aloe 19
27 Alstonia scholaris 20
28 Alumen 21
29 Alumina 22
30 Alumina silicata 24
31 Ambra grisea 24
32 Ambrosia 25
33 Ammoniacum doreina 26
34 Ammonium benz 26
35 Ammonium brom 26
36 Ammonium carb 27
37 Ammonium caust 28
38 Ammonium iod 28
39 Ammonium mur 28
40 Ammonium phos 30
41 Ammonium pic 30
42 Ammonium val 30
43 Ampelopsis 30
44 Amygdalus persica 30
45 Amyl nitrosum 31
46 Anacardium 31
47 Anagallis 32
48 Anatherum 33
49 Anhalonium 33
50 Anemopsis 33
51 Angustura vera 33
52 Anilinum 34
53 Anthemis nobilis 34
54 Anthracinum 34
55 Anthrakokali 34
56 Antimonium ars. 35
57 Antimonium crud 35
58 Antimonium sulph 36
59 Antimonium tart 36
60 Antipyrine 37
61 Apis mel 38
62 Apium grave 40
63 Apocynum andro 40
64 Apocynum can 40
65 Apomorphia 41
66 Aquilegia 41
67 Aragallus lambe 41
68 Aralia racemosa 41
69 Aranea diadema 42
70 Arbutus andra 43

71 Areca 43
72 Argemone mexi 43
73 Argentum met 43
74 Argentum nit 44
75 Aristolochia mil 46
76 Arnica 46
77 Arsenic alb 48
78 Arsenic brom 50
79 Arsenicum hydro 51
80 Arsenicum iod 51
81 Arsenicum met 52
82 Arsenicum sulph flav 52
83 Artemisia vul 52
84 Arum drac 53
85 Arum triph 53
86 Arundo 54
87 Asafoetida 54
88 Asaram europum 55
89 Asclepias syr 55
90 Asclepias tuber 55
91 Asimina tri 56
92 Asparagus off 56
93 Aspidosperma 56
94 Astacus fluv 57
95 Asterias rub 57
96 Astragalus moll 58
97 Aurum met 58
98 Aurum mur nat 60
99 Avena sativa 61
100 Azadirachta ind 61
101 Bacillinum 61
102 Badiaga 62
103 Balsamum peru 62
104 Baptisia 63
105 Barasoma crenata 64
106 Baryta acetica 64
107 Baryta carb 64
108 Baryta mur 66
109 Baryta iodata 67
110 Belladona 67
111 Bellis perennis 69
112 Benzenum 70
113 Benzoicum acid 70
114 Berberis aquifolium 71
115 Berberis vulgaris 72
116 Beta vulgaris 73
117 Betonica 73
118 Bismuthum 73
119 Blatta americana 74
120 Blatta orientalis 74
121 Boletus laricis 74
122 Boricum acid 74
123 Borax 75
124 Bothrops 75
125 Bcthulinum 76
126 Bovista 76
127 Brachyglottis 77
128 Bromium 77
129 Bryonia 78
130 Bufo 81
131 Butyric acid 82
132 Cactus grand 82
133 Cadmium sulph 83
134 Cahinca 83
135 Cajuputum 84
136 Caladium seg 84
137 Calcarea acetica 85
138 Calcarea ars 85
139 Calcarea carb 86
140 Calcarea fluor 89
141 Calcarea iod 89
142 Calcarea lactica 90
143 Calcarea phos 90
144 Calcarea silicata 91
145 Calcarea sulph 91
146 Calendula off 92

147 Calotropis ... 93
148 Caltha palustris ... 94
149 Camphora ... 94
150 Camphora mono bromata ... 95
151 Canchalagua ... 96
152 Cannabis indica ... 96
153 Cannabis sativa ... 97
154 Cantharis ... 97
155 Capsicum ... 99
156 Carbo animalis ... 100
157 Carbo vegetabilis ... 101
158 Carbolicum acid ... 103
159 Carboneum hydro ... 104
160 Carboneum oxy ... 104
161 Carboneum sulph ... 104
162 Carcinosin ... 105
163 Carduus mar ... 106
164 Carlsbad ... 106
165 Cascara sagrada ... 107
166 Cascarilla ... 107
167 Castanea vesca ... 107
168 Castor equi ... 107
169 Castoreum ... 108
170 Catarea nepeta ... 108
171 Caulophyllum ... 109
172 Causticum ... 110
173 Ceanothus ... 111
174 Cedron ... 111
175 Cenchris contortrix ... 112
176 Cereus bonplandi ... 112
177 Cerium oxal ... 112
178 Chamomilla ... 113
179 Chaparro amargoso ... 114
180 Chelidonium majus ... 115
181 Chenopodium anthel ... 116
182 Chenopodi glauci ... 117
183 Chelone ... 117
184 Chimaphila umb ... 117
185 Chininum ars ... 118
186 Chininum sulph ... 118
187 Chionanthus ... 120
188 Chloralum ... 121
189 Chloroform ... 121
190 Chlorum ... 122
191 Cholesterinum ... 122
192 Chromicum acid ... 123
193 Chrysarobinum ... 123
194 Cicuta virosa ... 124
195 Cimex ... 124
196 Cimicifuga ... 125
197 Cina ... 126
198 Cinchona off ... 127
199 Cineraria ... 128
200 Cinnabaris ... 129
201 Cinnamonium ... 129
202 Cistus can ... 129
203 Citrus limon ... 130
204 Citrus vul ... 130
205 Clematis ... 131
206 Cobaltum ... 131
207 Coca ... 132
208 Cocaine ... 133
209 Coccinella ... 133
210 Cocculus ... 133
211 Coccus cactl ... 134
212 Cochlearia armo ... 135
213 Codeinum ... 135
214 Coffea cruda ... 136
215 Colchicum ... 137
216 Collinsonia ... 138
217 Colocynthis ... 139
218 Comocladia ... 141
219 Condurango ... 141
220 Conium ... 142
221 Convallaria ... 143
222 Copaiva ... 144

223 Corallium 145
224 Cornus circinata 146
225 Corydalis 146
226 Cotyledon 147
227 Crataegus oxy 147
228 Crocus sativa 148
229 Cromicum kali sulph 149
230 Crotalus hor 149
231 Croton tig 150
232 Cubeba 151
233 Cucurbita citr 152
234 Cucurbita pepo 152
235 Cuphea 153
236 Cuprum acet 153
237 Cuprum ars 154
238 Cuprum met 155
239 Curare 157
240 Cyclamen 157
241 Cypripedium 158
242 Daphne Indica 159
243 Digitalis 159
244 Dioscorea 161
245 Diphtherinum 161
246 Dolichos 162
247 Doryphora 162
248 Drosera 163
249 Duboisia 163
250 Dulcamara 164
251 Echinacea 165
252 Elaps cor 166
253 Elaterium 166
254 Epigea repens 167
255 Epihysterinum 167
256 Epiphegus 167
257 Equisetum 168
258 Erechthites 168
259 Erigeron 169
260 Eriodictyon 169
261 Eryngium aqua 169
262 Eschscholtzia cal 170
263 Eucalyptus 170
264 Eugenia jambos 172
265 Euonymus 172
266 Eupatorium arom 173
267 Eupatorium perf 173
268 Eupatorium purp 174
269 Euphorbia lath 174
270 Euphorbium 174
271 Euphrasia 175
272 Eupion 176
273 Fabiana imbr 176
274 Fagopyrum 176
275 Fel tauri 177
276 Ferrum met 177
277 Ferrum magnet 180
278 Ferrum phos 180
279 Ferrum pic 181
280 Ficus religosa 182
281 Filix mas 182
282 Fluoricum acid 183
283 Formalin 184
284 Formica rufa 184
285 Fragaria 186
286 Franciscea 186
287 Fraxinus americana 187
288 Fuligo ligina 187
289 Fucus vesiculosis 187
290 Fuchsina mag 187
291 Galium aparine 188
292 Gallium acid 188
293 Gambogia 188
294 Gaultheria 189
295 Gelsemium 189
296 Gentiana lutea 191
297 Geum rivale 191
298 Ginseng 192

299 Glonoine 192
300 Glycerinum 193
301 Gnaphalium 193
302 Gossipium 194
303 Granatum 194
304 Graphites 195
305 Gratiola 196
306 Grindelia 197
307 Guaco 198
308 Guaiacum 198
309 Gun powder 199
310 Hamamelis 199
311 Hekla lava 201
312 Helleborous 202
313 Heloderma 203
314 Helonias 203
315 Hepar sulph 205
316 Hippomanes 206
317 Hippozaenium 207
318 Hoang nan 207
319 Homarus 208
320 Hydrangea 208
321 Hydrastis 209
322 Hydrocotyle 211
323 Hydrocyanic acid 212
324 Hydrophobinum 212
325 Hyoscyamus 213
326 Hypericum 214
327 Iberis 215
328 Ichthyolum 216
329 Ignatia 217
330 Ilex aquifolium 220
331 Indigo 220
332 Indium 221
333 Indol 221
334 Influenzinum 221
335 Insulin 222
336 Inula 222
337 Iodoformum 222
338 Iodum 223
339 Ipecacuanha 226
340 Iridium 227
341 Iris tenax 228
342 Iris versicolor 228
343 Jacaranda 229
344 Jalapa 229
345 Jatropha 230
346 Jequirity 230
347 Jonosia asoka 231
348 Juglans cinerea 232
349 Juglans regia 233
350 Justicia adhatoda 233
351 Kali arsenic 234
352 Kali bichrom 235
353 Kali brom 237
354 Kali carb 238
355 Kali chloricum 240
356 Kali cyanatum 240
357 Kali hydriodicum 241
358 Kali mur 242
359 Kali nitricum 243
360 Kali permanganicum 244
361 Kali phos 245
362 Kali sulph 246
363 Kalmia latifolia 247
364 Kaolin 248
365 Kousso 248
366 Kreosotum 249
367 Lac can 250
368 Lac def 251
369 Lachesis 251
370 Lachnantes 253
371 Lactic acid 254
372 Lactica virosa 255
373 Lapis albus 255
374 Lappa arcticum 256

375 Lathyrus 256
376 Lactrodectus mac 257
377 Laurocerasus 257
378 Lecithin 258
379 Ledum 258
380 Lemna minor 259
381 Leptandra 260
382 Liatris spicata 260
383 Lilium tig 260
384 Lithium carb 261
385 Lobelia infl 262
386 Lolium temul 263
387 Lycopodium 263
388 Lycopus virginicus 267
389 Magnesia carb 268
390 Magnesia mur 269
391 Masgnesia phos 269
392 Magnesia sulph 270
393 Magnetis poli ambo 271
394 Magnetis polus arcticus 271
395 Magnetis polus australis 272
396 Malandrium 272
397 Mancinella 272
398 Manganum acet 273
399 Mangnifera ind 274
400 Medorrhinum 274
401 Medusa 276
402 Melilotus 276
403 Melitagrinum 276
404 Menispermum 277
405 Mentha piperita 277
406 Menyanthes 277
407 Mephitis 278
408 Merc perennis 279
409 Mercurius hydrargyrum 279
410 Mercurius cor 281
411 Mercurius cyanatus 283
412 Mercurius dulcis 283
413 Merc proto iodide 284
414 Mercurius iod ruber 284
415 Mercurius sulph 285
416 Methylene blue 285
417 Mezereum 286
418 Millefolium 287
419 Mitchella 287
420 Momordica 288
421 Morbillinum 288
422 Morphinum 289
423 Moschus 290
424 Mucuna urens 290
425 Murex 291
426 Muriatic acid 292
427 Mygale lasiodora 292
428 Musa 293
429 Myrica cerifera 293
430 Myristica sebi 294
431 Naja tripu 295
432 Naphthaline 296
433 Natrum ars 296
434 Natrum carb 297
435 Natrum mur 298
436 Natrum nit 300
437 Natrum phos 300
438 Natrum salicyli 301
439 Natrum sulph 302
440 Niccolum 303
441 Nitric acid 303
442 Nitro muriatic acid 305
443 Nuphar luteum 305
444 Nux moschata 306
445 Nux vomica 307
446 Ocimum can 311
447 Oenanthe crocata 312
448 Oleander 313
449 Oleum animale 313
450 Oleum jecoris 314

451 Oleum santali 315
452 Onosmodium 315
453 Oophorinum 316
454 Opium 316
455 Origanum 318
456 Ornithogalum 318
457 Osmium 318
458 Ovigallinae pell 319
459 Oxallicum acid 319
460 Oxydendron 321
461 Oxytropis 321
462 Paeonia 321
463 Palladium 322
464 Paraffine 323
465 Pareira brava 323
466 Paris quadrifolia 324
467 Parotidinum 324
468 Parthenium 324
469 Penthorum 325
470 Pertussin 325
471 Passiflora 325
472 Petroleum 326
473 Petroselinum 327
474 Phaseolus 328
475 Phellandrium 328
476 Phlorizin 329
477 Phosphoric acid 329
478 Phosphorus 330
479 Physalia 332
480 Physalis-sol 333
481 Physostigma 333
482 Phytolacca 334
483 Picricum acid 336
484 Pilocarpus 337
485 Pilocarpinum 338
486 Pinus sylvestris 339
487 Piper methysticum 339
488 Piperazinum 340
489 Piper nigrum 341
490 Pituitary gland 341
491 Pix liquida 342
492 Plantago maj 342
493 Plantanus occi 343
494 Platina 343
495 Plumbum met 345
496 Podophyllum 346
497 Polygonum 347
498 Populus candicans 348
499 Populus tremul 348
500 Pothos foetidus 349
501 Primula obconica 349
502 Propylamin 350
503 Prunus spinosa 350
504 Psorinum 351
505 Ptelea 352
506 Pulex irritans 353
507 Pulmo vulpis 353
508 Pulsatilla 354
509 Pyrogenum 356
510 Quassia 357
511 Quercus 358
512 Quillaya 358
513 Radium brom 358
514 Ranunculus bulb 360
515 Ranunculus scel 360
516 Raphanus 361
517 Ratanhia 362
518 Rhamus 362
519 Rheum 363
520 Rhododendron 363
521 Rhus aromatica 364
522 Rhus glabra 364
523 Rhus tox 365
524 Rhus ven 368
525 Ricinus communis 368
526 Robinia 369

527 Rosa damascena 369
528 Rumex 370
529 Ruta grav 371
530 Sabadilla 372
531 Sabal serrulata 373
532 Sabina 373
533 Saccharum off 375
534 Salicylicum acid 376
535 Salix nigra 377
536 Salvia off 378
537 Sambucus 378
538 Sanguinaria can 379
539 Sanguinaria nit 380
540 Sanguisuga 381
541 Sanicula 381
542 Santoninum 383
543 Saponaria 383
544 Sarcolatic acid 384
545 Saracenia pur 384
546 Sarsaparilla 384
547 Scarlatinum 386
548 Scilla maritima 386
549 Scirrhinum 387
550 Scrophularia 387
551 Scutellaria 387
552 Secale cor 388
553 Selenium 391
554 Sempervivum 392
555 Senicio aureus 392
556 Senega 392
557 Senna 394
558 Sepia 394
559 Serum anguillar 397
560 Silicea 398
561 Silphium 401
562 Silphium 401
563 Simaruba 402
564 Sinapis nigra 402
565 Skookum chuck 403
566 Solanum lycopersicum 403
567 Solanum nigrum 403
568 Solidago virgo 405
569 Spartium scoparium 406
570 Sphingurus 407
571 Spigelia 407
572 Spiraea ulmaria 408
573 Spiranthes 409
574 Spongia 409
575 Squilla 411
576 Stannum 411
577 Staphisagria 412
578 Stellaria 415
579 Sterculla 415
580 Sticta pulmo 416
581 Stigmata 417
582 Stillingia 418
583 Stramonium 418
584 Strontium carb 419
585 Strophanthus 420
586 Strychninum 422
587 Succinic acid 423
588 Sulphonal 423
589 Sulphur 424
590 Sulphur iod 427
591 Sulphuric acid 428
592 Sumbul 429
593 Symphori carpus 430
594 Symphytum 430
595 Syphilinum 431
596 Syzygium jambol 433
597 Tabacum 434
598 Tanacetum vul 435
599 Taraxacum 436
600 Tarentula his 436
601 Tarentula cub 438
602 Tartaricum acid 438

603 Taxus baccata 438
604 Tellurium 439
605 Terebinthina 440
606 Teucrium 441
607 Thallium 442
608 Thaspium aureum 442
609 Thea 443
610 Theridion 443
611 Thiosinaminum 444
612 Thlaspi bursa pastoris 444
613 Thuja 445
614 Thymol 448
615 Thymus 449
616 Thyroidinum 449
617 Thyroiodinum 452
618 Titanium 452
619 Tribulus terrestris 452
620 Trifolium 452
621 Trillium 453
622 Triosteum 454
623 Triticum 455
624 Trychosanthes 455
625 Trombidium 456
626 Tuberculinum 456
627 Turnera 459
628 Tussilago 459
629 Upas tiente 459
630 Uranium nit 460
631 Urea 460
632 Uricum acid 461
633 Urinum 461
634 Urtica urens 462
635 Usnea barbata 464
636 Ustilago 464
637 Uva ursi 465
638 Vaccininum 465
639 Vaccinium myrt 466
640 Valeriana off 466
641 Vanadium 467
642 Vanilla panifolia 468
643 Variolinum 468
644 Veratrum alb 468
645 Veratrum vir 470
646 Verbascum 472
647 Vesicaria 473
648 Vespa crabro 473
649 Viburnum op 474
650 Viburnum prun 475
651 Vinca minor 476
652 Viola odorata 476
653 Viola tricolor 477
654 Vipera 478
655 Viscum alb 479
656 Wiesbaden 480
657 Wyethia 480
658 Xanthoxylum 480
659 Xerophyllum 481
660 Xray 481
661 Yohimbinum 482
662 Yucca flamentosa 483
663 Zincum acet 483
664 Zincum brom 483
665 Zincum cyanatum 483
666 Zincum iod 484
667 Zincum met 484
668 Zincum mur 486
669 Zincum oxy 486
670 Zincum phos 487
671 Zincum sulph 487
672 Zincum val 487
673 Zingiber 487

Therapeutic Index 489

◆◆◆

1. *Abies Canadensis*

Dyspepsia, Faint feeling in epigastrium, Gnawing hunger, Craving for meat, pickles and Coarse food, Rumbling of gas, Burning in rectum, Prolapse of uterus, Skin cold and clammy.

Mucus membranes are affected by Abies Can and gastric symptoms are most marked and a catarrhal condition of the stomach is produced. There are peculiar cravings and chilly sensation that are very characteristic, especially for women with uterine displacement, probably due to defective nutrition with debility, Respiration and heart action laboured, wants to lie down all the time, Skin cold and clammy, Hands cold, very faint, Right liver and lung, feel small and hard. Gnawing hungry, faint feeling at epigastrium, Tendency to eat far beyond capacity for digestion, distention of stomach and abdomen with palpitation.

Dose: 1-3 potency. *(Boericke)*

This remedy is indicated in cases of Dyspepsia when the patient is irritable and easily annoyed. The mouth is dry. There is a faint feeling in the epigastrium with gnawing hunger and craving for meats, pickles and coarse food and a tendency to eat beyond his capacity. Following the meal there is a rumbling of gas in the intestines. The bowels are constipated and there is often a sensation as of burning in the rectum. As a result of the gastric and intestinal derangement the general nutrition is impaired. The heart's action is disturbed by the accumulation of gas in the intestines. There is prolapsus of the uterus and a feeling of weakness in the pelvic region.

There is pain behind the right shoulder blade and a sensation as of cold water between the shoulders.

The skin is cold and clammy, the hands are cold and shrunken, the patient is greatly prostrated and desire to lie down.

Compare: Nux vomica, Abies Nigra, Helonias (Blackwood)

2. *Abies Nigra*

(Black Spruce)

A powerful and long acting remedy in various forms of disease, whenever the characteristic stomach symptoms are present. Many of the symptoms are associated with gastric disturbance. In dyspeptic trouble of the aged with functional heart symptoms, also after tea or tobacco constipation. Pain in external meatus.

Stomach: Pain in stomach always comes on after eating, sensation of a hard boiled egg lodged in the cardiac end of stomach. Heart's action, heavy and slow, tachycardia, bradycardia.

Dose 1-30 potency *(Boericke)*

Synopsis: Dyspeptic trouble with functional heart symptoms, also after tea or tobacco-sensation of a hard boiled egg lodged in the cardiac end of stomach.

3. *Abrotanum*

(Southernwood)

Synopsis: Marasmus, Lower extremities, Metastasis, Suppressed rheumatism, Nose bleed, Hydrocele, Oozing of blood from navel of new born, Pleurisy after Bryonia, Mumps changing to Testes, and mammae.

A very useful remedy in marasmus especially of lower extremities only yet with good appetite. Metastasis, Rheumatism following checked diarrhoea. Ill effects of suppressed conditions, especially in gouty subjects. Tuberculous peritonitis. Exudative pleurisy and other exudative processes. After operation of the chest for hydrothorax or empyema, a pressing sensation remains. Aggravation of haemorrhoids when Rheumatism improves. Nose bleed and Hydrocele in boys.

Face: Angioma of the face-stomach; feels as if swimming in water; Abdomen: distended; Extremities: Pain in wrists, ankles, Legs greatly emaciated.

Dose: 3rd to 30th potency *(Boericke)*

Artemisia Abrotanum-Lady's love-The most prominent symptom of "Abrot" is the wasting it causes, most marked in lower extremities. It has also-face wrinkled, pale, old looking, feels cold, blue rings around eyes. It is suited to affections of new born children and especially little boys, hydrocele, epistaxis, emaciation, oozing of blood and moisture from navel of new born.

(JHC)

Rheumatic conditions, with heart irritation, epistaxis, bloody urine, anxiety and trembling, when there has been a history of diarrhoea. Suppressed rheumatism. The emaciation being in the lower limbs and gradually spreads upwards, so that the face is last affected. Opposite to Lyco, Nat mur and Psorinum, it has cured pleurisy after Bryonia. Metastasis is a marked feature of Abrot-inflamn of parotid (Mumps) changing to Testes or Mammae is generally cured by Curb Veg. or Puls., but Abrot. has cured when these remedies have failed. Sensitive to cold air and cold damp weather. In boys it cures Hydrocele. *(Kent)*

4. *Absinthium*

(Common Worm Wood)

Synopsis: Epileptiform seizure, Nervous tremors, Hysterical and infantile spasms, Kleptomania, Vertigo with tendency to fall backward, Spasmodic facial twitching.

A perfect picture of Epileptiform is produced by this drug. Nervous tremors precede attack. Sudden and severe giddiness, delirium, with hallucinations and loss of consciousness. Nervous excitement and sleeplessness, Cerebral irritation, hysterical and infantile spasms come within the range of this remedy. Poisoning by mushrooms, Chorea, Tremor, Nervousness, Excitement and sleeplessness in children, Kleptomania.

Head: Vertigo with tendency to fall backward, Spasmodic facial twitching

Dose: 1-6 potency *(Boericke)*

The convulsions of Absinth are preceded by trembling, the patient makes grimaces, bites tongue, foams-Halbert regards "Absinth" as of special service in cases of minor epilepsy where consciousness is not entirely lost. Tremor is a marked feature of the remedy. Tremor of tongue and of heart.

(JHC)

The alcoholic solution of the oil of 'worm wood' is used in the preparation of the french liqueur under the name of 'Absinthe'.

This remedy is of service in case of epileptiform convulsions, Cerebral irritation and infantile hysterical spasm. Epilepsy that is preceded by nervous trembling when there is distortion of the features, the pupils are equally dilated and patient is obliged to walk about. Vertigo-tendency to fall backwards. Compare Artemesia Vulg, Hydrocyanic acid. *(Blackwood)*

5. *Acalypha Indica*

(Indian Nettle)

Phthisis with racking cough, bloody expectoration, Spluttering diarrhoea, pure blood in the morning and dark clotted blood in the evening.

A drug having a marked action on the alimentary canal and respiratory organs. It is indicated in incipient phthisis with hard racking cough, bloody expectoration, arterial haemorrhage but no febrile disturbance. Very weak in the morning gains strength during day. All pathological haemorrhages having notably a morning aggravation. Cough dry, hard, followed by haemoptysis, worse in morning and night. Abdomen-spluttering diarrhoea with forcible expulsion of noisy flatus.

Modality: Worse in morning.

Dose: 3-6 potency. *(Boericke)*

"Cupameni" Indian Acalypha - violent dry cough, followed by bloody expectoration. Expectoration of pure blood in the morning and dark clotted blood in the evening, cough most violent at night. Progressive emaciation. A proving of several Indian physicians has brought out a number of symptoms in the alimentary tracts characterised by burning sense of weight at stomach, flatulence and spluttering diarrhoea.

(JHC)

This remedy is indicated in the early stages of phthisis, with dry racking cough which is followed by haemoptysis.

There is constant severe pain in the chest. The blood is bright red and profuse in the morning but dark and clotted in the afternoon. It is of service in menorrhagia, when the blood is bright red and is worse during the morning. Compare-Millefolium, Phosphorus. *(Blackwood)*

6. *Acetanilidum*

(Anti febrinum)

Depresses heart, respiration and blood pressure, lowers temperature, cyanosis and collapse-increased susceptibility to cold. Destroys red blood corpuscles.

Used as a sedative and antipyretic for various forms of headache and neuralgia-in doses of one to three grains.

Homoeo. dose 3rd potency *(Boericke)*

This agent is employed to depress the temperature in fevers, to allay the pains in La grippe, acute articular rheumatism, lumbago, sciatica and nervous and neuralgic headaches. There is no doubt, but that its use is responsible for many of the cases of heart failure that are so common during recent years. *(Blackwood)*

Given as remedies for migraine and in order to reduce fever several cases of Thrombosis of the lower extremities from heart weakness have followed its use.

(JHC)

7. *Acetic Acid*

(Glacial Acetic Acid)

This drug produces a condition of profound anaemia, with some dropsical symptoms, great debility, frequent fainting, dyspnoea, weak heart, vomiting, profuse urination and sweat, haemorrhage from any part, especially indicated in pale lean persons with lax flabby muscles. Wasting and debility. Acetic acid has the power to liquefy albuminous and fibrinous deposits. Epithelial cancer, internally and locally (W.Owens), sycosis with nodules and formation in the joints. Hard chancre. The 1X solution will soften and cause formation of pus.

Face: Pale, waxen, emaciated.

Stomach: Salivation-fermentation-violent burning pain in stomach and chest, followed by coldness of skin and cold sweat on forehead, abdomen tympanitic, large quantities of pale urine.

Female: Haemorrhage after labour.

Respiratory: Difficult breathing, cough when inhaling.

Back: Pain relieved only by lying on abdomen.

Fever: Hectic, with drenching night sweats, red spot on left cheek. No thirst in fever, sweat profuse cold. Acetic acid is antidotal to all anaesthetic vapours-counteracts sausage poisoning.

Dose: 3-30 potency-not to be repeated often except in croup. *(Boericke)*

The leading features of acetic acid are excessive wasting and debility, Anaemia with waxy pallor of face, intense thirst, burning in throat, nausea, retching and sour rising as met with in cases of cancer and debility. There are gnawing ulcerative pains in stomach, pain and burning in abdomen. Profuse exhausting diarrhoea. It has been used in diabetes. It corresponds to putrid and hectic fevers with night sweats-Haemorrhage, Varicose swellings dropsies-equal parts of Vinegar and hot water make a refreshing sponge down for many conditions of fever, with or without perspiration. *(JHC)*

Haemorrhage from every mucous outlet, nose, throat, lungs, stomach, bowels, uterus, metrorrhagia, vicarious, traumatic epistaxis, marasmus and other wasting diseases of children, cannot sleep lying on the back-rests better lying on belly-follows well after Cinchona, in haemorrhage, after Digitalis in dropsy. *(HCA)*

Vinegar is an old remedy for bad effects of chloroform. It has cured diabetes, either with sugar in the urine or without where there is great thirst, weakness and pallor and loss of flesh. All substances abused as food, become great remedy, such as Vinegar, coffee, common salt etc. We should look to them more often than we do for the stubborn chronic cases. *(Kent)*

8. *Aconitum Nap.*

(Monkshood wolfsbane)

A state of fear, anxiety, anguish of mind and body, physical and mental restlessness. Fright is the most characteristic manifestation of Aconite. Acute, sudden and violent invasion with fever call for it. Does not want to be touched. Sudden and great sinking of strength. Complaints and tension caused by exposure to dry cold weather, draught of cold air, checked perspiration, also complaints from very hot weather, especially gastro-intestinal disturbances etc. First remedy in inflammation, inflammatory fevers. Serous membranes and muscular tissues affected markedly, burning in internal parts, tingling coldness and numbness, Influenza, Tension of arteries, Emotional and physical / mental tension explain many symptoms, when prescribing Aconite. Aconite causes only functional disturbance, no evidence that it can produce tissue change, its action is brief and shows no periodicity. Its sphere is in the beginning of the acute disease and not to be continued after pathological changes come. In Hyperaemia, congestion, not after exudation has set in. Influenza, great fear, anxiety, foreboding and fears, fears death, fears of future, restlessness. Head heavy, hot, bursting, worse on rising. Eyes feel dry and hot, lids swollen hard and red-reflection from snow, after extraction of cinders. Ears very sensitive to noises.

Nose: Smell acutely sensitive, pain at root of nose-mucus membrane dry, nose stopped up, dry or with scanty watery coryza.

On rising the red face becomes deathly pale or he becomes dizzy. Tingling-Neuralgia especially of left side with restlessness, tingling and numbness. Mouth dry, tongue tip tingles, gums hot and inflamed, tongue coated white. Throat red dry constricted. Vomiting with fear, heat, profuse sweat and increased urination, bitter taste. Abdomen sensitive to touch, colic. Stool-Green like chopped herbs. Urine scanty, red hot and painful, retention with screaming and restlessness. Menses suppressed from fright. After pain with fear and restlessness. Breathing oppressed, hoarse. Dry, croupy cough, shortness of breath, worse at night and after midnight.

Heart: Tachycardia, pain in left shoulder, palpitation with anxiety, pulse full, hard, tense and bounding. Extremities-numbness and tingling, hot hands and cold feet-anxious dreams. Skin-Purpura miliaris, pruritus relieved by stimulants.

Fever: cold waves pass through him.

Modalities: Better open air, Worse-warm room, evening, night, lying on affected side, music, from tobacco smoke, dry cold wind.

Dose-6th potency. (also 30th) *(Boericke)*

The Wolfsbane grows in the damp and covered parts of almost every mountainous country in north or middle of Europe, especially in the Jura, Switzerland, Germany and Sweden. Teste mentions that it has the reputation of being much more poisonous to carnivorous animals than to the herbivorous. Aconite is more closely associated with the rise and progress of homoeopathy than any other member of the materia medica. It was Aconite more than any other remedy which paved the way for the disappearance of blood letting from general medical practice. Hughes remarked that the condition to which Aconite is homoeopathic is one of tension. There is emotional and mental tension as shown in fright or fear and its consequences, anxiety and fear of death, tension of the systemic vessels, tension as it is tetanus. We think of Acon in sudden inflammation, especially if caused by cold, dry air, suppressing exhalation of the body. Aneurism had been diagnosed by leading physicians in England and on the mountains amongst which the plant flourishes, give the signature of this remedial action. The mental exaltation some time goes so far as to the predicting of the day and hour of death - clairvoyance. Everything tastes bitter, except water (China everything including water). Imagine they do all their thinking from the stomach. Acon is one of the great pain remedies, lying with Chamo and coffea in the intensity of the pain it causes. Cannot bear to be touched. Cannot bear to be covered. Acon has a very wide sphere of usefulness in affections of the eye. Inflammation of many kinds, from cold, injury, dust, surgical operations, scrofulous inflammation with enlarged glands all come with in its range- sudden blindness- the timing of the aggravation of Acon symptoms is chiefly at night and about midnight that Aconite is really without analogue. Comple: to coffee (in fever, sleeplessness, intolerance of pain) (Gels - effects of bad news, fright, anger) (Bry - effects of cold dry wind) Causation- Fear, Fright, Chill, Cold dry winds- Heat, especially of sun. *(JHC)*

Like a great storm it comes and sweeps over and passes away. Persons who come down with Aconite sickness are plethoric individuals, strong robust people, rugged children and infants become sick and suddenly seem to be threatened with a sudden and violent death, but recovery is quick- complaints that come on suddenly from the very cold weather of winter or from intensely hot weather of summer. Screams with pain. The pains are like knives, they are stinging, cutting, stabbing- vertigo that comes on from fear, from sudden fear- there is a remnant of that fear left, but it will lead you on more strongly towards Opium- Complaints from fear. Aconite has no result of inflammation. Oh what a comforting remedy it is for Toothache - but the violence of toothache, again the same old story from the dry cold winds, plethoric individuals- Aconite patients long for water- Burning is a symptom that runs all through the remedy. If he could only get something bitter, and yet his food tastes bitter- Most of the bowel troubles come on from intense heat in the children- Urine retention from shock. This retention from shock makes it one of our best remedies for retention in the new born- the child has not passed urine- Aconite cures most violent cases of Orchitis. Aconite is so often the infant's remedy because the infant is so often made sick from fright- New born children with difficulty of breathing, after the use of forceps or from tedious labor, the child is breathless- there is difficulty with the heart and in a few hours fever comes on- Aconite is a very simple remedy- Better during expiration- the spasm of the larynx often comes on during inspiration- Along nerves a sensation of heat- a sensation of cold- After Aconite, Arnica and Belladonna follow well. *(Kent)*

9. *Aconitinum*

(Alkaloid of Aconite Nap)

Ice cold sensation creeps up from his feet- Fear of death, anguish, intense chilliness, feeling of sickness- Twitchings and spasms over whole body, especially in face- all symptoms are Agg. by vomiting - All parts except head and stomach feel as if filled with lead — The symptoms of Aconitinum set in with great rapidity. *(JHC)*

10. *Actea Spicata*

(Baneberry)

Suited to men- Violent tearing pains run from decayed tooth to temples- Swelling of joints from slight fatigue- Rheumatic remedy- especially small joints- wrist rheumatism.

This is a Rheumatic remedy, especially of small joints. Tearing, tingling pains characterize it. Wrist rheumatism. Pulsation over whole body, especially liver and renal region, cardio vascular spasms. Pains worse from touch and motion.

Great oppression, shortness of breath on exposure to cold air. Rheumatic pains in small joints - ankles. Swelling of joints from slight fatigue. Wrist swollen. Paralytic weakness on hand.

Dose: 3rd Potency. *(Boericke)*

Especially suited to men (Actea Racemosa to women)- Rheumatism pains notably affecting small joints, wrists, fingers, ankles, toes. Violent tearing pains run from decayed tooth to temples- Swelling of joints from slight fatigue- throbbing in the region of kidneys- urinary calculi- lameness of right arm. *(Black wood)*

11. *Adonis Vernalis*

(Pheasant's Eye)

A heart medicine, after rheumatism or influenza or Bright's disease, where the muscles of the heart are in stage of fatty degeneration, regulating the pulse and increasing the power of contractions of heart, with increased urinary secretions. Most valuable in cardiac dropsy. Low vitality, with weak heart and slow weak pulse. Hydrothorax, Ascites, Anasarca.

Headache from occiput around temple to eyes. Heart: praecordial pain, palpitation and dyspnoea.

Dose: 5-10 drops of the tincture. *(Boericke)*

Like convallaria, Adonis is a popular heart remedy in Russia. It has not been proved but the indication for its use have been defined by experience as follows. Rapid and feeble action of the heart, dropsy, scanty urine with albumen and casts- Valvular disease and cardiac Asthma. There is no record of its use in the potencies- Gave great relief to a water logged patient of seventy four with Mitral regurgitation with one grain doses of Adonidin at eight hour interval after failure of Arsenic and Digitalis- Urinary secretion rose from half a pint to 2 1/2 pints in 24 hours- Breathing was relieved, sleep returned-

Relation: Digit, Conval, Strophanthus. (JHC)

This agent is a cardiac and arterial stimulant and a diuretic. By its direct action upon the heart it increases its rate, force and the blood pressure. It diminishes the frequency of the pulse and increases the force of the cardiac contraction, cyanosis gradually disappears, while dyspnoea is less marked. No cumulative effects were noticed.

It is useful in Hydrothorax, ascites and anasarca, when they are dependent upon a chronic dilation of the heart or Valvular disease. *(Blackwood)*

12. *Adrenalin*

(An internal secretion of supra-renal gland)

Acute congestion of lungs, Asthma, Graves' and Addison's disease, Arteriosclerosis, Angina pectoris, Aortites, rise of blood pressure, bronzing of skin and wasting.

Its chief therapeutic use depends on its vasoconstriction action, therefore a most powerful and prompt astringent and haemostatic and invaluable in checking capillary haemorrhages from all parts where local or direct application is feasible. Nose, ear, mouth, throat, larynx, stomach, rectum, uterus, bladder. Haemorrhagic condition not due to defective coagulation of the blood. Complete bloodlessness,

Ischaemia may be induced with impunity. Locally solutions 1:1,000-1:10,000 sprayed or applied on cotton have been very efficient in bloodless operation about the eye, nose, throat and larynx.

Therapeutically adrenaline has been suggested in acute congestion of lungs Asthma, Graves' and Addisons' disease, arteriosclerosis, chronic aortitis, angina pectoris, haemophilia, chlorosis, hay fever, serum rashes, acute urticaria etc.

Dr. P. Jousset reports success in treating homoeopathically cases of Angina and Aortitis (Sub acute and chronic). When adrenaline has been prescribed per 0s and in infinitesimal dose, the symptom guiding to thus is, sensation of thoracic constriction with anguish. This with vertigo, nausea and vomiting have been produced by the drug. Abdominal pain. Shock or heart failure during anaesthesia, as it causes very prompt rise of blood pressure by its action on nerve endings in vessel wall- For Homoeopathic use- 2x to 6x & 200c.

The leading feature of this affection may be taken as guides for its use, bronzing of skin, loss of strength, wasting, exceedingly rapid pulse-when injected to the circulation, blood pressure rises, the arteries being contracted. *(JHC)*

Adrenalin or Epinephrin, the active principle of medulla of the suprarenal gland, (Cortical secretion not as yet isolated), is employed as a chemical messenger in the regulation of the activities of the body; in fact, its presence is essential to the activity of the sympathetic nerve. Adrenalin action on any part is the same as stimulation of the sympathetic nerve endings thereto. Local application (1:1,000 solution) to mucous membranes promptly induces transient Ischaemia, seen in a blanching, persisting several hours from conjunctival instillation. Its action is very prompt, effective, evanescent, owing to rapid oxidation and therefore practically harmless, unless too frequently repeated, when atheroma and heart lesions-myocardial- in animals have been reported. Arteries, heart, supra-renal bodies and vasomotor system are prominently affected.

The main action of Adrenalin is stimulation of the sympathetic endings, notably the splanchnic area, causing contriction of the peripheral arterioles, with resulting rise in blood pressure. This is especially observed in stomach, intestines; less in uterus, skin; nil in brain and lungs. Furthermore, there is slowing of pulse, (medullary vagus stimulation) and strengthening of heart beat (increased myocardial contractility), resembling Digitalis; increased glandular activity, glycosuria; depression of respiratory centre; contraction of muscular tissue of eye, uterus, vagina; relaxation of muscular tissue of stomach, intestines, bladder.

Its chief therapeutic use depends on its vaso-constriction action. Externally, it has been used in neuritis, neuralgia, reflex pains, gout, rheumatism, as an ointment, 1-2m of (1:1,000) solution, along the nerve trunk at point of skin nearest its origin which could be reached. *(H.G. Carleton)*

Therapeutically, Adrenalin has been suggested in acute congestion of lungs, Asthma, Graves' and Addisons diseases, arteriosclerosis, chronic aortitis, angina pectoris, haemophilia, chlorosis, hay fever, serum rashes, acute urticaria, etc. Dr. P. Jousset reports success in treating, homoeopathically, cases of angina and of aortitis, sub-acute and chronic, when Adrenalin has been prescribed per os and in infinitesimal dose. The symptom guiding to this is sensation of thoracic constriction with anguish. This with vertigo, nausea and vomiting have been produced by the drug. Abdominal pain, Shock or heart failure during anesthesia, as it causes very prompt rise of blood pressure by its action on nerve endings in the vessel wall.

Dose: Internally, 5-30m of 1:1,000 solution.

For homoeopathic use 2x to 6x attenuation. *(Boericke)*

13. *Aesculus Hippocastanum*

(Horse chest nut)

The action of this drug is most marked on the lower bowel, producing engorged haemorrhoidal veins with characteristic back ache, with absence of actual constipation. Much pain but little bleeding, venous stasis general, varicose veins of purple colour, everything is slowed down, digestion, heart, bowels etc. Torpor and congestion of the liver and portal system with constipation. The back aches gives out and make the patient unfit for business. Flying pains all over. Fullness in various parts, dry swollen mucus membranes. Throat with haemorrhoidal conditions.

Head: Depressed and irritable.

Eye: With engorged blood vessels.

Nose: Nasal passage sensitive to it, coryza.

Throat: Dry, Veins in pharynx distended.

Rectum: Dry, feels full of small sticks, burning in anus with chills up and down back.

Female: Constant throbbing behind symphysis pubis - lameness of back across the sacro-iliac articulation.

Cough: depending on hepatic disorders.

Back: Backache affecting sacrum and hips, worse walking or stooping. Worse in morning, walking, from moving bowels. Better cool open air.

Dose: Tr. to 3rd potency. *(Boericke)*

Aescul. hip. is a great pile remedy. Follicular pharyngitis with dryness, burning roughness, contraction of throat. Feeling of dryness in rectum as if little sticks or splinters were pricking the folds of mucous membrane, with weak feeling in Sacro-iliac joints. Constipation, stools large followed by feeling of prolapse of rectum. General aching in lumbar and sacral regions with stiffness in the back, almost impossible to walk. Tearing in the small of the back and hips. Aesc. H. patients are as a rule despondent and irritable. Walking generally agg. all symptoms. *Amel:* Summer *Agg.* winter haemorrhoids.

Compare: Phytolacca (follicular pharyngitis). (JHC)

Vascular fullness which affects the extremities and the whole body- the conditions of Aesculus are worse during sleep, hence symptoms are observed on waking. He wakes up with confusion of mind useful in children that rouse up in sleep frightened and in confusion like Lycopodium. The symptoms pass away after considerable exertion, moving about, doing something, keeping busy relieves. Extreme irritability is the very general state from which ramify a great many mental symptoms. The remedy is full of headaches. As soon as the patient has swallowed the food, or a little while after, it becomes sour and he eructates it until after a while he has emptied the stomach of its contents. This remedy is often supposed to be suitable to haemorrhoids that do not bleed but it cures bleeding piles also. Constant dull backache, walking is almost impossible, scarcely able to rise or walk after sitting. *(Kent)*

Severe dull backache in lumbo sacral articulation. After Coll. has improved piles Aesc. often cures, useful after Nux. and Sulph. have improved but failed to cure piles. *(HCA)*

14.Aethiops Mercurialis

Minerales

This preparation is of use in scrofulous affections, ophthalmia, otorrhoea, painful, irritating, scabby eruptions, hereditary syphilis. Skin-Eruptions, flavus-like, scrofulous, herpetic and eczematous.

Dose: The lower triturations, especially the second decimal.

Compare: Calc, Sil, Psorin. (Boericke)

15. Aethusa cynapium

(Fools parsley)

The characteristic symptoms relate mainly to the brain and nervous system connected with gastro-intestinal disturbance. Anguish, crying and expression of uneasiness and discontent, lead to this remedy most frequently in disease in children, during dentition, summer complaint, diarrhoea, there is marked inability to digest milk and poor circulation, symptoms set in with violence.

Mind: Anxious, crying, inability to think, to fix the attention.

Head: Occipital pain, hair feels pulled, vertigo with drowsiness, with palpitation, head hot after vertigo ceases.

Eyes: Swelling of meibomian glands, eyes drawn backward.

Ears: Feel obstructed.

Nose: Herpetic eruptions.

Face: Puffed, linea nasalis marked.

Stomach: Intolerance of milk. Vomiting as soon as swallowed or in large curds. Regurgitation of food about an hour after eating. Vomiting with sweat and great weakness.

Stool: Undigested, thin, greenish, preceded by colic.

Skin: Surface of the body cold and covered with sweat. Lymphatic glands swollen. Itching eruption around joints.

Fever: Great heat, no thirst, must be covered during sweat.

Sleep: violent starting. After vomiting or stools, child is so exhausted, it falls asleep at once.

Mod: Worse 3-4 am, evening, warmth, summer, better in open air and company.

Compare: Athamantha, Antimon, Calc. ars, Cicuta-com, Calc.

Dose: 3-30c. *(Boericke)*

"Fools parsley" has not received its name for nothing- it is indeed a medicine for fools. There is great weakness of mind or body. One very characteristic symptom is inability to think or fix the attention. Guided by this symptom, I once gave it to an undergraduate preparing for examination, with complete success. He had been compelled to give up his studies but was able to resume them and passed a brilliant examination. Idiocy. Patient becomes more and more retired in his disposition and more inclined to weep. Intolerance of milk-vomiting-the child is so exhausted it falls asleep at once. It wakens hungry, eats and vomits again. Linea nasalis, a surface of pearly whiteness on upper lip bounded by distinct lines from wings of nose to angles of mouth. All symptoms agg. 3 to 4 am. The remedy is suited to teething children and cholereic affections of old age. *(JHC)*

Digestion has absolutely ceased from brain trouble. Sometimes the brain trouble does not affect the stomach but the child goes into convulsions. *(Kent)*

Especially for children during dentition in hot summer weather. Children who cannot bear milk-idiocy in children, incapacity to think. Confused. An expression of great anxiety and pain with a drawn condition and well marked "linea nasalis". Herpetic eruption on end of the nose. Complete absence of thirst. Intolerance of milk. Cannot bear milk in any form, it is vomited in large curds as soon as taken, then weakness causes drowsiness. Indigestion of teething children, violent sudden vomiting of a frothy milk white substance or yellow fluid, followed by curdled milk and cheesy matter. Regurgitation of food an hour or so after eating, copious greenish vomiting, epileptic spasm, with clenched thumbs, red face, eyes turned downwards, pupils fixed and dilated, foam at the mouth, jaws locked, pulse small, hard, quick. Weakness and prostration with sleepiness after vomiting, after stool, after spasm. Agg: after eating, drinking, after stool and spasm. *(HCA)*

16. *Agaricus Muscarius*

(Toad Stool-bug Agaric)

This fungus contains several toxic compounds. The best known of which is muscarin. The symptom of poisoning do not develop at once, usually 12-14 hours elapse, before the initial attack. There is no antidote treatment, entirely symptomatic. Agaricus acts as an intoxicant to the brain, producing more vertigo and delirium than alcohol, followed by profound sopor with lowered reflexes.

Jerking, twitching, trembling and itching are strong indications. Incipient phthisis, is related to the tubercular diathesis, anaemia, chorea, twitching ceases during sleep. Various forms of neuralgia and spasmodic affections and neurotic skin troubles are pictured in the symptomatology of this remedy. It corresponds to various forms of cerebral excitement, rather than congestion. In delirium of fevers, Alcoholism etc. General paralysis. Sensation as if pierced by needles of ice. Sensitivity to pressure and cold air. Violent bearing down pains, symptom appear diagonally eg. right arm and left leg. Pains are accompanied by sensation of cold, numbness and tingling.

Mind: Loquacity, delirium.

Head: Vertigo from sunlight, coldness like icy needles.

Eyes: Reading difficult as type seems to move, to swim, twitching of lids and eyeballs.

Nose: Nose bleed in old people.

Face: Facial muscles twitch.

Stomach: Gastric disturbance with sharp pains in the liver region.

Female: Bearing down pains especially after menopause.

Respiratory: Spasmodic cough at night after falling asleep, with expectoration of little balls of mucus.

Heart: Irregular tumultuous palpitation after tobacco.

Back: Sensitiveness of spine to touch, twitching of cervical muscle.

Extremities: Itching of toes and feet as if frozen.

Skin: Burning itching, redness and swelling as from frost bites.

Sleep: Paroxysms of yawning, starts, twitches and awakes often.

Modalities: Worse open air, cold, after eating, coitus, in cold weather, before a thunder storm, pressure on dorsal spine which causes involuntary laughter. *Better:* moving out slowly.

Dose: 3-200. In skin affections and brain exhaustions- Lower attenuation.

(Boericke)

As Agaricus is used in many parts for making an intoxicating drink, we find in alcoholism, a sphere for its action and also in all states of delirium, mania and even idiocy. To make verses and prophecy, also silly merriness and incoherent talk, with mania and kisses companions, general paralysis of all remedies, hilarity and excitement followed by depression, confusion and imbecility, constant impulse to fall backward, twitching about eyes and face, redness without heat puffy and distorted, ravenous appetite with bolting of food. Sexual appetite enormous and enthusiastic with relaxed penis and impotence. Throughout the body there are spasmodic twitchings, rolling of the head is a leading indication for brain affections and fever, muscular jerking and twitchings. Twitchings marked in the eyes, eyelids and facial muscles, pain as if touched or pierced by needles of ice. It has cured stitch in runners enabling them to run further. The symptoms appear at the same time on opposite sides of the body but diagonally, right upper and left lower or vice versa. Mushrooms are among articles of diet forbidden by Gran-Vogal to persons having the hydrogenoid constitution. Agg. in cold weather. All the symptoms of frost bite and chilblains (itching, redness and burning). Agaricus has been found specially useful by many practitioners

(JHC)

It is hardly confined to the skin. In the flesh a sensation as if ants is felt, itching of the skin all over, which changes place from scratching. No place is exempt from this. Agaricus also agg. after sexual intercourse especially in the symptoms of the spinal cord. It is useful for the symptoms which come on after coition in young married nervous women, hysterical fainting after coition, children with twitching and early fainting, nervous girls prior to puberty who have convulsions from being scolded, from excitement and shock, late in mental development, children who cannot remember, make mistakes and are slow in learning. Nervous patients who on going over their manuscripts, find out their mistakes in writing and spelling. In handling things she drops them, fingers fly open spasmodically while holding things. You will sometime cure 'Briget' in the kitchen with Agaricus or Apis, when the trouble is that she is continualy breaking the dishes by letting them fall. Agaricus must stay with fire, while Apis, she wants to get out of the kitchen. All jerking and twitching subside during sleep. Sensation as of a mist or cobweb before the eyes. Nose bleed profuse, foetid discharge from the nose. This remedy is a great antidote to alcoholic beverages. Agaricus has cured many cases of epileptiform convulsions, more commonly the hysteric epileptic type with frothing of the mouth- opisthotonos- those suffering from spinal affections have distress after the act of coition- leucorrhoea copious, acrid, it keeps the parts raw and irritated around the genitals and the patient cannot walk. Hering's observation of the relationship of Agaricus to the tuberculous diathesis is confirmed. *(Kent).*

17. *Agave Americana*

(Century plant)

Indicated in stomach ache and painful erections in gonorrhoea, strangury, Hydrophobia, scurvy, countenance pale, gums swollen and bleeding, legs covered with dark purple blotches, swollen, painful and hard, appetite poor, bowel constipated.

Compare: Anhalonium, Lyssin, Lach.

Dose-Tincture. *(Boericke)*

The plant has a reputation as a remedy for hydrophobia. A striking case is quoted by the 'H.Recorder' from 'El Siglo Medico'. A boy developed the classical symptoms of hydrophobia 4½ months after being bitten. Quarrelsomeness, excitement, fright, inability to swallow, small frequent pulse, great anxiety. Finally swallowing was impossible, restraint had to be used to prevent him biting his nurses in the hospital, when as a last resort a piece of Agave was offered to the boy by the doctor in attendance, cut from a hedge of the plant with which the hospital grounds were fenced. To the astonishment of all, the boy reached for it and ate it greedily, almost without chewing. By evening a decrease in the violence of the nervous attacks was manifested, though they remained as frequent as before. The improvement was slow but continued. On the fourth day he took some nourishment but also continued chewing Agave and swallowing the juice. On the fifth day he recovered consciousness but still demanded Agave. On the eighth day he said he did not want any more as it tasted too bitter and caused a burning in the mouth. He had no further symptoms of the disease.

(JHC)

18. *Agnus Cactus*

(Chaste tree)

The most effective point of attack of Agnus upon the organism is the Sexual organ. It lowers sexual vitality, with corresponding mental depression and loss of nervous energy. It shows the distinctive influence in both sexes but is more pronounced in Men. Premature old age from abuse of sexual power. History of repeated gonorrhoea. A prominent remedy for- sprains and strains, gnawing and itching in all parts especially eyes. Tachycardia caused by tobacco in neurotic young men.

Mind: Sadness with impression of speedy death.

Eyes: Pupils dilated.

Abdomen: Sensation as if intestines were pressed downwards.

Male: Yellow discharge from urethra, no erections, Impotence, parts cold, relaxed, desire gone, (Selen, Con, Sabal). Scanty emission without ejaculation.

Female: Agalactia.

Compare: Selen, Phos Ac., Camphor, Lycop.

Dose 1-6c.

Verbena Verticillata, Mental sphere, Great sadness with a fixed idea of approaching death. When this mental stage is found after confinement and the milk fails to appear Agn. c. is the remedy, it corresponds to lymphatic constitutions, sterility, Deficiency of milk with despair of recovery. *(JHC)*

It should come to mind for old sufferers who are broken from sexual excesses and secret vice. The pale sickly and sad mortals who lament over the mis-spent life. It is good for both sexes. Sexual weakness- relaxation of parts- perversion of all the functions. A woman who indulged extremely in secret vice, found after marriage that she had no sexual thrill, was cured by this remedy. Later she was confined and no milk came in her mammae, again 'Agnus' started the belated milk at the end of three weeks. When the milk ceases after it has started or becomes scanty, when the above history is known and the woman is sad, this remedy will, if not opposed, most likely cure. The vagina is much relaxed, there is often prolapsus and there is a copious white of egg like leucorrhoea. Young man who had gonorrhoea- relaxed and cold genitalia- prostatic discharge at stool- his young and beautiful wife excites no errection. *(Kent)*

Complaints of imaginary odor before the nose, as of herring or musk.

Relation: 'Calad' and 'Selen' follow well after Agnus in weakness of sexual organs or impotence *(HCA)*

Physiological action: This agent exerts a depressing action upon the sexual organs of both the male and female, even to complete extinction of the virility with a corresponding loss of energy. The chaste matrons at the feast of 'Ceres' strewed it upon their beds as did the medieval monks to repress carnal desires. *(Blackwood)*

19. *Agraphis Nutans*

(Blue bell)

A relaxed condition of the system generally and a proneness to take cold on exposure to cold winds.

Catarrhal condition, obstruction of nostrils, Adenoids, throat deafness, enlarged tonsils, Mucous diarrhoea from cold, chill from cold winds, Throat and ear troubles with tendency to free discharge from mucus membranes. Mutinism of childhood not connected with deafness.

Compare: Hydrast, Cepa, Calc. phos, Sulph, Iod, Calc iod.

Dose- 3c- Single dose of Tincture (Dr. Cooper) *(Boericke)*

It partakes of the characters of the lilies and corresponds to catarrhal conditions. Obstruction of the nostrils, especially from Adenoids and throat deafness, I have frequently seen relieved by this remedy. The action of it is felt towards the root of the nose. The plant grows in sheltered places and Dr. Cooper gives Amel. from shelter as a leading indication. It also corresponds to chill from cold winds and is very like silica in this. I regard it as one of the leading remedies in cases of Adenoids. Dr. Cooper gives in Adenoids with enlarged tonsils, frequently accompanying dentition. He has cured with it, mucous diarrhoea following a suppressed cold. *(JHC)*

20. *Ailanthus Glandulosa*

(Chinese Sumach)

This remedy shows by its peculiar skin symptoms, its pronounced power of disorganising the blood, causing conditions we meet with low fevers, low types of eruptive diseases, diphtheria, follicular tonsillitis, streptococcus infection. Haemorrhagic diathesis etc. The skin appears livid or purplish, face dark as mahagony, hot, sordes, throat swollen, purple, livid, semi-conscious, delirious, weak pulse, general torpor and prostration, Symptoms remarkably like malignant scarlatina. Diarrhoea, dysentery and great weakness are very marked. Adynamia characterises all its conditions. Lividity, stupor and malignancy. Mucous membranes haemorrhagic and ulcerative.

Head: Headache frontal, suffused dilated eyes. Thin copious ichorous bloody nasal discharge.

Throat: Much swelling, internal and external, neck tender and swollen, tongue dry and brown, teeth covered with sordes, pains while swallowing.

Skin: Irregular, patchy, livid eruption, disappearance on pressure.

Antidotes: Rhus, Nux.

Compare: Ammn carb., Bapt, Arn, Mur ac., Lach, Rhus.

Dose: 1-6c *(Boericke)*

Corresponds to conditions characterised by certain livid or purpled appearances of the skin. Rash coming out in patches. Eruptions which are slow in appearing. Low adynamic forms of disease with extreme prostration, torpor, vomiting- Prostration at the outset of disease is a leading indication for it. The patient is stupid, dull, delirious, weak. It has proved of signal service in cases of malignant and suppressed Scarlatina. The rash of Ailanthus often returns annually. A feeling of fullness every where and a sensation of passage of electric current from head into limbs are prominent in the provings. The throat is severely affected, thick, oedematous, dry, choky feeling. *(JHC)*

21. *Aletris Farinosa*

(Star grass)

An anaemic relaxed condition, especially of the female organism is portrayed by this remedy. The patient is tired all the time and suffers from prolapses, leucorrhoea, rectal distress etc., Marked anaemia, chlorotic girls and pregnant women.

Stomach: Disgust for food.

Rectum: Loads up with faeces, paretic condition.

Female: Premature and profuse menses with labor like pains (Bell, Cham, Kali. c, Plat.), retarded and scanty flow (Senecio), Uterus seems heavy, Prolapse with pain in the right inguinal region, leucorrhoea due to weakness and anaemia. Habitual tendency to abortion, muscular pain during pregnancy.

Compare: Helonias, Hydrastis, Tenacet, China.

Dose: Tincture to third potency.
(Boericke)

— Alet Far is said to be the most bitter of all plants. It is characterized by weariness of body and mind. Want of appetite, especially in connection with uterine disorders. The least food distends the stomach. There are fainting attacks with Vertigo. Emaciation is marked in some cases. Disgust for food, nausea, constipation. Obstinate vomiting of pregnancy. Many symptoms appear in the uterine sphere, Uterine atony, menses profuse and premature with labour like pains or amenorrhoea, debility from loss of fluids, protracted illness. Menorrhagia, black clots, fullness and weight. Leucorrhoea with debility, sterility, Habitual tendency to abortion, sensation of weight in occiput in girls and pregnant women. Weak emaciated people. *(JHC)*

If she becomes pregnant, there is a tendency to abort. It has been termed 'the china' of the uterine system.

(Blackwood)

22. *Alfalfa*

(Medicago Sativa, Californis clover Lucerne)

From its action on sympathetic system, Alfalfa favourably influences nutrition, evidenced in toning up the appetite and digestion resulting in greatly improved, mental and physical vigor, with gain in weight. Disorders characterised by malnutrition and mainly within the therapeutic range for example, neurasthenia, splanchnic blues, nervousness insomnia, nervous indigestion etc. Acts as a fat producer, corrects tissue waste, deficient lactation. Increases, quantity and quality of milk in nursing mothers. Its pronounced urinary action, suggests it clinically in diabetes insipidus and phosphaturia and it is claimed to allay vesical irritability of prostate hypertrophy. The rheumatic diathesis seems especially amenable to its action.

Stomach: Increased thirst, appetite impaired, but chiefly increases even to bulimia. He must eat frequently, so that he cannot wait for regular meals- hungry in forenoon. Much nibbling of food and craving for sweets.

Dose: The best results are elicited with material doses (5-10) drops of Tincture several times daily. Continue its use until tonic effects ensue.

Compare- Avena sat, Dipodium punet, Gels, Hydr, Kali phos, Phos ac, Zinc.

(Boericke)

Medicago sativa (Alfalfa) - The salts contained in this agent are lime, potash, magnesia, phosphoric acid and sulphur. After observations on seventeen provers, all except one, noted three things in particular, an increased appetite, an increase in the amount of urine and urea excreted and a general sense of well being.

This remedy is indicated in weak, delicate undernourished children, when the appetite, digestion and assimilation is below normal, the child is under size and undernourished.

It should be studied in polyuria and phosphaturia, when there is a weakened heart's action, the blood pressure is low. There is an increased amount of urine and an excess of phosphates.

It should be thought of in cases of uric acidaemia, especially in the aged. There are muscular pains, backache, with an excess of uric acid and urates.

There is apt to be irritation of the neck of the bladder. The appetite is impaired and there is much flatulence and abdominal distension.

It should be thought of in retarded digestion, when the appetite is impaired, the patient is emaciated, weak and complains of fermentation and flatulence in the line of colon. He is drowsy, dull, stupid, gloomy and irritable, especially in the evening.

Compare: Hydrastis Can, Kali phos, Avena sativa. *(Blackwood)*

23. *Allium Cepa*

(Red onion)

A picture of coryza with acrid nasal discharge and laryngeal symptoms, eye secretion bland, "singers cold", worse in warm room and towards evening, better in open air is presented by this remedy. Especially adapted to phlegmatic patients, colds in damp cold weather, neuralgic pains, like a fine thread, following amputations or injuries to nerves. Traumatic chronic neuritis. Burning in nose, mouth, throat, bladder and skin. Sensation of glowing heat on different parts of body.

Head: Worse in warm room.

Eyes: Sensitive to light, bland lachrymation.

Nose: Copious, watery and extremely acrid discharge.

Respiratory: Hoarseness, Hacking cough on inspiring cold air, tickling in larynx. Sensation as if larynx is split or torn, oppressed breathing.

Modalities: Worse evening, in warm room, Better in open air and in cold room.

Relation: Gels, Euph, and Kali hyd, Acon, Ipecac.

Complementary: Phos, Thuja, Puls.

Antidote: Arn, Cham, Verat.

Dose: 3c. *(Boericke)*

Allium Cepa covers more symptoms of common cold than any other remedy as the well known effect of Onions in producing tears would suggest. It will cure a large proportion of cases of cold in the head but the conditions which most particularly indicate it are, Cough or cold or headache agg. in warm room, amel. in open air, agg. again on returning to warm room. A raw onion eaten just before going to bed is a popular remedy for sleeplessness, followed by Calc. and Silic. in polypus. *(JHC)*

It is not strange that the old ladies used to bind onions on the ear for earache and around the neck for sore throats. Notice that the fluid from the nose is excoriating and the fluids from the eyes bland. In Euphrasia we will find just the opposite. Watery discharge from nose and the lachrymation is acrid. Troubles begin on the left side and go to right side- nasal discharge after damp cold winds. Every year in August morning coryza with violent sneezing, very sensitive to the odour of flowers and skin of peaches. With Pulsatilla, Chamomilla and Allium cepa one can cure the majority of earaches in children. We all know, what a flatulent vegetable the onion is. Hoarse, harsh, ringing spasmodic cough excited by constant tickling in the larynx- compel the patient to crouch from suffering and to make every effort to suppress the cough- Laryngeal cough makes the patient grasp the larynx, feels as if cough would tear it. *(Kent)*

24. *Allium sativum*

(Garlic)

Acts directly on intestinal mucus membrane, increasing peristalsis, colitis with pathological flora. Vasodilatory properties. Arterial hypotension begins usually within 30-45 minutes after twenty to forty drop doses of the tincture.

Adapted to fleshy subjects with dyspepsia and catarrhal affections. High livers, Patient who eat a great deal more, especially meat, than they drink. Pain in hip, pain in Psoas and iliac muscles. Pulmonary tuberculosis.

Cough and expectoration diminishes, temperature becomes normal, weight is gained and sleeps becomes normal.

Mouth: Tongue pale, red papillae.

Respiratory: Constant rattling of mucus in bronchi, cough in the morning after leaving bed room, with mucous expectoration, which is tenacious and difficult to raise sensitive to cold air. Dilated bronchi with fetid expectoration. Darting pain in chest.

Relation: Allium Sat, according to Dr. Teste belongs to the Bryonia, Lycopod, Nux, Colocy, Digital and Ignatia group, which affect deeply all flesh eating animals and hardly at all vegetarian. There is special applicability to meat eaters.

Compare: Capsicum, Ars, Senega, Kali nit.

Compl: Ars.

Anti: Lycopod.

Dose: 3-6c. In tuberculosis 4-6 grains divided dose. *(Boericke)*

Suited to persons, who are disposed to excesses at table, have strong constitutions, dark complexion, firm flesh though occasionally disposed to obesity. The All. Sat. patient is rather a gourmand than a glutton. Chronic bronchial catarrh with profuse mucous expectoration. Permanent dyspnoea- rheumatism of the hip- swelling of breasts after weaning- relieved with it- cases of diabetes mellitus. The pains of Allium Sat. are mostly pressive from within outward, distensive like those of Bry. Garlic has been used as condiment from ancient times and also as a remedy against worms and fevers. Sensation as if hair on tongue, copious sweetish saliva, the hip is the seat of rheumatic pains. Tearing in hip. *(JHC)*

This remedy is of service in cases of catarrhal affections of the lungs, when there is constant rattling of mucus in the bronchial tubes, also in cases of haemoptysis, when the garlic should be eaten in quantities of a drachm or more during the day. *(Blackwood)*

25. *Alnus Rubra*

(Red Alder)

Has some reputation as a remedy for skin affections, glandular enlargements. Indigestion from imperfect secretion of gastric juice. It stimulates nutrition and thus acts favourably upon stomach disorders, enlarged glands etc. Ulcerated mucus membranes of mouth and throat. Fingers covered by crusts, caused by pustules, disagreeable odour. Indigestion from imperfect secretion of gastric juice.

Skin: Chronic herpes, enlarged submaxillary glands. Eczema, prurigo, Purpura haemorrhagica, poison oak- use locally.

Dose: Tincture to 3rd potency. *(Boericke)*

This remedy should be studied in cases of scrofula, chronic skin diseases, rheumatism and syphilis, where there are glandular enlargements and skin presents an unhealthy condition, simulating eczema in the pustular stage. These cutaneous exhibitions often alternate with diseases conditions of the mucous membranes.

It is of service when the digestion is slow, due to a lack of gastric and intestinal secretions and as a result marasmus has developed for which it has been employed.

It has been employed in haematuria and in leucorrhoea which caused erosions and bleeding. *(Blackwood)*

26. *Aloe*

(Socotrine Aloes)

An excellent remedy to aid in re-establishing, physiological equilibrium after much dosing, where disease and drug symptoms are much mixed. There is no remedy richer in symptoms of portal congestion and none that has given better clinical results, both for primary pathological condition and secondary phenomena. Bad effects from sedentary life or habits. Especially suitable to lymphatic and hypochondriacal patients. The rectal symptoms usually determine the choice. Adapted to weary people, the aged and phlegmatic, old beer drinkers, dissatisfied, angry about himself, alternating with lumbago. Heat internally and externally. Has been used successfully in the treatment of consumption by giving the pure juice.

Head: Aches above forehead, with heaviness in eyes, must close them partially.

Eyes: Yellow vision, pain deep in orbits.

Lips: Marked redness, cracked and dry.

Abdomen: Abdomen feels full and heavy.

Rectum: Pulsation in rectum, sensation of plug, between symphysis pubis and os coccygis, sense of insecurity in rectum after stool, bleeding, burning in anus, Haemorrhoids protrude, lumbago, alternating with headache and piles.

Modality: worse early morning, better from cold open air.

Comple: Sulphur

Compare: Kali bich, lycop, allium sat.

Antidotes: Opium, Sulph.

Dose: 6th potency and higher

In rectal condition- A few doses of 3rd and wait. *(Boericke)*

Aloe is one of the oldest and most famous drugs. It is in worldwide use as purgative and forms a leading ingredient in a large number of patent medicines for regulating the bowels and menstrual functions- Sudden and continued desire to go to stool- desire for stool after each meal. The hard stool falls out without being noticed, urging to stool while passing water. A hard stool may be passed involuntarily. A child constipated from birth, screams all the time, he is being held to stool, cannot pass it, even after enema, yet when not trying, passes solid pieces in bed with out knowing- stools like mush, bright yellow, grey, hot, undigested- mucus and blood in faeces- profuse with jelly like lumps diarrhoea driving one out of bed very early in morning- Haemorrhoids protrude like a bunch of grape- constant bearing down in rectum.

Bleeding- Carrol Dunham has cured incontinence of urine in an old man with enlarged prostate with the Aloe diarrhoea- increased sexual desire in males with erections- diarrhoea *Agg.* in the early morning- It resembles sulphur in many symptoms and is of equal importance with 'Sul' in chronic diseases with abdominal plethora. *(JHC)*

Greatest disturbance is in the veins of the portal system - It has abdominal pains that drive him to stool like Nux vomica- Dysenteric and diarrhoeic troubles- there is gushing of thin yellow offensive excoriating faeces, which burn like fire and the anus is sore. He cannot let the least quantity of flatus escape, because with it there will be a rush of faeces- but if you notice, those who get sick, have a cholera like trouble from eating 'Oysters' in the hot season, you will find that, that is where 'Aloe' is the remedy- Agg. from heat and relief from cold runs through Aloe- he wants to be in cool room- he wants to be uncovered at night in bed, burning of the extremities- hot hands and cold feet, or cold hands and hot feet, these alternate- Bleedings are common in this remedy, venous oozings from the nose, the bowels, the bladder, bleeding in general- in person who have a diarrhoea every time they drink beer. It is pre-eminently a liver medicine- it is not as deep in its action as sulphur- feeling as if a plug was wedged in between symphyses pubis and os coccygis- urging to stool, only hot flatus passes, giving relief, but urging soon returns- the idea is that it compels him to go to stool, but when upon the commode nothing but wind passes. It is useful also in old chronic sufferers from this trouble- entire loss of sensation in the anus, an anaesthesia, no feeling during the passage of stool- much of the Aloe trouble is dysenteric in character, with a sharp inflammatory condition of the rectum and lower portion of the colon, bloody discharges and yellow jelly like mucus. Sometimes the Aloe patient will pass nothing, but large quantities of this catarrhal jelly like mucus- don't forget Aloe for haemorrhoids that form like a bunch of grapes. A common feature of Aloe is that ointments increase the burning. The sulphur patient also cannot bear any application. The stricture prevented nearly all the faecal matter from getting down to the anus, but the rectum would fill up three or four times a day and compel the patient to expel a quantity of jelly like mucus. *(Kent)*

Headache across the forehead *agg.* by every foot step (Bell, Bry) with heaviness on eyes and nausea. Headaches are worse from heat- better from cold application. *(HCA)*

Aloe has cured a chronic headache which is of the bilious type, and the distress is confined to the forehead. A sensation of pressing on the eyes from above that causes the patient to contract the eyelids in order that they may see. *(Blackwood)*

27. Alstonia Scholaris

(Dita bark - Growing in India)

Malaria disease with diarrhoea, dysentery, anaemia, feeble digestion are the general conditions suggesting this remedy. Characteristics are the gone sensation in stomach and sinking in the abdomen with debility. Atonic after exhausting fevers.

Abdomen: Dysentery, painless watery stools.

Dose: Tincture to 3rd potency. *(Boericke)*

Alstonia Constricta- Bitter bark- Growing in south wales and Queensland. This is exceedingly bitter- debility from lack of digestive power, in the stomach or general assimilative power- Tongue generally has a dirty white coat- especially at base- though it may be clean- the nausea is *Agg.* morning before breakfast or at irregular times, especially when depending on reflex irritation from disturbance of pelvic organs. Food seems to remain in stomach a long time undigested- diarrhoea of undigested food immediately after eating has to leave table before finishing a meal- leucorrhoea and bearing down- agg. by walking- swollen feeling in right ovarian region *(JHC)*

28. *Alumen*

(Alum)

The clinical application of this remedy points to its bowel symptoms, both in obstinate constipation and in haemorrhage from bowel in the course of typhoid- one phase of the paralytic weakness of the muscles in all parts of the body. Tendency to induration is also marked, a low form of tissue making is favoured. Hardening of tissues of tongue, rectum, uterus etc. Ulcers with indurated base. Adapted to old people, especially bronchial catarrhs. Sensation of dryness and constriction. Mental paresis, dysphagia especially to liquids. Tendency to induration, Scirrhus of the tongue.

Head: Burning pain as of weight on top of head better by pressure.

Throat Enlarged and indurated tonsils.

Heart: Palpitation from lying down on the right side.

Rectum: Constipation of the most aggravated kind, marble like masses pass, but rectum still feels full. Haemorrhage from bowels.

Skin: Ulcers with indurated base, scrotal eczema and on back of penis.

Extremities: Weakness of all muscles constricted feeling around limbs.

Dose: 1-30c, The very high potencies have proved efficacious. Powdered alum placed on tongue, said to arrest an attack of Asthma. *(Boericke)*

The well known astringent action of Alum gives a leading indication for its use in practice- sensation of dryness- frequently removed with it, constipation of the most aggravated type as in cases of cancer of uterus and rectum. Stools as hard as stone is the leading indication- no desire for stool for days- on the other hand it is equally available for the states of relaxation which correspond with its secondary action- sluggish action of muscles, haemorrhages of various kinds- relaxed Uvula, hoarseness and bronchial affections- diarrhoea. The Alum patient is very sensitive to cold- exposure to air roughens and chaps the skin- slight scratches bleed- bleeding after tooth extraction- scirrhous indurations- indurated glands. Many complaints come on during sleep- There is nightmare- sensitiveness to all sorts of weather changes and especially to cold- bronchitis characterised by scraping from upper sternum to throat- compare Fer. (relaxed abdominal walls, prolapsed uterus). *(JHC)*

Another peculiar condition running through the remedy is the tendency to induration, wherever there is an inflamed surface. All remedies that have this in their nature relate more or less to cancerous affections, because in cancer we have as the most natural feature a tendency to induration- we have in this remedy features like epithelioma and other cancerous affections. What is the scirrhus but a peculiar form of induration? Many of these indurations will have cancer as an ultimate induration of the neck of the uterus and the mammary glands- enormously enlarged and very hard tonsils.

Alumen is one of the cognates of Baryta carb- Pain on the top of the head. Burning palpitation is brought on from lying on the right side- there is no ability to expel the stool- He will strain a long time with no success and finally after many days the stool is passed and is an agglomeration of hard balls, large masses of little hard balls like marbles all fastened together- Stools less frequent, dryer and harder, large black, hard or in small pieces like sheep dung, no relief afterwards. Nasal polypus left side- lupus or cancer on the nose- face pale as a corpse, lips· blue-scirrhus of the tongue- the teeth decay and the gums recede from the teeth, the teeth become loose- mouth burning, ulcerated- offensive saliva. Uvula inflammed and enlarged- retraction of the abdomen and drawing in of the navel- Plumbum and this remedy antidote each other- Lead colic of the painters is relieved by Alumen and the painters go back to their business- coldness of the spine, a feeling as if cold water were poured down the back- The clumsiness of the fingers as seen in dropping things. *(Kent)*

29. *Alumina*

(Pure clay)

A very general condition corresponding to this drug is dryness of mucus membranes and skin and tendency to paretic muscular states. Old people with lack of vital heat or permanently old with debility. Sluggish functions, heaviness, numbness and staggering and the characteristic constipation find an excellent remedy in Alumina. Disposition to cold in the head and eructations in spare, dry, thin, subjects. Delicate children, products of artificial baby foods.

Mind: Hasty, hurried, variable mind.

Nose: Point of nose cracked, red, worse touch, scabs with thick yellow mucus, ozaena, atrophica sicca.

Throat: Dry.

Stomach: Potatoes disagree, can swallow, but small morsels at a time.

Abdomen: Left sided abdominal complaints.

Stool: No desire, rectum sore dry, even a soft stool is passed with difficulty, great straining evacuation preceded by painful urging long before stool and then straining at stool.

Urine: Must strain at stool in order to urinate.

Female: Menses scanty, pale, followed by great exhaustion, acrid, profuse, ropy.

Respiratory: Cough morning, hoarse, aphonia, wheezing, rattling respiration talking aggravates soreness of chest.

Extremities: Legs feel asleep, especially when sitting with legs crossed, staggers on walking, Heels feel numb, brittle nails.

Skin: Intolerable itching when getting warm in bed.

Mod: Worse afternoon, Potatoes, awakening in morning, warm room, Better open air, cold washing, alternate days in evening, damp weather.

Comple: Bryonia.

Anti: Ipecac, Chamom.,

Dose: 6-30c and higher. Action slow in developing. *(Boericke)*

Like its relative Alumen, Alumina produces irritation of mucus membranes with dryness or extreme secretion and paralysis of involuntary muscles, as those of the rectum and of the nervous and muscular systems generally. Alumina paralysis the bowels in the same way as lead to which it is an antidote. Even small and soft stools are passed with great difficulty. Pregnant women and children are liable to this kind of constipation. Teste groups Alumina with Sepia and copaiva. He considers it as the chronic of Sepia, as Silicea is of Puls- Drawing pains appear in the limbs, a sensation of constriction in several organs. Several painful symptoms show themselves after the midday meals and continue till evening, when they disappear or are replaced by others which begin only then. On the other hand, the pain which appear in the morning or in the evening are abated after eating. Trembling of convulsive movement of the limbs and head, spasms with tears and laughter alternately - There is exaltation of the whole nervous system - Trembling of the whole body with desire to lie down, which however agg. the fatigue. Great general fatigue even after a short walk but chiefly after speaking- Frequent stretching while sitting. The nates go to sleep while sitting- Drags legs- especially left. Many of the symptoms of locomotor ataxy are reproduced by Alumina- and it is one of the most useful remedies in that disease- can only evacuate bowels when standing- Causticum has defaecation only when standing, but the straining is less. Suicidal tendency- a sudden impulse from seeing blood on a knife- catarrh with dryness of mucus membranes. The throat looked parched and glazed. The nose is stopped, feels dry and the point of it is cracked- fish bone sensation in the throat on swallowing- leucorrhoea excoriating- itching eruptions *agg:* from warmth of bed- eruptions of all kinds- induration ulcers- granular eye lids- hair fall out all over body. The skin of the face feels as if covered with dried white of egg or as if a cob web was on it. There is a craving for dry rice and dry food. It has agg: from starch, especially the starch of potatoes. Agg: from salts, wine, vinegar, spirits, *agg:* on alternate days, in afternoon, at new or full moon agg: in the morning on waking. The action of Alumina is slow in developing and the remedy must not be changed quickly- *Comple- Bryonia. (JHC)*

This remedy comes in very nicely after 'Alumen' which has much Alumina in its nature and depends largely upon Alumina which is its base for its way of working. Feels as if another person had said it or as if he could transfer himself into another and only then could see. He is not exactly certain who he was, it seemed as though he were not himself. He gets into a hurry. Nothing moves fast enough, time seems so slow, everything is delayed, nothing goes right- When he sees sharp instruments or blood, impulses rise up within him and he shudders because of these impulses. Impulse to kill herself. Everything is slowed down. The conductivity of the nerves is impaired, so that a prick of pin upon the extremities is not felt until a second or so afterwards. Most of the symptoms are agg: on rising in the morning. It has a catarrhal state of the stomach, bowels and rectum, so that with the soft and difficult stool, there is often an accumulation of mucus. When gets warm at night, has to scratch until the skin bleeds- with the bleeding and moisture of the skin, there is relief of the itching- agg: from starch and potatoes- cannot pass urine without much straining. It is a very common medicine for constipation in infants, when you can find nothing else. The child will strain and strain and make every effort to press the stool out and upon examining the stool, it is found to be soft and should have been expelled easily- a constant dry hacking cough- cough soon after waking in the morning. From sensation of elongated uvula- pain in sole of foot on stepping- numbness of heel when stepping- limbs go to sleep when sitting. A striking feature of the remedy is the chronic dryness of the skin- sweat is rare and scanty. *(Kent)*

Adapted to persons who suffer from chronic diseases. The Aconite of chronic diseases. *(HCA)*

30. Alumina silicata

(Andalastite rock - Alumina 63, Silica 37 parts)

Deep acting remedy for chronic complaints of brain, spine and nerves, constriction is a marked symptom, also constriction of orifices. Venous distention, weakness especially spinal, aching and burning in spine, formication, numbness, pain in all limbs. Epileptiform convulsion, coldness during pains.

Mod: *Worse,* cold air, after eating, standing, better: warmth, fasting, resting in bed.

Dose: Higher potencies *(Boericke)*

31. Ambra Grisea

(Ambergris - A morbid secretion of the whale)

Suitable to excitable nervous children and thin nervous patients. Extreme nervous hypersensitiveness. External numbness of whole body in the morning and weakness. Nervous bilious temperament. Thin scrawny women. Adapted to hysterical subjects, or those suffering from spinal irritation, with convulsive cough, eructation etc. Also for patients weakened by age or over work, who are anaemic and sleepless. Great remedy for the aged with impairment of all functions, weakness, coldness and numbness, usually of single parts, fingers, arms, etc. One sided complaints call for it. Music aggravates symptoms. Ebulitions and pulsations after walking in open air. One sided complaints.

Mind: Music causes weeping.

Head: Tearing pain in upper half of brain. Senile dizziness. Hearing impaired.

Stomach: Distension of stomach and abdomen.

Urinary: Feeling in urethra as if a few drops passed out, urine turbid.

Female: Itching of pudendum with soreness and swelling. Discharge of blood between periods, at every little accident.

Male: Voluptuous itching of scrotum.

Respiratory: Nervous, spasmodic, barking cough, coming from deep in chest.

Heart: Palpitation, with pressure in chest as from a lump lodged there or as if chest was obstructed.

Sleep: Cannot sleep from worry, must get up.

Extremities: Cramps in hand and fingers.

Mod: Worse music, presence of strangers, from any unusual thing, morning warm room.

Better: Slow motion in open air, lying on painful side, cold drinks.

Relation: Oleum succinum (Hiccough), Sumbul, Castor, Asaf, Arocus, Lilium.

Dose: 2nd and 3rd potencies, may be repeated with advantage. *(Boericke)*

Ambra produces faintness, nervousness, jerks and twitches. The patient has an embarrassed air- the bashful state is very characteristic in certain connections- Embarrassed in company- cough worse when many people are present. There is voluptuous itching on the scrotum and some rawness below the thighs in the male- in the female there is discharge of blood between the periods at every little accident, as straining at stool or extra work. Severe itching on pudenda- During urination, itching, tickling, burning in vulva and urethra. Nymphomania with discharge of bluish white mucus. In childhood obstinate constipation and tenesmus with bashfulness- cannot make the attempt to stool, if any one is present, even the nurse. Cough excited by speaking- night cough- cough followed by copious belching- itching in chest- The limbs go to sleep easily- Dried up nervous persons- Thin scrawny women, Antidote to staph (especially the voluptous itching of scrotum). *(JHC)*

On looking over this remedy as a whole, it will appear to you that you have been studying the characteristics of one prematurely old- he jumps about from one topic to another- a state of senility- That state of senility- a state of mind belongs to modern society women in such great frequency that you will be astonished to note it - the 'belle' that could not darn the heel of her stocking- a kind of nervous sickness- Alternation of depression of spirits with vehemence of temper is another feature- Many of the symptoms are worse in the morning- non descript vertigo of old men- presence of other persons aggravates the symptoms, also marked Agg: from conversation- mental prostration- music is intolerable- numbness you will find running through the complaints- itching is felt all over the body- itching in all the little openings- pressing headache starting from both temples- drawing and tearing in the head to and fro. This remedy is full of bleeding- copious bleeding from the nose in the morning- inveterate constipation in old persons, and especially when it is impossible to have anyone near at the time of stool- sore rawness between the thighs. Voluptuous itching on the scrotum- copious discharge of blood between the menstrual periods- menses appear, seven days before time and then comes that horrible itching of the genitals- soreness and itching with swelling of labia- the limbs easily become numb- pressed upon in the slightest manner they go to sleep- go to sleep on being crossed- This remedy has cured the premature trembling that comes on in middle aged persons. *(Kent)*

Ambergris is an odorous waxy material of an ash gray colour and is found in the intestines and among the excreta of the Sperm whale. *(Blackwood)*

32. *Ambrosia*

(Ragweed)

A remedy for hay fever, lachrymation and intolerable itching of the eyelids. Some forms of whooping cough. Respiratory tract in its entire length stopped up. Many form of diarrhoea especially during summer months, also dysentery.

Nose: Watery coryza, sneezing, watery discharge.

Nose bleed, stuffed up feeling of nose and head, irritation of trachea and bronchial tubes, with asthmatic attacks. (Aral, Eucalypt)

Wheezy cough.

Relation: In hay fever, Sabadilla, Wyethia, Succin. ac, Ars iod, Arundo.

Dose: Tincture to 3rd potency: 10 drops in water during and after attack of epistaxis. In hay fever high potencies. *(Boericke)*

33. *Ammoniacum Doreina*

(Gum ammoniac)

A remedy for the aged and feeble, especially to chronic bronchitis. Ill humour. Sensitive to cold. Sensation of burning and scratching in neck and oesophagus.

Respiratory: Difficult breathing, chronic bronchial catarrh, large accumulation of purulent matter a nd feeble expectoration, worse cold weather. Mucus tough and hard. Heart beats stronger, extends to pit of stomach. Coarse rattling of chest in old people.

Relation: Bry, Arnica

Compare: Senega, Tartar emet., Balsam-peru.

Dose: 3rd Trituration. *(Boericke)*

Ill humour is the prevailing mental feature of Ammoniac. It acts prominently on mucous membranes, causing first diminished then increased secretion. There are stars and fiery points before the sight. Sees smoke in circles. Dim sight from a blow on the head. Dim sight from reading- hydrocele- Heart beat too strong *agg.* lying on left side. Great accumulations of mucus. Stitches are prominent in the provings- Stitches in the caecum at 7 pm. alternating with pains elsewhere. This should make appropriate in some cases of appendicites. There are many rheumatic pains in the limbs and loins. There is marked sensitiveness to cold and *Agg:* in cold weather. It is suited to bronchial affection in old people brought on by cold weather. *(JHC)*

34.*Ammonium Benzoicum*

(Benzoate of Ammonia)

One of the remedies for albuminuria especially in the gouty. Gout with deposits in joints. Urinary incontinence in the aged.

Tongue: Swelling under tongue like Runnel.

Urine: Smoky, scanty, albuminous and thick deposits.

Relation: Terebinth, Benz. ac., ammonia salts, caust.

In Albuminuria- Kalmia, Helon, Merc cor, Beriberi, Canth.

Dose: Second Trituration. *(Boericke)*

35. *Ammonium Brom.*

(Bromide of Ammonia)

Indicated in chronic, laryngeal and pharyngeal catarrh, neuralgic headaches and obesity, constructive pain in head, chest, legs etc. Irritable feeling under finger nails relieved only by biting them.

Throat: Smarting in the mouth, tickling in throat, with inclination to dry spasmodic cough, especially at night. Burning in fauces, white sticky mucus, chronic speakers catarrh.

Respiratory: Sudden short cough, strangling, tickling in trachea and bronchial tubes, wakes at 3 a.m. with cough. Feels suffocated, continuous cough, when lying down at night. Sharp pain in lungs, whooping cough, dry spasmodic cough on lying down.

Relation: Hydos, Con., Arg nit, Kali bich.

Dose: First potency. *(Boericke)*

The eyes and ovaries are markedly affected. In the morning the eyes are red and sore with mucus in corners. There is a pain in the left ovary, dull with hard swelling- chronic laryngeal catarrh of speakers. A sudden desire to cough- so sudden it causes- strangling- sudden short cough, when rising in morning from accumulation of mucus in throat- Cough at 3 a.m. The mucus of Am. Brom is stringy- there is an irritable feeling under finger nails. Amel, only by biting them- amel: by warmth, warm drinks, agg. open air, cold air- Many symptoms occur on waking at 3 a.m. Must walk about for fear of suffocation. *(JHC)*

It should be remembered in cases of epilepsy, when the prominent symptom is the intense cerebral congestion, also in cerebro spinal meningitis during the congestive stages. The cough returns at short intervals and may be almost continuous for hours, especially while lying down.

(Blackwood)

36. *Ammonium carb.*

(Carbonate of Ammonia)

The diseased conditions met by this remedy are such as we find often in rather stout women who are always tired and weary, take cold easily, suffer from cholera-like symptoms before menses, lead a sedentary life, have a slow reaction generally and are disposed to frequent use of the smelling bottle. Too frequent and profuse menses. Mucus membranes of the respiratory organs are especially affected. Fat patients with weak hearts, wheezing, feel suffocated. Very sensitive to cold air. Great aversion to water, cannot bear to touch it. Malignant scarlatina, with somnolence (sleepiness), swollen glands, dark red sore throat, faintly developed eruption. Uraemia, Heaviness in all organs. Uncleanliness in bodily habits. Swelling of parts, glands etc., acid secretion, prostration from trifles.

Mind: Gloomy during stormy weather, uncleanliness.

Nose: Discharge of sharp burning water, stoppage at night, with long continued coryza, cannot breathe through nose, snuffles of children, epistaxis after washing and after eating.

Mouth: Pressing teeth together, sends shock through head, eyes and ears.

Rectum: Bleeding piles, worse during menses.

Respiratory: Hoarseness, cough every morning about 3'o clock with dyspnoea, palpitation, burning in chest, worse ascending. Chest feels tired. Emphysema. Much oppression in breathing worse after any effort and entering warm room or ascending even a few steps. Asthenic pneumonia. Slow laboured stertorous breathing, bubbling sound. Winter catarrh with slimy sputum and specks of blood. Pulmonary oedema.

Heart: Heart weak.

Sleep: Sleepiness during the day.

Skin: Eczema in the bends of extremities, between legs, about anus and genitals.

Mod: *Worse* evening, from cold wet weather, wet applications, washing, 3-4 a.m., during menses.

Better: Lying on painful side and on stomach, in dry weather.

Relation: Inimical to Lachesis.

Antidotes: Arnica, Camphor.

Compare: Rhus, Muriatic acid, Tartar. emet.

Dose: 6th potency best for general use (Lower potencies deteriorate with age).

(Boericke)

Sal Volatile: Ammonium carb is a right sided remedy and a venous medicine. A condition of under-oxygenation, underlies a large proportion of symptoms. Chilly medicine agg: cold open air, wet stormy weather, from washing- amel: by warmth- stout women, take cold in winter agg: at night 3 a.m., haemorrhagic, bleeding gums, nose, especially morning on washing, bleeding piles, at every menstrual period bleeding from rectum- menses premature, copious, dark (colic and pains in loins or toothache accompanying) somnolence, bloody expectoration, cough, tickling cough, Asthma, cough from 2 to 5 a.m.- eyes, dryness, black spots, sparks, myopia, cataract, Pterygium. A curious symptom inability to blow the nose, in children, stuffed coryza agg: at night, breathes with mouth open, sore throat, heel painful on standing, sleepiness produced in the day time. Dr. Gallavardin has cured uncleanliness in bodily habits with Ammon. carb. Most of the carbonates are suited to states of corpulency- Nose bleed comes on when washing the face. *(JHC)*

37.Ammonium Causticum

This is a powerful cardiac stimulant. As such in syncope, thrombosis, haemorrhage, snake bites, chloroform narcosis, may be given by inhalation. The oedema and ulceration of mucus membranes produced by the powerful drug have been utilised as guiding symptoms for its use. Hence in membranous croup with burning in oesophagus, Aphonia, see causticum.

Respiratory: Loss of voice, burning rawness in throat.

Extremities: Excessive exhaustion, Rheumatism of shoulders, skin hot and dry.

Dose: 1-3rd potency, 5-10 minims well diluted with water. *(Boericke)*

The symptoms of Caustic ammonia, closely resemble those of the Carbonate. The caustic nature of the drug is exemplified in the burning sensation experienced especially in throat gullet and rectum. A good all round remedy in aphonia, oppression of breathing, Timidity. *(JHC)*

38.Ammonium Iodatum

Indicated, when iodine has but partially relieved in cases of laryngitis and bronchitis, catarrhal pneumonia, oedema of lungs.

Dose: Second and third trituration.

(Boericke)

39. Ammonium Mur

A state of prostration bordering on a typhoid state is produced by this remedy. All mucus secretions are increased and retained. It is especially adapted to fat and sluggish patients having respiratory troubles. Coughs associated with catarrhs and affections of liver. A tendency to irregular circulation, blood seems to be in constant turmoil, pulsation etc. Many group of symptoms are accompanied by cough, profuse glairy secretions. Its period of aggravations are peculiarly divided as to the bodily region affected, thus the head and chest symptoms are worse in mornings, the abdominal in the afternoon the pains in the limbs, the skin and febrile symptoms in the evenings 'Boiling' sensation.

Mind: Desire to cry.

Nose: Hot acrid watery discharge, corroding the lips, sneezing, loss of smell, obstructed stuffy feeling.

Throat: Viscid phlegm, so tough it cannot be hawked up.

Stomach: Thirst for lemonade.

Stool: Crumbly.

Female: Menses flow more at night.

Respiratory: Hoarseness and burning in larynx, worse lying on back or right side.

Back: Icy coldness between shoulders, not relieved by warm covering.

Extremities: Shooting and tearing in tips of finger and toes. Pain in heels. Contraction of hamstring tendons, worse sitting, better lying.

Fever: Chilliness evenings after lying down.

Mod: Better open air.

Antidotes: Coffea. Nux, Caust.

Compare: Calcarea, Senega, Caustic.

Dose: 3-6c potency. *(Boericke)*

Ammon Mur. is less prominently a right sided medicine than Ammn. Carb. Guernsey regards it as rather left sided, ulceration and ulcerative pains, tension as if tendons were contracted, Ammn carb. has greater sensitivity to cold and to damp weather than the Murate. Fear of darkness like stramonium. Ulceration in corners of mouth, shooting in scapula and ice cold sensation between scapulae, Unrelieved by external wraps. Constipation and piles with bleeding at stool. Sore smarting haemorrhoids, hard stool covered with mucus, Pain as from ulceration at tips of fingers. Ulcerative pain in heels. Sciatica pain as if tendons were too short- large buttocks. Fatty tumours, Obesity, legs thin (Ammn carb. fat all over). *(JHC)*

The patient frequently feels a boiling throughout the body as if in the blood vessel. Sensitive to cold. Many complaints increase while in the open air. Flushes of heat ending in sweat. Drawing or sensation of shortening of tendons. It cures capsular cataract when the symptom agree. The abdomen is fat, relaxed and heavy and the lower limbs are lean, Burning of the rectum and anus during and long after stool- hard crumbling stool- All the salts of ammonia, like this one have painful haemorrhoids- Menses black clotted- Coldness between the shoulders. *(Kent)*

1) Especially adapted to those who are fat and sluggish or body large and fat but legs too thin.

2) Watery acrid coryza, corroding the lip.

3) During menses-diarrhoea and vomiting bloody discharge from the bowels Neuralgic pains in the feet, flow more profuse at night.

4) Obstinate constipation accompanied by much flatus.

5) Hard crumbling stools require great

effort in expulsion, crumble from the verge of anus.

6) Haemorrhoids, sore and smarting, with burning and stinging in the rectum for hours after stool: especially after suppressed leucorrhoea.

7) Leucorrhoea like white of egg, preceded by griping pain about the navel, brown, slimy, painless after every urination.

8) Sensation of coldness in the back, between scapulae.

9) Hamstring feel painfully short when walking, tension in joints as from shortening of the muscles.

10) Offensive sweat of the feet. *(HCA)*

40. *Ammonium Phosphoricum*

A remedy for chronic gouty patients, uric acid diathesis, indicated in bronchitis and nodosities of the joints of the fingers and backs of the hands. Facial paralysis. Pain in shoulder joint. Tightness around chest, heaviness of limbs, unsteady tottering gait, coldness from least draft of air.

Head: Sneezing with excessive running from nose and eyes only in morning.

Dose: 3rd decimal trituration.

(Boericke)

41.*Ammonium Picratum*

A remedy for malarial fever and neuralgias and so called bilious headaches. Pain in occiput and mastoid region. Whooping cough.

Dose: 3rd Trituration. *(Boericke)*

42. *Ammonium valerianum*

A remedy for nervous hysterical people, suffering from neuralgia, headaches and insomnia, great nervous erethism is always present.

Heart: Pain in cardiac region, functional disturbances, tachycardia.

Dose: Lower triturations. *(Boericke)*

43. *Ampelopsis*

Renal dropsies, hydrocele, and chronic hoarseness in scrofulous patients have been benefited by this drug. Cholereic symptoms, generally worse about 6 p.m. Dilated pupils. Left costal region sore and sensitive. Elbow joints pain, back sore, soreness of all limbs. Vomiting, purging with tenesmus. Rumbling in abdomen.

Dose: Second to third potency.

(Boericke)

44. *Amygdalus persica*

(Peach tree)

A most valuable remedy in vomiting of various kinds, morning sickness, Irritation of eyes. Ischuria and haematuria. Gastric irritation of children, no form of food tolerated, loss of smell and taste. Gastric and intestinal irritation, when the tongue is elongated and pointed, tip and edges red. Constant nausea and vomiting.

Dose: Fresh infusion or mother tincture.

45. *Amyl Nitrosum*

On inhaling the drug, it rapidly dilates all arterioles and capillaries producing flushing of face, heat and throbbing in the head- superficial arterial hyperaemia. Palpitation of the heart and similar condition are readily cured by it, especially the flushings and other discomforts at climacteric. Hiccough and yawning. Often relieves temporarily epileptic convulsions, sea sickness.

Head: Anxiety, must have fresh air, surging of blood to head and face, flushings followed by sweat at climacteric.

Chest: Tumultuous action of heart.

Relation: Glonoine, Lachesis.

Antidote: Cactus, Strychnin, Ergot.

Dose: 3rd potency.

For palliations. In all conditions where the blood vessels are spasmodically contracted as in angina pectoris, epileptic seizure, megrim, accompanied by cold pallor etc., also in paroxysms of Asthma, chloroform asphyxia, inhalation of the Amyl nit. will give immediate relief.

For this non homoeopathic application 2-5 minims (put up in pearls) dropped in a handkerchief and inhaled as may be required. *(Boericke)*

The nitrate of Amyl was introduced into medicine by the old school as a remedy for angina pectoris and was supposed to act by lessening arterial tension- homoeopathic provings have shown that in some cases at any rate Amyl nit has a specific action. The most striking action of the drug is the deep facial flushing it causes and the pulsation all over the body- smacking of lips as if in an act of tasting- Minching movement of lower jaw as if chewing- Exophthalmic goitre from grief- Nash has cured with it chronic blushing on least excitement, mental or physical *(JHC)*

Rapidly dilates the arteries and accelerates but later weakens and retards the pulse- profound and repeated yawning- The cure more frequently depends upon the strength of the potency than many who have put it to the curative test imagine. *(HCA)*

46. *Anacardium*

(Marking nut)

The Anacardium patient is found mostly among the neurasthenics, such have a type of nervous dyspepsia, relieved by food, impaired memory depression and irritability, diminution of senses (smell, sight, hearing), Syphilitic patients often suffer with these conditions. Intermittency of symptoms. Fear of examination in students. Weakening of all senses, sight, hearing etc. Aversion to work, lacks self confidence, irresistible desire to swear and curse, Sensation of a plug in various parts- eyes, rectum, bladder etc., also of a band. Empty feeling in stomach, eating temporarily relieves all discomfort. This is a sure indication often verified. Its skin symptoms are similar to *Rhus.* and it has proved a valuable anti-dote to poison oak.

Mind: He is possessed of two persons or wills. Tendency to use violent language, Brain fag, impaired memory, absent mindedness, very easily offended.

Eyes: Objects appear too far off.

Face: Blue rings around eyes.

Stomach: Empty feeling in stomach. Eating relieves the Anacardium dyspepsia.

Rectum: Ineffectual desire, rectum seems powerless as if plugged up, soft stool will passes with difficulty. Itching at anus, moisture from rectum.

Male: Voluptuous itching, warts on palms of hands, vesicular eruption.

Skin: Intense itching (xerophyl, Grindel, Croton), Lichen planus.

Mod: Worse on application of hot water.

Better: Eating, lying on side, rubbing.

Antidote: Grindel, Coff, Juglans, Rhus, Eucalyptus.

Compare: Anacard occ., Anaesthetic variety of leprosy, warts, corns, ulcers, cracking of the skin on soles of feet- *Rhus, Cypriped, Cheledon, Xerophyl,* follows Platina well, swearing 'Serpentina'

Dose: 6-200c.

A very characteristic sensation is a pressing or penetrating pain as from a plug, which may occur in any locality in connection with neuralgias and ear affection, piles etc. Sensation of a hoop or band around the body or about any part is a leading symptom. The nut is heart shaped, hence its name and perhaps this may be taken as the sign of its courage imparting properties- examination funk- Loss of memory is very marked. Headache agg: by mental exertion, *Amel:* by eating- hearing voices of persons far away or dead- voices behind her- seems to have two wills, propensity to swear - irritability - tendency to commit suicide by shooting. Illusions of smell - The Anacardium indigestion contrasts with that of Nux in a striking way - with the Nux, the pain is worst for two or three hours after a meal, during stomach digestion and is Amel: when that is over, where as with Anac, it is just then (when digestion is complete) that the pain is worst, and it last until the next meal which again *Amel:* for a time- Anac is suited to affections of the palms of the hands- There are warts on the palms. *(JHC)*

The remedy is full of strange notions and ideas. He is in a continuous controversy with himself. He cannot decide, especially in an action of good or evil- Laughs when he should be serious, i.e. the internal will is in a turmoil over this external disturbance. Full of internal anxiety. Fears some dreadful thing will happen. Many symptoms are ameliorated by eating- it will be seldom used except for such mind symptoms- usually when the mental symptoms are strong, the physical are also covered by this remedy- Eruptions all over. *(Kent)*

Wants to pray continually (Stram.)- Great desire for stool but with the effort the desire passes away without evacuation, rectum seems powerless, with sensation as if plugged up- irregular peristaltic or over action (Nux) *(HCA)*

47. *Anagallis*

(Scarlet pimpernel)

Marked action on skin, characterized by great itching and tingling everywhere. Favours expulsion of splinters. An old medicine for hydrophobia and dropsy. Possesses power of softening flash and destroying warts.

Skin: Itching, dry bran-like eruption especially on hands and fingers. Palms especially affected.

Mind: Hilarity- Better from Coffee.

Compare: Cyclamen, Primula, Obcon.

Dose: 1st to 3rd potency. *(Boericke)*

48. *Anatherum*

(Cuscus- An east Indian grass)

A skin remedy of high order. Painful swelling of various parts, going on to suppuration. Glandular inflammation.

Skin: Diseased and deformed nails. Offensive foot sweat. Abscesses, boils, ulcers, Erysipelas, pruritus, herpes.

Relation: Staphys, Mercur, Thuja.

Dose: 3rd potency.

Compare: Sepia, Echinacea, Lappa, Hepar sulph. (Boericke)

49. *Anhalonium*

(Mescal button)

A cactus growing in Mexico.

Mescal is a strong intoxicating spirit distilled from 'Pulque fuerte'. Pulque is made from the Agave Americana of Mexico, locally known as Maguey and is the national beverage of Mexico. Indians call it Peyote. It weakens the heart, produces insanity. Its most striking effects appear in the auditory nerve for it makes each note upon the Piano a centre of melody, which seems to be surrounded by a halo of colour pulsating the Rhythm of the music (Hom. World). Causes a form of intoxication accompanied by wonderful visions remarkably beautiful and varied Kaliedoscopic changes and a sensation of increased physical ability. Also visions of monsters and various gruesome forms. A cardiac tonic and respiratory stimulant. Hysteria and insomnia. A remedy for brain fag, delirium, megrim, hallucinations with coloured brilliant visions. Motor incoordination. Extreme muscular depression, increased patellar reflex. Paraplegia.

Dose: Tincture.

Relation: Agave, Cannabis Indica, Oenanthe. (Boericke)

50. *Anemopsis Californica*

(Yerba mansa)

A mucus membrane medicine. Chronic forms of inflammation of the Schneiderian membrane with considerable relaxation and profuse discharge. Chief value in catarrhal states with considerable stuffy sensation in head and throat. Useful in cuts, bruises and sprains, and as a diuretic and in malaria. Not yet proven, but found useful in profuse mucous or serous discharges, in nasal and pharyngeal catarrh, diarrhoea and urethritis. Recomended in heart disease as a quieting agent, when unduly excited. Flatulence, promotes digestion.

Relation: Piper meth.

Dose: Tincture internally and locally as a spray. *(Boericke)*

51. *Angustura vera*

(Bark of Galipea - Cusparia)

Rheumatic and paralytic complaints- Great difficulty in walking. Cracking in all joints. The greatest craving for coffee. Caries of long bones, paralysis, tetanus, stiffness of muscles and joints oversensitive.

Extremities: Pain in knees, cracking in joints.

Relation: Nux ruta, Mercur, Brucea, Bark of nux vomica- Angustura falsa.

Dose: 6th potency.

52. *Anilinum*

(Coal tar product-Amidobenzene)

Marked giddiness and pain in head, face has a purple hue. Pain in penis and scrotum with swelling. Tumors of the urinary passages. Profound anaemia, with discolouration of skin, blue lips, anorexia, gastric disturbances, swelling of skin.

Relation: Arsenic, Antipyrin.

(Boericke)

The symptoms are in many respects like those of Arsenic. *(JHC)*

53. *Anthemis Nobilis*

(Roman chamomile)

This remedy is akin to the ordinary chamomilla. Gastric disturbance with coldness, sensitive to cold air and cold things.

Coryza with much lachrymation, sneezing and discharge of clear water from the nose. Symptoms worse indoors. Constriction and rawness of throat. Cough tickling, worse in warm room.

Abdomen: Chilliness inside of abdomen.

Dose: Use 3rd potency. *(Boericke)*

54. *Anthracinum*

(Anthrax poison)

This nosode has proven a great remedy in epidemic spleen diseases of domestic animals and in septic inflammation, carbuncles and malignant ulcers. In boils and boil like eruptions, acne. Terrible burning induration of cellular tissue, abscess, bubo and all inflammation of connective tissue in which there is a purulent focus.

Relation: Arsenic follows.

Compare: Pyrogen, Lachesis, Crotalus, Hippozen, Echinac, Silica, Tarentula cub. Tissues Haemorrhage, black, thick, tar like, rapidly decomposing from any orifice.

Glands swollen, cellular tissues, oedematous and indurated, septicemia, ulceration, sloughing and intolerable burning, Erysipelas, black and blue blisters, dissecting wounds, insect stings, bad effects from inhaling foul odors, gangrenous parotitis, secretion from boils, gangrene, foul secretions.

In the treatment of carbuncles, remember the prescription of the Prophet 'Isaiah' for king 'Hezekiah's' carbuncle i.e. apply the pulp of a fig placed on a poultice.

Dose: 30c. *(Boericke)*

Anthracinum is indicated in all conditions of boils and boil like eruptions. Hard stony swelling in region of right lower jaw and submaxillary gland- Anthrax quinsy. *(JHC)*

55. *Anthrakokali*

(Anthracite coal dissolved in boiling caustic potash)

Useful in skin affections, scabies, prurigo, chronic herpes, cracks and ulcerations. Papular like eruption with a vesicular tendency, especially on scrotum, also on hands, tibia, shoulders and dorsum of feet. Intense thirst. Chronic rheumatism. Bilous attacks, vomiting of bile, tympanic distension of abdomen.

Dose: Low triturations. *(Boericke)*

A very absurd combination says Herring proved on many people, but in a very superficial way. It has been principally used in skin affections, scabies, prurigo, chronic herpes and chronic cracks and ulceration of nostrils- Eruption decrease with the full moon. The intense thirst and diuresis suggest a place for the remedy in Diabetes.

(JHC)

56. *Antimonium Arsenicosum*

Synopsis: Emphysema, extreme dyspnoea, worse on eating and lying down, cardiac weakness, pleurisy, oedema of face.

Found useful in emphysema with excessive dyspnoea and cough with mucus secretion. Worse on eating and lying down. Catarrhal pneumonia associated with influenza. Myocarditis and cardiac weakness. Pleurisy, especially of left side with exudation and pericarditis, with effusion. Sense of weakness. Inflammation of eyes and oedema of face.

Dose: 3rd trituration. *(Boericke)*

This remedy is of service in cases of extreme dyspnoea and emphysema in those who are weak and prostrated. This is frequently observed during pleurisy and pericarditis, when attended with effusion. There is cough, the patient is worse after eating and while lying down.

(Blackwood)

57. *Antimonium Crudum*

(Black sulphide of Antimony)

For homoeopathic employment the mental symptoms and those of the gastric sphere determine its choice. Excessive irritability and fretfulness together with a thickly coated white tongue are guiding symptoms to many forms of disease calling for this remedy. All the conditions are aggravated by heat and cold bathing. Cannot bear heat of the sun. Tendency to grow fat. An absence of pain, where it could be expected, is not noticeable. Gout with gastric symptoms.

Mind: Child cannot bear to be touched or looked at. Angry at every little attention.

Head: Aching from bathing, from disordered stomach.

Eyes: Canthi raw and fissured, blepharitis.

Nose: Chapped and covered with crusts. Eczema of nostrils, sore, cracked and scurfy.

Face: Yellow crusted eruption on cheeks.

Mouth: Cracks at corners of mouth, tongue coated thick white as if white washed, canker sores.

Stomach: Loss of appetite, desire for acids, pickles, eructation tasting of ingesta, constant belching, bloating after eating.

Stool: Diarrhoea alternates with constipation. Hard lumps mixed with watery discharge, catarrhal proctitis.

Respiratory: Cough worse coming into warm room, itching of chest, voice harsh and badly pitched.

Extremities: Arthritic pain in fingers, feet very tender, corns.

Skin: Urticaria, warts, pustular eruption, itching worse at night.

Dose: 3rd to 6th potency.

Complementary: Sulphur- Anti: Hepar.

(Boericke)

Anti-crud corresponds in a sense to the race of swine, as Arsenic does to horses and pulsatilla to sheep- Rough scaling skin with horny patches- warts- Anti-crud 200 has cured many cases of these tendency of the nails to grow in splits- coated moist white tongue- Tendency to grow fat- Moist eruption behind ears, sentimental mood by moonlight- It cures many cases of mucous piles- continuous oozing staining linen- Sore cracked and crusty nostrils and corners of mouth- Moonlight agg: mental symptom, agg: from wine, especially sour wine from vinegar and acids (though tamarind water does not disagree), from fruits, pork bread and pastry. *(JHC)*

Centre about the stomach- it does not matter much, what kind of complaints he suffers from, the stomach takes part in it. It produces a very serious state in the mind and absence of the desire to live- 'Oh! doctor, if I could only die'. The medicine is thirstless, over excitable, intense, nervous, hysterical, ecstatic young girls and women are over come by mellow lights, such as flow through stained glass windows or the mellow light from the moon in the evening- sentimental mood in the moon light- a gouty or rheumatic state, worse in cold damp weather- Taking sour wine- A child with whooping cough will cough more after looking into the fire, such things are 'queer'-gout in the stomach- catarrh of the nose, stomach, rectum- As soon as he gets into an overheated room, his nose gets stuffed up- The whole tongue is covered with a milky- white coating- He hurries to stool and passes little lumps and some liquid and is soon hurried again to stool and more lumps and liquid are passed and this goes on in summer diarrhoeas and finally the bowel is emptied and then there is a great tenesmus- agg: sour wine or taking sour food- tendency to grow warts- callosities- bad nails and bad hair- hard horny excrescences grow under the nail. *(Kent)*

58. Antimonium sulphuratum auratum

(Golden sulphuret of Antimony)

A remarkable remedy for many forms of chronic nasal bronchial catarrh, Acne, Amaurosis.

Nose and throat: Nose bleeding on washing.

Respiratory: Increased mucus.

Dose: Second or third trituration.

(Boericke)

Its most notable effects were produced on the eye and chest- Amaurosis commencing- spots on cornea and hypopion- Acute and chronic nasal and bronchial catarrh- Acne- Nose bleed on washing. *(JHC)*

59. Antimonium tartaricum

(Tartar emetic. Tartar of Antimony and Potash)

Has many symptoms in common with Antimonium crudum but also many peculiar to itself. Clinically its therapeutic application has been confined largely to the treatment of respiratory diseases, rattling of mucus with little expectoration has been a guiding symptom. There is much drowsiness, debility and sweat, characteristic of the drug group which should always be more or less present when this drug is prescribed. Gastric affections of drunkards and gouty subjects, Cholera morbus. Sensation of coldness in blood vessels. Bilharziasis. Antimonium Tart is homoeopathic in dysuria, strangury, haematuria, albuminuria, catarrh of bladder and urethra, burning in rectum, bloody mucus stools etc. Ant. tart acts indirectly on the parasites by stimulating the oxidizing action of the protective substance. By effects following the injection for Bilharziasis. Chills and contractures and pain in muscles. Trembling of whole body, great prostration and faintness. Lumbago, chill contractures and muscular pains. Warts on glans penis.

Tongue: Coated and pasty, thick white.

Face: Pale covered with cold sweat. Incessant quivering of chin and lower jaw.

Stomach: Nausea, retching and vomiting. Thirst for cold water, little and often and desire for apples, fruits and acids generally.

Respiratory organs: Great rattling of mucus but very little is expectorated. Coughing and gaping consecutively. Oedema and impending paralysis of lungs.

Back: Violent pain in sacro-lumbar region. Sensation of heavy weight at the coccyx, dragging downwards all the time.

Skin: Pustular eruption, warts, small-pox.

Mod: Worse night, sour things, milk. Better- sitting erect, eructation and expectoration.

Antidotes: Puls., sepia.

Compare: Kali sulph, Ipecac.

Dose: 2nd to 6th Trituration. The lowest potencies some time aggravate.

(Boericke)

Anti tart was the favourite emetic of olden times and consequently, it is one of the best remedies in states on nausea. The nausea is as intense as that of Ipcc, but less persistent and is Amel: by vomiting. Nash has found it the nearest thing to a specific in cholera morbus, the indication being Nausea, vomiting, loose stools, child cough when angry is characteristic. The symptoms of which, disease are so closely reproduced in the proving that, it has been used instead of vaccine for inoculation purpose and prophylactic power has been claimed for it- the terrible back ache of small pox is paralleled by the back pains of Ant. tart. which I have found to correspond to more cases of lumbago, than any other remedy.

(JHC)

In the first state Anti-tart may not be indicated but Bry and Ipecac come in- It is the remedy that close out the scene with the severe cases of bronchitis, pneumonia- most of these cases die in an Anti tart state. The children that do not look sick, when they have cold, rattling in chest, but do not come down with weakness- they call for *Kali sulph-* Anti tart with its difficult breathing is sick at stomach, loathes every thing, loathes food, vomits even water- Then this gouty state affects the teeth. His teeth are all rheumatic- rheumatic pain in the teeth- with rheumatic pains in joints, teeth are sensitive, teeth covered with mucus- this remedy is thirstless- aversion to milk and every other kind of nourishment, but milk especially makes the patient sick causing nausea and vomiting. *(Kent)*

60. Antipyrine

(Phenazone- A coal tar derivative)

Antipyrine is one of the drugs that induces leucocytosis similar to ergotin, salicylates and tuberculin. Acts especially on the vasomotor centres, causing dilation of capillaries of skin and consequent circumscribed patches of hyperaemia and swelling. In large doses causes profuse perspiration, dizziness, cyanosis and somnolence, albumen and blood in urine. Acute erythema multiform.

Mind: Hallucinations of sight and hearing.

Head: Sensation of constriction, head ache under ears with earache.

Eyes: Lachrymation.

Ears: Tinnitis.

Mouth: Swelling of lips.

Skin: erythema, Eczema, pemphigus, intense pruritis, Urticaria appearing and disappearing suddenly with internal coldness. Angio neurotic oedema. Dark blotches on skin of penis, some times with oedema.

Dose: Second decimal potency.

(Boericke)

This remedy is of service in erythema which appears first upon the arms and extends to the legs, also chronic urticaria of women with great itching and bulbous eruptions. In these cases the intense itching has been a guiding indication.

(Blackwood)

61. Apis Mellifica

(The honey bee)

Acts on cellular tissues causing oedema of skin and mucous membranes. The very characteristic effects of the sting of the bee furnish unerring indications for its employment in disease. Swelling or puffing up of various parts, oedema red rosy hue, stinging pains, soreness, intolerance of heat and slightest touch and afternoon aggravation are some of the general guiding symptoms. Erysipelatous inflammations dropsical effusions and anasarca, acute inflammation of kidneys and other parenchymatous tissues are characteristic pathological state corresponding to Apis. It acts especially on outer parts, skin, coatings of inner organs, serous membranes. It produces serous inflammation with effusion, membranes of brain, heart, pleuritic effusion etc. Extreme sensitiveness to touch and general soreness is marked. Constricted sensations. Sensation of stiffness and as of some thing torn off in the interior of the body. Much prostration.

Mind: Awkward- drops things readily, whining tearfulness.

Eyes: Lids swollen, oedematus serous exudation, oedema and sharp pains, suppurative inflammation of eyes, intense chemosis of ocular conjuctiva, styes.

Nose: Red swollen, puffy, fiery red. Fiery red margin, thirstless, craving for milk, cholera infantum type.

Urine: Scanty high coloured last drop burn and smart.

Respiratory: Dyspnoea as if he could not draw another breath.

Skin: Sudden starting during sleep. Fever, afternoon chill with thirst, worse on motion and heat.

Modalities: Worse heat in any form, touch, pressure, late in afternoon after sleeping, in closed and heated rooms, right side. Better in open air, uncovering and cold bathing.

Relation: Comple.: Natrum mur, chronic: Apis, also Baryta carb, if lymphatics are involved.

Compare: Apium virus (auto toxaemia with pus products) zinc, canth, vespa, lachesis.

Dose: Tincture to 30th potency. In oedematous conditions the lower potencies. Some times action is slow, so several days elapse before it seems to act and then urine is increased.

Apium Virus- 6c *(Boericke)*

Honey bee poison- Tr. are made of the whole bee- The well known effects of a bee sting, burning, stinging and lancinating pain with excessive swelling give leasing key notes for its employment in a great variety of conditions. The burning symptoms of 'Apis' are distinguished from those of *Ars.* in being *agg:* by heat. Apis has slow action and must not be changed too soon- increased flow of urine shows it is having a favourable effect- The dropsies of Apis are characterised by a waxy hue of skin, whitish or yellowish, transparent swelling of eyelids, bag like swelling under eyes- in cardiac dropsy, the feet swell after walking and are intolerably sore and burning. Tension, swelling and stiffness of limbs- Aversion to tight things like Lach.- Sensitiveness to heat especially to heated rooms. Agg: in the night and sleep is disturbed by piercing cries or else by moaning and whining- Compare Acet. Ac. (dropsy) - Apo. can. (dropsy), Apis is right to left- Antidotes to medium doses and poisonings; Nat. mur in all forms, sweet oil, onions, Ammonia- Nat mur the chronic of Apis. Inimical: Rhus in eruptive diseases. Causation- Grief, Fright, Rage, Vexation, Jealousy, (The queen bee is the most jealous thing in nature). *(JHC)*

All over the body a thick rash, sometimes of a rose colour is found. In the extremities we have marked dropsy, swelling with pitting upon pressure. A general anasarca may appear. The face is greatly swollen at times. The eyelids look like water bags, the uvula hangs down like a water bag, the abdominal walls are of great thickness and pit upon pressure- puffing or oedema with pitting upon pressure is a general condition, that may be present in any inflammatory state- Amel: from cold and aggr: from heat- If the baby needs opium or Apis in congestion of the brain the fits become worse by bathing in hot water- Apis affects the thing that are external- it also affects the envelopes or coverings of organs for example the pericardium- inflammation of the membrane of the brain. Peritoneum- The symptoms themselves are- great sadness, constant tearfulness, without any cause, weeping night and day. Foolishly suspicious and jealous- Absolutely joyless- No ability to apply things that would make her happy herself- talking foolish things, such as a child would talk on serious occasions- child lying with eyes partly closed- meningitis- opisthotonus- Ailments from fright, rage, vexation, jealousy or hearing bad news. Apis is a great remedy for eyes- deep seated inflammatory complaints- White spots- opacities- enlarged blood vessels. Oedema of the lids, both upper and lower, burning and stinging like fire, better from washing, from cold applications. Whole conjuctiva inflamed, diphtheria, Uvula hangs down like a bag of water. The tongue swells until it fills the mouth. An adult who is shivering while covered up will kick off the covers. The abdomen is distended with gas. Great tension and fullness, hard and drum like- In the external abdomen there is an oedematous state- Dropsy sometimes alone, sometimes with anasarca- limbs swollen to the full extent- pitting upon pressure the feet and limbs swollen- with burning, stinging and numbness in the limbs. The anus protrudes with stool and seems to remain open- chronic diarrhoea, dysentery- the urine is scanty, coming only in drops- burning urine- the whole urinary tract is irritated very much like cantharis and these two medicines antidote each other - it is queer how the old women knew long before Apis was proved, that when the little new born baby did not pass its water they could find cure by going out to the bee hive and catching a few bees, over which they poured hot water and of which they gave the baby a tea spoonful- "Urine scanty and foetid, containing albumen and blood corpuscles"- genital organs of both male and female- swelling and oedematous. Apis is a great friend of women- inflammation of uterus and ovaries. Ovaries enlarged, dropsy of right ovary. *(Kent)*

62. *Apium Graveolens*

(Common celery)

Contains a soporific active principle. Obstinate retention of urine, throbbing headaches and heart burn have been produced by celery. Swelling of throat, face and hands. Rheumatic pain in muscles of neck, also in sacrum. Growing pains. Hungry for apples. Dysmenorrhoea, with sharp short pains better flexing legs.

Dose: 1-30c *(Boericke)*

63. *Apocynum Androsaemifolium*

(Dogbane)

The rheumatic symptoms of this remedy promise most curative result. Its pains are of wandering nature, with much stiffness and drawing. Every thing smells and tastes like honey. Worms, trembling and prostration. Swollen sensations.

Extremities: Pain in all joints. Pain in toes and soles. Swelling of hands and feet- Profuse sweat- with much heat in soles. Tingling pain in soles, toes. Cramp in soles. Violent heat in soles. (sulph.)

Dose: Tincture to 1st potency.

(Boericke)

Swelling sensation of face and body. Swelling of hands and feet, showing its relation to dropsical states like Apo. Can and Stroph- Heaviness with great desire to sleep- flying pains in different parts, itching of body and face. Acute rheumatism with great stiffness - General rheumatic pains. Hale has cured with it rheumatic gout. Acute pains in the joints attended with cramps, bilious stools and flying pains in the teeth- The tincture in drop doses has been known to expel ascarides and other worms. It has been called upon for expelling renal calculi and gravel. *(JHC)*

64. *Apocynum Cannabinum*

(Indian hemp)

Increases secretions of mucus and serous membranes and acts on cellular tissue producing oedema and dropsy and on skin diaphoresis. Acute hydrocephalus. A diminished frequency of pulse is a prime indication. This is one of the most efficient remedies in dropsies, ascites, anasarca and hydrothorax and urinary troubles, especially suppression and strangury. In the digestive complaints of bright disease with the nausea, vomiting, drowsiness, difficult breathing, it will be found of frequent service. The dropsy is characterised by great thirst and gastric irritability- Arrhythmia, Mitral and tricuspid regurgitation. Acute alcoholism. Relaxation of sphincters. Stool watery.

Urine: Hot urine with thick mucus burning in urethra, little expulsive power, dribbling, renal dropsy.

Respiratory: Short and unsatisfactory.

Heart: Irregular cardiac action, low arterial tension.

Mod: *Worse* cold weather, cold drinks, uncovering.

Relation: *Compare Apis, Arsenic, Digital, Hellab.*

Dose: Tr. (10 drops three times daily) and in acute alcoholism. 1 dram of decoction in 4 oz. water.

Cymarin active principle of Apocyn lowers pulse rate- increase blood pressure. *(Boericke)*

65. Apomorphia

(Alkaloid from decomposition of morphine by Hydrochloric Acid)

The chief power of this drug lies in the speedy and effective vomiting that it produces, which becomes a guiding symptom to its homoeopathic use. The vomiting is preceded by nausea, lassitude and increased secretion of sweat, saliva, mucus and tears. Pneumonia with vomiting. Combined alcoholism with constant nausea, constipation, insomnia.

Stomach: Nausea and vomiting of pregnancy, sea sickness.

Dose: 3rd to 6th potency. *(Boericke)*

66. Aquilegia

(Columbine)

A remedy for hysteria. Globus and clavus hystericus. Women at climaxis with vomiting of green substance, especially in the morning. Sleeplessness. Nervous trembling of body. Sensitive to light and noise. Dysmenorrhoea of young girls.

Dose: First potency. *(Boericke)*

67. Aragallus Lamberti

(White loco weed)

Acts principally on nervous system producing a bewildered confused state, symptoms of inco-ordination and paralysis. Locomotor ataxia, Tired in the morning.

Dose: 6-200C. *(Boericke)*

68. Aralia Racemosa

(American spikenard)

This is a remedy for asthmatic condition with cough aggravated on lying down, drenching sweat during sleep. Extreme sensitiveness to draughts. Diarrhoea, prolapse of rectum. Aching in rectum, extending upwards, worse lying on side lain upon first.

Respiratory: Dry cough coming on after sleep, about middle of night with spasmodic cough, worse after first sleep with tickling in throat, constriction of chest, feels as if foreign body were in throat. Obstruction worse in spring. Hay fever, frequent sneezing, Rawness and burning behind sternum. The least current of air causes sneezing with copious watery excoriating nasal discharge of salty acrid taste.

Mod: Worse about 11 p.m. (cough)

Relation: Pectin, Scallop (humid asthma), Ars iod, Naphthaline, Cepa, Rosa, Sabad, Sinapis.

Dose: Tincture to third potency.

(Boericke)

Aralia was used by the old herbalists and by eclectics as a remedy in phthisis and coughs and also for leucorrhoea and other complaints of women whose secretions are acrid or suppressed. The homoeopathic uses have been chiefly based on a proving by Dr. S.A. Jones, in whom it developed an attack of asthma. The symptoms were loud wheezing, respiration coming on immediately on lying down at midnight, and he particularly noted that inspiration was very loud and more difficult than expiration. The right lung appeared more affected than the left on turning to left side became quite free. As the attack passed off phlegm came more freely, had a salty taste, and felt warm in the mouth. The characteristic cough according to Burnett is a fit of coughing occurring before midnight, either immediately on lying down or more commonly after a short sleep- cough occurring at 11 p.m. After a short sleep- Profuse perspiration whist asleep. Dr. Jones also experienced diarrhoea and prolapse of rectum, soft yellow stools, after stool an aching pain in the rectum, extending upwards on the left side.

Compare: 'chlorium'(opp of Aral- inspiration easy, expiration difficult), Rumex (11p.m. cough)

(JHC)

69. *Aranea Diadema*

(Papal cross spider)

All spider poisons powerfully affect the nervous system. (see Tarentula, Mygale etc.). All symptoms of Aranea are characterised by periodicity and coldness and great susceptibility to dampness. It is the remedy for the constitutional favourable to malarial poisoning where every damp day or place favours chilliness. Patient feels cold to the very bones, coldness not relieved by anything. Feeling as if parts were enlarged and heavier. Wakes up at night with hands feeling twice their natural size. Spleen swollen. Hydrogenoid constitution i.e. abnormal sensitiveness to damp and cold, inability to live near fresh water, lakes, rivers etc. or in damp, chilly places. (Nat sulph., Thuja)

Head: Better by smoking in open air.

Female: Menses too early, too copious.

Fever: Coldness, with pain in long bones- chilly day and night.

Mod: worse damp weather. Better- smoking tobacco.

Relation: Heloderma, Cedron, Arsenic.

Dose: Tr. to 30th potency.

Aranearum Tela (cobweb)- Lowers the frequency of pulse, sleeplessness.

Aranea scinencia (Grey spider) Constant twitching of under eyelids.

Grauvogl is our chief authority for the use of Aranea- It is one of the leading remedies for the hydrogenoid constitution as described by him and for intermittent fevers and other intermittent affections. By hydrogenoid constitution he meant, abnormal sensitiveness to damp and cold and inability to live near fresh water, either rivers or lakes or in pamp., chilly places. This gives the agg. from bathing, from damp weather, damp localities or habitations agg. drawing in cold air, chill and neuralgic attacks at the same hour everyday, every other day- of coldness as if bones were made of ice- Toothache agg: night after lying down- on lying down in bed and touching bed clothes, weather linen or wool, has a chill.

(JHC)

This agent produces a coldness, similar to that of malarial poisoning that returns with marked regularity and renders the system very susceptible to dampness and cold changes. *(Blackwood)*

70. *Arbutus Andrachne*

(Strawberry tree)

A remedy for eczema, associated with gouty and rheumatic symptoms. Arthritis, especially larger joints, urine rendered more clear. Lumbago, symptoms shift from skin to joints. Vesical symptoms.

Dose: Tincture to 3rd potency.

Relation: Arbutine, Ledum, Bryonia, Kalmia. *(Boericke)*

This is one of Cooper's remedies. He cured several cases of eczema with it and observed that it produced pains in the joints of a gouty or rheumatic character. Hence he was led to give it in certain inveterate cases of Arthritis. In one case the patient noticed that it cleared his urine- Arbutin has a reputation among the allopaths as a urinary remedy- Arbutus is allied to 'Uva Ursi' which belongs to the Ericaceae. One patient who was benefited by the remedy had agg: in north east winds. The larger joints are principally affected and the slightest movement sets up inflammation. The tree sheds its bark annually, which gives the signature of its use in skin cases. *(JHC)*

71. *Areca*

(Betel nut)

The chief medical use of the Areca nut has been in helminthiasis in dogs but it is not without danger. The dose 1 grain each pound of dog's weight, it arrests the heart action in diastole in poisonous doses and in nontoxic doses, increases the amplitude without increasing the frequency. Contracts the pupil, Helminthiasis, Glaucoma, Salivation, contraction of intestine. *(JHC)*

Of use in Helminthiasis. Its alkaloid Areollin hydrobrom contracts the pupil, acting more promptly and energetically but of shorter duration than Eserine. Serviceable in glaucoma. Acts also as a salivatory like pilocarpin. Also increases the amplitude of pulsations of the heart and promotes the contractibility of the intestines. *(Boericke)*

72. *Argemone Mexicana*

(Prickly poppy)

Colicky cramp and spasm of bowels. Painful neuro-muscular conditions, preventing sleep. Rheumatic disease associated with bright's disease.

Mod: Worse at noon (Weakness)

Dose: 6c- Fresh juice is applied to ulcers and warts. *(Boericke)*

73. *Argentum Met*

(Silver)

Emaciation a gradual dry up, desire for fresh air, dyspnoea, sensation of expansion and left sided pains are characteristic. The chief action is centered on the articulations and their component elements, bones, cartileges and ligaments. Here the small blood vessels become closed up or withered and carious affections result. They come on insidiously, lingering but progressing. The larynx is also a special centre for this drug.

Head: Feels empty hollow.

Throat: Jelly like mucus, profuse and easy morning expectoration.

Respiratory: Hoarseness, easy expectoration, looking like boiled starch. Feeling of raw spot near supra-sternal fossa. Worse from use of voice. Cough from laughing. Great weakness of chest.

Urine: Profuse, turbid. Sweet odour.

Extremities: Involuntary contraction of fingers, writers cramp, Swelling of ankles.

Male: Seminal emissions, without sexual excitement.

Female: Eroded spongy cervix, leucorrhoea, climacteric haemorrhage.

Mod: Worse from touch, towards noon. Better:- in open air, cough at night when lying down (Opp Hyoscy)

Relation: Antidotes Merc., Puls.

Compare: Selen., Alum., Platina, Stannum, Ampelopsis.

Dose: 6x and higher- not too frequent repetition.

(Boericke)

He walks and walks- many symptoms are better from motion and especially walking. Pains are many times palliated by copious drafts of Coffee- A man of forty is like one of eighty- all these pains are better from motion. A super abundance of cartilaginous tissue, so that round about the joints the cartileges are thickened. It has cured all sorts of tumors, enlargement of ovary and infiltration of tissues, it is a chilly remedy- wants to be kept warm- hysterical itching and burning like frost bites. Scratching until bleeding in the ear. Now this itching involves the whole outside ear- thickening of the bones in the nose. It cures albuminuria, it cures diabetes, and sugar in the urine and many of the broken down conditions of the kidneys- A copious flow of urine. Crushed pain in the right testicle- The right testicle, the left ovary- women, prolapsus. Argentum is one of the medicines. It is a medicine of great use in horribly offensive leucorrhoea- where it was given in case of scirrhus of the uterus (it says)- in less than three days, foul smell was lost entirely- Loss of voices, with inflammation, from over-use of the voice, such as occurs in singers and talkers- Many of the complaints are increased during rest. All the nervous excitement that is possible in remedies comes up in this remedy.

(Kent)

This agent acts upon the larynx producing a sub-acute catarrhal condition, and upon the articulations, producing a condition that stimulates arthralgia and arthritis.

There is loss of voice in professional singers, or the quality of the voice is changed. It is if service in arthritis, especially of the elbow and knee, the legs are trembling and weak. Also in arthralgia, as coxalgia and hysterical joints.

(Blackwood)

74. *Argentum Nit*

(Nitrate of silver)

In this drug the neurotic effects are very marked, many brain and spinal symptoms presenting themselves which give certain indications for its homoeopathic employment, symptoms of in-coordination, loss of control and want of balance every where, mentally and physically, trembling in affected parts. It is an irritant of mucus membranes, producing violent inflammation of the throat and a marked gastroenteritis. Very characteristic is the great desire of sweets, the splincter like pains and free muco-purulent discharge in the inflamed and ulcerated mucus membranes. Sensations as if a part were expanding and other errors of perception are characteristic. Withered up and dried constitutions, present a favourable field for its action, especially when associated with unusual or long continued mental exertion. Head symptoms often determine the choice of this remedy. Pains increase and decrease gradually. Flatulent state and premature aged look. Explosive belching especially in neurotics. Upper abdominal affections brought on only by undue mental exertion. Paraplegia, Myelitis and disseminated sclerosis of brain and cord. Intolerance of heat. Sensation of a sudden pinch.*(Dudgeon)*

Destroys red blood corpuscles, producing anaemia.

Mind: Nervous, Melancholic, time passes slowly, impulsive, wants to do things in a hurry. Peculiar mental impulses.

Head: Headache with coldness and trembling sense of expansion, vertigo, enlarged feeling in corresponding eye, better on tight bandaging and pressure.

Eyes: Swollen and red, purulent ophthalmia discharge, abundant and purulent.

Mouth: Gums tender and bleed easily, taste coppery, like ink.

Throat: Thick mucus, sensation of splinter in throat. Strangulated feeling.

Stomach: Belching, painful swelling of pit, great craving for sweets.

Ulcerated pain in left side under ribs, desire for cheese and salt.

Abdomen: With much flatulent distention.

Stool: Green like chopped spinach, fluids go right through him.

Respiratory: High notes cough.

Sleep: Dreams of snakes and sexual gratification.

Mod: Worse sweets, left side, better cold.

Relation: Antidote: Nat mur.

Compare: Ars, Merc, Phos, Pulsat, Argent Cyanatum, Argent iodat., Argent Phos (An excellent diuretic in dropsy).

Dose: 3-30c.

Best form of an aqueous solution 1 to 9, two or three doses. This solution in water preferable to lower triturations. Unless fresh, these readily decompose into the oxide.

In ophthalmia, mother tincture one or two grains in one ounce of distilled water as eye drop. *(Boericke)*

It was the use of *Arg. nit.* in olden times in the treatment of epilepsy, which led to the production of the lamentable cases of lead coloured pigmentation of the skin called Argyria- Sensation of a splinter sticking in various parts. Irresistible desire for sugar. Fluids go right through him- Belching accompanies most gastric affections- Green stools are remarkable- Green mucus like chopped spinach in flakes- stool turning green after remaining on diaper- agg: sugar- At night or in morning on rising (epileptic attacks), Arg. Met. acts on cartileges, Arg. Nit. more on mucous membranes, skin, bone and periosteum and is suited to herpetic patients. *(JHC)*

Disturbance in the memory, disturbance of reason, does strange things and comes to strange conclusions- hurry and in a fidget- he goes out and walks and walks. The faster he walks, the faster he thinks- he must walk and he walks fatigued- when about to meet an engagement, he is anxious until the time comes- he is like a pulsatilla patient, he wants cold air, cold drinks, cold things, wants ice cream, wants the head in cold air, suffocates in a warm room- every where we find ulceration but particularly upon mucous membrane- the throat has ulcers in it- ulceration of the eye lids and of the cornea- ulceration of the bladder, ulceration of the uterus of the vagina and of the external soft parts. This tendency to ulcerate seems rather strange, peculiar. It has cured prolonged and most inveterate ulceration of the stomach, when there has been vomiting of blood- the most flatulent medicine in the book-cornea opaque-far sightedness-produce warts in the throat-felt as if he had a stick in the throat-stick in the throat like fish bones. Nit. ac, Hepar and Arg. nit have fish bone sensation- desires sugar, brings on eructation- increased flatulence- sour stomach- flatulence passes upwards- frequent eructations- Antidote is Nat mur- when you have the ulceration where the throat has been cauterised or the cervix uteri or eyelids have been cauterised by nitrate of silver study Natrum mur. *(Kent)*

Opthalmia neonatorum, profuse purulent discharges, cornea opaque, ulcerated, lids thick swollen agglutinated in morning. Boys complain after using tobacco. The 200th or 1000th potency in watery solution as topical application in ophthalmia neonatorum has relieved when the crude silver nitrate has failed. *(HCA)*

75.Aristolochia Milhomens

(Brazilian snake root)

Stitching pains in various parts. Pain in heels burning in anus and frequent irritation. Flatulence in stomach and abdomen. Pain in back and extremities. Stiffness of legs. Pain in tendo-achilles. Itching and swelling around the malleoli.

Relation: Compare- Aristolochia serpentaria.

Dose: Lower potencies. *(Boericke)*

76. Arnica

(Leopards bane)

Produces condition upon the system quite similar to those resulting from injuries, falls, blows, contusions, Tinnitus aurium, putrid phenomena, septic conditions, prophylactic of pus infection. Apoplexy red full face. It is especially suited to cases when any injury, however remote seems to have caused the present trouble. After traumatic injuries over-use of any organ, strains. Arnica is disposed to cerebral congestion. Acts best in plethoric, feebly in debilitated with impoverished blood, cardiac dropsy with dyspnoea. A muscular tonic. Traumatism of grief remorse or sudden realisation of financial loss. Limbs and bodyache as if beaten, joints as if sprained- bed feels too hard. Marked effect on the blood. Affects the venous system inducing stasis. Ecchymosis and haemorrhages. Relaxed blood vessels, black and blue spots. Tendency to haemorrhage and low fever states. Tendency to tissue degeneration, septic conditions, abscesses, that do not mature. Sore, lame bruised feeling. Neuralgias originating in disturbance of pneumo-gastric. Rheumatism of muscular and tendinous tissue, especially of back and shoulders. Aversion to tobacco. Influenza. Thrombosis, haematocele (diffusion of blood into a cavity).

Mind: Says there is nothing the matter with him- wants to be let alone- cannot bear pain- over-sensitive.

Head: Hot with cold body.

Mouth: Fetid breath, taste as from bad eggs.

Stomach: Longing for vinegar, distaste for milk and meat, canine hunger, feeling as if stomach were pressing against spine.

Stool: Straining of tenesmus in diarrhoea, offensive, bloody, dysenteric stools.

Respiratory: Violent spasmodic cough with facial herpes, pleurodynia (Ranunc., Cimic.)

Heart: Angina pectoris.

Skin: Black and blue, corps of small boil, Acne indurata. (Ichthyol & Sil)

Fever: Febrile symptom closely related to typhoid, nightly sour sweats.

Mod: *Worse:* least touch, Better: lying down- head low.

Relation: Antidotes- Camphor.

Comple: Aconite, Ipecac.

Compare: Acon, Bapt, Bellis, Hamam, Rhus, Hyperic.

Dose: 3rd to 30c- Locally tincture- should never be applied hot and not on abrasions and cuts. *(Boericke)*

Growing on the mountains Arnica may be said to possess a native affinity to the effects of falls. Trauma in all its varieties and effects, recent and remote is met by Arnica. Tumours in many parts, following injury, have been cured by Arnica, including scirrhous tumours of the breast- An odd symptom of Arnica is coldness of the nose- Patient had bitter taste- 'Usher' notes that the local use of Arnica, produced an extra ordinary growth of hair on a limb- This suggested the use of an oil mixed with Arn. 1x in a case of baldness, which was followed by marked success- Nash gives the following as leaders- Stupor with involuntary discharge of faeces and urine- Fears being touched or struck by those coming near him- Putrid smell from mouth- Bruised sore feeling in uterine region- cannot walk erect- while answering falls into a deep stupor before finishing. Head alone or face alone hot- rest of body cool- many small boils- painful one after another extremely sore- amel: lying down, and lying with head low- Arnica should not be used externally, where there is broken skin- Bap. Feels ill- Arn. feels well. Injuries- fright or anger. Excessive vinery. *(JHC)*

A sudden fear of death comes on at this time, rousing up in the night- he grasps at the heart, and thinks, he is going to die suddenly- when roused up, he looks at the doctor and says, I do not want you, I did not send for you, I am not sick, I don't need a doctor. It is a wonderful remedy, a misunderstood remedy, a misused remedy, because it is almost limited to bruises- it is one of the sheet anchors in certain seasons, in the malarial valleys of the west for intermittent fever- for many years, I practised among these cases and have seen numerous congestive chills and had no need for Quinine - the Sugar Pills cure safely, permanently and gently- while the Quinine never cures, but suppresses and there is nothing in the after history of that patient, drugged with Quinine and Arsenic but congestion and violence, so long as he lives- all over the body a feeling as if bruised. It is very foolish to put it on the outside and to rub it on in the form of tincture- The Rhus tox and Arnica patients get better from every little motion- the Arnica patient bleeds easily- there is not sufficient tone in the fibres of vessel to hold the blood with in the vessel walls and they ooze- A high potency of Arnica is most satisfactory in bruises, and when no decided contra- indication is present Arnica is the first remedy- but for the weakness of tendons, that follows such a condition, Arnica is not always sufficient and Rhus tox is its natural follower. If the weakness and tenderness remain in the joints follow the Rhus with Calcarea. Now and then we have to resort to causticum, staphysagria and other remedies, because of some peculiar feature in the case, but these remedies are all related more or less to Arnica, Rhus and Calcarea. For another class of injuries compare Ledum and Hypericum- Arnica has aversion to meat broth and milk- there is great thirst at particular times, for instance during the chill of intermittent fever he has thirst, while at other times he is thirstless- Do not forget the symptom of Arnica in appendicitis- you do not run for the surgeon for every case of appendicites, if you know *Bryonia, Rhus tox, Belladonna, Arnica* and similar remedies- the body is cold and the head hot- Most physicians will think of Belladonna which has such cold extremities and such a hot head. Do not forget Arnica especially in those children, who seem to have aversion to being touched and scream out every time the mother takes hold of the leg or arm.

(Kent)

77. Arsenicum Album

(Arsenious Acid- Arsenic Trioxide)

A profoundly acting remedy on every organ and tissue. Its clearcut characteristic symptoms and correspondence to many severe types of diseases make its homoeopathic employment constant and certain. Its general symptoms often lead to its successful application. Among these the all prevailing debility, exhaustion and restlessness with nightly aggravation are most important, great exhaustion after the slightest exertion. This with the peculiar irritability of fibre gives the characteristic irritable weakness. Burning pains. Unquenchable thirst. Burning relieved by heat. Sea side complaints (Natrum mur. Aqua marina). Injuries. Effects of fruits, especially more watery ones. Gives quiet and ease to the last moments of life when given in high potency. Fever, fright and worry, green discharges. Infantile Kala-azar *(Dr. Neatby)*

Ars. should be thought of in ailments from alcoholism, ptomaine poisoning, stings, dissecting wounds, chewing tobacco, ill effects from food or animal matter, odour of discharge is putrid, in complaints that return annually. Anaemia and chlorosis. Degenerative changes, gradual loss of weight from impaired nutrition reduces the refractive index of blood serum (also China and Ferrum phos). Maintains the system under the stress of malignancy regardless of location. Malarial cachexia. Septic infections and low vitality.

Mind: Great anguish and restlessness, changes place continually, fears, sensitive to disorder and confusion.

Head: Hemicrania, dandruff.

Eyes: Burning in eyes with acrid lachrymation. Oedema around eyes, burning hot, intense photophobia.

Ears: Thin, excoriating, offensive otorrhoea.

Nose: Thin watery excoriating discharge, sneezing without relief.

Face: Tearing needle like pains, lips black.

Mouth: Unhealthy easily bleeding gums. Ulceration of mouth, tongue clean, dry and red, gulping up of burning water.

Stomach: Cannot bear the sight or smell of food. Great thirst, drinks much but little at a time, burning pain, craves acid and coffee. Vomiting of blood bile, green mucus or brown black mixed with blood.

Abdomen: Liver and spleen enlarged and painful.

Stool: Smell offensive, dark and much prostration. Worse at night and after eating and drinking.

Urine: Albuminous, Diabetes.

Female: Menorrhagia.

Respiratory: Air passages constricted. Asthma worse midnight, darting pain through upper third of right lung, wheezing respiration.

Heart: Pulse more rapid in morning.

Skin: Dry, rough, scaly, worse cold, Psoriasis.

Fever: Periodicity marked with adynamia, intermittent paroxysms with marked exhaustion, Hay fever, ofter after Rhus. Worse after midnight.

Mod: Worse after midnight, cold drinks and food, seashore, Rt. side, Better heat, head elevated, warm drinks.

Comple: Rhus, Curb, Phos, Thuja, Secale.

Antidotes: Opium, Curb, China, Hepar, Nux.

Dose: 3-30c- The very highest potency often yields brilliant results. Low attenuations in gastric, intestinal and kidney diseases. Higher in neuralgias, nervous disease, and skin. But if only surface conditions call for it give the lowest potencies. 2x to 3x repeated dose advisable.

(Boericke)

Arsenic is the horses' remedy as Puls. is the sheep's and Anti crud. the pigs'. The Arsenic habit of the Styrian mountaineers has arisen from the discovery of its power of strengthening the muscles, both of the limbs and of the breathing apparatus, but in another way the horse typifies the Arsenic temperament- According to Teste Arsenic acts much more powerfully on vegetable eating animals, than on carnivora and it is suited to the effects of excess of vegetable diet, melons, strawberries and fruits in general especially watery fruits- The fine skin and glossy hair of the young women among the arsenic eating populations is remarkable and is comparable to the fine coats of arsenic fed horses. Restlessness is one of the grand characteristics of Arsenic- full of the fear of the death- Jerks and starts on falling asleep- irritability, desperately angry, almost furious, despair, hopelessness, unutterable misery- Burning is another of the leading characteristics of Arsenic. *Amel:* by heat- cold drinks agg: stomach irritations- the mouth is aphthous, ulcerated or gangrenous- prostration-exhausted from slightest exertion- exhaustion is not felt while lying still- must lie down- asthma. Acute coryza and hay fever- corrosive, reddening the upper lip- *agg:* out of doors- amel: by warmth- predominantly right sided- darting pain in apex and through upper third of right lung- many dropsical conditions are controlled by Arsenic- agg: 1 a.m.- puffiness is one of its characteristics and from this to dropsy- the skin is cold and clammy- scurfy eruptions, bran coloured scales- epithelioma of the lips- cancerous diathesis. Many cures of cancer have been reported under its use- both in crude and in potencies- when the subjective symptoms of Arsenic are present, it will cure in the potencies- when the homoeopathicity is more crude the lower potency will be required- in this case the Arsen appears to act directly on the cancerous tissue and cancerous elements in the system- the fear of death is not that of Acon, but is an anxiety and a feeling that, it is useless to take medicine as they will surely die. *(JHC)*

Anxiety, restlessness, prostration, burning and cadaveric odours- burning is amel: heat- amel, all complaints of the body by wrapping up amel complaints of internal head by cold but external head are amel. complaints amel: wrapping up and heat- All night itching and burning alternate- the secretion and excretions of Arsenic are acrid, tendency to bleeding- bleed from any place- lungs, throat etc.- The only distinguishing feature between secale and Ars. is that secale wants cold and Ars. wants heat- thirst for small quantities often- Bry. has thirst for larger quantities- Ars. little and often or violent unquenchable thirst- thoughts of death. Thirsty stage goes on to another in which there is aversion to water and hence we see that in chronic diseases Ars. is thirstless. Many complaints come on in the evening as darkness is coming on- it is full of dyspnoea, cardiac dyspnoea and varying forms of Asthma- Ars. is full of puffiness and dropsy, oedematous condition of extremities- dropsy of the cavities- swelling about eye lid rather than the upper- while in Kali Carb. the swelling is more in the upper eye lid than the lower, between the lid and the brow- there is periodicity- useful in malarial affections- there are dreadful occipital headaches- headache from walking and becoming heated- agg: walking in the sunlight and noise-amel: lying in a dark room, lying with the head on two pillows- many headaches after noon meal- often attended with pallor, nausea and prostration during sweat, thirst for large drinks- oversensitiveness of all the senses. Ars. patient is an extremely fastidious patient- the gold headed cane patient- sensitive to disorder and confusion- the eye symptoms of the remedy are prominent- baggy lids and little bags forming under the eyes- sneezing and coryza with inflammatory conditions through the whole nasal cavity, throat, larynx and chest- striking tendency to ulcerate- extreme irritation of the stomach- vomiting everything, even a tea spoonful of water taken- stools burn as though there were coals of fire in the rectum burning all the way through purging, little spurts with flatus, mucus, slimy, whitish stools- haemorrhoid. Protrude- Ars. and Merc cor. are the two leading medicines for spreading ulceration- genitals swollen- Ferrum and Ars. are two strong drugs for anaemia- wonderful palliative in cancerous affections, such as in uterus and mammary glands- heart becomes weak, pulse thread like, patient pale and cold, covered with sweat- dropsy of pericardium- A striking feature of the Ars. time of chill is its irregularity- coming not twice alike- coming at any time. It has afternoon chill and after midnight chill, sometimes in the morning, sometimes at 3 or 4 p.m., sometimes at 1 p.m. It has a striking periodicity in its nature. Hence it has an intermittent nature. *(Kent)*

78. *Arsenic Brom*

(Bromide of Arsenic)

Has proven a great anti-psoric and anti-syphilitic remedy. Herpetic eruptions, syphilitic excrescences, glandular tumors and indurations, carcinoma, locomotor ataxia and obstinate intermittents and diabetes are all greatly influenced by this preparation.

Face: Acne Rosacea in young people.

Dose: Tincture 2-4 drops daily in water. In diabetes, three drops three times a day in a glass of water. *(Boericke*

79. Arsenicum Hydrogenisatum

(Arseniuretted Hydrogen)

The general action of Arsenic more accentuated. Anaemia, Anxiety, despair. Haematuria with general blood disorganisation. Haemorrhages from mucus membranes. Urine suppressed followed by vomiting. Prepuce and glans covered with pustules and round superficial ulcers, collapse, coldness, prostration, sudden weakness and nausea, skin becomes dark brown.

Dose: 3rd potency. *(Boericke)*

80. Arsenic Iodatum

(Iodite of Arsenic)

It is to be preferred for persistently irritating corrosive discharges. The discharge irritates the membrane from which it flows and over which it flows. The discharge may be fetid, watery and the mucus membrane is always red, angry, swollen, itches and burns, influenza, hay fever, old nasal catarrh and catarrh of middle ear. Swelling of tissues within the nose. Hypertrophied condition of eustachian tube and deafness. Senile heart, myocarditis and fatty degeneration. Pulse shotty, chronic aortitis, epithelioma of the lip, cancer of breast after ulceration has set in.

It seems probable that in arsenic iodum, we have a remedy most closely allied to manifestation of tuberculosis. In the early stage of tuberculosis, even though there is an afternoon rise in temperature Ars iod is very effective. It will be indicated by a profound prostration, rapid, irritable pulse recurring fever and sweats, emaciation, tendency to diarrhoea, chronic pneumonia with abscess in lung. Hectic, debility, night sweats.

This remedy is also to be remembered in phthisis with hoarse cough and profuse expectoration of purulent nature and attended with cardiac weakness, emaciation and general debility in chronic watery diarrhoea in phthisical subjects, in cases of emaciation with good appetite, in amenorrhoea, with anaemic palpitation and dyspnoea. In chronic pneumonia when abscess is about to form. Great emaciation. Arteriosclerosis, myocardial degeneration and senile heart. Threatened pyaemia (Pyrog, Methyl blue).

Head: Vertigo.

Nose: Thin watery, irritating, excoriating discharge from anterior and posterior nares, sneezing, chronic nasal catarrh, membrane sore and excoriated.

Eyes and Ears: Burning.

Fever: Drenching night sweats.

Skin: Marked exfoliation of skin in large scales, ichthyosis, enlarged scrofulous glands, venereal bubo.

Relation: Tuberculinum, Antimonium Iod, aralia, Naphthalin, Rosa, Sang. nit.

Dose: Second and third trituration.

(Boericke)

Chronic inflammatory states of the lungs and bronchial tubes, with profuse, greenish, yellow, pus-like expectoration and short breath are especially relieved- Many skin affections have been remedied by it, particularly dry, scaly, burning and itching eruptions as Psoriasis, tinea, impetigo, pityriasis- in several persons taking low attenuations, I have observed headaches. *(JHC)*

Extreme anaemia, such as belongs to tuberculous subjects. The patient craves open air, when not too cold, wants the window open, is sensitive to a closed room, complaints are worse from bathing, takes cold from bathing. Some are sensitive to cold like Arsenicum, and others to heat like Iodine. The symptoms predominate on the right side. He is impatient and in a constant state of hurry, he becomes indifferent to his friends, to happiness and to his surroundings- Aversion to work- He seems to be going towards insanity- very talkative at times. Inflammation of the conjuctiva and of the Iris. The lids are swollen and oedematous. The ears discharge an excoriating foetid pus- Most stubborn nasal catarrh with bloody, acrid, copious, excoriating, greenish, purulent, thick, yellow or yellow greenish discharge. In hay fever much sneezing, bluish lips and bluish circles about the eyes- twitching of the face- the gums bleed easily- and the tongue is cracked- coated brown or white- many complaints of the liver- troublesome constipation- diarrhoea alternating with constipation- urine is albuminous, cloudy, dark- itching of the penis and glans- perspiration of the genitals- ulcers on the penis- leucorrhoea acrid, bloody, burning, copious, growth of ovarian tumors, respiration is fast and asthmatic. *(Kent)*

81. Arsenicum Met.

(Metallic arsenic)

Arouses latent syphilis, periodicity very marked, symptoms recur every two and three weeks, weakness, swollen feeling of parts.

Mind: Desire to be alone.

Dose: 6th potency. *(Boericke)*

82. Arsenicum Sulfuratum Flavum - Arsenic Trisulph.

(Yellow sulphuret of Arsenic Orpiment)

Needle pricks from within outwards in chest, also on forehead, right side. Sticking behind ear. Difficult respiration. Skin chafed about genitals.

Leucoderma and squamous syphilides. Sciatica and pain around the knee.

Relationships: *Ars sulph. rub* (influenza with intense catarrhal symptoms, great prostration and high temperature, purulent discharges, psoriasis, acne and sciatica. Chilly even before a fire. Itching in various parts. Pellagra.

Dose: Third trituration. *(Boericke)*

83. Artemisia Vulgaris

(Mugwort)

Has some reputation as a remedy for epileptic conditions and convulsive diseases of childhood and girls at puberty. Locally and internally is injurious to eyes. Petit mal Epilepsy without aura, after fright and other violent emotions and after masturbation. Several convulsions close together. Somnambulism. Gets up at night and works, remembers nothing in the morning. (Kali phos.)

Eyes: Coloured light produces dizziness.

Fever: Smelling like garlic-sweat.

Relation: Absinth, Cina, Cicuta.

Dose: 1-3rd potency. Said to act better when given with wine. *(Boericke)*

Convulsive diseases indicated where the patient is excitable and irritable before attack of epilepsy- Epilepsy after fright or grief, after a blow on the head, with menstrual disturbances, with teething. Attack accompanied or followed by profuse offensive sweat, seminal ejaculations. Worms. *(JHC)*

84. *Arum Dracontium*

(Green Dragon)

A remedy for pharyngitis with sore, raw and tender throat.

Dose: First potency. *(Boericke)*

Great diminution, mostly an entire absence of sexual desire. Penis flacid and relaxed- Fine shooting pains in course of left spermatic cord. Chronic pruritus Scroti. *(JHC)*

85. *Arum Triphyllum*

(Jack in the Pulpit)

Arum maculatum, Italicum, Dracontium have the same action as the Triphyllium. They all contain an irritant poison causing inflammation. of mucus surfaces and destruction of tissue. Acridity is the keynote of the kind of action characteristic of Arum.

Nose: Acrid excoriating discharge. Nose obstructed, must breathe through mouth. Burning in the nose. Constant picking at nose until it bleeds.

Mouth: Raw feeling at roof and palate, corners of the mouth sore and cracked.

Throat: Constricted and swollen, burns, hoarseness.

Skin: Raw bloody surface anywhere.

Mod: Worse north west wind, lying down.

Comp: Ammon carb, Ailanthus, Cepa.

Antidotes: Butter milk, Acet acid, Puls.

Dose: 3-30c. *(Boericke)*

Scarlatina of malignant type in which it has met with great success- Raw, bloody surfaces appear on lips, on mouth, on nose etc.- Picks lips till they bleed, corners of mouth sore, cracked and bleeding- picking ends of fingers and boring nose- Tongue cracked and bleeding- it should not be given low or repeated often- hoarseness as that of public speakers, prominently affects the left side. *(JHC)*

It is manifested to a great extent in these associated symptoms- there is such a painful tingling in the nose and lips that the patient persists in boring the fingers into the nose. Manipulating and pinching the lips, picking the lips- It is altogether a different symptom that occurs in delirium of a low muttering type, which we call carpholigia, picking the bed clothes, picking all the time, picking and handling the clothing, a busy low form of muttering, must be doing all the time, groping around with the fingers and feeling for something. They come into the office with a sore, raw nose and it tingles and tickles and he cannot let it alone. Fluids run down over the lip and excoriate- the glands of the neck are often enlarged. *(Kent)*

86. *Arundo*

(Reed)

A remedy for catarrhal states. Hay fever.

Nose: Itching of palate, annoying itching in the nostrils and root of mouth. Itching of the nostrils.

Dose: 3-6c *(Boericke)*

Arundo has cured a case of hay fever, the symptoms beginning with burning and itching of palate and conjuctiva. *(JHC)*

87. *Asafoetida*

(Gum of the Stinka)

The flatulence and spasmodic contraction of stomach and oesophagus with reverse peristalsis are the most marked symptoms. In its selection, its relation to the hysterical and hypochondriacal patients must be borne in mind. Besides these superficial symptoms it has been found to affect favourably deep ulcerations, caries of bones, especially in the syphilitic organism, here the extreme sensitiveness and terrible throbbing, nightly pains, guiding to its use.

Head: Pressive pain from within outward.

Nose: Caries of nasal bones (Arum).

Throat: Globus hystericus.

Stomach: Flatulence and regurgitation of liquid. Pulsation in pit of stomach.

Female: Mammae-deficient milk.

Rectum: Diarrhoea, extremely offensive with meteorism.

Chest: Spasmodic tightness.

Mod: Worse at night, rest. Better open air, motion.

Relation: China, Mercur antidotes.

Compare: Moschus, China, Mercur, Aurum.

Dose: 2nd to 6th potency. *(Boericke)*

Asafoetida presents an almost perfect picture of hysteria of the flatulent order. Many of the discharges of Asaf are fetid watery stools of most disgusting order- profuse and greenish, fetid flatus- eructations smelling like garlic- Hiccough- like contractions of diaphragm. Asaf affects the left side generally- left side of abdomen- left hypochondrium- left side of neck and nape- the fetid smell of the drug may be regarded as one of its signatures- Multiple nodes on roof of mouth, discoloured, bone deeply involved- deficient milk with oversensitiveness after confinement- nervous and hysterical people. *(JHC)*

These cases that come into your office with puffed, venous purple faces, they have an appearance of plethora, the face looks puffed, bloated and dropsical at times, it is a dark red, dusky face. Such a face, we shall cure sometimes with Asafoetida- Carb-an. Aurum, Carb veg and Pulsatilla are also related to this kind of face- Patients often say, I get no sympathy when I am sick, because I look so well, fat, flabby and purple- It is full of discharges, catarrhal discharges, discharges from ulcers, watery discharges from different places and even watery stools.

It also seems as if the atmosphere were filled with little floating black flies- you have looked into the air and seen little gnats and mosquitoes- offensive discharge comes from the nose- numbness is great feature of this remedy- hiccough- like contractions of the diaphragm- Liquid stools of most disgusting smell- women who are not pregnant, some times have the breasts fill up with milk- a wonderfully annoying thing and few remedies have it. This is one of the few. It has also deficiency of milk- ten days after delivery milk diminished- Anti syphilitic remedies- Mercurius, Stapisagria, Hepar, Nitric acid. *(Kent)*

88. Asarum Europum

(European snake root)

A remedy of nervous affections, loss of energy, with excessive erethism. Scratching on silk or linen or paper unbearable. Pains and spasmodic muscular actions. Nervous deafness and asthenopia. Cold shivers from any emotion. Feels as if parts were pressed together. Tension and contractive sensations. Always feels cold.

Mind: Sensibility increased even from mere imagination.

Stomach: Desire for alcoholic drinks; smoking tobacco tastes bitter.

Rectum: Undigested stools.

Modality: Worse cold weather, penetrating sounds. Better from washing, in damp wet weather.

Dose: 3-6c. (A popular remedy in Russia for drunkards) *(Boericke)*

89. Asclepias Syriaca-Cornuti

(Silkweed)

Seems to act especially on nervous system and urinary organs. A remedy for dropsy, hepatic, renal, or cardiac and post scarlatinal, causes diaphoresis and augments the urinary secretions. Acute Rheumatic inflammation of large joints. Intermittent pressing down uterine pains.

Head: Feels as if sharp instrument were thrust through from temple to temple, increased urine with increase of specific gravity.

Dose: Tincture. *(Boericke)*

This remedy is indicated in cases of cardiac and renal dropsy, when the amount of urine and perspiration is diminished and the solids of urine are not being eliminated.

There are several headaches, with a sensation as though a sharp instrument were thrust from one temple to the other which are the result of suppression of the perspiration or a defective elimination of solids. They are followed and relieved, by profuse diuresis, the specific gravity of the urine being increased.

It is of service in uraemia that is preceded by profuse, then scanty, or suppressed, urination and attended with severe headache. *(Blackwood)*

90. Asclepias Tuberosa

(Pleurisy-root)

Its action on the chest muscles is most marked and has been verified. Sick head with flatulence in stomach and bowels. Dyspepsia. Bronchitis and pleurisy come within its range. Catarrhal states from cold and damp weather. Irritation of larynx with huskiness, grip, and pleuritic pain.

Rectum: Catarrhal dysentery with rheumatic pain all over.

Dose: Tincture to First potency.

(Boericke)

This remedy is of service in cases of pleurisy when there are acute pleuritic pains attended with a dry, hacking cough or a scanty mucous expectoration. The intercostal spaces close to the sternum are sensitive to pressure. Sub-acute rheumatic pericarditis is benefitted by it, with pain beneath the soft nipple, palpitation of the heart and dyspnoea, also in pleuro-pneumonia.

It is indicated in bilious diarrhoea in which the stools are preceded by rumbling in the abdomen, and followed by urging, also cases of autumnal dysentery and diarrhoea and subacute mucous enteritis when there is soreness of abdomen following the passage from the bowels. *(Blackwood)*

91. Asimina Triloba

(American papaw) (Custard apple)

Throat sore, itching pimples. Produces a series of symptoms much like scarlet fever, vomiting, scarlet eruption, tonsils and submaxillary glands enlarged, with diarrhoea, fauces red and swollen, face swollen, desire for ice cold things. Hoarseness. Languid, drowsy, irritable.

Acne: Itching in evening on undressing.

Relation: Compare- Capsic, Bellad.

(Boericke)

92. Asparagus officinalis

(Common garden Asparagus)

Its marked and immediate action on the urinary secretion is well known. It causes weakness and cardiac depression with dropsy. Rheumatic pains. Especially about left shoulder and heart.

Heart: Palpitation, with oppression of chest.

Relation: Anti-Acon, Apis.

Dose: 6c *(Boericke)*

Like other Liliaceous plants 'Aspar' acts on the heart, kidneys and dropsical effusions- Severe coryza and nasal catarrh, with profuse secretion of thin, whitish fluid from left nostril, afterwards right- Frequent violent sneezing, copious discharge of tenacious mucous from the throat, not easily loosened but brought up by hawking or paroxysms of cough. Frequent urination with fine stinging in the meatus follcwed by stitches out of the urethra. After urinating burning in urethra with sensation, as if some were still passing, increased urine, beer brown, without sediment. Urine strong smelling, odour peculiar. Deposits greasy sediment on sides of vessel, gravel, prurigo pudendi. Fullness in chest, hydrothorax. Visible violent palpitation, increased by motion or ascending, with oppression of chest. Pulse weak, slow, irregular. Pain at left acromion process, under clavicle and down left arm. Constant desire to be carried about in the arms.

(JHC)

93. Aspidosperma

(Quebracho)

The Digitalis of the lungs. Removes temporary obstruction to the oxidation of the blood by stimulating respiratory centres, increasing oxidation and excretion of carbonic acid. Pulmonary stenosis. Thrombosis of Pulmonary artery. Uraemic dyspnoea. An effective remedy in many cases of Asthma.

It stimulates the respiratory centres and increases the oxygen in the blood. 'Want of Breath' during exertion is the guiding symptom of "Cardiac Asthma".

Relation: Compare- Coca, Arsenic, Coffea, Catalpa. (difficult respiration).

Dose: First trituration or Tincture or Aspidospermin hydrochloride. 1-grain of 1x trit. every hour for a few doses. *(Boericke)*

Quebracho is a Brazilian fever remedy from which the alkaloid Aspidospermine has been isolated. This is in small, very brilliant, white crystals, sparingly soluble in water, readily soluble in alcohol and ether. Hale says Queb. produces in animals respiratory paralysis, slow heart and paralysis of extremities. It relieves dyspnoea in phthisis and pleurisy, but without influencing the fever. The 1x relieved asthma with cyanosis. Hale gives these cases as relieved by it (1) Mitral incompetence and stenosis with severe nocturnal dyspnoea (2) Fatty heart (Queb. had no influence on the oedema, which was removed by Dig.). *(JHC)*

This remedy is indicated in cases of dyspnoea of functional origin, also when it is dependent upon emphysema. The face is pale, anxious and livid, the lips are cyanotic, the pulse is small, irregular, compressible and soft. In cardiac asthma and dyspnoea of the aged it is of service, as well as in cases of bronchitis, and simple asthma when there is depression of heart action. It will not relieve asthma with good heart action, but when it is associated with Emphysema. *(Blackwood)*

94. Astacus Fluviatilis-Cancer Astacus

(Crawfish)

Skin symptoms most important. Urticaria.

Skin: Nettle rash over whole body. Itching, crusta lactea, with enlarged lymphatic glands. Erysipelas and liver affections with nettle rashs swelling of cervical glands. Jaundice.

Relation: Compare Bomby- Caterpillar-itching of whole body (urticaria).

Apis, Rhus, Nat mur, Homar.

Dose: 3-30c. *(Boericke)*

The well known effects of shell fish, as well as other fish in producing nettle rash are exemplified in 'Astacus' beyond all other varieties. The lacquer workers of east have discovered in the river crab, the best antidote to the effects of Rhus which they employ in their craft. The liver is markedly affected and a great characteristic is 'nettle rash with liver complaint'. Jaundice of children. Itching of various parts. Crusta lactea with large lymphatic glands. Enlarged glands of neck in children and old people. Pain and tenderness of liver, jaundice, stools of pipe clay colour. Inward chilliness, nervous crawls over body. Tumours, recent, gout of drinking people. Stinging pains are in various parts. A notable remedy. *(JHC)*

95. Asterias Rubens

(Red star fish)

A remedy for the sycotic diathesis, flabby with red face. Lancinating pains, nervous disturbances, neuralgias, chorea and Hysteria, come within the range of this remedy. Has been used for cancer of the breast and has an unquestioned influence over cancer disease. Excitement in both sexes.

Head: Heat in head as if surrounded by hot air.

Face: Disposition to pimples at adolescence.

Breast: Left breast feels as if pulled inward. Cancer mammae in ulcerative stage, acute lancinating pain. Axillary glands swollen, hard and knotted.

Antidotes: Plumb, Zinc.

Compare: Common, Carb, Ars, Condurango.

Incompatible: Nux, Coffea.

Mod: *Worse* coffee, night, cold damp weather, left side.

Dose: 6th potency. *(Boericke)*

The star fish was used by Hippocrates in Uterine diseases. This shows its pathogenetic relationship to sepia and Murex. It is also an ancient remedy for epilepsy. It powerfully affects the mind and head, producing symptoms strongly suggesting apoplexy. The face is red and there is strong congestion to the head, which is hot and feels as if surrounded with hot air, certain forms of cerebral congestion with obstinate constipation. Electric shocks in the head. Nightly lancinating pains in the breast have led to its successful use in cases of mammary cancer. Petroz used Aster. R. successfully in old skin affections, old ulcers, and in cancers. The found that it only acted on the latter when on the left side (I have a case- probably not cancerous of tumour of the left breast, diminishing under this remedy, but I have also seen it act well on the right breast.)

Sexual desire increased. A pushing out sensation in womb, impeding walking, recalling Sepia. H.C. Allen mentions it as a remedy for acne having small red bases- Great desire for cold drinks. Coffee *Agg:* all symptoms excites them anew several days after they have disappeared. Ast. r. is a very important remedy too, seldom used. *(JHC)*

96. Astragalus Mollissimus

(Purple or Wooly Loco-weed)

Affects animals, like effects of alcohol, tobacco and morphine in man. First stage, period of hallucination or mania with defective eye sight during which the animal performs all sorts of antics. After acquiring a taste for the plant it refuses every other kind of food. Second stage brings emaciation, sunken eyeballs, lustreless hair and feeble movements after a few months dies from starvation (U.S. Depot agriculture). Irregularities in gait- paralytic affection. Loss of muscular co-ordination.

Dose: 6th potency. *(Boericke)*

97. Aurum Met

(Metallic Gold)

Given full play, Aurum develops in the organism, by attacking the blood, glands, and bone, conditions bearing striking resemblance to mercurial and syphilitic infections and it is just for such deteriorations of the bodily fluids and alterations in the tissues, that Aurum assumes great importance as a remedy. Like the victim of syphilis, mental states of great depression are produced by it. Hopeless, despondent and great desire to commit suicide. Every opportunity is sought for self destruction. Exostosis, caries, nightly bone pains, especially cranial, nasal and palatine. Glands swollen in scrofulous subjects, palpitation and congestions. Ascites often in conjunction with heart affections. Frequently indicated in secondary syphilis and effects of mercury.

This use of gold as an anti-venereal and anti-scrofulous remedy is very old but has been well-nigh forgotten by the old school until rediscovered and placed on its scientific basis by homoeopathy and now it can never be lost again. When syphilis is implanted on thee scrofulous constitution, we have one of the most intractable morbid conditions and gold seems to be especially suited to the vile combination. Ennui (weariness). Ozaena, sexual hyperaesthesia. Arteriosclerosis, high blood pressure, nightly paroxysm of pain behind sternum. Sclerosis of liver, arterial system, brain. Pining boys, low spirited, lifeless, weak memory.

Mind: Disgust of life, talks of committing suicide. Constant rapid questioning without waiting for reply, oversensitiveness to noise.

Head: Violent pain in head, worse at night.

Eyes: Extreme photophobia, upper half of the object invisible, vascular cornea, stitching pain inward.

Ears: Obstinate fetid otorrhoea.

Nose: Ulcerated, painful. Putrid smell from nose.

Male: Swelling of testicles. Atrophy of testicles in boys- Hydrocele.

Heart: Sensation as if the heart stopped beating for two or three seconds. Pulse rapid, feeble, irregular, high blood pressure (Aurum 30).

Mod: Worse in cold weather, in winter from sunset to sunrise.

Relation: Aur ars, Aur brom, Aur mur, Aur mur kali, Aur iod, Aur sulph, Asaf, Syphilin, Kali iod, Hepar, Merc, Mez, Nit ac, Phosp.

Anti: Bell, Cinch, Cupr, Merc.

Dose: 3-30. (30 for high B.P.)

(Boericke)

Uterus prolapsed and indurated, the weight of it causes prolapse. The chloride of gold and sodium acts more powerfully in these conditions- thick leucorrhoeal discharges, not offensive, white or yellowish, occasionally profuse agg: by walking- Perspiration in the morning hours, mostly on and around the genitals- agg: from sunset to sunrise is a leading condition of Aurum-paralytic drawing in the limbs in the morning when awaking and on getting cold- Agg: at night, in morning, on getting cold, by rest. Shivering on getting into bed *Amel:* by moving, walking, getting warm.

(JHC)

Sometimes the following state comes on and no disturbance in the man's intellectual nature has been observed, it is intact, it is sound. He has been sound in business affairs, he has been a good father, he has been observed by those around him to be intelligent, but he has silently brooded over his state and his hatred of the world, he has told nobody of it, and then he has been found hung in his room-Ailments from grief, disappointed love, fright, anger, contradiction, mortification. The remedy is full of rheumatic symptoms, with swelling of the joints, affections of the cartilages and bone, inflammation of the periosteum- induration of the glands- induration of the cartilages about the joints- bones are breaking down in any part of the body- the skin bones, nose bones, earbones, any of the small bones, complaints agg: at night- dropsy is presented throughout the remedy, oedema of the extremities, with pitting upon pressure. Cardiac affection, with marked oppression behind the sternum with dyspnoea on walking fast or going upstairs. Boring in bones 'Pains drive to despair'- the pains drive the patient out of bed at night and make him walk. This medicine wonderfully affects the glands, about the groin, parotid glands, the lymphatic in the abdomen, the glands everywhere- The mammary glands, the testes and ovaries are involved, and undergo states of hardness, infiltration etc. Tumors in these glands, of cystic character have been cured by Aurum. Desire for open air., generally amel: growing warm- This is in connection with headaches. Cold water amel: pain in eyes. Averse to uncover- but he desires open air like Pulsatilla- warm air agg: Asthma- many symptoms appear after washing- especially cold washing- by gas light a number of bright floating specks and dots are seen- Enlargement of the thyroid gland with rapid and full pulse- Exophthalmic goitre has been cured by *Aurum and Nat. mur.*- inflammation of the conjunctiva, choroid, iris, and retina. Opacity of the cornea, caries of the mastoid process, obstinate otorrhoea- dropsical condition of the abdomen- inguinal hernia. All sorts of disturbances of the sexual organs, menses too late and scanty- leucorrhoea thick white- the symptoms of asthma and of difficult breathing, you would naturally expect to be associated with the cardiac affection in Aurum- Extreme oppression in the region of the heart on walking fast and going upstairs with oedema of the lower limbs. *(Kent)*

Foul breath in girls at puberty- Aurum follows and is followed well by syphilinum. *(HCA)*

Melancholia, suicide, obesity, syphilitic, caries, salivation, induration of testicles sexual desire diminished, detached retina, religious melancholy. *(Blackwood)*

98. Aurum Muriaticum Natronatum

(Sodium Chloroaurate)

This remedy has a most pronounced effect on the female organs and most of its clinical application has been based there on. Has more power over uterine tumours than any other remedy (Burnett). Psoriasis syphilitica. Periosteal swelling on lower jaw. Swelling of Testicle. High blood pressure due to disturbed function of nervous mechanism. Arteriosclerosis, syphylitic ataxia.

Dose: 2nd and 3rd Trituration.

(Boericke)

Symptoms agg: cold wet weather- warts on tongue- white stools (jaundice), bright's disease, chancres, ulcers, warts, bubo, enormous induration of one part, softening of another part of the uterus- corrosive leucorrhoea. Pustules on genitals. Scirrhus or carcinoma of breast or uterus. According to Hale- this is the most active of all the preparations of gold. In toxic doses it causes violent gastro- enteritis. The constipation is like that of Hydrastis, being accompanied with catarrh- Hale states that the primary effect of the salt is to cause congestion, irritation of uterus and ovaries, subacute metritis, ovaritis, profuse and premature menses habitual abortion, nymphomania, ulceration of uterus, endocervicitis. For these the attenuations are suitable. Burnett considers it to have more power over uterine tumours than any other gold preparation *(JHC)*

Suited to curb-nitrogenoid and mercurio-syphilitic constitutions. Boring pains in bones generally- Boring pains in left eye, skull, chest, tibae- chancres, ulcers, warts. Warts on tongue. Ulcers on foreskin of penis, warts around them, ulcers of glans eating deeply- very efficacious in uterine tumors- enormous induration of an ovary-chronic metritis and prolapsus, ulcers and induration of uterus- Scirrhus of uterus and mammae- ulceration of neck of the womb and vagina. Ovaries indurated and ovarian dropsy- leucorrhoea corroding the parts-Given to syphillitic mothers, it prevents the disease in her offspring. Intolerable itching all over the body. Syphilitic ataxia. Swelling of testicles. *(HCA)*

99. *Avena Sativa*

(Common Oat)

Has a selective action on brain and nervous system favourably influencing their nutritive function. Nervous exhaustion, sexual debility and morphine habit call for this remedy in rather material dosage. Best tonic for debility after exhaustive disease. Nerve tremors of the aged, chorea, paralysis agitans, epilepsy. Post diphtheritic paralysis, rheumatism of heart.

Colds: Acute coryza (20 drop doses in hot water hourly for a few doses).Alcoholism, sleeplessness, especially of alcoholics. Bad effects of Morphine habit. Nervous state of many female troubles.

Male: Spermatorrhoea, impotence, after too much indulgence.

Mind: Inability to keep mind on any one subject.

Dose: Tincture 10-20 drops doses preferably in hot water *(Boericke)*

100. *Azadirachta indica*

(Margosa bark) (Neem)

An afternoon fever and rheumatic pains in various parts are caused by this remedy. Pain in sternum and ribs, in back and shoulders and extremities. Heat, pricking and aching in hands, especially palms, fingers, also soles of feet, appearing in the afternoon.

A poultice of flowers is said to kill lice. A kind of oil is prepared from the seeds of ripe fruits which is said to cure lepra, eczema and some other malignant disease.

Relation: Arsenic Alb, Cedron, China, Ipecac, Nat mur, Pulsatilla, Rhus tox and Sulphur.

Dose: 6, 30, 200 potencies. *(Boericke)*

101. *Bacillinum*

(A maceration of a typical tuberculous lung introduced by Dr. Burnett)

Has been employed successfully in the treatment of tuberculosis, its good effects seen in the change of the sputum, which becomes decreased and more aerated and less purulent. Many forms of chronic non-tubercular disease are influenced favourably. Dyspnoea is present. Respiratory pyorrhoea. The patient expectorates less.

Bacillinum is specially indicated for lungs of old people, with chronic catarrhal condition and enfeebled pulmonary circulation, attacks of suffocation at night with difficult cough. Suffocative catarrh. Tubercular meningitis. Favours falling off of tartar of teeth. Constant disposition to take cold.

Respiratory: Oppression, catarrhal dyspnoea. Humid asthma, bubbling rales and muco-purulent expectoration.

Skin: Ringworms, glands of neck enlarged.

Mod: *Worse* night, early morning and cold air.

Relation: Antimon Iod, Lach, Ars iod. Myosotis, Levico 5-10 drops follows as an intercurrent where much debility is present.

Compli: Calc phos, Kali carb.

Compare: Its effects seem to be identical to that of Koch's Tuberculinum. Both are useful in the tubercular diathesis before phthisis has developed. In the early stage of Tubercular disease of glands, joints, skin and bones, Psorinum seems to be its chronic equivalent. Bacillin testicum acts especially on lower half of the body.

Dose: The dose is important, should not be given below the 30th and not repeated frequently. One dose a week is sufficient to bring about reaction. It is rapid in action and good results ought to be seen soon, otherwise there is no need of repetition.

(Boericke)

102. *Badiaga*

(Fresh water sponge)

Soreness of muscles and integuments, worse motion and friction of clothes with sensitiveness to cold. Glands swollen-general paresis, Basedows disease Lues, Bubo, Roseola.

Feelings of enlargement, pain and fullness of the head, pain extending to the eyeballs, coryza, sneezing, watery discharge from the nose with difficult breathing. Twitching of left eye lid, intermittent pain in the eyes at 3 p.m. Dandruff, stiff neck.

Modality: Worse by cold, better by heat.

Relation: Compare Merc- (Similar but opposite modalities), Spongia, Kali hyd, Phytol, Conium.

Comple: Sulph., Merc., Iod..

Dose: 1-6c. *(Boericke)*

This remedy is of service in cases of indurated buboes, in forcible palpitation of the heart from unpleasant news, in headaches, when the pain is in the forehead and extends to the eyeballs.

It should be remembered in whooping cough, when the expectoration is thick and flies out of the mouth and nostrils.

It should be suited in myalgia when the muscles are sore and painful, as if beaten.

(Blackwood)

103. *Balsamum Peruvianum*

(Peruvian Balsam from Myroxylon Pereirae)

Peruvian Balsam has been chiefly used empirically in catarrhal phthisis or bronchial catarrh with copious purulent expectoration. Sputa thick, creamy, yellowish white, loud rales, night sweats hectic. Hale has used it with success in chronic purulent fetid anterior or posterior nasal catarrh with or without ulceration. He says that a Cereate of Balsam is the best application next to glycerole of Aloes for indolent ulcers, cracked nipples, crack in fingers and palmar surfaces of hands or fissured and chapped lips.

Dose: 1st attenuation. *(Boericke)*

The Balsam is also used externally for killing the acarus of itch. All parts affected are gently rubbed with it at night and a bath taken in the morning- A single application is sufficient. It has been proved by Lembke. *(JHC)*

104. Baptisia

(Wild Indigo)

The symptoms of this drug are of an asthenic type, simulating low fevers, septic conditions of the blood, malarial poisoning and extreme prostration. Indescribable sick feeling. Great muscular soreness and putrid phenomena are always present. All the secretions are offensive- breath, stool, urine, sweat etc. Epidemic influenza. Chronic intestinal toxaemia of children with fetid stools and eructations.

Baptisia in low dilutions produce a form of anti-bodies to the bacityphosus, viz. the agglutinins. Thus it raises the natural bodily resistance to the invasion of the bacillary intoxication, which produces the typhoid syndrome. Typhoid carriers. After inoculation with anti-typhoid serum, intermittent pulse, especially in the aged.

Mind: Thinks he is broken or double and tosses about the bed trying to get pieces together. Falls asleep while being spoken to.

Face: Besotted look.

Mouth: Breath fetid, tongue feels burned, surface cracked and sore. Can swallow liquids only.

Throat: Constriction and contraction of oesophagus, contraction of cardiac orifice.

Stomach: Sinking feeling at stomach.

Stool: Offensive, thin dark bloody.

Extremities: In whatever position the patient lies, the parts rested upon feel sore and bruised.

Mod: Worse humid heat, fog, indoors.

Relation: *Bry, Ars,* may be needed to complete the favourable reaction.

Ailanthus differs being more painful- Baptisia more painless-

Compare: Rhus, Mur acid, Ars, Bry, Arnica, Echin, Pyrogen.

Echinacea is perhaps its nearest natural analogue.

Dose: Tincture to 12c has rather short action. *(Boericke)*

Another disease in which it has proved specific in a large number of cases is epidemic influenza. On being spoken to, confused as if drunk- cannot keep his mind together, a wild wandering feeling. Scattered feeling is exemplified in the illusion that the body is double, limbs separated and conversing with each other, can't sleep because body seems scattered about and cannot collect pieces. There is a dull heavy sensation in head with drowsiness and heavy eye lids. Frontal head ache with pressure at root of nose. The neck is tired, cannot hold head in any position- the eyes cannot bear light, burn, are weak- painful on reading, weight on eyes, eyeballs sore, lame on moving, bleary eye lids partially paralysed, an illusion of smell as of burnt feathers, has been caused and cured by it. Pain in left parotid gland. Flat bitter taste, tongue swollen, feels numb, speech difficult- is coated whitish yellow and feels burnt or scalded- dry parched, brown centre- cracked and ulcerated- can only swallow liquids. *(JHC)*

It brings on this state more rapidly than most other remedies. He is increasing his prostration more rapidly than usual. It is not a gradual decline of days and weeks. He goes into a state of stupor when aroused, he takes on delirium- it does not matter, whether it is scarlet fever or typhoid fever, or a septic surgical fever or puerperal fever or what- All of the discharges are putrid- the odour is cadaverous, pungent, penetrating- Ulceration runs all through the remedy- aphthous patches- These little ulcers that start no bigger than a pin head become black and are so offensive and run together so that the whole mouth will be in a state of ulceration- Bleeds much from the mouth, throat and nose, thick oozing, putrid- Baptisia has cured the ulcerated sore throat of young mothers and nursing sore mouth in children- now with all this trouble, saliva pours into the mouth, is thick and ropy and runs all over the pillow, like we find in mercury- the oesophagus feels as if constricted from above down to the stomach. *(Kent)*

105. Barasoma Crenate

(Buchu)

Marked specific effects on genito-urinary system muco-purulent discharges, irritable bladder with vesical catarrh, prostatic disorders, Gravel, Leucorrhoea.

Relation: Copaiva, Thuja, Populus, Chimaph.

Dose: tincture or tea from leaves.

(Boericke)

106. Baryta Acetica

(Acetate of Barium)

Face: Feeling of cobweb on face.

Produces paralysis beginning at the extremities and spreading upward. Pruritus of aged.

Dose: Second and third trituration.

(Boericke)

107. Baryta Carb

(Carbonate of Baryta)

Specially indicated in infancy and old age. This remedy brings aid to scrofulous children, especially if they are backward mentally and physically dwarfish, do not grow and develop, have scrofulous ophthalmia, swollen abdomen, take cold easily and then always have swollen tonsils. Persons subject to quinsy which is prone to suppurate, gums bleed easily. Diseases of old men, when degenerative changes begin- cardiac, vascular and cerebral — who have hypertrophied prostate or indurated testes, very sensitive to cold, offensive foot sweats, very weak and weary, must sit or lie down or lean on something, very averse to meeting strangers, catarrh of posterior nares with frequent epistaxis. Often useful in the dyspepsias of the young who have masturbated and who suffer from seminal emissions together with cardiac irritability and palpitation.

Affects glandular structures and useful in general degenerative changes especially in coats of arteries, aneurysm and senility. Baryta is a cardio-vascular poison acting on the muscular coats of heart and vessels. Arterial fibrosis. Blood vessels soften and degenerate, become distended and aneurysms rupture and apoplexies result.

Ears: Glands around ears painful and swollen.

Nose: Coryza with swelling of upper lip and nose.

Throat: Tonsils swollen, takes cold easily with stitches and smarting pain, Quinsy, suppurating tonsils from every cold.

Abdomen: Hard and tense, distended.

Heart: Blood pressure increased. Suppressed foot sweat- Fetid foot sweats.

Back: Swollen glands in nape of occiput- Fatty tumors about neck.

Sleep: Talking in sleep.

Mod: Worse while thinking of symptoms, from washing, lying on painful side- Better- walking in open air.

Relation: Compare- digit, Radium, Aragallus Oxytrop, Astrag. Incompatible, Calc.

Antidote: Epsoms salts.

Dose: 3-30c-the latter removes the predisposition to quinsy. Baryta is slow in action, bears repetition. *(Boericke*

Many cases of aneurism have been cured with Baryta. Old people who are fat. It corresponds to the atheromatous condition. A paralytic conditions runs throughout the pathogenesis. There is a paralysis of mind and body- fetid foot sweat- deficient memory- children cannot remember and learn- baldness of young people- enlarged glands in occiput and neck- on face there are rough, dry and herpetic eruptions. Painful swelling of parotid and submaxillary glands- the sense of smell is very acute- salivation- saliva runs out during sleep- the digestion is weak, after eating, pressing in stomach, the pain is hard, swollen abdomen, habitual colic of children- piles protrude with urination as well as during stool- haemorrhoids, burning and soreness. Soreness and moistening between scrotum and thighs- enlarged prostate- there is a spasmodic cough like whooping cough- cough agg: evening till midnight- Baryta carb are met with in many cases of aneurysm and atheroma and no remedy has a better record here- Bar. carb has cured tumours of several kinds. Fatty tumours, especially about the neck, swelling and induration of glands. Cold feet. Fetid respiration of feet- Corns with burning and stinging, itching, sore and humid skins, warts. (Calc iod-large tonsils) (Silicea- glands, fetid foot sweat, but Bar C. lacks the head sweat of Silic which has self-will instead of the weak-mindedness of Bar C.) Incompatible - Calc. *(JHC)*

Baryta Carb is an interesting study, because it is fully proved and a constitutional remedy- dwarfishness- (late walking is Calc- late learning to walk is Baryta carb)- knotty chains form in the neck- has cured fatty tumours, encysted tumours- general state agg: cold- but headache amel: by cool air. Eruption upon the head. Baldness. Full of eye symptoms. Coarse rattling in the chest of old people (Compare senega, Ammoniacum and Bar. mur), gagging and choking with a little food. Inveterate constipation- stool hard and insufficient- a lack of action in the rectum- haemorrhoidal protrusion during stool and urination - impotency - relaxed penis - diminished sexual desire- hypertrophied prostrate- atrophied testicles. Numbness of the genitals- Female, sterility, dwindling of the ovary- passive leucorrhoea about a week before the menstrual period- Voice lost- hoarseness and huskiness- chest full of mucus but unable to expectorate it- night cough with asthmatic breathing- coughs and coughs, no relief until he lies on abdomen- muscle tension of the back- swelling of the glands of back and neck- swelling of the cervical glands- fatty tumours upon the back. The pains are of a gouty, rheumatic character agg: from cold and cold weather- offensive perspiration of the feet- checked foot sweat. *(Kent)*

Haemorrhoids protrude every time he urinates. Throat affections after checked foot sweat- frequently useful before or after *Psor-sulph* and *Tuberculinum-* After Bar. C., Psor will often eradicate the constitutional tendency of quinsy. *(HCA)*

108. Baryta Mur.

(Barium chloride)

The different salts of Baryta are called for in organic lesionS of the aged and dwarfish, both mentally and physically. Arterio-sclerosis and cerebral affections due to the condition. Headache, but without acute crisis occurring in old people. Heaviness rather than pain. Vertigo due to cerebral anaemia and noises in ears. Acts on lower alimentary canal, especially rectum, on muscles and joints, giving stiffness and weakness as from over walking. The white blood corpuscles increased. Hypertension and vascular degeneration. Increased tension of pulse. Arteriosclerosis (Aurum, secale) where a high systolic pressure with comparative low diastolic tension is attended with cerebral and cardiac symptoms.

This remedy has induration and narrowing of the cardiac orifice with pain, immediately after eating and epigastric tenderness which has been repeatedly verified, also its use in aneurysm and chronic hypertrophy of the tonsils. Nymphomania and satyriasis, convulsions. In every form of mania when sexual desire is increased. Icy coldness of the body with paralysis. Multiple sclerosis of brain and cord. Voluntary muscular power gone but perfectly sensible. Paresis after influenza and diphtheria. General feeling of lassitude in the morning especially weakness of the legs with muscular stiffness, children who go around with their mouth open and who talk through their nose, stupid- appearing, hard of hearing.

Throat: Tonsils enlarged.

Respiratory: Bronchial affections of old people with cardiac dilation, facilitates expectoration.

Stomach: Gone feeling in epigastrium.

Urine: Great increase in Uric acid.

Abdomen: Induration of Pancreas.

Relation: Plumbum met, Plumb iod, also Aurum mur.

Dose: 3rd trituration- Bears repetition of dosage well. *(Boericke)*

Convulsions are more marked in the Muriate- Periodical attacks of convulsions with excessive restlessness of the limbs, Mania with increase of sexual desire, in every form of mania as soon as the sexual desire is increased- offensive otorrhoea. Parotid glands hard and swollen especially right. It has cured whizzing and buzzing in ears, noises on chewing and swallowing- tonsillitis. There is great indigestion. Induration of pancreas. Many cases of aneurysm have been benefited by Bar. mur, Baryt mur acts on parotid glands and pancreas. The earache is amel: by sipping cold water. *(JHC)*

Convulsions with full consciousness, with electric shocks, clonic spasms, it has cured most stubborn cases of Epilepsy- formication all over the body- induration of glands- inflammation and swelling of glands. Pulse fast, 120, full, hard, small, rising up brings on many symptoms, electric shocks with convulsions. It is the natural complement of Common in glandular affections and it is very similar, but much deeper acting- it is useful in children who are slow to learn or understand, children who do not desire to play like other children- concentration impossible- insanity where the sexual excitement becomes strong- mania in every form when sexual desire is increased- it is a remedy of great usefulness in eruptions of the scalp- thick offensive crusts. Eczema of the whole top of the head, extending to sides and occiput- copious pus. Agglutination of the lids in the morning, discharge of mucus and pus from the eyes- itching and smarting- pressing pain in eyes. Paralysis of upper lids. Ulceration of the cornea- discharge from both ears- copious offensive- like spoiled cheese- dryness in the nose- epistaxis- frequent sneezing- swelling of the glands of neck and jaw- very hard- right parotid bleeding gums- cracked tongue- white tongue- odour from mouth- inflammation of the throat and tonsils- enlarged tonsils- elongation of the uvula with sore throat- appetite ravenous. Desires dry wheat bread- distension of the stomach. Constipation, difficult stool, no desire for stool, stool hard and covered with mucus, generally painless diarrhoea, bloody mucus, jelly like stools- frequent, generally painless- external piles- protrude during urination- itching of the anus- burning during and after stool- worms with stool- urination difficult- frequent at night- chronic gonorrhoea, induration of ovaries- leucorrhoea- menses too often, copious, painful- catarrh of larynx and trachea- voice is hoarse- husky and weak- chronic dry cough of scrofulous children, from irritation- cold hands and feet- cramps in the toes, drawing up the limbs ameliorates- hot hands- itching of the limbs- the thighs- perspiration of the feet- suppressed foot sweat- swelling of hands- lower limbs- knees, feet, tension in knees, eruption, eczema, herpes all over body, pimples- scabs- yellow scales- stinging urticaria- unhealthy skin. *(Kent)*

109. *Baryta Iodata*

(Iodide of Baryta)

Acts on lymphatic system. Indurated glands especially tonsils and breasts, strumous ophthalmia with tumefaction of cervical, glands and stunted growth. Tumours.

Relation: Acon, Lycotonum (swelling of cervical axillary and mammary glands) Lapis, Con, Merc, Iod, Curb an.

Dose: Second and third trituration.

(Boericke)

110. *Belladonna*

(Deadly night shade)

Belladonna acts upon every part of the nervous system, producing active congestion, furious excitement, perverted special senses, twitching convulsions and pains. It has a marked action on the vascular system, skin and glands. Belladonna always is associated with hot red skin, flushed face, glaring eyes, throbbing carotids, excited mental state, hyperaesthesia of all senses, delirium, restless sleep, convulsive movement, dryness of mouth and throat with aversion to water, neuralgic pains that come and go suddenly

(Oxytropis). Heat, redness, throbbing and burning, great children's remedy. Epileptic spasms followed by nausea and vomiting. Scarlet fever and also prophylactic. Here use the thirtieth potency. Exophthalmic goitre. Corresponds to the symptoms of 'air sickness' in aviators. Give as preventive. No thirst anxiety or fear. Belladonna stands for violence of attack and suddenness of onset. Bell- for the extreme of thyroid toxaemia- use 1x. *(Beebe)*

Mind: Acuteness of all senses, visual hallucinations, desire to escape, sees monsters, hideous faces.

Head: Painfulness especially in forehead, worse- light, noise, jar, lying down and in afternoon.

Face: Bluish red, swelling of upper lip.

Eyes: Pupils dilated, staring brilliant, red, burn, diplopia.

Ears: Otitis media, pain causes delirium, child cries out in sleep.

Nose: Bleeding of nose.

Mouth: Grinding of teeth.

Throat: Red, worse on right side, tonsils enlarged. Feels constricted, difficult deglutition, spasms.

Stomach: Averse to meat and milk. Great thirst for cold water, spasmodic hiccough.

Urine: Retention, dark and turbid, frequent and profuse.

Male: Nocturnal sweat of genitals.

Female: Sensation as if all the viscera would protrude at genitals. Menses bright red, too early, too profuse. Haemorrhage hot. Menses and lochia very offensive and hot mastitis.

Respiratory: Dryness in nose, fauces, larynx very painful, high piping voice, moaning at every breath.

Extremities: Cold.

Back: Swelling of glands of neck.

Skin: Hot and dry, glands, swollen tender, red boils, alternate redness and paleness of the skin.

Fever: Burning, pungent, steaming heat, no thirst with fever.

Sleep: Starting when closing the eyes or during sleep.

Mod: Worse, jar, touch, noise, draught, afternoon, lying down- Better semi-erect.

Relation: Calcarea is often required after Bel. Atropia (alkaloid of Belladonna) covers the more neurotic sphere of the Belladonna action. Everything appears large (Platina opposite).

Antidote: Camph, Coff., Opium, Acon.

Complementary- Calc (Bell contains lime).

Incompatible: Acet acid.

Dose: 1-30 (Must be repeated frequently in acute diseases). *(Boericke)*

On goats and rabbits, it has no poisonous action whatever. On carnivorous animals it acts with moderate intensity- it is a chilly medicine sensitive to changes from warm to cold, to draught of air, to damp weather, to chilling from having the head uncovered or having the hair cut, better from being wrapped up warmly in a room- congestion of blood to the head. Vertigo, mostly at night on turning over in bed, or when getting up in the morning, also when walking and on every change of position- Headache with flushed face and brilliant eyes, dilated pupils. Feeling in brain like swashing of water. It has cured a very severe headache in a nervous man occurring whenever he was exposed to tobacco smoke- In the mental sphere are mania, rage, disposition to bite, scratch and tear things- Fantastic illusions when closing eyes- Dull and sleepy- half asleep and half awake- spasms and twitchings are very marked- Many disorders of vision- Rheumatism agg: by motion, sweat on covered parts only- in cases of worm fever- Cina 200 has ameliorated- Bell-CM and 1M cured permanently- starting, twitching or jumping in sleep- sweat on covered parts only, is also marked symptom of Bell- Bell is predominantly a right sided medicine- symptoms are agg: afternoon, 3 p.m., 11 p.m. after midnight, draught of air, cold application, having hair cut, looking at shiny things, drinking, sleeping lying down, lying on affected side- It grows in dry lime stone soils and is the acute correlative of Calc. c. *(JHC)*

It is especially suitable to plethoric, vigorous individuals and intellectual people- when you put your hand upon a Bell. subject, you will suddenly withdraw it, the heat is so intense; the memory of the heat is carried in the hand and fingers for some time- the idea of that heat must be well fixed in the mind- heat, intense heat, violent heat- we have three leading features- heat, redness and burning- it is one of the most painful remedies- it may be in the cystic duct, that the circular fibres, clutch that little bit of stone and will not let it through- there is never a failure in homoeopathic prescribing in gall stone colic- the symptoms are not always Bell- but in this instance, where that horrible sensitiveness is present, it is Bell. The Bell. subject as an individual like Bry. is worse in his all complaints from motion- the delirium and excitement are very commonly ameliorated by eating a little food- Full of imaginations, sees ghosts and spirits and officers and wild things- Dreams horrible things, hammering in the head- patient will bite the spoon, will bark like a dog- will do all sorts of violent things- we notice it particularly in the woman. She cannot have the hair bound up- the reaction to medicine is so quick and so sudden. Drawing the head back often ameliorates the violent headaches- expansive sensation, as if the head were enlarged- Great dryness, dryness in the nose, mouth, tongue, in the throat, dry cough- unconquerable craving for lemons and lemon juice. Bell. is a remedy in appendicitis. Haemorrhoids painful, much burning. Whole urinary tract is in a state of irritation- wets the bed on going to sleep. More troubles in the woman than man, related to female sexual organs, parturition, breasts, gestation, nervous sensitive women, women of irritable fibre- copious flow of bright red fluid mixed with clots is the characteristic of the Belladonna flow. Sensitive to touch, jar, nervous excitement manifested both when awake and in sleep- violent dysmenorrhoea- pain like labour pains- uterus congested, enlarged and heavy, bearing down sensation as if the uterus would escape- prolapsus as if the whole inner parts were coming out. Dry spasmodic cough, whooping cough- with spasms of the larynx which cause the whoop- this remedy cures pneumonia and pleurisy. *(Kent)*

111. *Bellis perennis*

(Daisy)

Traumatism of the pelvic organs, auto-traumatism, expresses the condition calling for this remedy; ill effects from masturbation. Excellent remedy for sprain and bruises. Complaints due to cold food or drink, when the body is heated and in affections due to cold wind. Externally in naevi. Acne, Boils all over, sore bruised feeling in the pelvic region. Exudation, stasis swelling come within the range of this remedy Rheumatic symptoms, does not vitiate the secretions. It is a princely remedy for old labourers, especially Gardners. *(Burnett)*

Head: Bruised soreness.

Female: During pregnancy, inability to walk, uterus feels sore as if squeezed.

Abdomen: Soreness of abdominal walls and of uterus.

Skin: Boils.

Relation: Arnica, Arsenic, Staphis, Hamamelis, Bryonia, Vanadium. (Degenerative Stasis).

Dose: tincture to third potency.

(Boericke)

The old name of 'wound- wort' or 'bruise wort' shows one of the main spheres of the action of Bellis and allies in its action with its fellow compositae, Arnica and Calendula. The daisy is a flower which is repeatedly trodden upon and always comes up smiling afterwards and being the days 'Eye' may be the sign of its too early waking propensities- It acts very much like Arnica- tumours originating in a blow. Fagged womb- Varicose Veins, it has marked action on female sexual organs, especially on engorged uterus and breasts. It relieves troubles of pregnancy, inability to walk, varicose veins, Fag from masturbation. Burnett has generally given it in the 'Q' tincture- pre-eminently left side medicine- Acne, Boils, rheumatic pains, giddiness. A leading indication is found in its causation- ill effects of cold or iced drinks when heated, dyspepsia, amenorrhoea. Skin affections including a striking case of psoriasis- near and remote effects of blow, falls, accidents (trauma)- acute attacks of gout. Burnett gives it a very high place, classing it with Vanadium- it is not to be given near bed time, as it is apt to cause sleeplessness waking at 3 a.m. and conversely 'waking up too early' in the morning and cannot get to sleep again is a leading indication for its use. Causation- injuries. Effects of cold drinks when over heated- wetting when over-heated.

(JHC)

112. Benzenum

(Coal Naphtha)

The most striking fact in the proving of Benzol seems to be the influence it had on the circulatory system. It caused a slowing of the pulse stream which in the guinea- pigs brought about the formation of infarcts. In the human provers it results in a decrease of the red and increase of white cells (R.F. Rabe M.D.) It ought to be of use in leukaemia. Eye symptoms striking. Hallucinations. Epileptiform attacks, coma and anaesthesia.

Mod: Worse night, right side.

Dose: 6th potency. *(Boericke)*

113.Benzoicum Acidum

(Benzoic acid)

The most marked characteristic pertains to the odour and colour of the urine. It produces and cures symptoms of a Uric acid diathesis with urine highly coloured and very offensive and gouty symptoms.

Renal insufficiency. Child wants to be nursed in the arms, will not be laid down. Pains suddenly change their locality. Antisycotic, Gouty and asthmatic.

Urine: Repulsive odour, Enuresis, offensive urine of old men.

Extremities: Joints crack on motion, tearing with stitches- Pain in tendo-Achilles, Rheumatic gout, nodes very painful, gouty deposits.

Ganglion: Swelling of the wrist, pain and swelling of the knees, bunion of great toe, tearing pain in great toe.

Mod: worse open air, uncovering.

Relation: Useful after Colchic. Fails in gout, after Copaiva in gonorrhoea.

Compare: Nitric Acid, Ammon Benz, Sabina, Tropaeolum, Garden Nasturtium in fetid urine.

Antidote: Copaiva.

Incompat: Wine- which aggravates urinary gouty and rheumatic affections.

Dose: 3rd to 6th potency.

(Boericke)

Strong smelling urine, generally also dark- joints crack when moving. If he saw any one deformed, it made him shudder. Tongue spongy on surface with deep cracks, and spreading ulcers- enuresis nocturna, urine dark, strong smelling like horses' urine, shivering before stool. Ganglion of wrist and bunion of great toe, I have frequently cured with Benz. ac. Most of the symptoms appear on the left side, but many subsequently come on the right. *(JHC)*

It has a strong smelling urine, the urine is pungent and it sometimes becomes so strong that it smells like hippotic acid. It has cured many times wetting the bed, involuntary urination in sleep, when the bed that has been wetted, several times becomes uncleanable. Inclined to dwell on unpleasant things. If he saw anyone deformed, it made him shudder. Stool copious watery- the white stool, like soap suds is a strong symptom. The urinous odour of the body and especially that peculiarly pungent, intense smell of urine- Rheumatic complaints in the heart. The extremities are full of rheumatic affections- all gouty affections belong to this remedy- Benzoic acid patient sweats without relief, copious exhaustive sweat and profound sleep, but there is no relief. *(Kent)*

114. *Berberis Aquifolium-Mahonia*

(Mountain grape)

A remedy for the skin, chronic catarrhal affections, secondary syphilis. Hepatic torpor, lassitude and other evidences of incomplete metamorphosis stimulates all glands and improves nutrition.

Skin: Pimply, dry, rough, scaly, eruption on scalp extending to the face and neck. Tumour of breast with pain. Psoriasis. Acne, dry eczema, pruritus, glandular induration.

Relationship: Carbol acid, Euonym, Berb. Vulg., Hydr.

Dose: Tincture in rather material dose. 5-10 drops. *(Boericke)*

It has been used by eclectics in chronic syphilis, chronic skin diseases, in scrofulous cachexia and for removing pimples from the faces of girls. Berb. aq. has a reputation for making a new man of an old one. This agent acts upon the glandular system as a stimulant, assisting digestion and absorption, upon the skin, relieving eczematous, herpetic and syphilitic exhibitions. This remedy is indicated in chronic skin affections of a scaly and pustular character, that are dependent upon a constitutional dyscrasia, as syphilis, with pain in the muscles and bones, and a cutaneous, exhibition of this disease, especially psoriasis, pityriasis, pimples, roughness of the skin and chronic dermatisis in general. It should be thought of in glandular induration and chronic ulceration, both of a scrofulous and syphilitic character, also soreness in the region of the spleen. It is useful in persistent acne, pimples and roughness of the skin of the face, that are not dependent upon uterine or ovarian irritation- In eczema capitis of the genitals with pruritus and in scaly eczema and in chronic cases of 'Scald head' it has acted very kindly- In every, rough, scaly skin, it has given favourable results.

(Blackwood)

115. Berberis Vulgaris

(Barberry)

Rapid change of symptoms- pains change in regard to place and character, thirst alternates with thirstlessness, hunger and loss of appetite etc. Acts forcibly on venous system, producing pelvic engorgements and haemorrhoids.

Hepatic and rheumatic affections, particularly with urinary, haemorrhoidal and menstrual complaints. Old gouty constitutions, pain in region of kidneys is most marked, hence its use in renal and vesical troubles, gall stones and vesical catarrh. It causes inflammation of kidneys with haematuria. Pains may be felt all over the body, emanating from small of back. It has also marked action on the liver, promoting the flow of bile. Often called for in Arthritic affections with urinary disturbances. Wandering radiating pains. Acts well in fleshy persons, good livers, but with little endurance. Spinal irritation. All Berberis pains radiate, are not worse by pressure but worse in various attitudes especially standing and active exercise.

Head: sensation of a tight cap pressing upon the whole scalp.

Mouth: Diminished saliva, sticky, frothy, saliva like cotton.

Stomach: Nausea before breakfast.

Stool: Fistula in ano.

Urinary: Urine with thick mucous and bright red mealy sediment- pain in the thighs and loins on urinating.

Extremities: Neuralgia under finger-nails with swelling of finger joints.

Skin: Itching- worse scratching- Eczema of anus and hands. Circumscribed pigmentation.

Mod: worse- motion, standing. It brings on increased urinary complaints.

Antidotes: Camphor, Bell.

Dose: Tincture to 6th potency.

Relation: Similar to- *Canth, Lyco, sars, tab.* in renal troubles. *Arn, Bry, Kali bi, Rhus, Sulph,* in rheumatic affections.

(Boericke)

Berberis produces both constipation (sheep dung stools) and diarrhoea and a number of symptoms of the anus- Haemorrhoids, with itching or burning, particularly after stool which frequently is hard and covered with blood. Fistula in ano with painful pressure in perineum- The emission of urine is frequently accompanied by pains in thighs and loins- Many cases of (especially right) renal colic have been cured by it (Kent says for left side). During urination burning in urethra, or bladder, pressure in bladder, cutting burning, or stitches in urethra- 'Stuart Close' records the cure with Berberis 200 of a woman who had cutting, burning pains in the balls of the feet on stepping- On rising in the morning, sensation in soles as if stepping on needles. Guernsey admirably sums up the remedy as follows: Affects particularly the lumbar region, kidneys, uterus. *(JHC)*

Benzoic Acid, it fits into the gouty and rheumatic sphere- Berberis- gouty deposits to the finger joints, wandering around through the economy- It cures gall stone colic when these little twinges go in every direction, from that locality. As to the heart, the pulse becomes slow, very often it is slowed down astonishingly- A feeling in the head as if it was becoming larger is a peculiar symptom. One grand feature about Berberis, that it has no particular direction and has all directions. Anything that is spasmodic can be relieved instantly- patient becomes constipated- stool is white or very light coloured- Herpes around anus. Fistula in ano- the remedy that is indicated for the patient will cure the patient and fistula. It is a dangerous thing to operate upon a fistula in ano- burning and soreness in the region of the kidneys- great urging with pain in the neck of the bladder with burning scanty urine. Formation of little calculi in the pelvis of the kidney- little stones like pin heads- you will be astonished to know how quickly Berberis will receive this particular kind of renal colic. Woman tired, gouty constitution, though not old, physically tired, so that all of her domestic affairs fret and tire her. Coition becomes painful and she has an aversion to it. Violent cutting tensive pain deeply seated in left side of bladder. *(Kent)*

116. Beta Vulgaris

(Beet Root)

Influenza, chronic catarrhal states and tuberculosis. The salt Betanium Hydrochloricum obtained from the beet root itself seems to be the best adapted to phthisical patients. Children yield very quickly to the action of the remedy.

Dose: Use about the 2x Trit.

(Boericke)

117. Betonica

(Betony wood)

Pains in various parts.

Produces pain in various parts.

(Boericke)

118. Bismuthum

(Precipitated, sub-nitrate of Bismuth)

Irritation and catarrhal inflammation of the alimentary canal is the chief action of this drug.

Mind: Desire for company, Anguish.

Mouth: Gums swollen, black borders on gums and loosening of the teeth.

Stomach: Water is vomited as soon as it reaches the stomach. Burning, feeling of a load. Better cold drinks- but vomiting when stomach becomes full.

Relation: Antidotes- Nux, Capsi, Calc.

Compare: Antimon, Ars, Bellad, Kreosot.

Dose: 1-6th potency. *(Boericke)*

119. Blatta Americana

(American cockroach)

Dropsy, Yellow complexion, pain in urethra while passing urine. Ascites, various forms of dropsy, yellow complexion. Extreme weariness. Pain in urethra on urinating. Weariness on going upstairs.

Dose: Sixth potency. *(Boericke)*

120. Blatta Orientalis

(Indian cockroach)

A remedy for asthma. Especially when associated with bronchitis. Indicated after Arsenic when there is insufficient cough with dyspnoea in bronchitis and phthisis. Acts best in stout and corpulent patients- much pus-like mucus.

Dose: General- Lowest potencies during an attack. After the spasm, for the remaining cough use the higher. Stop with improvement to prevent aggravation. *(Boericke)*

Found accidentally to relieve Asthma in a patient who took tea in which a beetle had been infused. It has since proved to have a wide range in asthmatic cases. In the acute attack it acts better in low potencies, the higher being given in the more chronic stages, agg: rainy weather.

Why should any patient of Asthma die or suffer so long as there is Blatta in the Phial? Blatta is a unique remedy for Asthma. During paroxysm of asthmatic dyspnoea first use Passiflora Incarnata- ɸ- 60 drops mixed with Blatta orientalis 10 drops in an oz. of hot water. This will act like a magic, suffocative dyspnoea will at once disappear and the patient will enjoy a sound refreshing sleep. For a week repeat this process every night at bed time- then select suitable constitutional remedy such as Sulphur, Bacillinum, Psorinum in high potencies. *(Dr. Yadubir Sinha- Bihar)*

121.Boletus Laricis - Polyporus Officinale

(white Agaric)

Quotidian intermittent fever. Sweat is light and without relief. Night sweat, phthisis.

Fever: Chilliness along spine, with frequent hot flushes. Yawns and stretches when chilly. Severe aching in shoulders and joints and small of back. Profuse perspiration at night with hectic chills and fever.

Characteristics: But proved the crude substance and the 3rd trituration.

The gastro-enteric irritation common to the fungi was very well marked.

Dose: First attenuation. *(Boericke)*

122. Boricum Acidum

(Boracic acid)

Used more non homoeopathically as dusting powder- antiseptic lotion etc. Vagina cold as packed with ice. Coldness is a prominent feature, such as cold saliva.

Used as an antiseptic disinfectant, since it arrests fermentation and putrefaction. **Non-homoeopathic use:** A teaspoonful to a glass of hot milk, taken internally for chronic cystitis. Boro-glyceride in solution (1:40) is a powerful antiseptic. Styes 15 gr to 1 oz water externally. As a dusting powder on ulcerated surfaces. In cystitis as an irrigating fluid.

Dose: 3rd trituration. *(Boericke)*

123. *Borax*

(Borate of sodium)

Gastro-intestinal irritation. Salivation, nausea, vomiting, colic, diarrhoea, collapse albuminuria, casts and vesical spasm. Delirium, visual changes, haematuria and skin eruptions have all been observed from over-dosing. Dread of downward motion such as rocking- being carried downwards, in nearly all complaints. For homoeopathic purposes the peculiar nervous symptoms are very characteristic and have frequently been verified especially in the therapeutics of children, of much value in epilepsy. Aphthous ulceration of mucus membranes. Sensitive to sudden noises.

Mouth: Aphthae, white fungus-like growth, mouth hot and tender, ulcers bleed on touch and eating, painful gum boil, crying when nursing. Taste bitter. *(Bry, Puls, cup).*

Stool: Loose, pappy, offensive stool in children.

Female: Galactorrhoea, pain in opp: breasts, on nursing. Menses too soon, profuse, membranous dysmenorrhoea.

Respiratory: Stitches in chest.

Extremities: Stitches in soles.

Skin: Psoriasis.

Better: Evening, cold weather, pressure.

Relation: Acetic acid, vinegar, and wine are incompatible.

Antidote: Cham., Coffea.

Compare: Calc, Bry., Sanicula, Sul-ac.

Dose: 1st to 3rd Trituration.

In skin diseases continue its use for several weeks. Locally pruritus pudendi. A piece of Borax, the size of a pea, dissolved in the mouth acts magically in restoring the voice, in cases of sudden hoarseness, brought on by cold and frequently for an hour or so, it renders the voice silvery and clear.

(Boericke)

Sea sickness, every time the ship goes down everything in me comes up. *(JHC)*

Borax, in its proving produces aphthous conditions of the mouth, which extend to the throat and even into the stomach. It cures where the genitalia and anus are covered with these aphthous appearances - all complaints are aggravated from downward motion. It has been said in routine practice, that in all cases of sore mouth in children, when the child is worse from downward motion - the child screeches and screams when it is handled and tossed up and down - *Agg:* from mental exertion, from noise, from excitement, from downward motion, we get mental aspect of Borax. This remedy has a good deal of vertigo. Eye lashes turn inward, towards eye and inflame it. Aphthae in mouth and on tongue, in this condition sulphuric acid is also indicated, red blisters on tongue. Child screams on passing urine. Leucorrhoea like the white of eggs and sterile condition of the women due to this trouble. *(Kent)*

124. *Bothrops Lanciolatus -*

Lachesis Lanciolatus.

(Yellow Viper)

Its venom is most coagulating (also Lachesis). We should expect to find under these remedies, the symptomatology of thrombosis, also thrombotic phenomena as hemiplegia, aphasia, inability to articulate *(Linn-Boyd).*

Broken down haemorrhagic constitutions, septic states. Great lassitude, and sluggishness, haemorrhages from every orifice of the body, black spots. Hemiplegia with aphasia. Inability to articulate, without any affection of the tongue. Nervous trembling, pain in right big toe. Diagonal course of symptoms, pulmonary congestion.

Mod: Worse - Right side.

Dose: Sixth to thirtieth potency.

The most peculiar symptoms of Bothrops for which "Ozanam" is the authority are these Amaurosis, Blindness from haemorrhage into retina - Day blindness.

(Boericke)

125. *Botulinum*

(Poisoning of canned spinach)
(Toxin of Bacillus Botulinum)

Food poisoning from canned spinach produced a clinical picture, suggested in a bulbar paresis.

Eye symptoms - Ptosis, double vision, blurred vision.

Difficulty in swallowing and breathing, choking sensation, weakness and uncertainty in walking, "blind staggers", dizziness, thickening of speech. Cramping pain in stomach.

Mask-like expression of face due to weakness of facial muscles. Severe constipation

Dose: Higher Potencies. *(Boericke)*

126. *Bovista*

(Puff Ball) (Fungus)

Has a marked effect on the skin, producing eruption like eczema, also upon the circulation predisposing to haemorrhages. Marked languor and lassitude. Adapted to stammering children, old maid with palpitation and tottery patients. Stage of numbness and tingling in multiple neuritis. Asphyxia due to charcoal fumes.

Mind: Enlarged sensation, everything falls from hands.

Head: As if head were enlarging-stringy discharge from nose-stammering (Stram-Merc.).

Face: Ache due to use of cosmetics.

Female: Diarrhoea, before and during menses, worse night, cannot bear tight clothing around waste (Lach). Traces of menses between menstruation.

Abdomen: Colic, relieved by eating.

Extremities: Drops things from hands Sweat in axillae, onion smell. Tip of coccyx itches intolerably.

Skin: Urticaria on excitement, Eczema, itching on getting warm.

Relation: Bovista antidotes tar application, after Rhus in chronic urticaria.

Compare: Calc., Rhus., Sepia, Cicuta.

Dose: 3rd to 6th potency. *(Boericke)*

This globular fungus, which according to report is eaten in Italy before it is ripe, becomes filled while ripening, with a blackish dust that breaks the husk which contains it, with a slight noise. Corresponding to this signature, 'Bloatedness', puffy condition of body surface and a sense of 'enlargement', flatulent distension and noisy passage of flatus are leading features of the Bovista pathogenesis. Bovista has cured cases of ovarian cyst and also warts and corns with shooting pains. The corners of the mouth are broken out - There is stuttering and stammering speech relaxation of entire capillary system - the puffy, expanding properties of the remedy are shown in a puffy condition of the body surface, instruments (eg. Scissors) indent the fingers in an unusual degree. The heart feels enormously large. Bovista has colic like Colo., causing the patient to bend double, but it differs from 'Colo' by amel: by eating and is sometimes accompanied by voiding of red urine. 'Itching at tip of Coccyx' We may always think of Bovista when we see a very tottery person, one who has tetters here and there all over the body - Agg: at full moon - effects of tar applied locally - Teste puts Bovis in his sulphur group. *(JHC)*

127. Brachyglottis

(Puka-Puka)

Fluttering sensation (Caladium). Kidney and bladder symptoms predominate. Produces symptoms of albuminurea. Itching in ears and nostrils. Brights disease. Oppression of chest, writers' cramp.

Urinary: Pressure in neck of bladder, urging to urinate - Urine contains mucous corpuscles and epithelium, albumen, and casts.

Extremities: Cramps in fingers, thumb and wrist when writing. Soreness extending along flexor carpi Ulnaris.

Relation: Compare - Apis, Helonias, Merc-cor., Plb.

Dose: 3rd potency. *(Boericke)*

128. Bromium

(Bromine)

Most marked effects are seen in the respiratory symptoms, especially in larynx and trachea. It seems to effect especially scrofulous children with enlarged glands. Blonde type. Enlarged parotid and goitre, tendency to spasmodic attacks. Left sided mumps. Sense of suffocation. Excoriating discharges. Profuse sweat and great weakness. Complaints from being over heated. Tendency to infiltrate, glands become hard, but seldom suppurate.

Nose: Coryza, Tickling, smarting, as from Cob webs.

Respiratory: Whooping cough, (use persistently for about ten days). Dry cough with hoarseness, pain behind sternum, spasmodic cough with rattling of mucus. Hoarseness, croup, cold sensation when inspiring. Laryngeal diphtheria; better at sea, of sea faring men when they come to land. Fibrinous bronchitis great dyspnoea, bronchial tubes feel filled with smoke.

Skin: Acne, pimples, pustules, boils on arms and face, glands stony hard especially on lower jaw. Hard goitre. (Spongia)

Mod: *Worse* - evening to midnight, warm room damp weather, lying on left side - *Better* - motion, exercise, at sea.

Relation: Antidotes - Ammon carb; camph, salt inhibits the action of Brom.

Compare: Conium, Spongia, Iod, Aster, Arg-nit.

Avoid milk when taking bromium.

Dose: First to 3rd attenuation must be prepared fresh as it is liable to rapid deterioration. *(Boericke)*

It is predominantly a left sided medicine - the glands (thyroid, testes, maxillary, parotid) are swollen and indurated, there is much anxiety of mind, a fear of ghosts or visions when in the dark - it has Amel. at the sea side (opp. Nat. mur.), but agg: in sailors when coming ashore. Migraine chiefly left side. Agg: from stooping especially after drinking milk. Agg: at the sight of running water or putting his foot on a bridge agg: in damp weather. A very peculiar symptom is - loud emissions of air from the vagina. The cough is agg: entering warm room. Headache agg: from drinking milk - sailors coming ashore suffer from asthma, which is relieved when they go to sea again. *(JHC)*

It is indicated also in complaints that come on in the night after a very hot day in the summer - if the mother has the baby out in a dreadfully cold dry day and towards midnight it wakens with spasmodic croup, you know that it is more likely to call for Aconite than any other medicine. Hoarseness coming on from getting over heated - It is very similar to these enlarged hard scrofulous glands, that we find in the neck, enlargement of the parotid and submaxillary. It has cured enlargement and great hardness of the thyroid gland. Swelling and hardness of the left parotid gland - the ovaries, testes, etc. are all affected by Bromium - Sensation of coldness as if the mucus membrane of the nose were cold from inhaling cold air, Bromium fits the most malignant types of diphtheria - the membrane grows like a weed, shuts off breathing, closes up the larynx - Ulcers of the stomach - Haemorrhoidal tumors - induration of the left testicle - left ovary - loud emission of flatus from the vagina - the air breathed feels cold, just like it was the air blown off from snow or ice - sensation as if the air tubes were full of smoke - some patients will describe that as sulphur fumes or as of smoke from tar - the cough gets- immediately worse from dust - Handling of old books from the shelf agg.: sneezing, hoarseness, irritation of the respiratory tract from picking up and handling dusty things. *(Kent)*

129. Bryonia

(Wild hops)

Acts on all serous membranes and the viscera they contain. Aching in every muscle. The general character of the pain here produced is a stitching, tearing, worse by motion, better rest. The characteristic stitching pains, everywhere but especially in the chest, worse pressure. Mucous membranes are all dry. The Bryonia patient is irritable, has vertigo from raising the head, pressive headache, dry parched lip, mouth, excessive thirst, bitter taste. Sensitive epigastrium and feeling of a stone in the stomach. Stools large, dry. Dry cough. Rheumatic pains and swelling, dropsical effusions into synovial and serous membranes.

Bryonia affects especially the constitution of a robust, firm fibre and dark complexion with tendency to cleanness and irritability. It prefers the right side, the evening and open air, warm weather after cold days to manifest its action most markedly.

Children dislike to be carried or raised, 'physical weakness', all—pervading apathy complaint apt to develop slowly.

Mind: Irritable, talks of business.

Head: Burning, splitting headache.

Nose: Frequent bleeding of nose when menses should appear.

Mouth: Lips parched, dry, cracked, dryness of mouth, tongue and throat with excessive thirst.

Stomach: Nausea and faintness when rising up - vomiting of bile and water immediately after eating, stomach sensitive to touch. Pressure in stomach after eating as of a stone.

Abdomen: Stitching pain, worse pressure, coughing, breathing.

Stool: Constipation, stools hard, dry, as if burnt.

Menses: Suppressed with vicarious discharge or splitting headache. Breast hot and painful, hard. Menstrual irregularities inter-menstrual pain, with great abdominal and pelvic soreness.

Respiratory: Cough dry at night, must sit up, worse after eating or drinking with stitches in chest and expectoration of rust coloured sputa. Coming into warm room excites cough. Angina Pectoris. (Use tincture)

Back: Stitches and stiffness in small of back.

Extremities: Knees stiff and painful-Joints red, swollen, hot.

Skin: Seborrhoea, hair very greasy.

Modality: *Worse* - warmth, motion, morning, eating, hot weather, exertion, touch.

Better: Lying on painful side, pressure, rest, cold things.

Complementary: Upas when Bryonia fails. Rhus, Alumina, Illecebrum.

Antidotes: Acon., Cham., Nux. v.

Compare: Asclep., Tub., Kali mur., Ptelia.

Dose: First to twelfth attenuation.

(Boericke)

Bryonia alba is one of the polychrest remedies of the homoeopathic materia medica - it not only disorders the circulation but alters the blood itself. It corresponds to fevers of almost all kinds, especially rheumatic typhoid, bilious and remitting. In these, as in all other complaints, the exquisite sensitiveness of the drug to movement of all kinds is a leading characteristic - lying on the painful part. (keeps the part at rest) - amel: from hard pressure and cold applications. Agg: moving - decided thirst, generally for large quantities at long intervals. The lips are dry and cracked - the mucous membranes are dry, especially those of the mouth and stomach, deficient secretion. Nose bleed, consequent on suppression of the menses is characteristic. Food lies at the epigastrium like a stone *Amel:* bringing up wind - there is intolerance of vegetable food. Everything tastes bitter. Eructations of tasteless gas is characteristic - sour stomach - diarrhoea occurs in the morning as soon as he moves - the usual Bry state is one of constipation, there is usual dryness of mucous membranes atony of the bowels, stool large, dry, hard, brown or black as if burnt or chassed crumbling stool smell of old cheese - mastitis hard, tender. left ovarian pain. Dropsical swellings - swelling of the legs, sensitive to touch - joints red swollen, stiff with stitching pain from slightest motion, synovial swellings - speech is hasty - frequent desire to take a long breath, must expand the lungs - those who overeat or eat excess of meat - persons accustomed to rich living with rich blood, form resisting flesh - Teste regards the digestive canal and more particularly the stomach as the principal seat. Complaints when warm weather sets in after cold days - Sweat profuse night and morning, sour or oily - Brẏ and Calc. c should never be given one after the other without an intercurrent remedy between (Nat. m. headache in morning, oily, sour sweat on face) (Bry. on head generally, cracked lips) Bry and Nat. m. go well together and are often complementary - Nit-ac. and Nux. to epicures but Bry. to gourmands, is followed well by Alum, Ars., Kali. c., Nux. v., Phos., Puls., Rhus., Sul.

Complementary: Alum and *Rhus* - *Alumina* is the chronic. *(JHC.)*

Its complaints develop slowly i.e. slowly for acute conditions, its complaints are continuous, remittent and occasionally intermittent - the slightest inclination to move resisted with a feeling of anger. Bryonia is often indicated in injuries of joints where Arnica would be a failure - there is an extreme state of irritability in Bryonia, every word which compels him to answer a question or to think will aggravate him - catarrhal fever may be covered by Bryonia. This sluggish state of the mind, in them is the state of Bryonia, not an excitable state as in Coffea, Nux vom., and Ignatia - thinks he is always away from home and wants to be taken home - The acute mental state manifests its symptoms on rising - in the morning he wants something and he knows not what (a very important symptom of Bryonia) - Bry to be ameliorated from cool air and from cool applications. Rheumatic complaints of Bry which are better from heat and under these circumstances he is better from continued motion. I sometimes wonder whether Bry. has a greater element of relief from heat or greater element of relief from cold - Most of the head complaints, that are of congestive character are better from cool applications, from cold air etc. - Yet there are some of the Bry head complaints, that are relieved by hot applications and these seem to have no accompanying cerebral congestion. So that 'Bry' has opposite modalities. In a damp climate Bryonia is one of the most frequently indicated remedies, but in the clear climates, where the thermometer runs low 'Aconite' will be indicated more than Bryonia. Often he wants the room dark - Bryonia patients are nearly always worse from visitors - persons who are subject to Bryonia conditions suffer in church, at the opera, in close warm rooms like Lycopodium - girls that faint every time they go to church, are relieved by Ignatia - the head feels so full, she wants to press it with hand, or tie it up, tight pressure over the whole skull - worse after eating. The head- aches are often accompanied by nose bleed. Constipation. Sluggish heart. Poor circulation, yet apparently plethoric, apparently rugged. Dandruff is common. Bryonia is ameliorated in all its complaints as soon as the perspiration becomes free and general. Arthritic sore eyes which means sore eyes in a gouty constitution. Many of the complaints of 'Bry' commence in the nose. Red eyes, lachrymation, aching through the nose, eyes and head the first day - then the trouble goes down into the posterior nares, the throat, the larynx with hoarseness and then a bronchitis comes on and if not checked it goes into pneumonia and pleurisy - Frequent sneezing, sneezing between coughs - loss of smell - during menstruation there is epistaxis - Great dryness of the lips - the lips parched and dry - children pick the lips - lips cracked and bleeding - Bryonia has tooth ache - worse - from warmth, toothache amel. from smoking - Bryonia has inflammation of the liver and many other liver symptoms. Bryonia furnishes many symptoms in connection with the stool and rectum - it has constipation and it has dysentery - stool is dry, hard as if burnt no desire for stool, but after going for many days there are passages of little hard pieces as if they had been burnt - it has

also diarrhoea, that drives the patient out of the bed in the morning - a yellow mushy stool - sometimes inter-mingled with mucus and slime, sometimes with blood - has cured many cases of chronic diarrhoea, where this yellow mushy discharge was present, and frequent, several times a day but more frequent in the morning he has stools several times in the morning that will satisfy for the whole twenty-four hours - during the night no stool at all - painful menstruation, dysmenorrhoea, pain in the ovaries during menstruation. In inflammatory conditions of the breast one of the most striking things is the stony hardness of the breast prior to menstruation - loss of voice with rawness in the trachea and great soreness in the chest - dry hacking cough as if the chest would burst from coughing. Bryonia prefers the right side when the condition is pneumonia - Bryonia patient lies upon the side that is affected in order to diminish the motion. Asthma worse in a warm room - wants cool air to breathe. Dry spasmodic cough, whooping cough - shaking the whole body.
(Kent)

In intermittent fevers the chills commence at the lips, the tips of the fingers, and toes, there is thirst during all stages. The perspiration in all fevers is sour or oily.
(Blackwood)

130. *Bufo*

(Poison of the Toad)

Acts on the nervous system and skin. Uterine symptoms marked. Lymphangitis of septic origin. Symptoms of paralysis agitans, Striking rheumatic symptoms.

Arouses the lowest passion, causes a desire for intoxicating drink and produces impotence.

Of use in feeble-minded children-prematurely senile. Epileptic symptoms. Convulsive seizures occur during sleep at night. More or less connected with derangements of the sexual sphere, seem to come within the range of this remedy. Injuries to fingers. Pain runs in streak up the arms.

Mind: Desire for solitude.

Ears: Music is unbearable.

Heart: Sensation of heart swimming in water.

Female: Epilepsy at time of menses.

Male: Disposition to handle organs.

Skin: Patches of skin lose sensation.

Relation: Compare - Baryta carb, Asterias, Salamand (Epilepsy and softening of brain)

Modalities: Better putting feet in hot water.

Dose: 6th potency and higher.
(Boericke)

Desire to solitude in order to practice masturbation - Adult people who act as if they were children - An aspect of child-like simplicity is present and the mind returns to a state of child-like innocence - This mental symptom is especially found under 'Baryta Carb' in adults who have never developed beyond child-hood but we do not prescribe this remedy on account of the epilepsy the child has not developed properly and the epilepsy is one of the manifestations - the old routinists have said of those people who are prematurely old or have taken on senility, that they need 'Baryta carb'. This medicine also stands out in bold type for those prematurely senile, the man at fifty acts like an old broken down man of eighty - Titters and says foolish things. Again, its action on the circular fibres of the abdominal aorta furnishes a key — note in epilepsy — an awful sensation of anxiety is felt in the abdomen and then there is a sudden loss of consciousness, the aura or warning is first felt in the abdomen. Stuttering and stammering, gets angry when incoherent speech is not understood - spasms or epilepsy come on during coition - burning pains or cramps in uterus - carcinoma of the uterus - offensive leucorrhoea. Cancer of the mammae for the burning pains and for the blisters that form round about - this is one of the remedies that you will need to use for the development of feeble minded children, whether there are spasms or not. *(Kent)*

131. Butyric acid

(A volatile acid obtained chiefly from butter)

Head: Constant state of fear and nervousness.

Stomach: Much gas in stomach and bowels. Cramps in pit of stomach.

Skin: Profuse offensive sweat of feet.

Dose: Third attenuation. *(Boericke)*

132.Cactus Grandiflorus

(Night-blooming cereus)

It is the heart and arteries especially that at once respond to the influence of Cactus, producing very characteristic constrictions of an iron band. This sensation is found in various places-oesophagus, bladder, etc. The mental symptoms produced correspond to those found, when there are heart affections, sadness and melancholy. Haemorrhage, constrictions, 'periodicity' and spasmodic pains, body feels as if caged, each wire being twisted tighter. Atheromatous arteries and weak heart. Congestions, irregular distribution of blood. Favours formation of clots speedily, Great periodicity. Toxic goitre with cardiac symptoms. Cactus is pulseless, panting and prostrated.

Head: Sensation as of a weight on vertex, congestive headache. Right sided prosopalgia.

Stomach: Constriction.

Female: Dysmenorrhoea.

Chest: Constriction in chest, as if bound, hindering respiration. Heart constriction as from an iron band.

Heart: Endo-Carditis with mitral insufficiency together with violent and rapid action. Tobacco heart. Violent palpitation, worse lying on left side, at approach of menses. Angina pectoris, pulse, feeble, irregular, quick. Low blood pressure.

Extremities: Oedema of hands and feet - subnormal temperatures.

Modalities: Worse 11 a.m. and 11 p.m. - Better open air.

Relation: Antidotes: Acon., Camph., China.

Compare: Digital, Spigel, Convallar, Kalmia, Naja, Magnol.

Dose: Tincture (Best made from flowers) 3rd attenuation. Higher in nervous palpitation. *(Boericke)*

Given as an organ remedy, it will benefit a large number of cases of weakened and painful heart sander considers - 'Cactus' specially indicated where the heart is weak and the arteries atheromatous. Many symptoms are Agg: at night (night blooming 'Cereus') - Chill at same hour every day 11 a.m. or 11 p.m.

It is the nature of Cactus to constrict, to cause constriction, in places where it has never been felt and never been thought of. "Congestion, Constriction and Contraction" - suppose you should tie a tape round a violently congested organ and tie it tighter and tighter - It seems to me that it is the suffering the patient has with that construction of a congested organ. That is not surprising. Any medicine that has such cardiac conditions and such vascular conditions will at times have more or less relaxation of blood vessels - Bleeding haemorrhoids - Constriction of anus - constipation - paralytic weakness of the bladder - retention of urine - urination prevented by clots. *(Kent)*

Functional irregularity of the heart from gastric irritation, neurasthenia, cigarette smoking in boys, the tobacco heart, masturbating and excessive bicycle riding.

133. *Cadmium sulph*

(Cadmic Sulphate)

Its pathogenesis gives symptoms corresponding to very low forms of disease, as in cholera, yellow fever, where with exhaustion, vomiting and extreme prostration, the disease runs deathward. Important gastric symptoms. Carcinoma ventriculi; persistent vomiting.

The attack is on stomach more especially. Patients must keep quiet.

Chilliness and coldness even when near the fire.

Eyes: Opacity of cornea.

Face: Facial paralysis.

Stomach: Nausea, black vomit, coffee ground vomiting.

Stool: Bloody, black and offensive.

Urine: Mixed with pus and blood.

Fever: Icy coldness, yellow fever.

Dose: 3rd - 30th potency. *(Boericke)*

The nasal symptoms are very important, no remedy has served me better in cases of ozaena and polypus. Compare Zn. (But in Zn. the action is primarily on brain - in Cadm primarily on stomach). Loss of breath on going to sleep, Carb. an., Carb. v., Op., Grind., Lach., Alet., - nausea of pregnancy. *(JHC.)*

Formication of the skin and deeper tissues - asleep sensation or like ants crawling in the extremities, deep in the muscles and the skin - Hyperaesthesia or anaesthesia - old nasal catarrh which has progressed till the nasal bones are being destroyed by caries - ulceration - pain in the bones, sneezing - coryza, boils, abscesses. It is a great remedy in the gastric irritation of carcinoma, a great palliative, coffee ground vomiting - Burning in the stomach extending up in the oesophagus, fluids burn all the way up into the mouth and throat, sour acid fluids. The main remedy in the hands of good prescribers. Draft causes a slight cold and on come sudden prostration, black vomit, death - in that state it competes with carbo veg. which used to be the main remedy in the hands of good prescribers. *(Kent)*

134. *Cahinca*

(Brazilian plant - Chiococca)

Synopsis: Dropsy, albuminuria, Dyspnoea at night, constant desire to urinate.

This remedy has been found of use in dropsical affections, its urinary symptoms are well marked. Albuminuria with dyspnoea on lying down at night.

Relation: Compare: Apocyn., Ars., Coffea.

Dose: 3rd potency or lower. *(Boericke)*

135. Cajuputum

(Oleum Wittnebianum)

(Cajuput oil)

A remedy for flatulence and affections of the tongue. Sense of enlargement. Causes copious diaphoresis. Retrocedent Gout. Neuralgic affections, not inflammatory. Nervous dyspnoea.

Mouth: Spasmodic stricture of oesophagus, constricted sensation on swallowing solid food. Tongue feels swollen, fills whole mouth.

Stomach: Hiccough on slightest provocation.

Abdomen: Flatulence, colic, urine smells like cat's urine. Spasmodic cholera.

Modalities: Worse 5 a.m. and night.

Relation: Compare - Bovista, Nux mosch., Asaf., Ign., Bapt.

Dose: 3rd potency. (5 drops of oil) *(Boericke)*

Smoking causes desire to vomit. *(JHC)*

136. Caladium Seguinum

(American arum)

This remedy has a marked action on the genital organs, and pruritus of this region. Coldness of single parts and inclination to lie down and aggravation on lying on left side. Slightest noise startles from sleep. Dread from motion. Modifies craving for tobacco, Tobacco heart. Asthmatic complaints.

Stomach: Stomach feels full of dry food, sensation of fluttering. Thirstless.

Male: Pruritus, sweating, skin of scrotum thick, impotency.

Female: Pruritus of vulva *(Ambra, Kreos.)* and vagina during pregnancy, (Hydrogen peroxide 1:12 locally) voluptuousness.

Skin: Sweet sweat attracts flies - Itching rash alternates with asthma.

Modalities: Better after sweat, after sleep in day time.

Worse: Motion.

Relation: Incompatible - Arum Triph.

Comple: Nitric acid, Capsic, Phos., Caust., Selen., Lyc., Ikshugandha, (Sexual weakness, emission, prostatic enlargement).

Dose: 3rd to 6th attenuation. *(Boericke)*

It is indicated in old debauches who are unable to perform the marital act. He has the most tantalizing craving for the opposite sex with no ability to perform coitus. Lascivious ideas - "such men stand on the street corner and feast upon the forms of passing girls and their semen dribbles away" - We may sum up the mental symptoms by saying he is extremely excitable things one done in great haste - Nervous excitement - the patient in general is - aggravated by warmth and the warm room - Yet he wants warm drinks in the stomach - effect of tobacco and cigarette smoking - removes the overwhelming craving that prevents smokers breaking off their habit. Itching is violent, especially about the genitals. It is useful in extremely nervous women who suffer from pruritus vulvae, keeping them awake at night, attended with abnormal excitement. Stools, soft, yellow, pasty, mushy. Violent sexual desire with relaxed penis - Impotency - Erections when half asleep in the morning, ceasing when fully awake. When the desire is most marked he has no ability - Caladium has cured as frequently as Thuja, itching eruption on the scrotum. The most striking symptom of the female sexual organs is the pruritus. She is compelled to scratch and the torment reduces her in body and mind. There are some strange sleep symptoms. Kept awake by crawling sensation sleeplessness from pruritus, especially in the genitals. Groans and moans anxiously in sleep, so that he wakens the neighbours. Restless sleep - anxious vivid dreams, which he remembers better than the things of the day - Fails asleep and continues to dream of the same subject where he left off. *(Kent)*

Common name: "Poisonous American Arum". This remedy is indicated in pruritus of Vulva and vagina during pregnancy; also in pruritus of the genitals of the male. The parts are oedematous or cold sweating and relaxed. It is of service in dyspepsia when the stomach feels as if full of dry food - Dosage of the Tr. 1 to 2 drops.

(Blackwood)

137. *Calcarea Acetica*

(Acetate of lime)

Has had brilliant clinical results in inflammations of mucous membranes characterised by a membranous exudation, otherwise its action and application is like the carbonate. Cancer pain.

Head: Senses obscure while reading, Megrim.

Respiratory: Cough loose with expectoration, of large pieces like casts of Bronchial tubes.

Female: Membranous dysmenorrhoea. (Borax)

Relation: Compare - Brom., Borax. (Calc. oxal. in excruciating pains of open cancer).

Dose: 3rd trituration. *(Boericke)*

This remedy has relieved Vertigo that is aggravated while walking in the open air, Migraine with coldness of the head and a sour taste in mouth - painless diarrhoea which does not exhaust the patient - itching of the anus. *(Blackwood)*

138. *Calcarea Arsenica*

(Arsenite of lime)

Epilepsy with rush, of blood to the head before attack. Aura felt in region of heart, flying sensation. Complaints in fat women around climacteric. Chronic malaria. Infantile enlarged liver and spleen. Nephritis with great sensitiveness in kidney region. Complaints of drunkards after abstaining, (Carbon sulph). Fleshy women at climacteric, slightest emotion causing palpitation. Dyspnoea with feeble heart, chilliness. Albuminuria, dropsy, affection of spleen and mesenteric glands. Haemoglobin and red corpuscles are low.

Dose: 3rd Trituration. *(Boericke)*

Headaches move from the side lain on to the side not lain on and continue to change about by changing position. Headache relieved during mental exertion. Loses the voice before an epileptic convulsion. Oedema of face, lids, temples and ears - eczema of face and scalp. *(Kent)*

139. *Calcarea Carbonica Ostrearum*

(Carbonate of lime)

This great Hahnemannian anti-psoric is a constitutional remedy par excellence. Its chief action is centered in the vegetative sphere, impaired nutrition being the key note of its action, the glands, skin and bones, being instrumental in the changes wrought. Increased, local and general perspiration, swelling of glands, scrofulous and rachtic conditions generally offer numerous opportunities for the exhibition of calcarea, incipient phthisis (Ars. iod., Tuberculin). It covers the tickling cough, fleeting chest pain, nausea, acidity and dislike of fat. Gets out of breath easily. A jaded state, mental or physical due to overwork. Abscesses in deep muscles, polypi and exostoses. Pituitary and thyroid dysfunction.

Raised blood coagulability (Strontium). Is a definite stimulant to the periosteum, is a haemostatic and gives this power probably to the gelatine injections.

Easy relapses, interrupted convalescence. Persons of scrofulous type, who take cold easily with increased mucous secretions, children who grow fat, are large bellied, with large head, pale skin, chalky look, the so-called leuco-phlegmatic temperament, affection caused by working in water. Great sensitiveness to cold, partial sweats. Children crave eggs and eat dirt and other indigestible things, are prone to diarrhoea. Calcarea patient is Fat, Fair, Flabby and perspiring and cold, damp and sour.

Mind: Apprehensive, fears, loss of reason, misfortune, forgetful.

Head: Icy coldness, and on the head, much perspiration, wets the pillow.

Eyes: Sensitive to light, spots and ulcers on the cornea, lachrymal ducts closed from exposure to cold, dimness of vision as if looking through a mist. Lachrymal fistula.

Ears: Inflammation with muco-purulent otorrhoea and enlarged glands.

Nose: Dry nostrils, sore, ulcerated, polypi, takes cold at every change of weather.

Face: Swelling of upper lip.

Mouth: Persistent sour taste, bleeding gums, delayed dentition.

Throat: Swelling of tonsils, Goitre.

Stomach: Craving for indigestible things, aversion to meat, boiled things, liking for chalk, coals, pencils, eggs, salt, and sweets - milk disagrees. Sour eructation, sour vomiting, dislike of fat. Loss of appetite when over worked.

Abdomen: Inguinal and mesenteric glands swollen, distention, gall stone colic.

Stool: sour, children's diarrhoea.

Male: Frequent emissions.

Female: Menses too early, too profuse, too long, cold damp feet, milky leucorrhoea, Polypi.

Respiratory: Painless hoarseness, suffocating spells, tightness, worse going upstairs, chest very sensitive to touch, percussion or pressure.

Back: Renal colic.

Extremities: Cold, damp, soles of feet raw.

Sleep: Some disagreeable idea always arouses from light slumber.

Fever: Chill at 2 p.m. begins internally in stomach region, fever with sweat over head in children, so that pillow becomes wet.

Skin: Petechial eruptions.

Modalities: Worse cold, water in any form, during full moon. *Better:* Dry weather, lying on painful side, sneezing.

Relation: Camph., Ipec., Nit. ac., Nux-v.

Comple: Bel., Rhus., Lycop., Silicea.

Calcarea is useful after Sulphur, where the pupils remain dilated.

Incompatible: *Bry.* (Sulphur should not be given after Calcarea)

Calcarea Calcinata: Calcined oyster shell - remedy for Warts.

Ova tosta: Toasted egg shells - Backache and Leucorrhoea.

Calcarea Lactic: anaemia, haemophilia, urticaria, where the coagulability of the blood is diminished.

Dose: 6x, 30, and higher potencies - should not be repeated too frequently in elderly people *(Boericke)*

Moreover, Calcarea is one of the Polychrest remedies and ranks with Sulphur and Lycopodium at the head of the anti-psorics - these three medicines should be thoroughly known; as these are in a sense, the standards around which the rest are grouped - it is a chilly remedy - Calc has cold clammy feet as if, there were damp stockings on - Sulph has characteristically hot sweaty feet. The sinking sensation common to all three is most marked with sulph at - 11 a.m. with Lyco at 4 p.m., with Calcarea at any time - Calcarea is closely allied to Belladonna, Nux., Puls. and Rhus in its action - It follows well sulph and Nit acid; to both of which it is complementary - It is inimical to, Bryonia and should not be given immediately before or after that medicine to persons of soft fibre with tendency to fat- Head sweats profusely, wetting the pillow for a space around the head. Child wakes at 2 to 3 a.m. screaming children are slow in teething and walk late - suppression of menses in women of - full habit after working in water - the sweat of the head must be remembered - it occurs chiefly on occiput and forehead (that of Sil. is all over). Burning in soles of feet at night, burning in back of hands - Calc. hand is soft, warm and moist, a boneless hand - there are copious night sweats, which may be sour or odourless. Foot sweat, sour or odourless - there is ravenous hunger, hunger and feeling of emptiness, immediately after a meal and in the early morning - sour body smell, milk disagrees - chronic disease of left tonsil, feeling a lump in left side of throat - crawling in rectum as from worms - burning in rectum - stools hard and pasty like chalk or clay, offensive undigested the cough is provoked by going into a cold room, by chilliness sensation of feather in throat a fat cough with easy expectoration - swelling of cervical and bronchial glands - scrofulous diseases of bones, spinal curvature, rickets. The skin is rough and scaly and inclined to chap - Rhagades - chapped hands - eruption behind right ear - warts and polypi - Calc. is an eminently sycotic medicine as the early morning aggravation would indicate - the epilepsy of Calc. has an aura spreading up from the solar plexus. Ascending causes great weakness. Calc is one of the remedies that has been used for the sensation of levitation - According to Guernsey Calc. is in general a right sided remedy - among the conditions of Calc., dread of the open air ranks most prominently, the least cold air goes right through - great sensitiveness to cold damp air - Also cannot bear sun - dread of bathing and water the Calc. patient generally feels better when constipated the diarrhoea of Calc. is generally Agg: in afternoon, at full moon, at new moon - "Teste" puts Calc. in the Pulsatilla group. *(JHC)*

They grow fat and flabby. They go into marasmus - Calcarea is full of congestions - cold feet, hot head tendency to attack glands, the glands of the neck, all the glands of the body, especially the lymphatic glands - cures many tumours-fatty, cystic, if the symptoms agree - polypi in the nose, ears, vagina, bladder and here and there - cystic growths - causes exostoses - chilly patient - tired patient - a big bellied child with emaciated limbs and emaciated neck - inability to prolong mental operation - thinks he is going insane - does carry on a conversation as ordinary people do - when he is alone, when he has nobody to talk with him he does strange things - right in the midst of his success he quits his business and goes home and leaves all. He has become so industrious that he has a mania for work. One of the most striking symptoms of the head of the Calcarea patient is the sweat - the sweat of the head upon the slightest exertion. Headache over the eyes - Congestion of the head, back of the head. Tearing headache above the eyes down to nose is a strong symptom of Calcarea - this is relieved by very hot application, in the dark, agg: day light - the headache continues to grow worse during the day until in the evening - it becomes so severe that it is attended with nausea and vomiting - periodicity, of seven to fourteen days, but again it comes on whenever he is exposed, by riding in the wind - he is a very chilly patient - Calcarea will again have cold head and icy cold feet when walking in cold weather, but as soon as the feet get warm they go to the other extreme and burn so that he puts them out of bed, this has often led inexperienced prescribers to prescribe "Sulph" because that is a key note of Sulph. The fontanelles remain open a long time - It has hydrocephalic conditions. In hydrocephalic children this sweating head is a common feature - the hair falls out but in patches here and there. It has eruptions upon the head and face - eczema that we find in children and infants - thick scabs on the head, with yellow pus, offensive eruptions. Eye comes in with a share of troubles - ulceration of the cornea - cannot even stand ordinary light - has cured cataract - on closing the eyes he sees the most horrible visions spectres, ghosts - wonderful remedy for eye strain - cured many cases of opacity of the cornea - an opacity itself is not a symptom but a result of disease. Thick yellow discharge from the ears. Whether the catarrh of the nose, the eyes or the ears, there will be headache - the catarrh of the nose is extremely troublesome - chronic sore throat, the uvula may be puffed or swollen. Food taken into the stomach turns sour - Milk sours Milk disagrees. Crave eggs - aversion to meat. Aversion to warm food pungent sour odor diarrhoea comes on, sour, watery diarrhoea, gradual emaciation. When constipation is present the stool is white or like chalk - calcarea babies are some times wormy. Menstrual period too soon, lasting too long, and profuse - leucorrhoea, dyspnoea - rheumatic conditions - enlarged joints - especially small joints of the toe and finger. The sleep is greatly disturbed - late going to sleep, sometimes not till 2, 3, or 4 o' clock - Full of ideas when closing the eyes, horrible visions. *(Kent)*

140. *Calcarea Fluorica*

(Fluoride of lime)

A powerful tissue remedy for hard stony glands, varicose veins and manifestation of bones. Hard knots in female breast. Goitre. Congenital hereditary syphilis, induration, threatening suppuration. Many cases of cataract have undoubtedly been influenced favourably by it. Congenital syphilis manifesting itself in ulceration of mouth and throat, caries and necrosis with boring pains and heat in parts. Arteriosclerosis, threatened apoplexy, Tuberculosis. Used after operations. The tendency to adhesions is reduced.

Mind: Groundless fears of financial ruin.

Eyes: Strumous phlyctenular Keratitis, subcutaneous, palpabral cysts.

Ears: Chronic suppuration of middle ear.

Tooth: Toothache with pain if any food touches the tooth.

Stomach: Acute indigestion from fatigue.

Anus: Fissure of the anus.

Male: Hydrocele, induration of the testicles.

Respiratory: Croup.

Circulatory: Varicose or enlarged veins.

Extremities: Lumbago Ganglia or encysted tumors at the back of the wrist. Chronic synovitis of knee joints.

Skin: Marked whiteness of skin, chaps and cracks - in the palms of the hands or hard skin - induration of stony hardness - swelling or indurated enlargements.

Modality: *Worse* during rest, change of weather.

Better: Heat, warm applications.

Relation: Con., Lapis., Baryta mur., Hecla., Rhus., Cacodylate of soda. (Tumours) - Calcarea sulph - Stibiata (acts as a haemostatic and absorptive in uterine Myoma) *Mangifera indica* - Varicose Veins.

Dose: 3-12 x.

Chronic remedy. Needs some time before manifesting its effects - should not be repeated too frequently. *(Boericke)*

Large indurated tonsils will be cured after Baryta Carb has failed - Hard nodules in mammae - It is similar to Silica in suppuration - *(Kent)*

Goitre and enlarged prostrate, exostosis and bony growth, early stage of aneurysm. *(Blackwood)*

141. *Calcarea Iodata*

(Iodide of lime)

It is in the treatment of scrofulous affection, especially of enlarged glands, tonsils etc. that this remedy has gained marked beneficial results. Thyroid enlargements about time of puberty. Flabby children, subject to colds. Secretion inclined to be profuse and yellow. Adenoids, uterine fibroids, croup.

Head: Polypi of nose and ear.

Throat: Enlarged tonsils are filled with crypts.

Skin: Indolent ulcers, accompanying varicose veins.

Relation: Agraphis. (Adenoids with enlarged tonsils).

Compare: Calc. fluor., Sil., Merc. iod.

Dose: 2nd and 3rd trituration.

(Boericke)

Calc. iod has a short proving, but it has been used mostly on indications, suggested by its two components. It is similar to Baryta iod in its action on enlarged glands and is specially indicated for enlarged tonsils honey combed with little crypts - a number of cases of breast tumors have been cured by 3x. *(JHC)*

142. *Calcarea Lactica*

Remedies for spine complaints are not very numerous and Calc Lact has been credited with cures of this troublesome complaint. It should be kept in mind. It has been prescribed in the crude, but homoeopathy may begin with eight grain doses of the 3X trit, three or four times a day. Migraine is another sphere of its action - A Danish writer C. I. Bastrup described a type in which he found Calc. Lact dramatically successful. It is accompanied by slight oedema affecting the eyelids, upperlip, or one hand - Bastrup suggests that the migraine may be due to an oedema of meninges. He gives 1 grain of Calc - lact once or twice a day for 3 weeks - It not only removes the headache but also to such troubles as vasomotor rhinitis. *(JHC)*

Anaemia haemophilia, urticaria, where the coagulability of the blood is diminished.

(Boericke)

143. *Calcarea Phos.*

(Phosphate of Lime)

One of the most important tissue remedies and while it has many symptoms in common with Calcarea Carb there are some differences and characteristic features of its own. It is especially indicated in tardy dentition and troubles incident to that period, bone disease, non-union of fractured bones and the anaemias after acute diseases and - chronic wasting diseases. Anaemic children who are peevish, flabby, have cold extremities and feeble digestion. It has a special affinity where bones form sutures or symphyses, and all its symptoms are worse from any change of weather. Numbness and crawling are characteristic sensations and tendency to perspiration and glandular enlargement are symptoms it shares with the Carbonate. Scrofulosis, chlorosis and pthisis.

Head: *Worse,* near the region of sutures, from change of weather. Adenoid growths.

Stomach: Craving for bacon, ham, salted or smoked meats - much flatulence.

Abdomen: At every attempt to eat, colicky pain in abdomen, sunken and flabby.

Stool: Green, slimy, hot, sputtering, undigested with fetid flatus.

Female: Menses too early, excessive and bright in girls with violent headache, leucorrhoea like white of egg.

Extremities: Cold numb feeling.

Relation: Ruta, Hepar.

Modality: *Worse* exposure to damp cold weather, melting snow. *Better* in summer, warm, dry atmosphere.

Dose: First to third trituration. Higher potencies often more effective. *(Boericke)*

Calc. carb has craving for eggs. Calc. phos has for salt or smoked meats, craving for fat, bacon in children, stool green and slimy or hot and watery with fetid flatus, weak memory, school headaches in children the patient is weak and consumptive, enlargement of tonsils, acute and chronic, defective nutrition, neck too thin and weak to support head, Diabetes when the lungs are affected, "Carb. An." contains Calc. phos and is the nearest analogue - in bone affections and Fistula, Berb., Calc., Calc. fl., Fluor acid., Ruta, Sil., Sul. - in joint affections Berb., Kali ph., Nat. m., - diabetes Kali ph., Nat ph. - Haemorrhoids, Ferr. ph. - worms, Nat phos - after operation of fistula "Berb". *(JHC)*

It has cured polypi of nose, rectum and uterus - It has cured enlarged glands of neck, groin and abdomen - Electric shock, so severe that the patient could not remain standing - Epileptic spasms. Convulsion of children. Dull headaches of school children. Always come home from school with headache, wants it washed in cold water - epistaxis - growing children suffer from chronic throat troubles - enlarged tonsils - crave salt, bacon and smoked meats - infants want to nurse all the time - cold drinks, ice cream, fruits disorder the stomach, causing pain or diarrhoea - constipation with difficult hard stool, bleeding from the rectum and anus during stool. Piles itch and burn and discharge yellow pus - itching of the anus in the evening - Boils and abscesses about and near the anus, discharging blood and pus. Fissured anus - this remedy has cured diabetes mellitus - sexual desire increased - the woman has no better friend than Calc. p. Her sufferings at puberty when she is slow in maturing are often met with by this medicine - prolapsus of uterus during stool and micturition - Uterine polypus leucorrhoea like white of egg day and - night - the most severe tearing, shooting pains are in the lower limbs - the probable reason for this is that the lower limbs are always cold to the knees and the cold parts are always the suffering parts in this remedy. *(Kent]*

144. *Calcarea Silicata*

(Silicate of lime)

A deep long acting medicine for complaints which come on slowly and reach their final development after long periods. Hydrogenoid constitution (Nat. sulph.), very sensitive to cold. Patient is weak, emaciated, cold and chilly, but worse from being over-heated. Sensitive generally. Atrophy of children.

Mind: Fearful.

Relation: Arsenic, Tubercul., Baryta Carb., Iod.

Dose: All potencies lowest to high. *(Boericke)*

145. *Calcarea Sulph*

(Sulphate of lime - Plaster of Paris)

Eczema and torpid glandular swellings cystic tumors. Fibroids. Suppurative processes come within the range of this remedy, after pus has found a vent. Mucous discharges are yellow, thick and lumpy. Lupus Vulgaris.

Eyes: Inflammation of the eyes, with discharge of thick yellow matter.

Nose: Yellowish purulent secretion, yellowish discharge.

Face: Pimples and pustules on the face.

Stool: Painful abscesses about the anus.

Extremities: Burning, itching of soles of feet.

Relation: Compare - Hepar, Silica.

Dose: 2nd and 3rd trituration. The twelth potency has been found effective in lupus. *(Boericke)*

Calcarea sulph. is closely related to Hepar sulph., Calc., which is an impure sulphide of Calcium - In the last edition of his (Schussler) Biochemic therapy he discards Calc. Sulph. because it is not an actual constituent of the tissues. It is indicated in all kinds of cases after pus has found a vent - it differs from Hepar in sensitiveness to air - Hepar cannot bear the slightest exposure - calc. sulph has amel. in open air-better walking in it - desire for it - Hansen recommends it in dry eczema in children - cystic tumours - fib - romata and polypi have been cured with Calc. sulph. *(JHC)*

The author frequently made use of Schussler's 12th potency, later the 30th and 200th, at present much higher potencies. - The tendency to the formation of abscesses in the body in any place is a strong feature of this remedy and is quite similar to pyrogen - the patient desires the open air. Always in a hurry, hysterical impatient - This remedy has partly cured several cases of cataract. Cracked lips and flushes of heat of the face - pale sickly pustules - scurfy eruptions - vesicles - itching of the face - pain in the face from becoming cold. Aversion to coffee, to meat and to milk. Desires fruit, cold drinks, acids, salt things, sweets. Fistula in ano - like sulphur it has cured morning diarrhoea - but has also an evening diarrhoea. Moisture about anus, prolapsus of the rectum - ineffectual urging to stool, can be in any form. It is an excellent remedy for impotency - itching of the genitals from leucorrhoea. Thick yellow bloody leucorrhoea - prolapsus of the uterus. Fibroid tumors of the uterus - cough is agg: in the evening and night amel: in cool air unlike Hepar - dry cough at night. Hacking cough - Hoarse dry cough - Loose rattling cough - the cough racks the whole body, short dry cough expectoration is copious in the morning - Gouty joints - awkward clumsy fingers from Gouty joints - Hip joint disease - itching of the skin of the extremities - often itching and burning - Burning of hands and feet - Burning palms and soles - pain in the shoulder, elbow, wrist and fingers - perspiration of the hands and feet - Oedematous swelling of the feet and legs - Tingling in the fingers as if asleep - perspiration at night - the perspiration is profuse and sour - there are numerous skin symptoms, as might be expected from a study of Sulphur and Calcarea - Burning and itching - desquamation - cracked skin - the skin is cracked after washing in winter - especially of the hands like we find in salt rheum - liver spots - pale skin and yellow skin - even to marked cases of jaundice.

Dryness of skin - the eruptions are boils, burning, moist or dry eczema - herpetic pustules - scabby scaly vesicles - this remedy cures Psoriasis when the symptoms agree - urticaria - excoriation and intertrigo - formication itching in bed, itching, burning, crawling - itching ameliorated by scratching. *(Kent)*

146. *Calendula officinalis*

(Marigold)

A most remarkable healing agent applied locally. Useful for open wounds, parts that will not heal, ulcers etc.

Promotes healthy granulations and rapid healing by first intention. Haemostatic after tooth extraction. Deafness. Catarrhal conditions. Neuroma. Constitutional tendency to erysipelas. Pain is excessive and out of all proportion to injury. Great disposition to take cold, especially in damp weather. Paralysis after apoplexy, for cancer as an intercurrent remedy. Has remarkable power to produce local exudations and helps to make acrid discharge, healthy and free. Cold hands.

Compare: Hamamel., Hyper., Symph., Arn. To deafness - *Ferr., Pic., Kali iod., Calc., Mag-c., Graph.*

Antidote: Chelidon., Rheum.

Comple: Hepar.

Dose: Locally Acqueous - Calendula, for all wounds, the greatest healing agent. Also as an injection in leucorrhoea, internally tincture to third potency. For burns, sores, fissures, and abrasions etc. use Calendula Cerate.

Locally - 1 dram mother tincture with an oz or two of water for wounds.

(Boericke)

The flowers of Calendula close when a dark cloud passes over - In Germany it is regarded as a cancer cure - His experience (C.W. a pharmacist) led him to conclude that Calendula has an action on spinal cord.

(JHC)

Helmuth speaking of the treatment of carbuncle says of late, "I have adopted a treatment which has been so successful, that I have been surprised at the results - it consists in applying over the parts, Four thickness of Lint, saturated with a solution of Calendula one part to Six of water, over this apply an oil silk and when it is dry to be resaturated with the Calendula solution." In connection with this he administered 5 grains of the 3x of the Arsenicum alb. every 2 hours.

(Blackwood)

147. *Calotropis*

(Madar Bark)

Has been used with marked success in the treatment of syphilis following mercury also in elephantiasis, leprosy and acute dysentery. Pneumonic phthisis, Tuberculosis.

Increases the circulation in the skin, has powerful effects as a sudorific. In the secondary symptoms of syphilis, where mercury has been used, cannot be pushed safely any farther, it rapidly recruits the constitution, heals the ulcers and blotches from the skin and perfects the cure. Primary anaemia of syphilis. Heat in stomach is a good guiding symptom. Obesity, while flesh decreases, muscles become harder and firmer.

Relation: Merc., Kali iod., Berb aqui., Sars., Ipec.

Dose: Tincture, 1-5 drops 3 times a day.

(Boericke)

Calotropis gigantica is possessed of great virtue in purifying blood and is very efficacious in curing syphilis in all its stages - Leprosy in feet around nails, fingers etc., in all kinds of putrid gangrenous ulcers. In these affections give Calotropis 1X, 1 drop, thrice daily and alternate it with Echinacea 1x, 3 drops twice daily

(Dr. Yudhbir Sinha)

The bark made into paste applied to the legs and scrotum in Elephantiasis to leprous ulcers and leucoderma.

The root bark reduced to a paste with sour Kanjee is applied externally over elephantiasis of the legs and scrotum. The powdered root bark is smoked like tobacco in syphilis.

According to Chevarse and others, forcing Madar juice down the throat is a common method of infanticide employed by castes among which female infanticide prevails. Madar juice is also given internally or applied locally to procure abortion like all other irritant vegetable juices. It is used locally, usually a stick smeared with the juice is pushed up into the Os uteri and left there until uterine contractions are induced. In some parts of India it is also used as a cattle poison.

(Dr. S.C. Gosh. Drugs of Hindoosthan)

148. *Caltha Palustris*

(Cow slip)

Pain in abdomen, vomiting, headache, singing in ears, dysuria and diarrhoea, anasarca, pemphigus.

Female: Uterine cancer.

Dose: Tincture. *(Boericke)*

149. *Camphora*

(Camphor)

Hahnemann says: The action of this substance is very puzzling and difficult for investigation, even in the healthy organism, because its primary action more frequently than with any other remedy, alternates and becomes intermixed with the vital reaction (after effects) of the organism. On this account it is often difficult to determine what belongs to the vital reactions of the body and what to the alternating effects due to the primary action of the camphor.

Picture a state of collapse. Icy coldness of the whole body. Sudden sinking of strength, pulse small and weak. After operations, if temperature is subnormal, low blood pressure - 3 doses Camph. 1x, 15 - minutes intervals. This condition is met with in cholera, and here it is that camphor has achieved classical fame. First stages of a cold, with chilliness and sneezing. Subsultus and extreme restlessness. Cracking of joints. Epileptiform convulsions. Camphor has a direct relationship to muscles and fascia. In local rheumatic affections in cold climates. Distension of veins. As a heart stimulant for emergency use, Camphor is the most satisfactory remedy. Drop doses on sugar as often as every five minutes.

It is characteristic of Camphor that the patient will not be covered, notwithstanding the icy coldness of the body. One of the main remedies in shock. Pain better while thinking of it. Very sensitive to cold and to touch. Sequelae of measles. Violent convulsion, with wandering and hysterical excitement. Tetanic spasms. Scrofulous children and irritable, weakly blondes especially affected.

Head: Sneezing, nose cold and pinched, fleeting, stitches in temporal region and orbits, Head sore, occipital throbbing synchronous with pulse.

Eyes: Sensation as if all objects were too bright and glittering.

Nose: Persistent epistaxis.

Face: Anxious, bluish, cold sweat.

Stomach: Coldness.

Stool: Asiatic cholera with cramps in calves, collapse.

Urine: Strangury.

Male: Priapism.

Respiratory: Breath cold.

Sleep: Insomnia.

Fever: Icy coldness of the whole body, congestive chill, tongue cold.

Skin: Cold.

Modalities: Worse motion, night, contact, cold air, better - warmth.

Relationship: Camphor antidotes or modifies the action of nearly every Vegetable medicine - Tobacco, Opium, Worm medicines etc.

Incompatible: Kali nitrate.

Complementary: Cantharis.

Antidotes: Opium, Nitr. sp., Dulc., Phos.

Compare: Carbo., Cuprum., Arsenic., Veratrum.

Dose: Tincture, in drop doses, repeated frequently or smelling of spirits of camphor. Potencies are equally effective.

Cholera: Use mother tincture 5 drop doses with sugar every few minutes until the reaction is set in. Camphor should not be given if there is sweat or it should be stopped as soon as sweat begins.

Note: For thought - All our progress as a school depends on the right view of the symptom obtained by proving with camphor and opium - Herring. *(Boericke)*

This medicine has Chill, cramp, convulsion with mental anguish - Feeling as if a cold wind were blowing over body - Camph. produces tetanic spasms, with showing of teeth by drawing up the mouth corners, like Nux-v. and Phytolacca, but the deathly coldness of Camph. distinguishes it from both. The cramps with icy coldness of limbs are characteristic of Camph. The coldness of Camph resembles that of Verat., but with the latter the discharges are copious and Camph. has marked nausea. Strangury and priapism are among its effects. Most pains are felt during a half-conscious condition, and disappear when thinking of them. Surface cold to touch, yet throws off all covering. In the form of the ordinary camphor pilule, I have found it an excellent remedy for simple sleeplessness. Teste notes that it acts much more powerfully on carnivorous animals than on herbivora, *(JHC)*

It has both sexual erethysm and impotency in its provings. I once knew a French woman who had an insane desire to keep her boys always at home with her, and she thought she could accomplish this if she could only keep them away from the girls, and to destroy their sexual desire she kept a bag of Camphor under their pillows. All of them were made impotent. But in some provers it establishes sexual erethysm. In camphor the coldness is relieved by cold, he wants more cold. *(Kent)*

150. Camphora Mono-bromata

(Mono - Bromide of Camphor)

Nervous excitability is the guiding condition. Suppression of milk.

Nightly emissions. Painful erections. Paralysis agitans, cholera infantum and infantile convulsions. Intensifies the action of Quinine and renders it more permanent. Directions appear reversed i.e. North seems South, and East seems West. Hysteria, weeping and laughing alternately, trance like state.

Dose: 2nd Trituration. *(Boericke)*

151. *Canchalagua*

(Erythrea Venusta - Centaury)

Used extensively as a fever remedy and bitter tonic (Gentiana) - Antimalarial and anti-septic, of use in severe type of intermittent fever in hot countries, also in influenza, sore as if bruised all over. Sensation of drops falling from and upon different spots. Skin wrinkled like a washer woman's, scalp feels tight as if drawn together by India rubber.

Dose: Tincture in drop dose. Must be made from the fresh plant. Its medicinal properties are lost in the dry.

(Boericke)

The skin presents a wrinkled, corrugated appearance - Leprosy. *(Blackwood)*

152. *Cannabis Indica*

(Hashish - Indian Hemp.)

Inhibits the higher faculties and stimulates the imagination to a remarkable degree, without any marked stimulation of the lower animal instinct. A condition of intense exaltation, in which all perceptions and conceptions, all sensation and emotions are exaggerated to the utmost degree.

Subconscious or dual nature state. Apparently under the control of the second self, but the original self prevents the performance of acts which are under the domination of the second self. Apparently the two natures cannot act independently, one acting as a check, upon the other, (Effects of one dram doses by Dr. Albert Schneider).

The experimenter feels ever and on that he is distinct from the subject of the hashish dreams and can think rationally.

Produces the most remarkable hallucinations and imaginations, exaggeration of the duration of time and extent of space being most characteristic. Conception of time, space and place is gone. Extremely happy and contented, nothing troubles. Ideas crowd upon each other. Has great soothing influence in many nervous disorders like epilepsy, mania dementia, delirium tremens and irritable reflexes. Exophthalmic goitre. Catalepsy.

Mind: Exuberance of spirits - Time seems too long, second seem ages, a few rods an immense distance. Very forgetful, cannot finish sentence. Uncontrollable laughter.

Head: Feels as if top of head were opening and shutting and as if calvarium were being lifted. Involuntary shaking of head.

Face: Grinding of teeth in sleep.

Urinary: Urine loaded with slimy mucus dribbling.

Heart: Pulse very slow.

Extremities: Pain across shoulders and spine, must stoop, can not walk erect. Entire paralysis of the lower extremities, very exhausted after a short walk.

Sleep: Very sleepy, but unable to do so. Obstinate and intractable forms of insomnia. Catalepsy. Dreams of dead bodies. Prophetic, nightmare.

Modalities: *Worse* - morning, coffee, liquor, tobacco, lying on right side

Better - from fresh air, cold water, Rest.

Relation: Bell., Hyos., Stram., Lach., Agar., Anhalon. (Time sense disordered, time periods enormously over estimated, thus minutes seem hours etc.

Dose: Tincture and low attenuation. *(Boericke)*

Horror of darkness, sensation of levitation, wants to sleep but cannot. *(JHC)*

The natural tendencies of the patient are exaggerated, the mild and gentle become more pleasant and agreeable, while the irritable become cross, vicious and violent. *(Blackwood)*

153. *Cannabis Sativa*

(European Hemp/
American Hemp)

Sensation of dropping water. Stuttering. opacity of cornea. Burning while urinating, inflammatory stage of gonorrhoea, cannot walk with legs together.

Seems to effect especially, the urinary, sexual and respiratory organs. It has a characteristic sensation as of dropping water on head. Great fatigue, as from over-exertion, weary after meals. Choking on swallowing, Things go down the wrong way. Stuttering, confusion of thought and speech, wavering speech, hasty, incoherent.

Eyes: Opacity of cornea, patient feels deeply approaching blindness.

Urine: Burning while urinating, extending to bladder. Gonorrhoea, walks with legs apart.

Respiratory: Palpitation, must stand up.

Modalities: *Worse* lying down, going up-stairs.

Relation: Antidotes: Camph., Lemon juice.

Compare: Hedysorum - Brazilian Burdock - (Gonorrhoea and inflammation of Penis), Canth, Apis, Copaiva, Thuja, Kali-nit.

Dose: Tr. to 3rd attenuation - In stuttering the 30th. *(Boericke)*

Cannabis sativa resembles closely Cannabis indica, but the mental symptoms and head symptoms are less pronounced and the eye and genito-urinary symptoms more so. Characteristic sensations are: As if hot water were poured over him, over heart. As if drops of cold water were falling, on head, from anus, from heart. As if pinched with pincers in back. Pressure as with a sharp point in coccyx. *(JHC.)*

This agent is quite similar to the Cannabis Indica in many particulars. It contains a greater amount of potassium nitrite than the latter and this has a more positive action upon the urinary organs. The Cannabis indica contains a greater amount of the Hashish which produces greater mental disturbance. It produces more smarting and burning in the urethra than does Cantharis but less tenesmus. It has been employed to remove corneal opacities following ophthalmia in scrofulous subjects. *(Blackwood)*

154. *Cantharis*

(Spanish fly)

This powerful drug produces a furious disturbance in the animal economy attacking the urinary and sexual organs especially perverting their function and setting up violent inflammations and causing a frenzied delirium stimulating hydrophobia symptoms (Anagallis). Puerperal convulsions. Produces most violent inflammation of the whole gastro-intestinal canal, especially lower bowel. Over-sensitiveness of all parts. Irritation. Raw burning pains. Haemorrhages. Intolerable constant urging to urinate is most characteristic. Gastric Hepatic and abdominal complaints, that are aggravated by drinking coffee. Gastric derangements of pregnancy. Dysuria, with other complaints. Increases secretion of mucous membranes, tenacious mucus. The inflammation Cantharis produces (Bladder, Kidney, ovaries, meninges, pleuritic and pericardial membranes) are usually associated with bladder irritation.

Mind: Acute mania, generally or sexual type.

Eyes: Fiery, sparking, staring look.

Throat: Burning in mouth, pharynx and throat. Great difficulty in swallowing liquids, very tenacious mucus.

Chest: Tendency to syncope, tenacious mucus.

Stomach: Burning sensation of oesophagus and stomach, aggravation from drinking coffee.

Stool: Shivering with burning. Mucous stool like scrapings of intestines, burning and tenesmus and shuddering after stool.

Urine: Intolerable urging and tenesmus, urine scalds and is passed drop by drop, constant desire to urinate.

Male: Strong desire.

Female: Nymphomania.

Heart: Pericarditis with effusion.

Skin: Vesicular eruptions, Burns, scalds, erysipelas.

Modalities: Worse from touch or approach, urinating, drinking water or Coffee.

Better: Rubbing.

Antidotes: Acon., Camph., Puls.

Compare: Cantharidin, Vesicaria, Fuschina, Androsace lactea, Apis, Ars., Merc. cor.

Complementary: Camph.

Dose: 6-30 c.

Bears repeated doses well. Locally in burns and eczema 1x and 2x in water or in a cerate.

Burns: Before blisters form and when they have formed. If the skin be unbroken apply an alcoholic solution of any potency and cover with cotton. This will promptly relieve pain and often prevent vesication. If the skin be broken use in boiled or distilled water and in each case give potency internally. *(Boericke)*

Cantharis belongs to the animal kingdom and finds its most prominent sphere of action in exciting the animal passions. The word irritation best expresses the totality of the Cantharis effects. There is also agg: from dazzling objects and by water - completing the hydrophobia picture. It may be well to remember in this connection the violent erotic action of Canth, for many have maintained that rabies only arises among domesticated animals where sexual functions are under more or less abnormal conditions. Guernsey gives it for the special indications in hydrophobia. Produces amorous frenzy unbounded sexual desire. Thirst with aversion to drinking. Dysenteric stools with tenesmus, urine can pass only a few drops, like molten lead. The sexual appetite is aroused to the point of mania. Coitus does not always reduce it. Vesication is the note of its effects on the skin and indicates its use in burns of the first degree, erysipelas, blisters. An ointment made with the 3x is a good application for herpes zoster. H.N. Guernsey observed that Canth. is almost always the remedy for whatever other sufferings there may be when there is as well frequent micturition with burning cutting pain, or if cutting burning pain attends the flow, even when micturition is not very frequent. Canth. expels moles, dead fetus, placentae, promotes fecundity. Agg. from coffee. *(JHC)*

It has been employed in eczema, elephantiasis and pemphigus when the surface is sore and burning and there is vesication. *(Blackwood)*

Haemorrhages from nose, mouth, intestines, genital and urinary organs. *(HCA)*

155. *Capsicum*

(Cayenne pepper)

Seems to suit especially persons of lax fibre, weak, diminished vital heat. A relaxed plethoric sluggish cold remedy. Not much reactive force. Such persons are not fat, indolent, opposed to physical exertion, averse to go outside of their routine, get homesick easily. General uncleanliness of body. Abstainers from accustomed alcoholics. It affects the mucous membranes, producing a sensation of constriction. Inflammation of petrous bone. Burning pain and general chilliness. Older people who have exhausted their vitality especially by mental work and poor living, bleary-eyed appearance, who do not react. Fear of slightest draught. Marked tendency to suppuration in every inflammatory process. Prostration and feeble digestion of alcoholics. Myalgia, aching and jerking of muscles.

Mind: Homesickness, delirium tremens.

Ears: Swelling and pain behind ears. Inflammation of mastoid, tenderness over the petrous bone.

Throat: Hot feeling in fauces, pain and dryness in throat, sore throat of smokers and drinkers.

Mouth: Herpes labialis, (Apply one drop of mother tincture) Stomatitis, disagreeable smell from mouth, fetid odour from mouth.

Stomach: Much thirst, but drinking causes shuddering.

Stool: Bloody mucus with burning and tenesmus. Thirst after stool, with shivering, bleeding piles.

Urine: Burning in orifice.

Male: Coldness of scrotum.

Respiratory: Constriction of the chest. Pain in distant parts on coughing.

Extremities: Sciatica, worse bending backward, *Worse* coughing.

Fever: Shivering after drinking.

Modalities: Better-while eating, from heat. *Worse* - open air, uncovering, draughts.

Relation: *Antidote - Cina, Caladium.*

Compare: *Puls., Lycop., Bell., Centaurea* (Surging of blood, home sickness, intermittent fever).

Dose: 3-6 c. In delirium tremens, dram doses of tincture in milk or tincture of Orange peel, equal parts of tincture of Capsicum and glycerine make an excellent liniment for external use in many cases of chronic rheumatism and neuralgia.

Natrum mur-is the chronic of Capsicum. *(Boericke)*

Capsicum corresponds especially to persons of light hair and blue eyes also to persons of lax fibre and muscles, obese, lazy, fat, unclean persons who dread the open air, clumsy children, awkward persons, haemorrhoidal troubles. The well known burning effect of red pepper is a leading indication for its use. The burning of Caps is agg: from cold water. Capsicum is among the remedies of the front rank in stomatitis, in inflammation of the middle ear, with involvement of mastoid cells. Amel: from heat is the most important modality. Patients who cannot get to sleep without a hot bottle at their back. *(JHC)*

The mother tincture is prepared of the ripe dried fruit and dilutions. Useful to those who are attempting to abstain from stimulants, when the digestive powers are weak and the absorption of food or medicine is practically stopped. In these cases 10 to 15 drops of the tincture in a cup of hot tea or other hot liquid food is of the greatest service.

If this is persisted in, it will help greatly in overcoming the desire for alcoholic stimulants.

It may be of use in suppuration of the middle ear with perforation of the ear drum, a thick yellow discharge of pus, with bursting headache and chilliness. It is also of service when an abscess of the mastoid is threatened. There is great tenderness and redness of the mastoid. *(Blackwood)*

The Capsicum mind is almost overwhelmed by persistent thoughts of suicide. He does not want to kill himself, he resists the thoughts and yet they persist, and he is tormented by these thoughts. There are persistent thoughts in many remedies, and it is necessary to distinguish between impulses and desires. *(Kent)*

156. *Carbo Animalis*

(Animal Charcoal)

Seems to be especially adapted to scrofulous and venous constitutions, old people and after debilitating diseases with feeble circulation and lowered vitality. Glands are indurated, veins distended, skin blue. Stitch remaining after pleurisy. easily strained from lifting. Weakness of nursing women. Ulceration and decomposition. All its secretions are offensive, cause local congestion without heat.

Mind: Avoids conversation.

Head: Cannot tell direction of sound.

Stomach: Weak digestion, Flatulence.

Female: Menses too early, frequent, followed by great exhaustion. Painful induration in breast.

Skin: Glands indurated.

Extremities: Night sweat, fetid and profuse.

Modalities: *Worse* after shaving, loss of animal fluids.

Relationship: *Carbon Tetrachloride* - is said to cause fatty liver. *(Phos, Ars, Chlorof.)* Paralysis of interosseus muscles of feet and hands. Wonderful clinical results in the treatment of Hookworm disease - See Thymol.

Complementary: Calc. phos.

Antidotes: Ars., Nux.

Compare: Badiaga, Sepia, Sulph., Plb-iod.

Dose: 3-30c. The third trituration for insufflation in Aural Polypi. *(Boericke)*

Copper coloured eruptions show the appropriateness of the drug to many cases of constitutional syphilis. Glands of stony hardness. Cancer of breast with burning, drawing pains through breast. Cancer of uterus, burning pains down thigh. Weeps when she eats. A feeling of looseness of eyes in sockets. Far-sighted (carb-v. is near-sighted). Aversion to cold (Carb-v. to heat). Carb. an. 3x trit has been used for insufflation in aural polypi. The leucorrhoea stains linen yellow. Sweat stains yellow. The pains in the coccyx are peculiar. It has cured many cases of injured coccyx and of neuralgia of the bone. There is an ichorous otorrhoea and swelling of the periosteum over the mastoid bone is very characteristic. *(JHC)*

It has been of service in induration of the uterus and right ovary especially. There is usually an offensive discharge from the vagina. The patient complains of a sensation of burning, tearing, heaviness and pressing downward. *(Blackwood)*

157. *Carbo vegetabilis*

(Vegetable Charcoal)

Disintegration and imperfect oxidation is the keynote of this remedy. The typical Carbo patient is sluggish, fat and lazy and has a tendency to chronicity in his complaints. Blood seems to stagnate in the capillaries causing blueness, coldness and Ecchymosis. Body becomes blue, icy cold. Bacteria find a rich soil in the nearly lifeless blood stream and sepsis and typhoidal state ensues.

A lowered vital power from loss of fluids after drugging, after other diseases, in old people, with venous congestions, states of collapse in cholera, typhoid, these are some of the conditions offering special inducements to the action of Carbo veg. The patient may be almost lifeless but the head is hot. Coldness, breath cool, pulse imperceptible, oppressed and quickened respiration, and must have air, must be fanned hard, must have all the windows open. This is a typical state for Carbo veg. The patient faints easily, is worn out and must have fresh air, Haemorrhage from any mucous surface. Very debilitated patient, seems to be too weak to hold out. Persons who have never fully recovered from the effects of some previous illness. Sense of weight, as in the head (occiput), eyes and eyelids, before the ears, in the stomach and elsewhere in the body, putrid (septic) condition of all its affections, coupled with a burning sensation. General venous stasis, bluish skin, limbs cold.

Head: Aches from any over-indulgence. Hair feels sore, falls of easily.

Nose: Epistaxis in daily attacks with pale face.

Mouth: Covered with aphthae.

Stomach: Eructations, heaviness, fullness and sleepiness. Contractive pain extending to chest, with distention of abdomen. Digestion slow, food putrifies. The simplest food distresses.

Abdomen: Abdomen greatly distended. Rectum and stool - acrid, corrosive moisture from rectum.

Male: Discharge of prostatic fluid at stool, itching and moisture at thigh near scrotum.

Respiratory: Hoarseness, worse evening, cough with burning in chest, must be fanned. Asthma in aged with blue skin.

Extremities: Limbs go to sleep, cold from knees down.

Skin: Blue, cold, echymosed, Itching worse on evening, when warm in bed, varicose ulcers.

Modalities: *Worse* evening, night and open air, cold, from fat food, butter, coffee, milk, warm damp weather, wine.

Better: from eructation, from fanning, cold.

Relation: Antidotes: Spirits nitre, Camph., Ambra., Arsenic.

Complementary: Kali carb., Dros.

Dose: First to third Trituration in stomach disorders. Thirtieth potency and high in chronic conditions and in collapse.

A Carbon ointment, made by carbonising a cork by plunging it into a clear fire and then, in its still glowing state into vaseline and mixing thoroughly is regarded as a sovereign remedy in anal irritation and haemorrhoidal troubles.

Carbo veg. is near sighted and Carbo an. is far sighted.

Carbo veg assists the action of Lycopodium.

Compare: Raphanus in flatulence.

Carbo. veg is sluggish. stout and lazy where as Nux is thin, spare, yellow, wiry. Carbo veg has aversion to milk - Lachesis craves milk. *(Boericke)*

Aversion to darkness. Fear of ghosts. Gas in stomach and intestines. Great desire for air, must be fanned. Varicose veins of arms, legs, vulva. Cold breath, collapse. Whooping cough with pain at base of brain. Desire for salt food sweetened with sugar. *(JHC)*

This agent has the property of absorbing gases which it does to an extent varying with the grade of charcoal and the gas absorbed - Generally speaking 1 volume of charcoal will absorb 10 volumes of oxygen, 35 volumes of carbonic acid gas, 55 volumes of hydrogen sulphide and 100 volumes of ammonia.

It is to be thought of in fermentative dyspepsia. There is an atonic condition, the slightest food disagrees and causes the stomach to become distended with gas to such an extent that it is distressing. The stomach refuses to digest the simplest articles of diet. This condition is often accompanied by diarrhoea rather than by constipation. It has been of service in relieving the symptoms attending dilation of the colon and Bulimia (Insatiable hunger). It has been found of service in respiratory diseases. The bronchitis of the aged when the expectoration is profuse yellow, foetid and yet difficult to raise, there is dyspnoea, rattling and a sensation of burning in the chest and indications of an impaired *circulation, and digestive disturbance,* also chronic aphonia, with a sensation of great roughness of the larynx with a deep rough voice which fails on the slightest exertion. *(Blackwood)*

Antipsoric - diseases come slow and insidiously - affects the heart, and the whole venous system - Veins are lazy, relaxed and paralysed - slow mind - Skin is lazy, itching and burning of skin-coldness and feeble circulation oozing of blood from the lungs, uterus, bladder, active gushing flow - blood vessel relaxed - feeble heart - The blood stagnates in the capillaries - gangrene, septic conditions - Dreams horrible visions, wakens in anxiety and covered with cold sweat - difficult to arouse - Headache occipital - like pounding with hammers - slow to learn and suffers from night terrors - will not sleep alone or go into a room without someone with them - Burning pain in the eyes - offensive discharge from ears, especially those dating back to malaria, measles or scarlet fever - Metastasis of mumps - will sneeze day and night - bleeding from the nose - rawness in the larynx, cough - The woman feels best when she has leucorrhoea - lips blue - cough, dyspnoea, copious expectoration, must be fanned - face flushes after a little wine - scorbutic and bleeding - gums - pain in the teeth from hot, cold or salt food - blood poisoning - Mouth aphthous - patches bleed easily, burn and sting. Blisters form. Smarting, dryness of the mouth with bleeding aphthous ulcers - Longing for coffee, acids, sweet, salty things, milk and meat causes flatulence - Burning in the stomach, eructation, flatulence - The pulse intermittent and thready - always belching, cramps in the bowels and stomach, burning pain, anxiety, distension - amel: belching or passing flatus - (China, agg: by belching) (Note: Lyco and China no relief from eructation). Ulceration of the stomach - Liver torpid and sluggish portal system engorged - putrid flatus - stool mixed with mucus - Excoriation about the anus, itching - relaxation and sweating of genitalia, dragging down of the uterus - haemorrhage from uterus-blood putrid black with small clots- metrorrhagia - (Nowadays we hear so much about this meddlesome mid-wifery, this curetting, and doing this, that and the other thing, that it makes a homoeopathic physician disgusted. Just as if those parts were not made by nature, and could not take care of themselves, as if they must be swabbed out and syringed out. Those injections and bichlorides, etc. to keep the germs out of a woman are all nonsense. A Homoeopathic physician can manage hundreds of these cases, and have no trouble.)

Carbo veg. is one of the greatest medicines we have in the beginning of whooping cough. Its cough has all the gagging, vomiting and redness of the face found in whooping cough. The carbo veg. patient suffers very much from difficulties of breathing. Sometimes it is due to cardiac weakness, and sometimes due to stuffing up of the chest. The latter is most common. Sometimes the difficulty is asthmatic. The remedy cures asthma. There has been hepatization in the lungs. There are bad places in the lungs and bronchial tubes, with weakness of the chest. Pulse irregular, intermittent, frequent. Blood stagnates in the capillaries. Indolent varicose ulcers upon the lower limbs - the legs above the ankles. There is no activity in these ulcers, there is watery discharge or it is thick, bloody and ichorous. Wants cold water during chill. *(Kent)*

158.Carbolicum Acidum

(Phenol - Carbolic acid)

Carbolic acid is a powerful irritant and anaesthetic. A languid, foul, painless, destructive remedy. Stupor, paralysis of sensation and motion, feeble pulse and depressed breathing, death due to paralysis of respiratory centers. Acts primarily on the central nervous system. Increased olfactory sensibility.

Produces mental and bodily languor, disinclination to study with headache like a band, very marked acuteness of smell is a strong guiding symptom. Stomach symptoms are also important. Pains are terrible, come and go suddenly physical exertion brings on abscess somewhere. Putrid discharges. Scarlet fever with marked tendency to destruction of tissue internally and fetid odour, spasmodic coughs, arthritis (See dose).

Headache: Better by green tea and smoking.

Nose: Smell very acute.

Throat: Burning in mouth, putrid discharge, diphtheria, fetid breath, regurgitation.

Stomach: Desire for stimulants and tobacco, vomiting, fermentative dyspepsia.

Stool: Constipation, with very offensive breath.

Extremities: Cramp, during walking.

Relation: Chrysorobin. (locally in ring worm of the scalp 5-10% in glycerine and alcohol-equal parts)

Antidote: Alcohol, vinegar, chalk, iod, glaubers salt in watery solution.

Incompatible: Glycerine and vegetable oils.

Dose: 3-30c. Phenol in Arthritis according to Goodno, must be absolutely pure-crystal solution (25%) in equal parts of water and glycerine - 20 minims well diluted 3 times daily. (Bartlett)

(Boericke)

159. Carboneum Hydrogenisatum

(Carburetted Hydrogen)

Synopsis: Apoplexy, Tetanus, Whooping cough.

Symptoms resemble an apoplectic attack, spasm as in lock jaw. Trismus, involuntary stool and urine. *(Boericke)*

160. Carboneum Oxygenisatum

(Carbon monoxide)

Synopsis: Herpes, pemphigus and trismus, cramps.

Herpes zoster, pemphigus and trismus are produced by this drug. Cramps.

Coldness, sleepiness loss of consciousness are marked. Vertigo.

Dose: 1st Attenuation. *(Boericke)*

The effects of Carb. ox. have been noted in persons poisoned by the gas. There is loss of consciousness, anaesthesia, cramps, sleepiness lasting for several days. On anaesthesia, the slightest touch with a hot iron recalls sensibility. *(JHC)*

161. Carboneum Sulph

(Alcohol Sulphuris - Bisulphide of carbon)

This drug has a deep and disorganizing action and an immense range of action judging from the symptomatology. Very useful in patients broken down by abuse of alcohol. Sensitive patients, worse cold, wasted muscles and skin and lack of vital heat, diarrhoea every four to six weeks, paralysis with intense congestion of nerve centers. Tabes, sensory difficulties in limbs, impotence, sciatica come within the therapeutic sphere of this remedy. Chronic plumbism, diminished sensibility of arms, hands and feet. Peripheral neuritis.

Head: Noises in head.

Ears: Tinnitus aurium, Menier's disease.

Abdomen: Wandering swellings as from flatus.

Extremities: Sciatica, flying pains, returning regularly, neuritis.

Dose: First attenuation locally in facial neuralgia and sciatica *(Boericke)*

Carbon. sulph., combines many characters of its two elements. It was first brought into notice by its effects on workers in rubber works. Persons employed in vulcanising works, exposed to the fumes. Carb. sul. has the flatulence of Carbo veg.

and the abdominal soreness of Sulphur. It produces eruptions of herpes and impetigo, discharges excoriating and producing violent itching. It corresponds to the herpetic diathesis. Agg: from warmth as in Carb. v. and Sulph. *(JHC)*

It is a remedy of great depth of action, frequently indicated and long neglected. Strong desire for open air and the open window - Better in the open air - Sensitive to warm damp weather - epileptic spasms - oedema of extremities - shrinking of all the muscles - Lymphatic glands are enlarged - Lassitude - worse during menses - pulse spasmodic and rapid, pulse slow 52/ min - Forgets things - Hysterical conduct - Imbecility and insanity - Weeping much - emptiness in the head - Eruptions, crusts, eczema, itching head - Discharge from ears - Coryza - sneezing - Acne rosacea on face - Comedones - Constant desire to hawk - Burning and spasms of the oesophagus - Enlarged thyroid gland - desire for cold drinks - empty eructations - flatulence - constipation and diarrhoea - bloody - intestinal parasites - stool like sheep dung - perspiration and itching of the genitals, scrotum - Leucorrhoea - Asthma - Bronchorrhoea - Constriction chest - aching in back in lumbar region, pain coccyx- between scapulae - Anaesthesia of arms and hands - coldness of limbs - Rheumatic shoulder, in elbow on motion, rheumatism in elbow, in hand-gout in hand. Pain in lower limbs, rheumatic, worse on motion, sciatica from taking cold - Pain in leg, rheumatic, in ankles in morning, in os - calcis on ascending steps - Profuse sweat during the night. Skin eruptions, herpetic, eczema, scaly, dry, oozing, chapping and cracks in winter - Itching at night, in a warm bed - Unhealthy skin, small wounds fester. *(Kent)*

162. Carcinosin

(A nosode from carcinoma)

It is claimed that carcinosin acts favourably and modifies all cases in which either a history of carcinoma can be elicited or symptoms of the disease itself exist.

Carcinoma of the mammary glands with great pain and induration of glands, of uterus. The offensive discharge, haemorrhage and pain are greatly relieved.

Indigestion, accumulation of gas in stomach and bowels, rheumatism, Cancerous cachexia.

Relation: Bufo, Conium, Phytolacca, Asterias.

Dose: 30 to 200, A dose every night or less frequently. *(Boericke)*

This is one of the principal nosodes of cancer and is one of Dr. Burnett's preparations. I use it more frequently than any other as a diathesic remedy. Burnett had a number of different cancer preparations and followed his instinct largely in their use and selection. In addition to Scirrhinum of which I have given an account in the dictionary, he had a preparation which he named Durum (Latinised form of Scirrhinum as I take it). This he used in treating deprived inherited conditions in children such as infantile self abuse, with good effects, which I have confirmed. I have met with a suicidal tendency in several cancer patients, so that the cancer nosodes may be appropriate in many mental cases, especially where the heredity points towards that.

Relation: Scirrhinum.

Compare: Scirrhinum. *(JHC)*

163. Carduus Marianus

(St. Marys Thistle)

The action of this drug is centered in the liver and portal system, causing soreness, pain, jaundice. Has specific relation to the vascular system. Abuse of alcoholic beverages, especially beer, varicose veins and ulcers. Diseases of miners associated with asthma. Dropsical conditions, depending on liver disease and due to pelvic congestion. Disturbs sugar metabolism. Influenza when liver is affected. Debility. Haemorrhages especially connected with hepatic disease.

Stomach: Taste bitter, aversion to salt meat. Nausea, retching, vomiting of green acid fluid, gall stone disease of enlarged liver.

Abdomen: Stools hard and knotty alternate with diarrhoea.

Chest: Asthmatic respiration.

Extremities: Pain worse from stooping.

Relation: Card - Benedictus, Chelidon, Chionanthus, Merc., Podo., Bry., Aloe.

Dose: Tincture and lower potencies. Give Carduus ϕ-5 drops thrice daily. In emergency case give every hour and often. *(Boericke)*

To Rademacher we are principally indebted for this remedy. It acts primarily on hepatic region - All its manifestations originating in some disorder of the liver. According to Burnett the greatest effect of Card. m. is felt on the spleen and liver, especially the splenic end of the liver. In the treatment of haematemesis, he says it is best to use a remedy that acts on the epigastric region without irritating the stomach and interfering with the healing of the lesion. Such a remedy he found in a decoction of the seeds of Card. mar. - An examination showed liver and spleen both very much enlarged so that they seem to fill the abdomen. Card. m. ϕ. Gtt. v. night and morning soon cured the patient. Card. m. incidentally cured at the same time some colossal varicose ulcers. *(JHC)*

The enlargement of the liver is more in the transverse than in the vertical diameter. It acts as a laxative producing catarrhal discharges from the bowels. The spleen is enlarged and sensitive and there is haematemesis and diuresis. The respirations are asthmatic. There is a severe cough so that the patient is obliged to sit up in bed. The expectoration is thick and tough and may consist of pure blood. *(Blackwood)*

164. Carlsbad

(The waters of the Sprudel springs)

Synopsis: Chief action is on the liver, Diabetes, obesity, itching, sweat on genitals.

Famous for its action on the liver and the treatment of obesity, diabetes and gout. In homoeopathic potencies useful in weakness of all organs, constipation, great liability to take cold. Periodicity, effects repeated after two to four weeks, Flushes of heat all over. Itching on various parts - urine passed only by pressing abdominal muscles.

Rectum: Faeces held back.

Relation: nat. sulph., Nux.

Dose: Lower potencies. *(Boericke)*

Carlsbad water is a very complicated solution containing the sulphite, bicarbonate and chloride of sodium in preponderating quantity, with carbonates, sulphates, phosphates, fluoride and oxides of calcium, magnesium, strontium, Ferrum, Manganum, Potassium, Aluminium, Silicon. and Carbon, with traces of iodide and Bromide of sodium, of Caesium, Rubidium, Lithium, and Boracic oxide. Its chief fame has been gained by its action on the liver, and in the treatment of obesity and diabetes. Crawling and prickling on various parts, with breaking out of sweat. Itching on various parts. Much itching and increased sweat of genitals.

(JHC)

165. Cascara Sagrada - Rhamnus Purchiana

(Sacred Bark)

Palliative for constipation, chronic indigestion with rheumatism of muscles and joints.

Introduced as a palliative for constipation (Non-homoeopathic), fifteen drops of fluid extract. Here it restores normal function by its tonic effects, but it has a wider sphere of action, as careful provings will show. Chronic indigestion, cirrhosis and jaundice. Haemorrhoids and constipation. Gastric headache, broad flabby tongue, foul breath.

Extremities: Rheumatism of muscles and joints with obstinate constipation.

Relation: Hyd., Nux-v. (rhamnus Californica. Tr. for constipation Lymphangitis and appendicitis and especially rheumatism)

Dose: Tr. to 6th potency.

(Boericke)

This agent stimulates the secretions of the intestinal tract, increases peristaltic action and relieves constipation by restoring the tonicity of the bowels. *(Blackwood)*

166. Cascarilla

(Sweet bark)

Constipation, stool covered with mucus, aversion to smell of tobacco, nausea and vomiting.

Acts on the digestive tract, constipation. Aversion to smell of tobacco. Inclination to vomit very marked.

Stomach: Nausea and vomiting.

Rectum: Constipation, stool hard, covered with mucus (Graph). Bright blood with stools, diarrhoea alternating with gripping. Grinding pain high up in the rectum.

Dose: 1-3c *(Boericke)*

167. Castanea Vesca

(Chest nut leaves)

A useful remedy in whooping cough especially in early stage, with dry ringing, violent spasmodic cough. Desire for warm drinks, very thirsty. Loss of appetite, diarrhoea, thick urine.

Lumbago, weak back, and can hardly straighten up.

Relation: Petrussin, Dros., Mephitis, Napthal, Ammon. brom.

Dose: Tincture *(Boericke)*

168. Castor Equi

(Rudimentary thumb nail of gorse)

Synopsis: Cracked and ulcerated nipple, wart on breast, coccygodynia, Epilepsy, nail affections.

General action on thickening of the skin and epithelium. Psoriasis linguae. The clinical experience of Herring and his fellow provers has shown this to be a highly useful remedy in cracked and ulcerated nipples. Affects principally female organs. Action on nails and bones, pain in right tibia and coccyx. Warts on forehead. Warts on breast. Chapped hands. Violent itching of breast.

Relation: Graphites, Hippomanes, Calc-oxal.

Dose: 6-12 c. *(Boericke)*

This is a blackish excrescence, found on the inner side of the fore and hind legs of the horse, above the knee and below the hock joints. *(Blackwood)*

This is a very ancient remedy, and was proved and introduced into homoeopathy by Herring. It especially acts on the nipples, the nails, and bones, especially causing pains in right tibia and coccyx. Burnett has cured with it a case of wart on forehead.

Back: Weak spine, pain in coccyx, Agg: every evening while sitting.

Skin: Warts, nails drop off, Brittle nails. *(JHC)*

169. *Castoreum*

(The Beaver)

Synopsis: Nervous women. Hysteria with painful cramps.

A great remedy for hysteria. Prostration marked. Hysterical symptoms. Day blindness, cannot endure the light. Nervous women who do not recover fully, but are continually irritable and suffer debilitating sweats. Spasmodic affections after debilitating diseases. Constant yawning. Restless sleep with frightful dreams and starts.

Relation: Ambra, Moschus, Mur. acid, Valeriana.

Antidote: Colch.

Dose: Tincture and lower potencies. *(Boericke)*

Castor, Beaver. The follicles connected with the external genital organs of the beaver, which contain a thick fluid secretion, are used. *(Blackwood)*

Castoreum when fresh is yellow and of the consistence of syrup, when dry it is dark red or brown and of the consistence of hard wax. Teste remarks that it has been regarded as a resinous substance, and he observes, moreover, that the beaver feeds almost entirely on the resinous bark of pine trees. In siberia beavers feed on the bark of the birch, which may make a difference on the effects of Castoreum from different countries. "Caspare" proved Russian Castor, Nenning that of southern Europe. Teste concluded from analogy that Castor would be an antisycotic, and he proved his point by initiating with it the cure of a case of pedunculated vegetations around the anus in a hysterical young woman. Thuja completed the cure. *(JHC)*

170. *Catarea Nepeta*

(Cat nip)

Children remedy for colic also for the nervous headache and hysteria, abdominal complaints, pain, flexing of thighs, twisting of body, crying similar to Chamomilla and Mag. phos.

Dose: 5 to 10 drops of Tr. *(Boericke)*

171. *Caulophyllum*

(Blue cohosh)

This is a women's remedy, want of tonicity of womb, during labour, when the pains are deficient and the patient is exhausted and fretful.

Besides it has special affinity for the smaller joints. Thrush, locally and internally.

Stomach: Cardialgia, spasms of stomach.

Female: Extraordinary rigidity of Os. Spasmodic and severe pains which fly in all directions, shivering without progress, false pains, revives labour pains and further progress of labour, after pains, leucorrhoea, with moth spots on forehead, Habitual abortion from uterine debility. Needle like pain in cervix. Dysmenorrhoea, with pains flying to other parts of body, Lochia protracted, great atony, menses and leucorrhoea profuse.

Skin: Discoloration of skin in women with menstrual and uterine disorder.

Extremities: Severe drawing erratic pain and stiffness in small joints, fingers toes, ankles, etc. Aching in wrists, cutting pains on closing hands. Erratic pains, changing place every few minutes.

Incompatible: Coffea.

Compare: Viola odorata (Rheumatic, carpal and metacarpal joints) - *Cimic., Sep., Puls., Gels.*

Dose: Tr. to 3rd attenuation.

(Boericke)

Caulophyllum the "Blue Cohosh" is closely related to Actea Racem. It acts most markedly on the female generative organs and on rheumatic states. The majority of the indications having been derived from tradition and clinical experience. It has been given with success for chloasma or pityriasis versicolor, curing incidentally dysmenorrhoea at the same time. Reflex symptoms having a uterine origin, headache, vomiting, hoarseness, rheumatism, cramps and spasms. No other drug produces uterine spasms so markedly except Secale. Bearing down pains. Paraplegia from disorders of the uterus. Left ovarian and left inflammatory pains. Leucorrhoea in little girls. The pains are intermittent and paroxysmal, and fly about from place to place, generally agg: at night. In rheumatic affections the special sphere of Caulo. is the small joints and muscles. Its special sphere in labour is: (1) when pains do not come regularly, (2) when they disappear from exhaustion, and (3) when they are too painful, Nash prescribed Caul. 3 for a lady of forty, seven months pregnant, who was attacked with severe pain and swelling of all the finger joints. *(JHC)*

There is great weakness in the upper eyelids, which are heavy and droop so that they must be raised with the finger. There are moth patches on the face. It is useful in acute and subacute rheumatism of the smaller joins, especially the hand.

(Blackwood)

Weakness in the reproductive system of the woman. From weakness she is sterile, or she aborts in the early months of gestation. During parturition the contractions of the uterus are too feeble to expel the contents, and they are only tormenting. Uterine haemorrhage from inertia of the uterus. She is hysterical, like Ignatia. She is fretful and apprehensive. She is rheumatic, like Cimicifuga, only the small joints are likely to be affected. She is sleepless, restless, and very excitable. This remedy has cured chorea at puberty when menstruation was late. *(Kent)*

172. *Causticum*

(Hahnemann's Tinctura
Acris Sine Kali)

Manifests its action mainly in chronic, rheumatic, arthritic and paralytic affections, indicated by the tearing, drawing pains in the muscular and fibrous tissues, with deformities about the joints. Progressive loss of muscular strength, tendinous contractors. Broken down seniles. In catarrhal affections of the air passages, and seems to choose preferably dark complexioned and rigid fibred persons. Restlessness at night with tearing pains in limbs and bones, and faint-like sinking of strength. This weakness progresses until we have gradually appearing paralysis. Local paralysis, vocal cords, muscles of deglutition, of tongue, eyelids, face, bladder and extremities. Children are slow to walk. The skin of causticum person is dirty, white, sallow with warts especially on the face. Emaciation due to disease, worry, etc., and long standing. Burning rawness and soreness are characteristics.

Mind: Intensely sympathetic.

Face: Warts.

Eyes: Cataract, ptosis.

Nose: Coryza with hoarseness, pimples and warts.

Taste: Greasy, aversion to sweets, acid dyspepsia.

Urine: Involuntary during first sleep at night.

Female: Uterine inertia during labour.

Respiratory: Hoarseness, aphonia, cough with raw soreness of chest, better by drinking cold water.

Extremities: Unsteadiness of muscles of forearm, contracted tendons, rheumatic tearing in limbs, better by warmth, especially heat of bed, restless legs at night.

Complementary: Carb., Petr.

Compare: Rhus t., Ars., Amm-ph. (Facial paralysis)

Modalities: *Worse* dry cold winds, in clear fine weather, cold air, from motion of carriage. *Better* in damp wet weather, warmth, heat of bed.

Dose: 3rd to 30th attenuation. In chronic ailments and especially in paralysis states. Higher potencies once or twice a week. *(Boericke)*

Causticum is one of the great polychrest medicines of chronic diseases. Paralysis, showing itself both involuntary muscles, weakness from grief of long standing or from disease. Constant sensation as if lime were burning in stomach. Itching scrotum. After - effects of burns and scalds. Fear of darkness. *(JHC)*

There is a hoarseness which is worst during the morning and again in the evening. Nocturnal enuresis. *(Blackwood)*

Joints ankylosed. Deformity of the joints. Causticum has cured insanity, not acute mania with violent delirium, but mental aberration of the passive kind, where the brain has become tired. Fear of death as if something will happen. Scalp contracts and tightens up in places. Torticollis - shortening of the muscle of the neck. Foggy vision, air seems full of black insects. Fissures about the lips, wings of the nose, corners of the eyes, of the anus, in the bends of joints, bleeding and ulceration of the gums, tearing in the roots of the teeth, stammering, tongue bites while chewing, seeing food appetite vanishes, nipples sore and crack. *(Kent)*

173. *Ceanothus*

(New Jersey Tea)

Splenic remedy, left sided, acute case of malaria. Liver and spleen are at fault. Chronic bronchitis with profuse secretion. Marked blood pressure reducing powers. Active haemostatic, materially reducing the clotting of blood. Splenitis, leukemia, dyspnoea, leucorrhoea, diarrhoea. Urine contains bile and sugar. Locally used as hair tonic.

Dose: ϕ 2-5 drops. TDS., preferably in alteration with Carduus ϕ in the same way. This remedy seems to possess a specific relation to the spleen. Ague cake of malaria, left sided remedy generally, anaemic patients where liver and spleen are at fault.

Abdomen: Enlargement of spleen, splenitis, pain all up the left side, leukaemia, violent dyspnoea, menses profuse. Yellow, weakening leucorrhoea. Unable to lie on left side, pain in liver and back.

Rectum: Diarrhoea, bearing down in abdomen and rectum.

Urine: Constant urging to urinate, green frothy, contains bile, sugar.

Compare: Berberis, Myrica, Cedron, Agaricus (Spleen).

Modalities: *Worse* motion, lying on left side.

Dose: First attenuation, locally as hair tonic. *(Boericke)*

Dr. Yudhbir Sinha: In the enlargement of spleen and liver Ceanothus is specific and has gained universal reputation. The more enormously large is the spleen, the more ceanothus is beneficial. It surpasses all other remedies in acute and chronic splenitis and a deep seated pain in the left hypochondrium. Give Ceanothus ϕ, 2 to 5 drops TDS, alternate it with Carduus ϕ in the sameway. In splenitis Ceanothus 1 drop TDS. Also paint one part of ϕ with 9 parts of olive oil on the region of spleen.

Dr. R.K. Ghosh has cured with it many cases of suppression of menses and leucorrhoea in patients from malarial districts. *(JHC)*

174. *Cedron*

(Rattle Snake Bean)

Periodicity is the most marked characteristic of this drug. Is particularly useful in tropical or in damp, warm marshy counties. It has been found curative in malarial affections, especially neuralgia. Adapted to persons of voluptuous disposition, excitable nervous temperament. Has powers of antidoting snake bites and stings of insects. Tincture of pure bean scraped on wound, Mania. Rapidity of action like Bell., strong sexual excitement.

Eyes: Pain in eyeball with radiating pain around eye, supra-orbital neuralgia periodic.

Fever: Chilliness towards evening numbness of limbs.

Relation: Antidote - Lach.

Compare: Ars., China.

Dose: Tr. to 3rd attenuation. *(Boericke)*

Petroz and Teste introduced Cedr. into Homoeopathic practice, having received the seed from Panama, with an account of its powers of antidoting snake bite when chewed immediately after being bitten, and also of its traditional reputation in intermittent fevers. The great characteristic of Cedron is a clock like periodicity. *(JHC)*

175.Cenchris Contortrix

(Copper-headed snake)

Like other snake poisons, dyspnoea, restlessness, thirst for small quantity of water, likes clothes loose, sexual desire in both sexes, amaurosis, heart affections, swelling over eyes, swelling of upper lip, general swelling, cold clammy sweat, below brow (eye) like an over hanging bag of water, must lie with head drawn back. Like the other snake poisons, it affects the system profoundly. Like Arsenic, it has dyspnoea, mental and physical restlessness, thirst for small quantities of water, necessity for having clothing loose like Lachesis, marked alternation of moods, vivid dreams. Is a wonderful restorative and deep acting remedy. Increased sexual desire in both sexes. Ineffectual desire for recline. Right ovarian region painful.

Modalities: Worse pressure, lying down, afternoon and night.

Relationship-Comparison: *Ars., Lach., Clotho Arictans., Puff. Adder.*

Dose: 6th potency. *(Boericke)*

Cenchris has the main features of all the serpent poisons, coma, semi-consciousness, insensibility of cornea, swelling of upper lip, a marked alternation of moods, and dreamy absent-mindedness. The dreams of Cenchris are very vivid and horrible, cannot be shaken off during waking hours, often lascivious. Swelling above eyes, below brow, like an over-hanging bag of water. *(JHC)*

176. Cereus Bonplandi

(A variety of Cactus grandiflora)

Desire to work and do some thing useful. Pain through globe of eyes, skin eruption, loss of weight. Heart affections.

Mind: Great desire to work and to do something useful.

Head: Pain through the globe of the eyes. The principal symptom of Cer. bon. are in connection with the heart as in the case of Cactus with which it must be compared. Itching in right popliteal space lasted eight or nine years after the proving. One prover lost 7 1/2 lbs.

Dose: 3-6 attenuations. *(Boericke)*

The symptoms are *Agg:* at night. Wants to be at work, on something useful. Pains through globe of eyes and orbit. Pain through heart, in left great pectoral muscle, left side of chest *(JHC)*

177. Cerium oxalicum

(Oxalate Cerium)

Vomiting of pregnancy (morning sickness), Dysmenorrhoea in fleshy robust women.

Spasmodic reflex vomiting and spasmodic cough are with in the sphere of this remedy. Vomiting of pregnancy and of half digested food. Dysmenorrhoea in fleshy robust women. Better when flow is established.

Relation: *Compare* - Ingluvin (made from gizzard of a fowl), vomiting of pregnancy, gastric neuasthenia. Infantile vomiting and diarrhoea.

Dose: 1st Trituration - 3x Trit. Amygdal, Lactic ac., Ip. *(Boericke)*

It should be thought of as a local gastric sedative in pyrosis, acid dyspepsia and catarrhal gastritis, especially if there are nervous complications. It has been employed in spasmodic cough as whooping cough when attended with haemorrhages, nausea and vomiting. *(Blackwood)*

178. *Chamomilla*

(German Chamomile)

Sensitive, irritable, thirsty, pain unbearable, child moans, impatient, earache, one cheek red and hot, other pale and cold, toothache, worse after warm drink, taste bitter, bilious vomiting, abdomen distended, griping pain, a flatulent and hepatic colic, stools hot, green, slimy, fetid, and watery, haemorrhages from uterus of clotted dark blood, nipples inflamed, irritable dry tickling cough, rattling of mucous in children, moaning in sleep with half open eyes, teething of children.

Complementary: Belladonna (Coffee drinkers and narcotic palliative). Patient insists the doctors should cure immediately. *Bell* - Cranial nerves

Chamomilla - Nerves of abdomen.

The chief guiding symptom belong to the mental and emotion group, which leads to the remedy in many forms of disease. Especially of frequent employment in diseases of children, where peevishness, restlessness and colic give the needful indications. A disposition that is mild, calm and gentle, sluggish and constipated bowels contra-indicate Chamomilla.

Chamomilla is sensitive, irritable and thirsty, hot and numb. Oversensitiveness from abuse of coffee and narcotics. Pains unendurable, associated with numbness, night sweats.

Mind: Whining restlessness, child can only be quieted when carried about and petted constantly, impatient, snappish, complaints from anger and vexation, mental calmness contraindicates chamomilla.

Ears: Earache, swelling and heat driving patient frantic.

Face: One cheek red and hot, the other pale and cold. Toothache worse after warm drink, worse coffee, distresses of teething children.

Abdomen: Griping in region of navel and pain in small of back.

Stool: Green, slimy, chopped white and yellow mucus, like chopped eggs and spinach.

Female: Dark blood with labor like pains.

Respiratory: Rawness of larynx, irritable, dry, tickling cough.

Back: Lumbago.

Extremities: Ankles give away in the afternoon.

Modalities: *Worse* by heat, anger, open air, wind, night.

Better: from being carried, warm wet weather.

Relation: Cypriped, Anthemis, Aconite, Puls., Coff., Bell., Staph., Ign.

Follows: Belladonna in diseases of children and abuse of opium.

Antidotes: Camph., Nux-v., Puls.

Complementary: Bell., Mag-c.

Dose: 3rd to 30. *(Boericke)*

There is a spiteful, sudden, or uncivil irritability. For coffee drinkers, and persons who have been treated with narcotic palliatives. The pains are unbearable and drive to despair. The patient insists that the doctor shall cure them at once. The toothache of Cham. comes on when entering a warm room or from drinking anything warm. Muscles of face and hands twitch. Twitching of hands and face. The Cham.

patient would rather die than suffer so. Arthritic diathesis. Useful in nerve storm when morphia is discontinued. Bell. in diseases of children (Cham. acts more on nerves of abdomen. Bell. more on cranial nerves). Ver. has maddening pains compelling to walk about, but there is none of the feverishness and excitement of Cham.

(JHC)

This agent produces a hyperaesthesia in both the mental and physical sphere. It acts upon the stomach producing excessive acidity, nausea and vomiting. This acidity extends to the small intestines, producing an acid diarrhoea with excessive, green, watery stools and severe gripping pains in the umbilical region. There is congestion of the liver with stitching pains in the hepatic region and vomiting of a bitter material. When this remedy is indicated there is over sensitiveness to pain, with irritability and peevishness, this applies to adults as well as to children. It should be remembered in neuralgia, earache, toothache, and headaches when there is intolerance to pain and heat. The patient must have instant relief. This mental condition has rendered this remedy of service excessive use of green tea and coffee and also to correct the morphine and bromide habit. *(Blackwood)*

It is useful in toothache, pain in the teeth ameliorated by cold, and made worse by heat. But the earaches and pains in the extremities are made better by heat. The patient seems to be driven to frenzy by the pains, and she forgets all about her prudence and her diplomacy, loss of generosity, she has no consideration for the feelings of others. She will simply enter into a quarrel or dispute regardless of the feelings of anybody. Inability to control her temper and the temper is aroused to white heat. The chamomilla infant will often hold a glass of cold water against the gums. The little one has inflamed gums, painful gums, the coming forth of the teeth is painful, and it seems to want to prolong the cold in the mouth. The aversion to coffee is a strange thing. The Chamomilla patient has violent retching. The child doubles up, and screams, and kicks, wants to be carried, is extremely irritable. Attack comes on in the evening. In adults, who have felt these symptoms, they are said to be cutting, burning, griping pains. Of course, such are the pains that are called colicky. Cramps in the bowels. Griping pains. Sometimes gripping as if must go to stool. The stool felt hot while it passed. It smells like sulphuretted hydrogen. Copious stool, scanty stool, with dysenteric straining. Watery diarrhoea, six or eight passages daily. Mucous diarrhoea. Green watery stool, faeces and mucus. Yellowish brown stool. Also constipation, with no ability to strain. A paralytic weakness of the rectum, inactivity of the rectum. She scolds everybody, drives the doctor out of the room, drives the nurse off, and then calls for her again. Most of the complaints oı Chamomilla are better after midnight. Burning of the soles at night, puts the feet out of bed. All the routine prescribers whenever the patient is known to put the feet out of bed give sulphur, yet there is a large list of remedies with hot feet, burning soles, and all of them will put the feet out of bed, of course, to cool them off. There is no reason why they should all get sulphur. *(Kent)*

179.Chaparo Amargoso

(Goat Bush)

Diarrhoea and Dysentery

Synopsis: Chronic diarrhoea, tenderness over liver, stools with little pain, but with much mucus. Dysentery. Acts as a tonic and antiperiodic.

Compare: Kali carb., Cup. ars., Caps.

Dose: 3rd attenuation - A teaspoonful of extract (infusion) 3 times a day for diarrhoea and dysentery. *(Boericke)*

Give ϕ 2 to 4 drops 3 to 4 times a day. *(Sinha)*

180.Chelidonium Majus
(Celandine)

A prominent liver remedy covering many of the direct reflex symptoms of diseased conditions of that organ. The jaundiced skin and especially the constant pain under inferior angle of right scapula are certain indications. Paralytic drawing and lameness in single parts. The great general lethargy and indisposition to make any effort is also marked. Ailments brought on or renewed by change of weather. Serous effusions, Hydrocele, Bilious complications during gestation.

Head: Feels heavy as lead, neuralgia over right eye.

Face: Yellow.

Stomach: Prefers hot food and drink, better very hot water. Eating relieves temporarily.

Stool: Constipation, stool hard, round balls like sheep-dung, bright yellow, pasty, alternation of diarrhoea and constipation.

Respiratory: Pain in right side of chest and shoulder.

Back: Fixed pain under inner and lower angle of right scapula.

Extremities: Icy coldness of tips of fingers.

Modalities: Worse, right side, motion, touch, change of weather, very early in morning.

Better: After dinner from pressure.

Complementary: Lyc., Bry.

Antidote: Cham.

Compare: Nux-v., Sulph., Bry., Lyc., Op., Podo., Sanguin., Ars.

Dose: Tr. and lower attenuation.

(Boericke)

Chelidonium is a poppy and therefore allied to Opium and sanguinaria, analogue to Lycopodium. The juice is yellow, resembling bile, given on the broad ground of organ homoeopathy. Acts on spleen and kidneys as well as liver, suggests cancer. Aversion to cheese. Pains particularly felt in the axilla and under the shoulder blade, dry racking, fatiguing cough night and day, outer ankle and lower leg become cyanotic, swelling, complaints lessen after dinner - Lyco has sour taste, Cheli. has bitter taste, tongue coated thickly yellow, gall stones. Ars., Lyco., and Sulph. follow well. Mouth - bitter taste, and odour from mouth, better after eating, desire for milk and hot water. Pain in the stomach relieved by eating.

(JHC)

This agent produces congestion and inflammation of the liver and jaundice, as a result of its action on the liver. The digestive organs are deranged, while the kidneys show indication of degeneration. There is a catarrhal inflammation of the bronchial mucous membrane. The lungs are congested, inflamed and hepatized, especially the right. *(Blackwood)*

Principally in gastric and intestinal catarrh, act throughout the system but almost always along with it the liver is involved, and it is suitable for what the old people and the doctors called biliousness. Inability to think and meditate, slow pulse. Dull aching pains under the right scapula, has cured gall stone colic in a few minutes. Has relieved that spasm, the little duct opens up and the stone passes out through the ductus communis choledochus. Every remedy that is indicated by the symptoms will cure gall stone colic.

Craves hot milk, hot fluids, eating warm food ameliorated the liver, the chest and stomach symptoms. Bilious diarrhoea along with jaundice, clay like, pale faecal, putty like stool, bileless stool, stool too light coloured. Stool quite white in children. Diarrhoea and constipation alternate. Itching of the skin, jaundice. It has cured old putrid ulcers. *(Kent)*

181. *Chenopodium Anthelminticum*

(Jerusalem Oak-Worm seed)

Characteristic pain in scapula very marked. Symptoms of apoplexy, right hemiplegia, and aphasia, stertorous breathing (Opium), sudden vertigo. Meniers diseases, affections of auditory nerves (natrum Salycyl). Oil of chenopodium for hook worm and thread worm. Pain below the angle of right scapula, analogous to chelidonium. Hemiplegia, aphasia, stertorous breathing, vanishing sight and roaring in ears. When given as a vermifuga it frequently produces, progressive and long lasting deafness. Hearing better for high pitched than low pitched sounds.

Dose: 3c. Oil of chenopodium for hookworm, 10 minims dose every 2 hours for 3 doses. Also Carbon tetrachloride. *(Boericke)*

Chenopodium: Ears serous or bloody effusion in the labyrinth, chronic otitis media, progressive deafness of the voice but sensitive to sounds or passing vehicles and other sounds, buzzing, absent or deficient bone conduction, a consciousness of the ear, hearing better for shrill, high pitched sounds than the low ones. (Boericke said this of Viola Odorata)

It has been employed extensively as a remedy for worms, and much of our knowledge of its toxic action is from the employment of large doses for this end.

The oil of Chenopodium has been employed extensively in the orient, especially Singapore and Sumatra, against the hookworm.

In Sumatra it is extensively employed in the treatment of round worm, tapeworm and whipworm.

There are two methods followed in those Oriental countries in its administration. In one the patient is given but light diet for the evening meal and no breakfast, ten to sixteen minims of the oil are placed on sugar, and this divided into three portions, one of which is taken each hour, two hours later a large dose of castor. oil and a full dose of chloroform is taken.

In the second method ten minims of the oil is given at a single dose in a capsule for three days, when a tablespoonful of castor oil is given. If these doses are followed there wili not result the nephritis and paralysis that has resulted when people have taken an "ounce and a half" as a single dose. *(Blackwood)*

182.Chenopodi Glauci Aphis

(Plant-lice from Chenopodium)

Partakes largely of the properties of the plant upon which the insect lives. Toothache relieved by general warm sweat, pain in region of lower inner angle of left shoulder blade.

Dose: 6-30 c. *(Boericke)*

183. Chelone

(snake head)

A remedy in liver affections with pain or soreness of the left lobe of the liver and extending downwards. Dumb ague. Soreness of external parts as if skin were off, debility, malaise following intermittents. Dyspepsia with hepatic torpor, jaundice, round and thread worm. It is an enemy to every kind of worm infecting the human body.

Dose: Tincture in one to five drop doses. *(Boericke)*

Cholagogue and vermifuge-organ remedy in liver affections - Quinine cachexia. *(JHC)*

It is indicated in dumb ague when there is an ill defined chill, aching, with fever and general distress. In the form of an infusion it is employed as an enemata for the relief of pin worms. *(Blackwood)*

184.Chimaphila Umbellata

(Pipsissewa)

Acts principally on kidneys and genito-urinary tract, affects also lymphatic and mesenteric glands and female mammae. Plethoric young women with dysuria. Women with large breasts. Hepatic and renal dropsies, chronic alcoholics. Incipient and progressive cataract. One of the remedies whose symptoms point to its employment in bladder affections, notably catarrh, acute and chronic. Scanty urine and loaded with ropy, muco-purulent sediment. Prostatic enlargement.

Burning and scalding during micturition and straining afterwards. Must strain before flow comes, prostatitis, feeling of a ball in perineum, sugar in urine, urination by standing with legs wide apart and body inclined forward. Painful tumor of mammae, not ulcerated, with undue secretion of milk, women with fiery large breasts, worse in damp weather, from sitting on cold stones. Inflammation of liver with ascites, abdominal and renal dropsies.

Dose: 10 drops of ϕ 4 hourly - same locally applied. *(Boericke)*

In dwindling and enlarged breasts give Chimaphilla 1x, one drop thrice daily. Alternate it with mammary 3x. two tabs. a dose thrice daily to restore the breasts to normal size, to make it firm, round, fleshy and light. Also Calcarea fluor 3x., 5 grs., twice daily and Alfalfa ϕ, one table spoonful after meals and see the result. *(Y. Sinha)*

Is used by many North American Indians in gravel and urinary disorders. Among the eclectics it is used as an alternative in skin affections, e.g., acne, herpes, eczema, in enlarged lymphatic glands in articular rheumatism. It is said by them to act mainly as an eliminative through the bowels and kidneys. They use it in cases of chyligerous urine, cystitis, strangury, smarting, burning pains on urination, turbid urine and frequent micturition, and diabetes. Constant desire to urinate, must rise several times in the night. Rapid atrophy of breasts, or tumours. Tumour in left breast, hard, movable, sharp pains at site. For months, under Arn., Ars., Cicut., Thuj, the tumour increased, skin became contracted, nipple drawn it. In eight months in broke out into an irregular ulceration with lacerated edges, fetid discharge. Axillary glands swollen. Chim. um. ϕ 10 drops every four hours was given, and the same locally applied. The pains diminished, swelling decreased, and in six months the patient was well. *(JHC)*

185. *Chininum Arsenic*

(Arsenite of Quinine)

The symptoms of general weakness and prostration produced by the drug have been utilised in prescribing it homoeopathically as a general tonic often with very marked beneficial and prompt effect. In diphtheria with great prostration, cases that are prolonged, especially and in malarial affections, neuralgia. It has been found curative in asthmatic attacks, which recur periodically, with great prostration. Icy skin. Pressure in the solar plexus, with tender spine on the back of it.

Bitter taste, no appetite, hyperchlorhydria. Anorexia. Eggs produce diarrhoea. Heart suffocative attacks, must have open air, sleeplessness due to nervous causes (single dose of 5th to 6th potency), coldness of hands and feet, knees and limbs.

Dose: 2nd and 3rd trituration.

(Boericke)

The Arsenite of Quinine combines many of the properties of its two components, sleep after nausea and vomiting, agg: at rest, in the morning - when the stomach is empty, agg: by motion (Vertigo) and by eating (Gastralgia). It corresponds to tobacco intoxication and its effects. Causation-tobacco.

(JHC)

186. *Chininum Sulph*

(Sulphite of Quinine)

A dose of Chinin sulph in high potency sometimes arouses suppressed malaria and brings back the paroxysm. Apart from its undoubted influence over malaria, it is indicated homoeopathically, whenever there is marked periodicity and spinal sensitiveness. Acute articular rheumatism. Polyarticular gout, pruritus and congested conditions of the rectum, symptoms of chronic interstitial nephritis, retro-bulbar neuritis with sudden loss of sight. Thready vessels. Hiccough.

Rapid decrease in red blood cells and reduction in haemoglobin - Amaurosis - ringing, buzzing and roaring in ears with deafness relieved by pressure - great sensitiveness of the dorsal vertebrae - urine bloody, turbid, slimy, clay-coloured, greasy sediment, albuminuria. Skin-itching urticaria, vesication, pustules. Fever, chill daily at 3 p.m., painful swelling of various veins during a chill. Shivering even in a warm room. Anguish, subnormal temperature.

Red rash all over body, with severe stinging followed by desquamation.

Dose: 1st to 3rd triturations, also 30th potency.

(Boericke)

This agent externally and locally is an antiseptic, preventing putrefaction and fermentation by its power of destroying fungi and infusoria in solution of from 1/250 to 1/10000 dependent upon the organism. According to Binz when given in the proportion of 1 part to 20,000 of blood, the white cells in the vessels cease to migrate. Small doses 2 to 3 grains increase the phagocytic power of the blood, while larger doses, more than four grains circulating in the blood, decrease this power, medicinal doses increase the number of red blood corpuscles, while toxic doses inhibit the oxygen bearing powers of the red corpuscles. Small doses increase the force and frequency of the heart's action, while larger doses slow and weaken it, and in children often cause an intermittent pulse. Toxic doses paralyze the heart arresting it in systole, small doses elevate, while large doses depress cardiac action.

Taken internally it has a bitter taste even in a proportion of 1 to 10,000; under small doses the appetite and digestion are improved. The secretions from the salivary and gastro-intestinal glands are increased, peristalsis is stimulated and the blood supply to the stomach is increased. Large doses disturb the digestion, cause nausea with possible vomiting and diarrhoea. It is absorbed from the stomach, not from the intestines. Its presence may be detected in the urine fifteen minutes after the ingestion of a full dose, but it is many hours or even days before it is finally excreted. Fully 90 percent, can be recovered in the urine. Small doses stimulate the cerebrum, while large doses occasion cerebral congestion, a sensation of dizziness, fullness in the head and unconsciousness. Small doses slightly increase the respirations, while large doses depress the respiratory movements and death may be due to respiratory paralysis. This may be accompanied by paralysis of the heart and vagus.

It is powerful antipyretic in malarial fever, but has little influence on the temperature in health. Excessive doses and the long continued use produce a group of symptoms known as cinchonism, in which there is a sensation of fullness in the head, ringing or buzzing in the ears with a varying degree of deafness, headache, disturbance of the vision, vertigo, muscular weakness, at times delirium, enlarged spleen, a disposition to shiver, great debility, a periodicity which is well marked and frequently haematuria. While there are no indications that it is an abortifacient, it does appear to stimulate the uterine contractions after the inception of labour.

This remedy is indicated in diseases that are characterized by a periodicity that is usually dependent upon a malarial infection when there is a distinct clear cut chill, fever, sweat, and apyrexia that returns with marked regularity. The type of the fever is not so important if the various stages are regular and well defined, the sweat is debilitating and relieves all the symptoms except the headache.

The beneficial influence of this remedy is not always in proportion to the size of the dose. A large dose may abort a chill if given during its course or the course of the fever, but is liable to increase the nervous erethysm and the temperature, while small doses administered during the intermission from one to three hours preceding the attack or when the temperature is at its lowest point, will give positive results. When these patients relapse, the cause is either an improper use of the remedy or the parasite has become immune to the remedy.

In these cases another remedy must be selected. Ehrlich tells us that an injection of neosalvarsan will at once cure the patient.

In continued remittent fever and in intermittent fevers this remedy is indicated when the stages are clear cut. The remedy should be administered during the remissions. This is also true of congestive chills, of the more malignant type of malaria.

It should be thought of in Bro ague, dumb ague and neuralgia when of malarial origin. The pains return with marked regularity. The patient feels weak, nervous and exhausted and slight exercise produces palpitation of the heart. In some cases it is a spinal irritation that is complained of when there is great sensitiveness of the last cervical and dorsal vertebrae to pressure, the pain extending to the head and neck.

It should be remembered in diarrhoea and dysentery in malarial subjects when the evacuations are copious and soft with borborygmi in the abdomen and abundant emissions of wind, pop-like, the stool may be attended with cutting pain and contain much blood. High rectal injections of this agent in the strength of 1/3000 are of service in amoebic dysentery as this agent destroys the amoeba coli. As it produces haematuria it should be remembered in this condition.

It has been employed in erythema scarlatiniforme, especially when the eruption is over the head, neck and upper portion of the body. There is severe itching and pricking sensation and it is attended with marked desquamation of the skin, also in the erythema nodosum when the arthritic complications are more marked and the process is intermittent in character.

It is an important remedy in Menier's Vertigo, the patient is worse from walking or standing, deafness and buzzing in the ears and more or less loss of consciousness. It should be remembered in nervous deafness when this is attended with ringing in the ears.

It is an important remedy in suppurative nephritis when the fever is intermittent in character, ushered in by severe chills and followed by profuse sweats.

Jousset gives it an important place in the purulent diathesis, it is indicated when the regular return of chills and the difference between the morning and evening temperature give to the disease the aspect and type of an intermittent fever. In this case it should be given in the first trituration 1-grain dose, in a very short time, two hours or more, after the paroxysm. *(Blackwood)*

187. Chionanthus

(Fringe tree)

This remedy is often of service in many types of headache, neurasthenic, periodical, sick, menstrual and bilious. Taken for several weeks, drop doses, will often break up the sick headache habit. The pain in the forehead, chiefly over eyes. Eyeballs very painful, with pressure over root of nose. Hepatic derangements, jaundice. Enlarged spleen (Ceanoth). Jaundice with arrest of menses. A prominent liver remedy. Gall stones (berberis, Cholest, Calc). Diabetes mellitus. Paroxysmal, abdominal pain.

Chion. acts powerfully on the liver and is indicated in hypertrophy: obstructed liver in malarious districts - sensation of contraction of stomach as if something alive moving in it. One observer who gave Chio. to a nursing woman who had liver disorder with jaundice noticed that whilst rapid improvement of the liver symptoms occurred, at the same time the milk disappeared and the menses returned. The medicine was stopped. Sabal Serr. given and the milk returned.

Dose: Tr. to 1st attenuation.

(JHC)

Gall stone colic. It gives instant relief and ensures radical cure in Gall stone colic. Give chionanthus. ϕ - 10 drops in an ounce of cool water every hour and more often during paroxysm of pain. To check the formation of stones and recurrence of pain give Cheo. ϕ-5 drops TDS in an Oz. of cool water and Carduus. ϕ-5 drops in an Oz. of cold water B.D. *(Sinha)*

188. *Chloralum*

(Chloral Hydrate)

This drug used in physiological doses is a powerful hypnotic and cardiac depressant. It has a marked effect on the skin, producing erythema, ecchymosis etc. These symptoms have been utilised homoeopathically with much success, especially in the treatment of hives. Emotional excitability, hallucinations, night terror in children, muscular prostration.

Urticaria, worse spirituous liquors. Surface of body stone cold, wheals come on from a chill, better warmth.

Luminal: Sleeplessness with skin symptoms in migraine, lethargy like epidemic encephalitis. *(Dr. Royal)*

The brain tissue is probably congested in the same way as the skin in the urticaria of the drug. Urticaria gives a good illustration of the effect of the drug on the minute tissues. Night terrors in children have been cured with it.

Dose: First trituration in hives, otherwise higher potencies, locally, in offensive foot sweat, bathe with one percent solution. For its physiological effects, five to 20 grains, use cautiously. *(Boericke)*

Night terrors in children have been cured with it. The brain tissue is probably congested in the same way as the skin in urticaria. Urticaria gives a good illustration of the effect of the drug on the minute tissues. Asthma and wheezing respirations are probably due to an urticarious condition of the lung tissue. A symptom that is very significant in this: when lying on back, inspiration was through the nose, while expiration was blown from the lips as in apoplexy. *(JHC)*

It should be remembered in chorea, hysteria, night terrors of children, insomnia and neuralgia, when ten grains may be put in an ounce of water, a teaspoonful given every hour or less until relief is obtained.

It is employed by many in urticaria, erythema and ecchymosis. When there is violent stinging over the whole body, wheals come on suddenly after a chill. In these cases one grain is given every three hours.

It is an important remedy in puerperal convulsions when it should be dissolved and carried high into the rectum which has been previously cleansed by a warm enema.

It is of service in severe cases of whooping cough and in spasmodic asthma, when dependent upon nerve irritation when it should be given in small doses, repeated. *(Blackwood)*

189. *Chloroformum*

(Chloroform)

General anaesthetic, antispasmodic, complete muscular relaxation, weak and quick pulse, shallow or stertorous breathing, convulsions, nephritic or biliary colic, gastralgia. Symptoms obtained by Dr. D. Macfarlan with the 6th potency.

Great weakness, especially on right side. Limbus with tired feeling from knee down. Much perspiration all over face and chest, drowsy and dizzy, dry lips and throat, dry tickling cough at night. Flatulence, food regurgitates, sore and bruised feeling in stomach, catching pain around heart. Sharp pain in right chest, when he takes long breath, shortness of breath on exertion.

Dose: Higher attenuations or 6th. Phosphorus is the remedy to give in narcosis of chloroform. *(Boericke)*

Its most note-worthy effect is complete relaxation of all the voluntary muscles of the body. It may cause death by paralysing the respiration or the heart. It is especially indicated in delirium where excitement and violence predominate, desire to kill. Paralysis of voluntary and involuntary muscles and special senses. Chloroform will dissolve gall stones and cases have been treated by the injection of chloroform into the gall bladder. Antidoted by Brandy and Ice in Rectum. *(JHC)*

190. Chlorum

(Chlorine gas in water)

The marked effect on the respiratory organs producing spasm of the glottis is the chief symptom of the drug. Asthma to relieve the spasm of glottis. Useful externally and internally in gangrene.

Marked loss of memory especially for names. Constriction with suffocation, spasm of the glottis - sudden dyspnoea from spasm of the vocal cords - inspiration free-with obstructed expiration (Mephit) - chlorum has been proved in the form of chlorine water.

Dose: Chlorine water, when required of full strength, must be freshly prepared. Fourth to sixth potency. *(Boericke)*

191. Cholesterinum

(The proximate principle-furnished by the epithelium lining of gall bladder and large ducts).

For cancer of the liver-obstinate hepatic engorgements. Burning pain inside, on walking, holds his hands on side, it hurts him so. Opacities of vitreous. Jaundice, gall stones, cholesterine is the physiological opponent of Lecithin. Both seem to play some unknown part in the growth of tumours. Gall stones and insomnia.

(Boericke)

Cholesterine is a substance crystallising in leaflets with a mother of pearl lustre and fatty feel. It is soluble in alcohol and ether. It occurs in the blood and brain, yolk of eggs, seeds and buds of plants but most abundantly in the bile and biliary calculi. Ameka, who did much to introduce the proximate principles of the tissues as remedies, anticipating the practice now so much in vogue in the old school, recommended, cholesterine as a remedy in cancer of the liver. Burnett has recently adduced conclusive evidence in support of the correctness of this assertion, and I have myself (J.H. Clarke) cured mainly with this, a case described to me. I did not see the patient a man over 50, was in the last stage of liver disease. He had been given up by his medical attendant, who ordered him to make his will without delay. Burnett uses the 3x of the 3rd trit. and substantial doses. He commends it in obstinate hepatic engorgements, which by reason of their obstinancy make one think interrogatively of cancer, also in cases in which there appears to be a semi-malignant affection, involving the left lobe of the liver and what lies between it and the pylorus and the pancreas. In such cases Burnett gives alternately cholest. 3x and Iodoform 3x. It has been used with success in the removal of opacities of the vitreous. *(JHC)*

192.*Chromicum Acidum*

(Chromic acid)

Diphtheria, post nasal tumors and epithelioma of the tongue have been benefitted by this drug. Bloody foul smelling lochia. Symptoms come and go suddenly and return periodically, offensive discharges. Chromium sulphate (in locomotor ataxia, goitre, prostatic hypertrophy. Herpes preputialis. Wry neck. Also exophthalmic, inhibits the vagus, relieving tachycardia, acts like a nerve tonic where there is a lack of nervous tone. Fibroid tumours, infantile paralysis.

Dose: For adults 3 to 5 grains after meals and at bed time. *(Boericke)*

193. *Chrysarobinum*

(Goa powder - Andira araroba)

Acts as a powerful irritant of the skin and used successfully in skin diseases especially in ring worm, psoriasis, herpes tonsurans, Acne rosacea. Vesicular or squamous lesions, associated with foul smelling discharge and crust formation tending to become confluent and to give the appearance of single crust covering the entire area. Violent itching in thighs legs and ears. Dry scaly eruptions especially around eyes and ears, scabs with pus underneath (Mezer).

Ears: Eczema behind ears, filthy scabby condition with tendency to form thick crust. While ear and surrounding tissue appears to be one scab.

Dose: Locally, as a cerate 4-8 grains to the ounce of vaseline, internally 3-6 potency, used externally should be used with caution on account of its ability to produce inflammation.

Chrysarobinum, contains chrysophan which is rapidly oxydised into chrysophanic acid. This is also contained in Rhubarb and Senna.

Seen ring worm disappear rapidly from a few applications of the ointment. (Boericke)

An organic acid obtained from rhubarb and some lichens. A constituent of Goa powder. Tried as a local application in the form of ointment in bad cases of psoriasis on one limb Chry. ac. has caused the disappearance of the eruption on the other limb as well, showing a constitutional action. It has been used with some success in the lower triturations internally in psoriasis, ringworm, and other skin affections, also as a local application in ringworm. It is a powerful irritant of the skin and mucous membranes. Given internally in crude form it has caused nausea, vomiting, and purging. Used locally Gr. iv to gr. viii with vaseline z. i, or internally, or both, it is a magnificent remedy in eye and ear cases where a filthy, scabby condition exists, and a tendency to form thick crusts. Cases in which the whole ear and surrounding tissue appeared to be one great scab from the centre of which oozed the pus which came from a suppurative otitis media cleared up in two or three weeks under internal and external use of Chry. ac.; also cases where a similar condition of eyelids and skin of face obtained. *(JHC)*

It relieves blepharitis, conjunctivitis, and keratitis, also an eczematous condition about the ears. *(Blackwood)*

194. Cicuta virosa

(Water Hemlock)

The action of the nervous system, producing spasmodic affections viz., hiccough, trismus, tetanus and convulsions, give the pathological picture calling especially for this remedy, whenever this is further characterised. Among these are the bending of the head, neck and spine backwards and the general action of the patient is violent, with frightful distortions, violent strange desires. Sensation of internal chill. Moaning and howling. Does absurd things. Marked action on the skin. Head turned or twisted to one side. Cerebrospinal meningitis. Cervical muscles contracted - stares persistently at objects. Convulsions from concussion of brain. Eyes pupils dilated, insensible, strabismus, haemorrhage from ears. Skin - pustules which run together forming thick yellow scabs on face and head, corners of the mouth and chin with burning pain - Red face - Trismus - disposition to grind teeth. Hiccough - Indigestion with insensibility frothing at mouth. Back bent backward like an arch. Skin - Eczema - hard lemon coloured crust - chronic impetigo.

Worse: From touch, draughts, concussion, tobacco smoke. *(Boericke)*

It chief influence is excited on the Medulla oblongata, the gastro - intestinal tract, and the skin. Twitching and spasmodic jerks are a keynote of Cicuta. Bending the head backward is very characteristic. The remedy has cured many cases of cerebro-spinal meningitis, the opisthotonous being the leading indication. Violence is a leading feature, violent spasms; moans and howls; great agitation; makes gesticulations; odd motions; strange desires, as to eat coal. Head turned or twisted to one side is no less indicative of the drug in convulsions of children or adults. It corresponds to falls and the effects of concussions. Utter prostration follows the convulsive attacks - sudden rigidity, then jerks and violent distortions, then prostration. Jerking of the left arm all day is a very characteristic symptom. *(JHC)*

195. Cimex-Acanthia

(Bed bug)

Of use in intermittent fever, with weariness and inclination to stretch. Hamstrings feel too short. Flexors mostly affected. Sensation of retraction of arm tendons. Stretching.

Chilliness of whole body. Sensation of wind blowing on knees. Pains in all joints as if tendons were too short. Musty offensive sweat. Constipation, faeces dry and in small balls.

Dose: Sixth to 200c. *(Boericke)*

Cimex is an ancient remedy for intermittent fever. A characteristic symptom is, weariness and inclination to stretch. The flexors are most affected. Pains in all joints as if tendons were contracted and too short, every motion or stretching of arms or legs causes tightening pain in them. Irresistible sleepiness. Frequent yawning. Sensation as of a cold wind blowing on knees. A.W.K. Choudhry relates a case of intermittent fever (quotidian) cured with Cimex 30, the chief indications being: chill slight, thirst some days, none other days, shiverings, passed water twice during chill, chill agg: by lying down, increase of cough if he drinks water during chill. *(JHC)*

The Bedbug is a well known insect of the order Hereroptera and family Cimidae. The tincture is prepared from the live insects; and dilutions from the tincture. *(Blackwood)*

196. *Cimicifuga Racemosa*

(Actea Racemosa) - (Macrotys)

(Black snake root)

Had a wide action upon the cerebro-spinal and muscular system, as well as upon the uterus and ovaries. Especially useful in rheumatic, nervous subjects with ovarian irritation, uterine cramps and heavy limbs. Muscular and crampy pains, primarily of neurotic origin, occurring in nearly every part of the body, are characteristic. Agitation and pain indicate it. Pains like electric shocks here and there. Migraine. Symptoms referable to the pelvic organs prominent. It lessens the frequency and force of the pulse, soothes pain and allays irritability.

Dreams of impending evil. Fears riding in a closed carriage, of being obliged to jump out.

Head: Waving sensation or opening and shutting sensation in brain, pressing out-ward, shooting pains in eyes, intense aching of eyeball, pain from eyes to top of head.

Stomach: Gnawing pain.

Female: Menses profuse dark coagulat-ed, pain across pelvis from hip to hip, intolerance to pain.

Respiratory: Tickling in throat, dry short cough.

Worse: Speaking and at night, cough when secretion is scanty, spasmodic dry with muscular soreness and nervous irrita-tion.

Heart: Irregular, slow trembling pulse. Angina pectoris, stiffness and contraction in neck and back, intercostal rheumatism.

Extremities: Pain in lumbar and sacral region, down thighs and through hips, crick in back, muscular soreness, sleeplessness.

Worse: Morning, during menses, the more profuse the flow the greater the suffering.

Better: Warmth, eating.

Dose: 1st - 30c (Third most frequently used). *(Boericke)*

Gloom and dejection - Incessant talking, changing from one subject to another. Head-ache reflected from pelvic organs. It has also ensured living births to women who have previously borne only dead children from no discoverable cause - given in daily doses of 1x for 2 months before term. Rheumatism affecting the vertebral joints and especially in the neck. It is suited to the climacteric period, to nervous persons to children during dentition. Causation - Anxiety, fright, disappointed love, business failure, over exertion, child bearing.

Sensation as if a heavy black cloud had settled all over her-illusion of mouse running from under her chair - excessive muscular soreness after dancing, skating or other violent muscular exertion - similar to *Caul., Puls.,* in uterine and rheumatic affections.

Actea spicata - especially suited to men - rheumatism, pains notably affecting, small joints, wrists, fingers, ankles, toes.

It is also very useful remedy for the rheumatism of the abdominal muscles and fleshy parts of the body-worse on motion. *(JHC)*

Cimicifuga-ϕ. It is a boon to despondent mothers who give birth to dead children only. Let the expectant mother take 5 drops of cimicifuga Φ once a day since the 5th month of pregnancy and she is sure to give birth to live children. Aggravation of all complaints with the increase of menstrual flow - Give 1 drop every 3 hours. *(Sinha)*

197. Cina

(Worm seed)

This is a children's remedy - big, fat, rosy, scrofulous, corresponding to many conditions that may be referred to intestinal irritation, such as worms and accompanying complaints. An irritability of temper, variable appetite, grinding of teeth, and even convulsions, with screams and violent jerkings of the hands and feet, are all within its range of action. The Cina patient is hungry, cross, ugly and wants to be rocked. Pain in shocks. Skin sensitive to touch. Child very cross, desires every thing but rejects everything offered. Pulsation of super-ciliary muscles - yellow vision. Nose-wants to rub it. Face pale, dark rings around eyes, white and bluish around the mouth, grinds teeths during sleep, choreic movements of face. Stomach hungry. Abdomen - twisting pain about navel-itching of anus - gurgling from throat to stomach after coughing. Extremities - twitching - sudden inward jerking of fingers of right hand - child stretches out feet spasmodically - troubles with yawning. In Cina fever, face is cold and hands warm.

Urine milky - wetting the bed - in sleep crying out as if in delirium - getting on hands and knees in sleep - causation - worms. Yawning.

Canine hunger - hungry soon after a full meal, craving for sweets and different things, refuses mothers milk-Santonine sometimes cures in worm affections when cina seems indicated but fails.

Dose: 30-200c. *(Boericke)*

Cina — The unexpanded flower - heads (commonly called seeds) of several varieties of Artemisia maritima. Semen cinae. Flores cinae. Artemisia contra. Worm seed.

Cina is the source of the alkaloid Santoninum. It is pre-eminently a worm medicine, as it causes all the symptoms which characterise Helminthias - mental, nervous, and bodily. It corresponds more to the effects of lumbrici than to those of other worms. Nothing pleases them for any length of time, grinding teeth during sleep, wetting the bed when accompanied by picking nose, great hunger, restless sleep, tossing all about the bed in sleep, crying out as if in delirium. Getting on hands and knees in sleep.

But Cina is much more than a mere worm medicine. Many symptoms appear to be reflex from abdominal irritation. *(JHC)*

This agent is indicated in those who present a pale, sickly looking face, with dark rings about the eyes. The child is fretful and cross, desires to be carried, but this gives no relief, it will not be reconciled, and though weak and cross, it is obstinate and strikes in anger at every one near it.

It should be remembered in those who are suffering from the presence of round, seat or pin worms. The child is fretful, has a ravenous appetite and swollen abdomen, there is itching of the nose and anus, frequent micturition, restless sleep and twitching of various parts of the body. This remedy will relieve this group of symptoms whether worms are present or not. It is to be studied in convulsions when they are dependent upon ascaride as well as twitching of the muscles of the face and about the eyes. There is a ravenous hunger that occurs after the meal, in other cases a watery diarrhoea, the stools contain pieces of white mucus like popped corn. These conditions are frequently associated with worms. *(Blackwood)*

198. *Cinchona Officinalis*

(Peruvian bark - China)

Debility from exhausting discharges, from loss of vital fluids together with a nervous erethysm calls for this remedy. Periodicity is most marked. Sensitive to draughts. Seldom indicated in the earlier stages of acute diseases chronic gout, chronic suppurative pyelitis. Post operative gas pains, no relief from passing it.

Intense throbbing of head, black specks, bright dazzling illusions, spots before eyes, pressure in eyes, amaurosis, ringing in ears, violent dry sneezing, bitter taste, food tastes too salty, slow digestion, weight after eating. Flatulence; belching of bitter fluid or regurgitation of food gives no relief, hiccough, bloatedness, better by movement, tympanitic abdomen, gall stone colic, stool undigested, frothy yellow, painless, worse at night, from fruit, milk, beer. Menses - dark clots and abdominal distension. Rattling in chest, suffocative catarrh, violent hacking cough after every meal, pains in limbs and joints, worse slight touch, hard pressure relieves. Coldness - one hand ice cold and other warm. Dermatitis. Fever intermittent, returns every week, chill generally in forenoon, thirst before chill and little and often debilitating night sweats.

Dose: Tr. to 30. *(Boericke)*

Kina is the Peruvia name for bark and Kina-Kina is the Bark of Barks. The story of its introduction into European medical practice is one of its many tragedies. According to Humboldt, writes Teste, about 500,000 lbs. of this bark are annually exported to Europe for the purpose of being converted into sulphate of quinine. Well may Teste add the exclamation, "Poor patients. As with almost every other good thing that comes into its hands, allopathy has contrived to do an infinity of harm with quinine to make up for the good. Some forms of intermittent fever it will cure."

China is placed by Teste in the Ferrum group with Plumb, Phos, Carb. an., Puls, Zinc and others, which have the property of remaking the altered blood, or increasing for the time being in a healthy person, the relative amount of haematin, globulin, fibrin, etc.

The glory of Hahnemann and the interest of homoeopaths are inseparably bound up with the history of this drug. It was the first medicine Hahnemann proved, and the one that opened up to his mind the idea of homoeopathy. Cinchona bark was to Hahnemann what the falling apple was to Newton, and the swinging lamp to Gallileo. Dissatisfied with the explanations of the action of Bark in curing ague that were current in his time, Hahnemann took the powdered Bark himself, being in health, and lo! an ague attack ensued. A repetition of the experiment produced the same result. Further experiments revealed that action of Bark which is the opposite of tonic-positively debilitating, in fact - already referred to.

The tincture of China is antiseptic, destroying amoeboid motion and retarding tissue change. It weakens the heart and impairs the circulation, produces congestions and haemorrhages, anaemia and complete relaxation and collapse.

Everything tastes bitter, even water. There is a desire for suicide, intolerable anxiety about 8 p.m. and 2 a.m. He springs out of bed and wishes to take his own life, but does not go near the window or take a knife.

The digestion of China is slow. China is one of the most flatulent of medicines. Fermentation in bowels, frothy, sour diarrhoea. Yellow, watery, undigested diarrhoea with much flatus and no pain. Diarrhoea of dark, inky fluid, stools frequent at night, only after food during the day. Leucorrhoea before period, painful.

It may be mentioned here the effect the tincture of China has in removing the craving for alcohol in drunkards who wish to reform. Ten to thirty drops two or three times a day is the usual dose for this, though where the general symptoms correspond the potencies would probably do better. *(JHC)*

The action of this agent has so many features in common with its alkaloid Chininum sulphuricum that its physiological action is considered under that heading.

It is useful in the anaemia and debility that follows the loss of a vital fluid, as a haemorrhage, prolonged and excessive lactation, diarrhoea, suppuration or sexual excesses. The face presents a pale, hippocratic expression, the eyes are sunken and surrounded by dark rings.

Flatulence is corrected by it when belching brings no relief. It is made worse by eating fruit, at times it is associated with abdominal colic that occurs periodically, and is worse at night and after eating.

It is of service in insomnia and unrefreshing sleep. It has some reputation in controlling the formation of gall stones.

(Blackwood)

199. Cineraria
(Dusty Miller)

Has some reputation in the cure of cataract and corneal opacities. Is used externally by instilling into the eye one drop four or five times a day. This must be kept up for several months, Most effective in traumatic cases.

Compare: In cataract, Phos., Plat., Cann., Caust., Naph., Led., Nat-m., Sil.

(Boericke)

I have seen no reports of cure by internal use of this remedy alone, but in some cases, it was given internally as well as used externally. Generally the patients have received specific homoeopathic treatment, internally at the same time. *(JHC)*

Habitate, Venezuela and other parts of tropical America. The expressed juice of the wild plant is used. When injected into the eye it is given in doses of 1 or 2 drops at a time.

This agent is employed in the treatment of cataract and corneal opacities. One drop is instilled in the eye four or five times a day for several months. *(Blackwood)*

200. *Cinnabaris*

(Merc-sulph)

(Mercurius sulphuratus ruber)

For certain forms of ciliary neuralgia and ulceration upon a syphilitic base, this remedy is most effective. Sleepless during night.

Eyes: Pains from lachrymal duct around eye to temple, from inner canthus across brows to ear. Severe shooting pains in bones or orbit, especially running from inner to outer canthus in the bone, redness of whole eye.

Male: Prepuce swollen, warts on it which bleed easily.

Skin: Very, fiery, red looking ulcers.

Mod: Worse, lying on right side.

Dose: 1st - 3rd Trituration.

(Boericke)

In warts on the prepuce it is more specific than Thuja, especially for fan shaped warts - left leg feels shorter than right whilst walking - Jerking in Penis occurring during sleep. *(JHC)*

201. *Cinnamonium*

(Cinnamon)

Cancer where pain and fetor are present. Best when skin is intact. Its use in haemorrhages has abundant clinical verification. Nose bleed. Haemorrhages from bowels, haemotysis etc. A strain in loins or false step brings on a profuse flow of bright blood. Post-partum haemorrhage. Flatulency and diarrhoea. Feeble patients with languid circulation. Menses early, profuse, prolonged, bright red.

Dose: Tincture to 3rd potency. For cancer; strong decoction, one half pint in a day. Oil of Cinnammon in aqueous solution best local disinfectant. 3-4 drops in two quarts of water as a douche whenever a germicide and disinfectant is needed. Three drops on sugar for hiccough. *(Boericke)*

A leading feature of Cinnamon is haemorrhage. The haemorrhage is bright red and clear and *agg:* by any physical exertion. Cinnamon also causes gastric disturbance and hysterical attacks. Pains in bones and in muscles and great weakness as after loss of fluids. *(JHC)*

Habitat, Ceylon. A small evergreen tree of profuse foliage. Mother tincture is prepared from the cinnamon bark.

This remedy is indicated in post partum and other uterine haemorrhages. The flow is profuse, the extremities are cold and the surface of the body is pallid. The menses are early and profuse, the blood is of bright colour. While its principal action is upon the uterine haemorrhage, yet it controls haemorrhage from other parts to a limited extent. It also has some reputation in cancer when pain and foetor are present. *(Blackwood)*

202. *Cistus Canadensis*

(Rock Rose)

A deep acting anti-psoric remedy, with marked action in glandular affections, herpetic affections, chronic swellings, when patient is extremely sensitive to cold. Sensation of coldness in various parts. Scrofulous ophthalmia. Poisoned wounds, bites, phagadenic ulcers. Malignant disease of the glands of the neck. Cistus has affinity for naso-pharynx, aborts colds that center in posterior nose. Sniffling.

Mouth feels cold, pyorrhoea (Merc cor., Caust., Staph., Kreos.) hurts, to protrude the tongue, Throat, very dry. Cold air passing over parts causes pain, sore throat from inhaling the least cold air, cool feeling, cool feeling in whole abdomen, the neck is studded with tumors, cannot sleep from coldness in throat. Skin itching all over, glands inflamed and indurated, worse slightest exposure to cold air.

Dose: 1st to 30c. Locally as wash to arrest fetid discharge *(Boericke)*

Cistus is a very ancient remedy, sensitive to cold air, runs through the pathogenesis and also feeling of coldness of which its peculiar property of favouring the formation of ice about its roots in early winter is strangely suggestive. *(JHC)*

Common name, frostwort. It is of service in catarrhal conditions of the throat, where the throat feels cold, and it becomes sore from inhaling the least cold air.

(Blackwood)

203. *Citrus Limonum*

(Lemon)

In the observations with this plant the expressed juice of the fruit has been used containing citric acid. Lemon juice and citric acid are traditional remedies for and preventives of scurvy. That their action is homoeopathic has been proved by the occurrence of scurvy from the excessive use of the acid when taken for other purposes. Used as a local application (in one part of citric acid to eight of water) it has relieved the pains of cancer. It has a powerful effect on the circulation and on the blood itself, producing faintness, weak pulse, haemorrhages and dropsies. Inflammation and painful enlargement of the spleen, dyspnoea. Daily headache. Stiffness in the joints, particularly in the fingers, bruised feeling particularly in the feet. Herpetic eruptions. *(JHC)*

204. *Citrus Vulgaris*

(Bitter orange)

Headache with nausea, vomiting and vertigo. Facial neuralgias, mostly right sided. Thoracic oppression. Frequent and irresistible yawning. Disturbed sleep.

All forms of Dropsy are benefitted with citric acid and lemon juice, table spoonful every 3-4 hour - Pain from cancer of tongue, used as a local application and mouth wash - one dram to 8 ozs of water. For cancer pains generally, often effective.

It antidotes snake bites and all animal poison.

Citrus decumana (Grape fruit) Tinnitus, noises and ringing in ears. Sensation of pressure in the temporal region.

Aurantium - Orange. Neuralgic and skin symptoms. Itching, redness and swelling of hands. Diseases of the aged with coldness and chilliness. Boiled dried orange peel excites the intestine in a manner similar to other forms of cellulose or agar. There is an increased flow of bile which continues for hours.

It unites both a cholagogue action with a mechanical stimulus to peristalsis.

Citrus Limonum (scorbutus, sore throat and cancer pains, checks excessive menstruation).

Citric acid: Useful in scurvy and chronic rheumatism and haemorrhages.

All forms of Dropsy are benefitted with citric acid and lemon juice, Tablespoonful every 3-4 hours. *(Boericke)*

The tincture of the peel is used as a pleasant bitter tonic in the old school practice. On sensitive individuals oranges in any form produce pathogenetic effects. One patient of my own could never eat an orange without experiencing a fearful taste at the back of the nose and throat, lasting many days and causing choking sensations and faintness. Nervous affections predominate, neuralgias of various kinds. The skin is the seat of many symptoms. *(JHC)*

205. *Clematis Erecta*

(Virgins bower)

Scrofulous, rheumatic, gonorrhoeal and syphilitic patients. Acts especially on skin, glands and genito urinary organs especially testicles. A remedy of much importance in disturbances of sleep and neuralgic pains in various parts. Many of these pains are relieved by perspiration. Muscles relaxed or twitching. Great emaciation. Great sleepiness. Distant pulsation in whole body. Confused feeling. Better in open air - Eyes sensitive to air-sensitiveness to cold. Toothache, worse at night and from tobacco - Teeth feel too long. Male - Testicles indurated and bruised feeling - Swelling of scrotum - right half only - urine interrupted flow. Skin-scaly, scabby, itches terribly, worse washing in cold water, scalp around occiput, glands swollen.

Modalities: Better open air, worse at night and warmth of bed (washing in cold water), new moon (Monthly aggravation).

Dose: 3-30c. *(Boericke)*

Clematis, like other Ranuncule, is a direct irritant of the skin producing, inflammation and vesication. It was used by Storeck before Hahnemann's time in cancerous and other foul ulcers, inveterate skin eruptions, syphilis, and rheumatism.

There is mucus in the urine, but not pus. Flow of urine by fits and starts, or has to wait a long time before he can urinate, with intense pain along fore part of urethra.

In men it is of service in ilio-scrotal neuralgia, the testicles are indurated and have a bruised sensation. The right one is usually the worst. There are pains along the spermatic cord.

It should be remembered in eczema and pustular eruptions, when the skin is red, burning, and itches severely. The glands are swollen, hot, and painful. The parts are worse from bathing in cold water.

(Blackwood)

206. *Cobaltum*

(The metal cobalt)

Adapted to neurasthenic spinal states. Sexual disturbances. Fatigue, agitation and bone pains, worse in morning.

Headaches: Worse bending forward.

Rectum: Constant drooping of blood from the anus.

Male: Emissions without erections, brown spots on genitals and abdomen.

Back: Pain in back and sacrum, worse while sitting, weak knees, foot sweat mostly between toes, disturbed by lewd dreams, skin dry and pimply.

Dose: 6-30c. *(Boericke)*

Other symptoms are, frequent nocturnal emissions, with lewd dreams with partial or no erections, impotence. Itching of the skin when warm in bed at night. Pain in hollow of tooth, which feels too long and is sensitive to touch. Tongue thickly coated white, cracks across middle. Warmth of bed causes itching all over. *(JHC)*

This remedy is indicated in sexual irritation of the male and in neurasthenia. In the male there is pain in the back and sacrum, which is aggravated while sitting, it is somewhat relieved while walking and lying. There are emissions without erection. The sleep is disturbed by lewd dreams, and is unrefreshing. *(Blackwood)*

207. Coca

Erythroxylon Coca

The divine plant of the Incas - But the spanish priests denounce it as "Undelusio del demonino". The mountaineers remedy. Useful in a variety of complaints incidental to mountain climbing such as palpitation, dyspnoea, anxiety and insomnia. Exhausted nervous system from physical and mental strain. Caries of teeth. Loss of voice.

Dose: Give 5-6 drops every half hour, two hours before expected demand on voice. Nocturnal enuresis, emphysema (Quebracho).

Head: Noises in ears, headache of high altitude, peppery sensation in mouth, longing for alcoholic liquors and tobacco, no appetite but for sweets.

Heart: Palpitation.

Male: Diabetes with impotency (Phos. ac.).

Respiratory: Hoarseness, want of breath, short breath, asthma, better from wine.

Dose: Tr. to 3c. *(Boericke)*

A characteristic symptom of cocaine poisoning is a sensation as if small foreign bodies were under the skin, generally like grains of sand, or as of a worm under the skin. This is undoubtedly the key-note symptom of coca. It is known as "Magnas symptoms named after the eminent neurologist who first described it. His description is: "a sensation as if foreign bodies were under the skin generally small round substances like grains of sand."

Cold, gone, relaxed feeling about the external genitals and a sensation as if the penis were absent. Compare this with the experiences of R.K. Gosh with Coca. ϕ. (which he finds in drop doses act better in such cases than in the potencies) in palpitation and dyspnoea on ascending, when arising from nervous causes, especially self abuse, in complaints from self abuse generally, excessive secretion of urine with or without sugar, enuresis nocturna, nymphomania after child birth, during menses, from irritation of eczema, or other affections of the vulva. In satyriasis, the homoeopathicity of Coca in enuresis is shown by its effect in relaxing the sphincters in one of the cases named above.

Mother tincture is prepared from the dried leaves and dilutions.

The tincture may be given in doses from 5 to 30 drops.

This agent in large doses produces delirium, hallucination and cerebral congestion. Medium doses act as a stimulant, increasing the bodily temperature, pulse rate and respirations, while moderate doses calm the nervous system and render the performance of muscular exertion easier.

It is of service in those who are performing acts and feats requiring great strength, also for mountain climbers, where it relieves dyspnoea, palpitation of the heart and controls haemoptysis. *(Blackwood)*

208. *Cocaine*

(An alkaloid from Erythroxylon - Coca)

Besides the great usefulness of Cocaine as a local anaesthetic, it has specific homoeopathic uses, though the symptoms are mainly clinical only. Sensation as if small foreign bodies or worms were under the skin.

Mind: Talkative, constant desire to do something great, to undertake vast feats of strength, sees and feels bugs and worms, moral sense blunted. Thinks he hears unpleasant remarks about himself, jealousy.

Head: Pupils dilated.

Stomach: likes sweets, haemorrhages.

Dose: Lower potencies. *(Boericke)*

This remedy is of service in delirium tremens, when the subject sees and feels bugs and worms over him. The moral sense is lowered and he neglects his personal appearance.

It is useful in chorea and paralysis agitans and senile trembling and in the persistent vomiting of pregnancy and sea-sickness it is used to allay the irritation.

The great use of this agent has been in the field of surgery as a local anaesthetic.

(Blackwood)

209. *Coccinella Septempunctata*

(Lady bug)

This remedy to be remembered in neuralgias, teeth, gums, mouth etc. Is awakened by profuse accumulation of saliva. Uvula feels too long. Symptoms of hydrophobia, worse by any bright object.

Throbbing toothache, cold sensation in teeth and mouth-Back pain in region of kidney and loins.

Dose: 3rd potency. *(Boericke)*

Lady bird - Sunchafer - crushed beetles.

It has been used in hydrophobia and there its action would appear to be analogus to that of Cantharis. *(JHC)*

210. *Cocculus*

(Indian cockle)

Within the sphere of action of Cocculus are many spasmodic and parotic affections, notably those affecting one half of the body. Affects the cerebrum (will not cure convulsive seizures proceeding from the spinal cord (A.E. Hinsdale). Painful contracture of limbs and trunk, tetanus. Many of the evil effects of nightwatching are relieved by it. It shows a special attraction for light haired females, especially during pregnancy, causing much nausea and backache. Unmarried and childless women. Sensitive and romantic girls. All its symptoms are worse riding in a carriage or on shipboard, hence its use in seasickness. Sensation of hollowness, or emptiness, as if parts had gone to sleep. Feels too weak to talk loud. Time passes too quickly, inclination to sing irresistible, profound sadness, vertigo, nausea, especially when riding, headache in occiput, worse opening mouth, paralysis of facial nerve - Aversion to food, metallic taste, seasickness (Resorcin 1x). Smell of food disgusts (Colch). Abdomen as if full of sharp stones, when moving. Pain in abdominal ring, Abdominal muscles weak. Purulent gushing leucorrhoea between menses, very weakening, paralytic pain in small of the back, pain in shoulder and arms as if bruised, knees crack on motion, chilliness with perspiration and heat of skin.

Compare: Morning sickness Symphoricarpus, Petrol., Puls., Ign.

Dose: 3 to 30c. *(Boericke)*

Cocculus has been used from ancient times as a poison for stupefying fish and making them easy to catch. It is commonly used as an adulteration of beer to heighten its intoxicating properties. A decoction of Cocculus is a domestic remedy and locally used for destroying head or body lice.

(JHC)

Adapted to hook worms. Sensitive romantic girls, with irregular menstruation, rates, onanists, and persons debilitated by sexual excesses. Nausea or vomiting from riding in carriage, boat or rail - road car (Arn., Nux m.) or even looking at a boat in motion, sea - sickness.

Has cured umbilical hernia with obstinate constipation, after Nux failed.

(H.C. Allen)

Diarrhoea, with emission of flatulence before the stool. Loose evacuation of a putrid smell. Faeces soft and yellow, which cause burning in the anus.

Itching in the scrotum. Great itching, esp. in the evening, or when undressing or at night in bed. *(JHC)*

There is a metallic taste in the mouth with a great afflux of saliva. Violent attacks of gastralgia, with cramping pain in stomach. There is great accumulation of flatulence, but this flatulence is not due to defects in decomposition of food as it is in Carbo veg, but mostly to retention of flatus, which when incarcerated, causes extreme distention of abdomen and great uneasiness. This diarrhoea in Cocculus is also peculiar in as much as it occurs mostly in daytime. Throughout the night there is absolutely no disturbance, but it comes on directly after rising from bed. Certain amount of urgency is noticeable as he has scarcely any time to undress; stools are soft, yellow, and faecal; prolapsus recti after stool is as much a feature of Cocculus as of Podophyllum. *(N.M. Choudhury)*

211. *Coccus Cacti*

(Cochineal)

The clinical application of the symptoms of this remedy, place it among the medicines for spasmodic and whooping cough and catarrhal condition of the bladder, spasmodic pain in kidneys, with visceral tenasmus. Anuria, anasarca, ascites.

Sensation of a foreign body between upper lid and eyeball. Constant hawking from enlarged uvula, accumulation of thick viscid mucus. Tickling in larynx, brushing teeth causes cough, whooping cough attacks end with vomiting of tough mucus. Urinary brick red sediment, urinary calculi, haematuria, urates and uric acid. Menses profuse, black, thick, dark clots, large clots escape when passing water, labia inflamed agg: after sleep, brushing teeth.

Dose: Lower triturations. *(Boericke)*

An insect infesting Cactus plants. The dried bodies of the female insects are used for making a tincture or trituration. They also constitute a well known dye. It compares with cantharis in its action on the renal organs and with cactus in causing haemorrhages in disturbing the heart and in causing lancinating, stitching and pricking sensations.

The cough exactly corresponds to the whooping cough type, there is no remedy which has a wider ranger in this affection. Cough *agg:* in morning, the child awakens and is immediately seized with a paroxysm of coughing ending in vomiting clear, ropy mucus hanging in long strings from the mouth. *(JHC)*

A small, red, gnat—like insect of the order Hemiptera, and the family coccidae. It is useful in nephritic colic, vesical and urethral irritation with pains that extend from the kidneys to the bladder. There is frequent urging to urinate. The urine is copious and clear as water. It may contain blood or deposit a brickdust sediment on standing. *(Blackwood)*

212.Cochlearia Armoracia Or

(Armoracea sativa)

Frontal bones and sinus, antrum and salivary glands are specially affected by this drug. Bloated sensation. Raises vital forces. Used as a gargle in scorbutic gums and sore throat, hoarseness and in relaxed conditions of the fauces. Internally in gonorrhoea. Useful as a condiment in enfeebled states of the stomach. An infusion of the root in cider for dropsy causes copious diuresis. Locally cures dandruff.

Eyes: Sore and scrofulous. Traumatic inflammation of eyes. Violent cramp from stomach through both sides around to back, gripping around navel, pain in back as from incarcerated flatulence from abdomen through to back and down into sacrum. Dry hacking laryngeal cough, throat feels rough and hoarse, frequent urination.

Dose: 1 to 3c. *(Boericke)*

This has the anti-scorbutic properties of the other cruciferae and is specially efficacious in scurvy from eating salt. The essential oil is said to be identical with that of sinapis. *(JHC)*

Armoracia sativa. This remedy is indicated in disease of the urinary organs and intestines, and in cases of rheumatism. In nephritis the urine is increased in quantity, is pale, and contains albumin. In the inflammatory stages of gonorrhoea, there is violent burning and difficult micturition; the discharge from the urethra is scanty. It is of service in abdominal cramps when the pains start from the region of the stomach and pass around both sides to the back. The stools contain an excess of mucus and at times there is involuntary passage of mucus from the bowels.

Dose: 1 to 60 drops of mother tincture. *(Blackwood)*

213. Codeinum

(An alkaloid from opium)

Trembling of whole body. Involuntary twitching of muscles of arms and lower limbs. Itching with feeling of warmth, numbness and pricking, diabetes.

Eyes: Involuntary twitching of lids. (Agaricus).

Stomach: Great thirst, with desire for bitter substances.

Dose: One quarter of a grain dose to 3x. *(Boericke)*

Codein possesses many of the properties of opium, from which it is derived but it has characters sufficiently distinctive to entitle it to a separate description, great degree of the exhilarating properties, itching with warmth, itching and heat of face and head. Codein has in many cases controlled diabetes. *(JHC)*

Codeinum is one of the alkaloids existing in Opium. The hydrochlorates of both Morphine and Codeine are obtained together in the process of extracting the Morphine. It occurs in white or yellowish white rhombic prisms.

It is of service when there is a general itching, with warmth and trembling of the whole body.

Also in cases when there is severe pain following attacks of neuralgia, in insomnia, especially if it is induced by attacks of coughing, which are constant, short, and irritating as is seen in phthisis. It has been employed in painful disorders of the Abdomen, such as Enteralgia. In diabetes it is also of service. *(Blackwood)*

214. Coffea Cruda

(Unroasted coffee)

Stimulates the functional activity of all organs, increasing the nervous and vascular activity. The drinking of coffee by the aged is likely to increase production of Uric acid, causing irritation of kidneys, muscle and joint pains and with the increased susceptibility of old people to the stimulating action of coffee and tea, their use should be curtailed or carefully watched.

Great nervous agitation and restlessness. Extreme sensitiveness characterises this remedy. Neuralgia in various parts, always with great nervous excitability and intolerance of pain driving to despair. Unusual activity of body and mind. Bad effects of sudden emotions, surprises, joy etc. Nervous palpitation. Coffea is specially suited in tall, lean, stooping persons.

Sensation as if a nail were driven in head, sensitive hearing. Toothache temporarily relieved by holding ice water in the mouth, hasty eating and drinking, delicate taste, hypersensitive vulva and vagina, voluptuous itching, sleeps till 3 a.m. after which only dozing. Sleepless on account of mental activity. Rapid, high tension pulse and urinary suppression.

Modalities: Worse excessive emotions (joy) narcotics, strong odors, noise, open air, cold night.

Better: Warmth, from lying down, holding ice in mouth.

Antidote: Nux-v., Tabac.

Dose: 3 to 200c. *(Boericke)*

The effects of coffea cruda have to be considered separately from those of Coffea tosta, since the roasting converts much of the coffeine into Coffeine or Methylamine, which gives to coffee its aroma. Coffee belongs to the same family as China, Ipecac and like these remedies has many symptoms of intermittent fever. It has been noticed that Coffee drinkers who do get ague are more difficult to cure than those who do not drink coffee. Sight is improved, fine print can be read easily, hearing is more acute and noises are intolerable. Teste remarks that dynamised Coff. Cruda prevents or neutralises in many persons the effects of roasted Coffee, dynamisations of many other drugs being antidotal to secondary effects of the crude substances. Hahnemann describes the migraine of Coffee - drinkers thus: it comes in the morning after waking, increasing little by little - patients look exhausted, retire to dark places. If the attack is very violent, a vomiting of mucus takes place. This kind of Megrim, scarcely ever leaves before evening. If the paroxysm is less violent, a little strong coffee, which was the first cause of such a headache will produce a temporary palliation of the pain, but the disposition to relapse becomes so much greater. The attacks comes irregularly and quite suddenly. It is well to enquire carefully into the dietary habits of patients who come complaining of headaches of this kind. The pulse is slowed. Insomnia is common. Diarrhoea in housewives who have much care and trouble in managing their households. The symptoms are *agg:* by warmth and *agg:* in open air, though in toothache warm drinks aggravate, cold drinks ameliorate. Wine drinkers should take coffee. Beer drinkers should take tea. *(JHC)*

Coffea tosta - In addition to opium and its derivatives, it counteracts the effects of Nux vom., Bell., Narcotic mushrooms, poisonous Sumach, Tobacco, bitter almonds, prussic acid, Coloc., Valer., Cic., Cham., salts of antimony, lead, phosphorus, Phosphoric acid. On account of its extensive antidotal properties coffee has largely been condemned by homoeopathic practitioners, but it should be remembered, that it does not antidote all other medicines and it is questionable if it counteracts the effects of many of the above named drugs, when they are given in high potencies. In any case it is desirable to forbid its use when Bel., Cham., Coloc., Ign., Lyc., and Nux v. are being given. I have several times cured a toothache like this with Coffea. c.30. Other indication for its use are: tense arteries, periodic headaches in hysterical women, nervous and gastric headaches - vomiting on least exertion - Diarrhoea from over work and too much care - Gout and Rheumatism with tendency to form Chalk stones.

Coffeinum is an alkaloid obtained from coffea arabica - A proving has brought out no symptoms not included in the pathogenesis of Coffea. *(JHC)*

Mix 1 part of Caffein with 9 parts of sugar of milk and get it well triturated and the 1x is prepared. Caffein in 1x is a great heart stimulant. Use it in cases of threatening heart failure due to frequent motions in 1 Gr. dose every 10-15 minutes. *(Yudhubir Sinha)*

It is of service in insomnia when the ideas roll upon the mind, and he is wide awake, ecstacy, full of ideas and there is no sleep.

It is of service in neuralgia, which may appear as a toothache, when there is extreme restlessness and complaining, with entire relief of the pain for a time from holding cold water in the mouth.

(Blackwood)

215. Colchicum

(Meadow saffron)

Affects markedly the muscular tissues, periosteum and synovial membranes of joints. Has specific power of relieving the gouty paroxysms. It seems to be more beneficial in chronic affections of these parts. The parts are red, hot, swollen. Tearing pains, worse in the evening and at night and from touch. Stubbing the toes hurts exceedingly. There is always great prostration, internal coldness and tendency to collapse. Effects of night watching and hard study. Shocks as from electricity through one half of body. Bad effects from suppressed sweat. — Dreams of mice.

The smell of food especially fish causes nausea, even to fainting. Great coldness in stomach, craving for various things but is averse to them. When smelling them, seized with nausea. Burning or icy coldness in transverse colon, abdominal distention, stools contain white shreddy particles. Pruritus of genitals, sensation of swelling in vulva and clitoris. Pulse thread like, pulse of low tension, sharp pain down left arm, pins and needles in hands and wrist, finger tip numb, joints stiff and feverish, shifting rheumatism, pain worse at night, inflammation of great toe, gout in heel, cannot bear to have it touched or moved, tingling in finger nails, oedematous swelling and coldness of legs and feet, worse sunset to sun rise, smell of food. Better - stooping.

Dose: 3rd to 30th attenuation.

(Boericke)

Ailments from grief or misdeeds of others (Staph), smell painfully acute, nausea and faintness from the odour of cooking food, especially fish, eggs or fat meat. Affected parts very sensitive to contact and motion. Arthritic pain in joints, patient screams with pain on touching a joint or stubbing a toe. *(H.C. Allen)*

Colchicum is best known as a remedy in gout and rheumatism, and the provings show its specific relation thereto. It acts on muscles, bones, and joints. It causes extreme relaxation of the muscular system - the head falls forward on the chest or falls back when the patient is raised from the pillow; arms fall helpless by the side.

It corresponds to the gouty constitution; leuco-phlegmatic and melancholic temperament, venous constitutions, uric acid diathesis, the sediment being pale yellow and rather like fine flour than sand. Also, urine black as ink, urine loaded with albumin and casts.

Colch. dysentery and rheumatism are exceedingly painful. Very sensitive and irritable. Cannot endure strong smells. Gouty diabetes, the uric acid reappearing as the sugar disappears. The heart is affected like other muscles. Oppression and anxiety amel. by walking.

She was unable to brush her own hair not so much from the pain as from the extreme weakness and powerlessness of the parts affected. T.F. Allen gives tingling in finger nails as characteristic of Colch., no other remedy has it. *(JHC)*

It is of service in hydrothorax, when there is marked dyspnoea and oedema of the extremities. This is often dependent upon disease of heart and kidneys.

(Blackwood)

216.Collinsonia Canadensis

(Stone root)

Pelvic and portal congestion, resulting haemorrhoids and constipation especially in females. Depressed arterial tension, general atony of muscular fibre, chronic, nasal, gastric, and pharyngeal catarrh, due to portal obstruction. Dropsy from cardiac disease. Pruritus in pregnancy with piles. Constipation of children from intestinal atony. Said to be of special value, when given before operation for rectal diseases. Sense of weight and constriction. Venous engorgement. Sensation of sharp sticks in rectum. Sense of constriction. Dry faeces.

Most obstinate constipation. Painful bleeding piles, dysentery with bleeding piles. Alternate constipation and diarrhoea, itching of anus. Pruritus of vulva, prolapse of womb, cough from excessive uses of voice, ministers' sore throat, better heat.

Dose: Tincture to 3rd attenuation. Higher potencies where there is organic heart affection. *(Boericke)*

Collinsonia is native to North America. It has a root very tough, hard and knotted. The legs felt light as if he could run like a deer. As a domestic remedy and among the eclectics it is known as a remedy for chronic catarrhal conditions especially of stomach, bowels and bladder, also of nose, pharynx and larynx and in tubular and capillary bronchitis. It is useful in heart affections alternating with suppressed haemorrhoidal bleeding, constipation with hard light stools. Stools or mucus and blood. Prolapse of the rectum with piles. Nash differentiates between Aesc. h. and Collins. Both have sensation as if rectum was full of sticks. Aesc. has sense of fullness in rectum which Collins does not. Aesc. piles do not bleed as a rule; those of Collins bleed persistently, Collins has more persistent constipation with colic because of it. Aesc. may have constipation or may not. Collins. has shown marked power of disturbing the circulation and causing haemorrhage.
(JHC)

The slightest mental emotion or excitement aggravates the symptoms.

(H.C. Allen)

This agent has a pronounced action on the veins and venous radicles leading to irritation and catarrhal states of the mucous surfaces, haemorrhoids and resulting constipation. In small does it stimulates the stomach and causes diuresis.

This remedy is indicated where there is venous stasis, dilated veins, with blueness and dark discoloration of the membranes, showing an imperfect venous capillary circulation. *(Blackwood)*

217. *Colocynthis*

(Bitter cucumber)

Often indicated in the transition season when the air is cold, but the sun is still powerful enough to heat the blood. Develops most of its symptoms in the abdomen and head causing intense neuralgia. It is especially suitable for irritable persons, easily angered and ill-effects therefrom. Women with copious menstruation and sedentary habits. Persons with a tendency to corpulency. The neuralgic pains are nearly always relieved by pressure. Cramps and twitching and shortening of muscles. Constrictions and contractions. Cystospasm following operation on orifices (Hyper.) Urinous odour of perspiration. (Berb., Nit-ac.) Agonizing pain in abdomen causing patient to bend double is most characteristic. Sensations: cutting, twisting, grinding, contracting and bruised, as if clamped with iron bands.

Vertigo when turning head to the left. Eye pains sharp, boring, better pressure. Gouty affections of eyes, violent pain in eyeballs precedes the development of Glaucoma.

Face: Neuralgia with chilliness, sounds re-echo in ears, very bitter taste, tongue rough as from sand and feels scalded.

Abdomen: Cutting agonizing pain in abdomen causing patient to bend over double. Sensation as if stone were being ground together in the abdomen, and it would burst.

Intestines feel as if bruised. Dysenteric stool renewed each time by the least food or drink, jelly like stools. Female - Boring pain in ovary. Must draw up double with great restlessness - Round, small cystic tumors in ovaries or broad ligaments, wants abdomen supported by pressure. Bearing down cramps causing her to bend double (Opium) - Pain on urinating, over whole abdomen, contraction of muscles, cramp like pain in hip, pressure and heat.

Modalities: *Worse* from anger and indignation-Better doubling up - hard pressure, warmth, lying with head bent forward.

Dose: 6 to 30 c. *(Boericke)*

The strongest characteristic, pain in abdomen causing the patient to bend over double. Relief is obtained by motion, such as twisting, turning and wriggling around and the motion is kept up steadily while the pain lasts. According to Nash - Mag. phos. comes nearest to it in colic and neuralgic affections - Veratrum has colic amel. bending double, but it has also cold sweat - Dioscorea has wind colic but is amel. by stretching out. The Stannum child wants to be carried with the abdomen on the mothers shoulder. The nearest analogue to Colocynthis in its entire action on the human body is its botanical congener Bryonia - Griping pain of coloc. forcing the patient to bend double may be accompanied by cramps in other parts which may occur with or without stool - if a stool occurs it gives immediate relief - sensation as of hard stones or potatoes in the body. Coloc has like Lyc., Hell., and Causticum a 4 p.m. aggravation. One prover had 4 p.m. colic coming on six days in succession.

(JHC)

Compare with Staph. in ovarian or other diseases, from bad effects of anger, reserved indignation or silent grief. *(HC Allen)*

Mother tincture from the dried fruit, freed from the outer rind and seed; and dilutions.

It should be studied in Enteralgia, whatever, the cause, when the pains are violent and griping in character and are relieved by pressure, heat, bending double, the passage of stool and the escape of flatus. The patient is often of the gouty or rheumatic type, there may be a history of the partaking of undigestible food, exposure to cold or some violent emotion, as a fit of anger. There may be a diarrhoea or cholera morbus present, which is attended with severe agonizing, twisting pains about the umbilicus. The patient finds relief by bending double and pressing firmly upon the abdomen. The pains are more severe every few minutes, are worse from partaking of food or drink; there is temporary relief from a discharge of flatus and stool. The pain is of a nervous, rather than inflammatory origin.

It should be studied in dysentery, when the stools are bloody and mucus, are worse after eating and drinking and there is the characteristic colic present. It is to be remembered in menstrual and vesical colic, when much the same group of symptoms is present.

It is indicated in sciatica when the pain is excruciating, paroxysmal; tearing, shooting, boring in character. There is relief from heat, pressure and flexing the thigh on the abdomen. Should the paroxysm come when the patient is walking, he will grip the thigh just above the popliteal space.

It is an important remedy in diseases of women, suppression of the menses due to fits of anger or chagrin; also dysmenorrhoea, when there are violent paroxysms of pain which are benefitted by firm pressure and from heat. It has cured cysts of the broad ligament and ovaries when the symptoms requiring the remedy are present. *(Blackwood)*

218.*Comocladia Dentata*

(Guao)

Important eye and skin symptoms. Affection of antrum - Sacroiliac and abdominal pain. Throbbing pains - worse by heat - pain in joints and ankles.

Eyes: Ciliary neuralgia with eyes feeling large and protruded, especially right, worse near warm stove, feels as if pressed outward, sees only glimmer of light with left eye, Glaucoma, Sense of fullness. Eye balls feel too large, motion of eye agg.

Face: Swollen with eyes projecting.

Skin: Itches, red and pimples, redness all over, like scarlatina; erysipelas, deep ulcer with hard edges, leprosy, red stripes on skin, Eczema papular of the trunk and extremities, also pustular type.

Modalities: Better open air, scratching, by motion. *Worse:* Touch, warmth, rest, night.

Dose: 1st to 30. *(Boericke)*

Guao (Cuba) - Tincture of leaves and bark of Comocladia - shows its botanical affinity with the Rhus family by the virulence of its effects on the skin, the slightest contact, and at times even walking in the neighbourhood of the growing tree, being sufficient to cause violent inflammation. The trunk and branches of the tree contain a milky fluid turning black on exposure to sunlight, discolouring the skin, linen etc. (Compare the marking nut. Anacardium). The plant causes tormenting itching, swelling, redness, vesication, ulceration. *(JHC)*

219. Condurango

(Condur plant)

Stimulates the digestive functions and thus improves the general health. Allays the pains in gastralgia accompanying cancer of stomach. Modifies secretions of digestive glands. Varicose ulcers. Lupus. Painful cracks in corners of mouth is a guiding symptom of this drug. Chronic gastric catarrh, syphilis and cancer.

Tumors: Stricture of oesophagus. The active principle (Condurangin) produces locomotor ataxia.

Painful affections of the stomach, ulceration, vomiting of food and indurations, constant burning pain. Stricture of oesophagus with burning pains behind sternum, where food seems to stick. Vomiting of food and indurations in left hypochondrium with constant pain.

Fissures from about the muco-cutaneous outlets, epithelioma of lips or anus. Ulcerative stage of Carcinoma, cutis when fissures form.

Dose: Tr. of bark, 3 grain doses before meals in water. Also the thirtieth potency in tumours. *(Boericke)*

It produced a painful crack in the right corner of the mouth. These cracks were seen produced in several patients who were taking the drug and has cured similar cracks with it. Regard them as a key note indication. Has cured patients of tumors, some undoubtedly cancerous, who had that symptom as a concomitant.

A hard tumor the size of an egg on the outer side of the nipple was the centre of lancinating pains radiating from it, the whole breast being very tender to touch. The tumour increased steadily under

Headrest, Phytolacca, and was only checked temporarily by Conium. Under Condur. It entirely disappeared. *(JHC)*

This remedy is of service in Carcinoma, especially of the stomach and in gastric ulcers, with catarrhal gastritis, atonicity and threatened ulceration.

220. Conium

(Poison hemlock)

An old remedy, rendered classical by Plato's graphic description of its employment in the death of Socrates. The ascending paralysis it produces, ending in death by failure of respiration, shows the ultimate tendency of many symptoms, produced in the provings for which Conium is an excellent remedy. Difficult gait, trembling, sudden loss of strength while waking, painful stiffness of legs etc. Such a condition is often found in old age, a type of weakness, languor, local congestion and sluggishness. This is the special environment that Conium chooses to manifest its action. It corresponds to the debility, hypochondriasis, urinary troubles, weakened memory, sexual debility found here. Troubles at the changes of life, old maids and bachelors. General feeling as if bruised by blows. Great debility in the morning in bed cancerous diathesis. Arteriosclerosis, caries of sternum. Enlarged glands. Acts on the glandular system engorging and indurating it, altering its structure like scrofulous and cancerous conditions. Tonic after grippe. Insomnia of multiple neuritis.

Vertigo, when lying down and when turning over in bed - worse after a meal.

Eyes: Photophobia and excessive lachrymation. The slightest ulceration or abrasion will cause the intense photophobia.

Nose: Nose bleed easily - becomes sore - polypus.

Stomach: acrid heart burn worse on going to bed - *Amel.* from eating and agg. a few hours after meals.

Stool: tremulous weakness after every stool.

Urine: flows and stops again - interrupted discharge.

Male: Effects of suppressed sexual appetite - Mammae lax and shrunken, hard, painful to touch. Stitches in nipples. Breasts enlarge and become painful - effects of repressed sexual desire.

Dry cough caused by dry spot in larynx - itching in chest and throat, when lying down.

Extremities: Muscular weakness - perspiration of hands - putting feet on chair relieves pain.

Skin: auxillary glands pain, with numb feeling down arm - glands enlarged and indurated - tumors, piercing pains - sweat as soon as he sleeps.

Modalities: Worse, lying down, turning or rising in bed; celibacy, before or during menses.

Better while fasting, in the dark, from letting limbs hang down; motion and pressure.

Compare: Scirrhinum (Cancer nosodes - cancerous diathesis; Enlarged glands; cancer of breast; worms).

Dose: Best in higher potencies given infrequently especially for growths, paretic states etc - otherwise 6 to 30c. *(Boericke)*

The primary action is one of rigidity, condensation and constriction of fibres with swelling of glands and diminution of the senses - persons of a lively quick sanguine disposition, with a marked development of the glandular system - it is to the glands and capillary system, what Aconite is to the heart and arterial system - in many cases Conium may be regarded as the Aconite of chronic diseases - Another symptom is yellow nails - Stools cold - I have used this remedy with very great good result in numerous cases of weakness from masturbation in men and youths - Emission on the slightest stimulus such as merely being in the society of women - Many engaged young men have been helped by this remedy. Obstinate constipation of long standing - stool (once in 7 days) large hard followed by tremulous weakness. Accumulation of ear wax. Craving for salt, coffee, and sour things. Paroxysms of hysteria and hypochondriasis from abstinence from sexual intercourse. I have some times found conium disagree with patients who had been taking psorinum. *(JHC)*

The balm of Gilead for diseases of old maids and women during and after climacteric - especially for diseases of old maids, old bachelors, with rigid muscular fibre, persons with light hair, who are easily excited, strong persons of sedentary habits - Morose, easily vexed, domineering, quarrelsome, scolds, will not bear contradiction, excitement of any kind causes mental depression - Dreads being alone, yet avoids society - Vertigo especially when lying down or turning in bed - sweat day and night as soon as one sleeps or even when closing the eyes - patients requiring Conium often improves from wine or stimulants, though persons susceptible to Conium cannot take alcoholic stimulants when in health. *(H. C Allen)*

This agent acts upon the motor nerves, producing paralysis which begins in the extremities. There is congestion and induration of the glandular structures.

This remedy is indicated in the diseases of old men, old maids, and in persons with light hair who are easily excited, and those with rigid fibres.

It is of service in glandular indurations when they are as hard as a stone, and especially if this induration is traceable to an injury or contusion; also in tumors and engorgement of the female breast. These tumors may only appear during the menstrual period.

It should be remembered for the pernicious effects of celibacy, as well as over indulgence; when there is hypochondriasis, mental depression, timidity, aversion to society, and dreams of being alone.

It is useful in tracheo-bronchial catarrh when the cough is spasmodic, and appears to be dependent upon a dry spot in the larynx or from itching in the throat or chest. It is worse at night when lying down and during pregnancy. It has been employed in cancer of various parts when the growth is of a stony hardness with sharp, lancinating pains.

In vertigo it is of service when the patient is unable to turn the head to either side.

It is useful in paresis and paralysis that extends from below upward, gradually involving new structures. There is giddiness, with debility and prostration, especially of the arms and legs. When walking he staggers as though drunk. *(Blackwood)*

221.*Convallaria Majalis*

(Lily of the valley)

A heart remedy, increases energy of heart's action, renders it more regular. Of use when the ventricles are over distended and dilation begins, and when there is an absence of compensatory hypertrophy and when venous stasis is marked. Dyspnoea, dropsy, aneuric tendency. Anasarca.

Sees imaginary gray spot about 3 inches square - grating of teeth in the morning, coppery taste - Great soreness in uterine region with sympathetic palpitation of heart - sensation as if heart ceased beating, then starting very suddenly.

Relation: *Digitalis, Crat., Lil., Adonis* (feeble heart action due only to functional disturbance)

Dose: Third attenuation. ϕ for symptoms of heart failure. Tincture 1-15 drops. *(Boericke)*

Convallaria is a popular remedy in Russia for heart affections and it has been introduced into old school medicine principally as a heart remedy. It compares closely in its action with Lilium tigrinum, and also resembles its other botanical relatives Aloe, Allium cepa and allium sativum. It is strongly purgative and causes morning vomiting. It has been proved and the symptoms produced show that its nearest analogue is Lilium tig. Nash has used it in 30th with very satisfactory results in women, complaining of great soreness in uterine region with sympathetic palpitation of the heart. In the case of convallaria when lying on back - sleepiness accompanies many symptoms. *(JHC)*

Convallaria corrects irregularities of the heart due to valvular diseases especially mitral, pericardial adhensions etc. rather than tissue degeneration. It calms the heart renders its movement, rhythmical and slows the pulse. It cures dropsy caused by the sluggish action of the heart. It cures palpitation, dyspnoea, diminished secretion of urine, oedema of the feet etc. due to inability of the circulatory system. Give convallaria ϕ 5 drops in an ounce of cool water thrice daily and crataegus oxy. ϕ. 5 drops twice daily. *(Yudhbir sinha)*

This remedy is indicated in organic weakness of the heart, and upon the gastro-intestinal tract, producing emesis and purging. At first it slows the contractions of the heart, while later the cardiac pulsations are quickened and the arterial pressure is further increased.

It should be studied when the heart's action is rapid, the pulse feeble and irregular, both in rhythm and force; with a condition of dropsy present.

It is of service in rheumatic carditis and endocarditis when there is a sensation as if the heart beat throughout the chest, with extreme orthopnoea, and at times anginal pains. It is of service in cardiac paresis when attended with palpitation, in mitral stenosis and insufficiency when accompanied by a failing compensation, resulting in pulmonary congestion and dyspnoea. It assists in controlling cardiac dilatation with or without hypertrophy. It affords great relief to those suffering from tobacco heart and from cigarette smoking, also in hearts that have been overstrained.

It relieves the asthmatic breathing that is dependent upon a feeble heart's action. It has a most favourable action in restoring the right heart, following pulmonary congestion and inflammation. *(Blackwood)*

222. *Copaiva*

(Balsam of Copaiva)

Acts powerfully on mucus membranes, especially that of the urinary tract, the respiratory organs and the skin, producing a well-marked nettle rash, colds and catarrhs.

Burning and dryness in nose, crush on turbinated bones - food seems too salty - Gastric troubles - gastric trouble during menstruation or following urticaria - gas and intestinal flatulence - urging to stool and difficult passage with pain. Urinary - burning, pressure, painful micturition - by drops - retention with pain in bladder - anus and rectum - catarrh of bladder - dysuria - swelling of orifice - constant desire to urinate - urine smells of violets - Greenish turbid colour - peculiar pungent odour. Rectum - mucus colitis. Testicles sensitive and swollen. Itching of vulva and anus with bloody purulent discharge. Skin - hives with fever and constipation, Roseola, erysipelatous inflammation, especially around abdomen - circumscribed lenticular patches, with itching, mottled appearance - chronic urticaria in children - Bulbous eruptions.

Dose: 1-3 c *(Boericke)*

Copaiva is an old world remedy for gonorrhoea and it has been used for other blenorrhagic conditions. The chief incidence of the drug's action is on the genito urinary organs and rectum, urethra - discharge milky, corrosive, meatus tumid and inflamed. It affects the skin and mucus membranes generally. He (A.P. Bowie) recommends also an ointment of Gtt x of balsam to 3j of vaseline to relieve the burning and itching at the anus caused by piles. *(JHC)*

This agent applied to the skin is mildly irritating; when taken internally produces a warmth in the stomach, causes offensive eructations and may excite nausea and vomiting. It deranges the appetite and produces diarrhoea.

Its special action is on the mucous membrane of the genito-urinary tract, producing inflammation of the kidneys, with bloody urine, pain in the bladder, strangury, and an increase of the secretions. It is a powerful diuretic, being eliminated by the kidneys, bronchial mucous membranes and skin. A rash frequently appears while it is being taken.

This remedy is indicated in chronic catarrhal affections, in gonorrhoea when the acute symptoms have subsided, in gleet and chronic urethritis when there is burning along the urethra in the region of the prostate, especially upon urinating. The testicles may be swollen, the urine has the odour of violets and may contain blood, the infection may have extended to the bladder and a cystitis resulted, the urine is scanty, its passage being attended with pain. It is frequently the most serviceable remedy in the irritation of the neck of the bladder and urethra in aged women. It should be studied in chronic bronchitis, bronchial catarrh and bronchorrhoea when attended with a profuse, greenish - gray, offensive expectoration. It relieves a mucus colitis when the stools are covered with mucus, this is most pronounced during the morning and evening, the passage being attended with colic and chilliness. Some of these cases are complicated by acne, urticaria and erythema, with violent itching. This is frequently observed following the ingestion of lobster and other rich foods. *(Blackwood)*

223. *Corallium*

(Red Coral)

The proving of Coral develops much coryza and epistaxis and even ulceration within the mouth. It is to be thought of for whooping and spasmodic cough, especially when attack comes on with a very rapid cough and the attacks follow so closely as to almost run into each other. Often preceded by sensation of smothering followed by exhaustion. Congestion of face after dinner. Patient becomes purple in face. Violence of paroxysms even with expectoration of blood. Feeling as if cold air were streaming through skull and air passages. One is too cold when uncovered and too hot when covered - relieved by artificial heat.

Nose: Odors of smoke, onions etc - Painful ulcer in nostrils - Post nasal catarrh - profuse secretion of mucus dropping through posterior nares.

Mouth: Food tastes like Saw dust - bread tastes like straw - beer tastes sweet - craves salt.

Respiratory: Hawking of profuse mucus - throat very sensitive especially to air - profuse secretion of mucus dropping through posterior nares - dry, spasmodic, suffocative cough, very rapid cough, short barking - air feels cold on inspiration. Continuous hysterical cough, feels suffocated and greatly exhausted after whooping cough.

Male: ulcers on glands and inner prepuce with yellow ichor - Emissions and weakened sexual power - profuse perspiration of genitals.

Skin: Red flat ulcers - Coral coloured then dark red spots - changing to copper coloured spots - psoriasis of palms and soles.

Modalities: *Worse* in open air - Changing from a warm room to cold room.

Dose: 3-30c. *(Boericke)*

Red coral, the product of a coralligene zoophyte, contains Carbonate of lime, oxide of iron (whence its colour) Gelatin and other elements. In old physic it was considered to have strengthening properties and to be astringent, sudorific diuretic and absorbent. In homoeopathic practice Corallium corresponds to a combination of syphilis and Psora. Is suited to persons of nervous temperament, nervous coughs. It causes eruptions which are for the most part of its own colour coral red - cough in "minute gun" paroxysms - crowing inspiration. There is much drowsiness with Coral - whooping cough or any other kind of cough, when the attack comes on with a very rapid cough and the attacks follow so closely as to almost run into each other. *(J.H. Clarke)*

224. *Cornus Circinata*

(Round leaved Dogwood)

Chronic malaria, hepatitis, jaundice, weakness in morning - Pain in pit of stomach - with distended abdomen - Vesicular eruption associated with chronic liver disease or aphthous stomatitis.

Dose: Tincture to 6th. *(Boericke)*

A popular remedy for aphthous and ulcerated conditions of mucous membranes. *(JHC)*

225. *Corydalis*

(Turkey Pea)

Syphilitic affections. Ulcers of mouth and fauces. Cancer cachexia pronounced - Gummata and night pains - Chronic disease with atony. Tongue clean, broad and full - Tissues flabby - doughy - cold - gastric catarrh (Hydrast).

Skin: Dry scaly scabs on face of old people - lymphatic glands swollen.

Dose: Tr 20 drops. TDS. *(Boericke)*

This is an unproved remedy, but clinical experience has revealed a specific relation to the manifestations of Syphilis : Hunterian chancre, syphilitic nodes, falling of the hair, syphilitic and scrofulous ulcerations of scalp, syphilitic and nonsyphilitic ulcerations of fauces - all these have been reported cured by it. Hale also commends it in. *(JHC)*

226. *Cotyledon*

(Pennywort)
(Navel Wort)

Marked action on heart, fullness in throat. Epilepsy. Numb aching in muscular and fibrous tissue. Sciatica. Well marked pains through the breast to scapula. Catarrh of larynx and trachea. Hysterical joint. Could not articulate for some time on awaking. Feeling as if a part of the body is absent. *(Boericke)*

Cotyledon has had a considerable proving, but I am not aware of any clinical experience with it having been recorded.

The whole houseleek family are deserving of careful study by homoeopathists. Among the most peculiar symptoms of Cotyl, are a feeling as if some part of the body - a foot or the head - were absent. *(JHC)*

This remedy has been employed in epilepsy, in catarrhal states of the larynx and trachea, in hysterical joints, and in neuralgic pains extending from the left nipple to the scapula. *(Blackwood)*

227. *Crataegus Oxy*

(Hawthorn berries)

Produces giddiness, lowered pulse, and air hunger and reduction in blood pressure. Acts on muscles of heart and is a heart tonic. No influence on endocardium. Myocarditis - Failing compensation. Irregularity of heart, Insomnia of Aortic sufferers - anaemic-oedema cutaneous chilliness - High arterial tension - is a sedative in cross, irritable patients with cardiac symptoms. Chronic heart disease with extreme weakness. Very feeble and irregular heart action. General anasarca - very nervous with pain in back of head and neck. Collapse of typhoid. Haemorrhage from bowels - cold extremities - pallor - irregular pulse and breathing-painful sensation of pressure in left of chest below the clavicle. Dyspepsia and nervous prostration with heart failure. In the beginning of heart mischief - after rheumatism - Arteriosclerosis. Said to have solvent power upon crustaceous and calcareous deposits in arteries.

Urinary: Diabetes, especially in children.

Head: Cardiac dropsy - Extreme dyspnoea on least exertion - without much increase of pulse - Pain in region of heart and under left clavicle. Heart dilated. First sound week. Pulse accelerated. Irregular - feeble intermittent - Valvular murmurs. Angina pectoris - cutaneous chilliness. Blueness of fingers and toes. All aggravated by exertion or excitement. Sustains heart in infectious disease.

Skin: Excessive perspiration - Skin eruptions.

Worse: In warm room.

Better: Fresh air, quiet and rest.

Dose: Fluid extract or tincture one to 15 drops - must be used for some time in order to obtain good results. *(Boericke)*

Crataegus was introduced in medicine as a heart remedy by Dr. Greene of Ennis

Ireland and it has been used empirically with much success in cases of heart failure. It has usually been given in 5 drops doses of the tincture. The drug may cause nausea when given in the tincture, unless given during or immediately after a meal - Crataegus is the nearest approach to a positive heart tonic that I know of. *(JHC)*

Crataegus Oxyacantha - Mother tincture prepared from the ripe berries and dilutions. This agent acts upon the heart as a restorative tonic. Produces a quieting and strengthening influence, and imparts tone and force to the cardiac contractions. It is solvent and absorptive to the disease accumulations, and tonic and stimulative to its nutritive nerve supply.

It should be remembered in all cases of failing compensation with dilation of the heart, also, in fatty hearts where it frequently gives relief when Digitalis and the other cardiac stimulants have failed. The patient is gloomy, despondent, apprehensive, there is great pallor of the skin, with a rush of blood to the head, there is dyspnoea with extreme and irregular breathing, which is aggravated by moving about.

It is of service in dilatation of the heart, the first sound being absent, weak, prolonged or replaced by a murmur, the pulse is accelerated, often intermittent, and irregular. It is useful in angina pectoris when there is sudden and terrible pain in the left breast, the pain radiating over the heart and down the left arm, accompanied with fear, apprehension and a sense of impending calamity. It is also of value in cardiac hypertrophy, in failing or broken compensation, and threatened heart failure during acute diseases. It acts favourably in functional diseases of the heart, palpitation and tachycardia when dependent upon anaemia. It should be studied in renal hyperaemia when the urine is diminished in quantity, contains traces of albumen and an excess of phosphates. The extremities are cold, oedematous, and evidence of general anasarca may be present.

Compare - Digitalis, Adonis vernalis, Strophanthus hispidus. *(Blackwood)*

228. Crocus Sativa
(Saffron)

Is a remedy often useful in haemorrhages that are black and stringy. Tingling in various parts - Chorea and hysterical affections. Frequent and extreme changes in sensation and mental conditions. Anger with violence followed by repentance. Laughing mania. Drowsiness and lassitude better by literary labour.

Mind: Vacillating, pleasant mania, sings and laughs - Happy and affectionate, then angry. Sudden changes from hilarity to melancholy. Vivid recollection from music heard.

Eyes: Feeling in eyes as after violent weeping. Eyes feel as if in smoke - Sensation as if cold air was rushing through eyes.

Nose: dark stringy clotted strings of dark blood hanging down the nose.

Abdomen: Obstinate constipation due to portal stagnation. Sensation of something alive in abdomen, stomach etc.

Female: When haemorrhage is dark and stringy. Menses dark, viscid, too frequent and copious, black and slimy - clots with long strings. Cracking in hip joint and knees.

Dose: Tr. to 30c. *(Boericke)*

Crocus has three characteristics, which clearly call for its use when met with. The first is haemorrhage from various parts (nose, uterus, etc.) when the blood is black, viscid, clotting, forming into long black strings, hanging from the bleeding orifice. The second is a peculiar sensation, as if something alive were moving about in the abdomen or chest. This may be a definite sensation or it may be a hallucination or fixed idea. A curious circumstance in this connection is the fact that Crocus has often been successfully given to pregnant women, who have complained of violent foetal movements as well as in cases of imaginary pregnancy. The remaining characteristic is at mental level. It is a rapid alternation of mental conditions anger with violence rapidly followed by repentance, laughter quickly followed by tears. Hysterical laughter is one of the affects observed by older physicians - Sensitive to music involuntarily joins in on hearing anyone sing (It is a domestic remedy for bringing out the eruption of measles). *(JHC)*

Excessively happy, affectionate, wants to kiss everybody - the next moment in a rage - Compare in menstrual derangements (Ust.) *(H.C. Allen)*

Mother tincture prepared from the dried stigmas of the flowers.

This agent in small doses so exhilarates the spirits that the subject ascend to the heights of happiness, while presently they are in the deepest rage.

Large doses induce headache, intoxication, delirium and stupor, doses of from two to three drachms have resulted in death.

It has relieved chorea and spasmodic twitching of the single set of muscles.

(Blackwood)

229. *Cromicum Kali Sulph*

(Chromic Alum)

Most valuable remedy for hay fever that we possess. 6th trituration - and downwards. Because it some times succeeds in the 3x and even the 1x when higher numbers fail. I generally give eight grains of the 5x to begin with 3 - 4 times a day. It can be used on general indications for coughs and catarrhs which its constituents will readily suggest. *(JHC)*

Alum of Chrome - 3x (produces in the nasal passages very fine threads from septum to external wall, affections of nasal fossae and hay fever - chronic colds - Sneezing red watery eyes, irritation of mucous membrane).

Compare : Puls , Kali bich, Nat. m.
(Boericke)

230. *Crotalus Hor*

(Rattle Snake)

Snake poisons are supposed to be chemically - Cyan-Hydrates of Soda and other salts. Alcohol is the natural solvent of these salts and is an antidote. Has a profound trophic action - Old age nutritional troubles - Lower septic states. General disorganisation of blood. Haemorrhages and jaundice. A crotalin injection decreases the rate of Coagulation of the blood. In epilepsy the average rate is far greater than the normal conditions. Blood decomposition, haemorrhages (dark fluid that forms no clots), tendency to carbuncles, malignant scarlatina, yellow fever, the plague, cholera, give opportunity to use this remedy. Haemorrhagic diathesis. Acts as a sedative. Sleeps into his symptoms. More right sided in his action

Eyes: Very sensitive to light, especially lamp light. Yellow colour of eyes. Illusions. Blue colors. Ciliary neuralgia. For absorption of intraocular haemorrhages into the vitreous but particularly for non-inflammatory retinal haemorrhages. Diplopia.

Ears: Blood oozes from ears.

Nose: Epistaxis, blood black and stringy.

Stomach: Bilious vomiting, vomiting of blood, black or coffee ground vomiting, gastritis in chronic alcoholism. Hungry craves stimulant, sugar. Averse to meat.

Extremities: Rightsided paralysis.

Fever: Malignant fevers of a haemorrhagic or putrescent character.

Skin: Yellow color of the whole body - great sensitiveness of skin of right half of body. Purpura haemorrhagica.

Sleep: Dreams of dead, starting in sleep.

Dose: 3-6c. *(Boericke)*

Trituration of sugar of milk saturated with solution of the venom in Glycerine.

It causes bleeding from all orifices and surfaces and it corresponds to the haemorrhagic diathesis. The crotal patient is readily moved into tears. Weeping mood. *(J.H. Clarke)*

This agent when introduced into the system at once produces an increase in the pulse rate which may rise to 150. There is soon a slowing to 75 and again a rise to 100. During this time there are pains in the body which are speedily followed by sensations of cold chills. The tissues about the wound become oedematous, the skin changes to a red color, while later it is of a purple hue. There is great muscular debility and a gradually developing state of coma. The blood is rapidly decomposed and will not coagulate. There are haemorrhages from all the orifices of the body, the finger and toe nails become discolored and blood flows underneath them. There is a bloody greenish froth upon the lips, and death ensues.

This remedy is indicated in adynamic conditions that are characterised by a haemorrhagic tendency. There is great prostration with low delirium, and vomiting of bile and blood and haemorrhages from any or all orifices. It is useful in pyaemia and septicaemia, and all forms of blood poisoning and septic conditions, as well as in purpura haemorrhagica and where there is a tendency to gangrene.

Compare: Ars, Carbo veg., Lachesis, Naja. *(Blackwood)*

231. *Croton Tiglium*

(Croton oil seed)

It is a valuable remedy in diarrhoea, summer complaint and skin affections. These may alternate with each other. Feels tight all over. It is one of the antidotes to Rhus poisoning as is evident from its wide and intense action upon skin and mucous surface, causing both irritation and inflammation with formation of vesicles and mucus discharges. Has elective affinity for skin of face and external genitals - Burning in the oesophagus.

Eyes: Feel drawn backward - Tensive pain above right orbit.

Abdomen: Copious watery stools with much urging, always forcibly shot, with gurgling in intestines.

Chest: Drawing pain through the left chest into back - Asthma.

Female: Nursing women, every suck the child gives, produces pain from nipple back - inflamed breasts.

Skin: Feels hide-bound. Intense itching, but scratching is painful. Pustular eruptions especially on face and genitals with fearful itching followed by painful burning - Vesicles confluent oozing herpes zoster - Stinging - Smarting pains of eruptions.

Dose: 6-30c. *(Boericke)*

Croton oil is best known in its uses as a powerful purgative, and as an irritant of the skin. The characteristic stool of Croton is a sudden evacuation in one gush, like a shot, followed by great prostration. Colic before stool, constant urging, Agg: from eating and drinking and from every movement. The evacuation is yellowish or yellowish green. On the skin Croton produces erythema, erysipelas, eczema, herpes pustules. The antidote to Croton is Ant. tart. Croton antidotes Rhus tox. Writhing in transverse colon. The face and the scrotum especially have been thus attacked. The eruptions in which it succeeded were, urticaria, large copper coloured spots almost like liver spots, small red blotches, not very apparent, in thighs, abdomen and genitals of fifteen years standing - all accompanied with intolerable itching.

Stool: Urgent inclination to go to stool, with rumbling and pinching in the abdomen, as from heat and agitation in the abdomen, with pressure on the anus, as in diarrhoea in the morning in bed, and after getting up, stool, followed by excoriating pain in the anus, sudden, immediately after rising or commencing exercise, so pressing that the closet cannot be reached soon enough.

Tetter like eruption on the Scrotum. Herpetic eruption on the Scrotum. *(JHC)*

This agent when applied to the skin causes irritation, inflammation, and a papular eruption which later becomes pustular. When taken internally it produces a congestion of the gastro-intestinal tract with copious watery stools, and peritonitis and death may result. There is hyperaemia of the glandular systems, and eruptions of the skin.

This remedy is indicated in choleric diarrhoea. The movement are forcible, coming out like a shot, or as water from a hydrant. The movements are worse from eating and drinking. The stools consist of a yellow watery material and between the stools there is a constant urging.

It should be remembered in eczema of the face and external genitals, when attended with intense itching, but owing to the tenderness the patient is unable to scratch the parts, gentle rubbing, however, relieving it.

It is of service in nursing women when the breast becomes tender, a pain extending from the nipple to the shoulder blade when the child nurses. *(Blackwood)*

232. *Cubeba*

(Cubebs)

Mucus membranes generally but especially that of the urinary tract are chiefly affected by this remedy. Frequent urination of a nervous origin. Leucorrhoea in little girls.

Urinary: Urethritis, with much mucus especially in women - Cutting after urination with constriction - Haematuria - Prostatitis-with thick yellow discharge cystitis.

Dose: 2-3c. *(Boericke)*

Cubeba corresponds to catarrh - It is an old world remedy for gonorrhoea and gleet but it affects the mucous membranes of the nose, air passage and intestines as well as that of the Urino-genital tract. It acts well in persons of bilious temperament with tendency to constipation.

Nash defines its place in gonorrhoea, after the inflammatory stage is passed under the usual remedies for that stage - if there is still burning in urethra after micturition and the discharge remains thick yellow or pus like. *(JHC)*

Habitate: Jaws, Bornea and other islands of the Indian ocean.

Mother tincture of the dried berries.

This remedy is indicated in urethritis, catarrh of the respiratory passages and in dysentery. In urethritis when the acute stage is passed and there is a chronic state present. There are cutting pains upon urinating, and the urine may contain blood. It is useful in prostatitis with a thick yellow discharge and cystitis with nocturnal enuresis, or spermatorrhoea, and in the leucorrhoea of children, also in urethro-vaginitis of long standing with abundant discharge.

In dysentery it has been of service when the stools are colorless and are mingled with particles like rice. *(Blackwood)*

233. *Cucurbita Citrullus*

(Seeds of Water Melon)

Infusion for painful urination with sense of constriction and backache. *(Boericke)*

234. *Cucurbita Pepo*

(Pumpkin seed)

Intense nausea immediately after eating. Vomiting of pregnancy, Sea sickness. One of the most efficient and least harmful of Tenia fuges.

Relation: Filix cuprum oxide nig.

Dose: Tincture.

The seeds are valuable remedy for tapeworm. Scald the seed and peel off the outer skin when softened. The green inner pulp being the part used.

Dose: 2 ozs of seed, yielding one of pulp. May be mixed with cream and taken like porridge. Take in morning after 12 hours fasting and follow two hours later by castor oil. *(Boericke)*

An excellent remedy for tape worm which may be given with safety to children. The seeds are scalded. The outer skin being softened is peeled of, the green inner pulp being the part used. Two ozs of seeds yielding one Oz of the pulp should be used for each patient. The pulp should be rubbed in a mortar or some other vessel to make a smooth mass. It may be mixed with milk or cream and sweetened and taken like porridge. It should be taken in the morning after a 12-16 Hrs fast and followed 2 hours later by a castor oil purge. Hales method is as follows. The patient to eat but little of the lightest food all day, taken no supper, and on going to bed eat one Oz. of the peeled seeds, bruised with milk or cream. In the morning on waking to take a tablespoonful of castor oil mixed with a half teaspoonful of pure sulphuric Ether. No breakfast to be taken. Only a cup of tea or coffee. In 2 or 3 hours the oil will operate, expelling the worm. Hansen mentions that millionaires find the mother tincture of great use in sea sickness and vomiting of pregnancy. Bonino records that Cucurb. P. 3 cured salivation and vomiting in women in whom the menses were absent and who was erroneously supposed to be pregnant. L.E. Griste records the following case. A woman four months pregnant had vomitted almost from conception and for six weeks had not retained a meal. "I am almost starved to death", she said, was pale haggard, tongue clean. Soon after eating or drinking anything she became intensily nauseated. The doctor got a fresh Pumpkin stem, cut in into thin slices and covered them with Alcohol. At the end of 1/2 an hour, he poured off a little and made a 1x dilution and directed 1/2 a drachm to be put in half a tea cup full of water, a tea spoonful every two hours. There was no further vomiting. Dr. Griste's indication is intense nausea immediately after eating. *(JHC)*

235. *Cuphea*

(Flux-weed)

Vomiting of undigested food-Cholera infantum. Much acidity, frequent green watery acid stools, tenesmus with great pain. High fever, restless and sleepless - obstinate constipation.

Dose: Tincture. *(Boericke)*

Dr. Roth gave 5-10 drops doses, according to age. The two chief forms on which it is successful are (1) cases arising from acidity of milk or food, vomiting of undigested food or curdled milk, with frequent green watery acid stools, varying in number from 5-30 a child, fretful and feverish, can retain nothing on stomach, foods seem to pass right through the child, (2) stools decidedly dysenteric, small, frequent, bloody and tenesmus and great pain, high fever, restlessness and sleeplessness - Dr. Brown says if you have a child that is fretful and feverish, vomits curdled milk, from a hyper - acidity of the stomach, has frequent green watery acid stools, or even the stools are dysenteric; with great tenesmus and colic, high fever and restlessness, give Cuphea.

Compare: Aethusa. *(JHC)*

This remedy is of service in cases of cholera infantum arising from acidity of the milk, or food. There is vomiting of undigested food or milk with green, watery, acid stools. The child is fretful and feverish. There may be traces of blood in the stools with tenesmus and great pain, high fever, restlessness and insomnia. *(Blackwood)*

236. *Cuprum Aceticum*

(Acetate of Copper)

Hay fever, burning excoriations, paroxysmal cough, tough tenacious mucus and fear of suffocation. Protracted labor. Chronic prosriasis and lepra.

Head reels when in high ceiling room. Vomiting, slimy, brown diarrhoea, violent tenesmus. Cholera. Attacks of angina pectoris, coming on when excited. Violent spasmodic cough, short difficult respiration. Spasmodic constriction of chest. Dyspnoea - Skin leprous like eruption, without itching over whole body in spots of various sizes.

Relation: Acts similarly to cuprum met but is more violent in action.

Dose: Third to sixth trituration. *(Boericke)*

Cupr. acet produces the leading features of Cupr. met - cramps, griping pains, spasms, paralytic affections and convulsions. Attacks come on suddenly and periodically. It corresponds to results of repelled eruptions. In poisoning cases it is antidoted by sugar or white of egg given freely. *(JHC)*

237. *Cuprum Arsenicum*

(Arsenite of copper - Scheele's Green)

A remedy for symptoms depending on deficient kidney action, various intestinal affections, cholera morbus and infantum; enter - colitis, diarrhoea, and dysentery, Gastro-intestinal disturbances of influenza and typhoid. Uraemic convulsions, headache, vertigo and unconscious conditions resulting from brain oedema. Nephritis of pregnancy. Convulsions preceded by gastrointestinal symptoms, chlorosis, Bronchial asthma with emphysema, purulent endocarditis (Royal) painful neurosis, enteroptosis. Delirium and tremor cordis.

Urine: Garlicky odor, Diabetes, urine of high specific gravity, increased acetones and diatetic acid.

Male: Perspiration of scrotum, is constantly damp and moist. Boils on Scrotum. Purulent discharge of a white color from urethra, tingling and burning in urethra. Pain in prostate. Pains in penis.

Extremities: Cramps in calves of legs, worse after midnight, only relieved by getting out of bed and standing, ulcers, gangrene.

Skin: Icy cold sweat and skin even when dry, cold clammy perspiration of an intermittent nature. Acne, pustules, on face and in the uro-genital region; ulcers look like chancre, Gangrene. Carbuncles.

Dose: 3rd trituration. *(Boericke)*

Cupr- ars. combines the characters of its two metallic compounds. Intense neuralgic pains in abdomen, awful distress in epigastric region, burning along oesophagus in urethra, numbness, creeping, itching and chilly sensations. According to J.N. Majumdar who gives a case, the great characteristic of cupr. ars. in choleraic conditions is icy coldness of the whole body with cramps and an obstinate hiccough. *(JHC)*

This agent in from 1/100 to 1/200 of a grain daily in broken doses is a gastro-intestinal irritant, stimulates the flow of the gastric and intestinal juices, increases the peristalsis and improves the digestive and nutritive function. In medium doses its action is on the gastro-intestinal tract to a great measure and produces nausea with vomiting with profuse evacuations of the bowels. There is distress in the epigastrium which is characterized by remittent exacerbations, burning and weight which stimulates neuralgia of the abdominal viscera. The epigastrium is sensitive to pressure. When large doses are taken there is excessive nausea with vomiting, purging and sensitiveness, increased permeability of the walls of the capillaries in the splanchnic area takes place, giving rise to a gastro-enteritis which closely resembles cholera. The epigastric and abdominal regions are distended, tympanitic, and extremely sensitive; there are cramps in the extremities which extend even to the fingers and toes. The patient passes into a state of semiconsciousness. The lungs are hyperaemic and oedematous. The urine is partially suppressed, contains albumin and epithelia. The urea is diminished and the phosphates are absent. The tongue is dry and shows a red streak down the centre.

This remedy is indicated in disease of the gastro-intestinal tract, in defective elimination of the kidneys, and in neurotic affections. Cases in which there is a profuse diarrhoea with violent vomiting of large quantities of watery material which is accompanied by sharp cutting colicky pains. The stools are usually offensive and tinged with green.

It should be remembered in enterocolitis, cholera infantum and in the diarrhoea of childhood when the stools are watery, offensive, and of a greenish color, and are attended with spasmodic pains and cramps in the extremities causing the patient to scream out. It is frequently of service in cases of dysentery and typhoid fevers when the gastric and abdominal symptoms correspond.

It should be remembered in acute catarrhal enteritis and cholera morbus when the pains are excruciating and the above symptoms are present.

It is to be remembered in the gastralgia enteralgia and nervous dyspepsia of neurotic subjects. There is frequently a history of an improper diet. The pains are excruciating in character.

In the gastrointestinal symptoms of phthisis it frequently controls the nausea, vomiting, cramps and diarrhoea resulting from indigestion. Through its action upon the cells of the mucous membrane of the intestine it assists absorption and in this manner has been of service in marasmus.

In bronchial asthma and the asthma that accompanies emphysema in neurotic subjects it should be remembered. While the distress is constant, it is subject to periods of aggravation. It will be of service in this class of subjects when hay-fever is the diagnosis.

It should be studied in case of acute uraemia, when it will relieve the convulsions, and in acute diffuse nephritis, when their are indications of oedema of the gastro-intestinal mucous membrane, and the urine is greatly decreased in quantity or wholly suppressed. This may be dependent upon exposure to cold or to an embarrassed activity of the skin following extensive burns.

In these cases a two-grain powder of the third decimal every half hour to every hour will be of service.

In the chronic type of uraemia when the urea is low and the patient suffers from the effects of the its retention its administration for a time will frequently bring the urea up to normal.

In delirium and tremor cordis it is frequently of service. There are pronounced variations of both-the cardiac rhythm and force, without any abnormal findings on percussion or auscultation. If the urine is observed for a time, defective elimination will be found.

It should be studied in cases of neuralgia of the abdominal viscera.

Compare: Arsenicum album, Cantharis, Cuprum. *(Blackwood)*

238. *Cuprum Met*

(Copper)

Spasmodic affections, cramps, convulsions beginning in fingers and toes, violent, contractive, and intermittent pains are some of the marked expressions of the action of Cuprum and its curative range therefore includes tonic and clonic spasms, convulsions, and epileptic attacks. Chorea brought on by fright. Nausea greater than in any other remedy. In epilepsy aura begining at knees, ascends to hypogastrium, followed by unconsciousness, foaming and falling. Symptoms disposed to appear periodically and in groups. Complaints — in left side (Lachesis). Tape worm (Colloidal Cuprum 3x).

Where eruptions strike in, as in scarlet fever, complaints may result, such as excessive vomiting, stupor, convulsions, which come within the sphere of this remedy. The pains are increased by movement and touch.

Face: Bluish - Contraction of Jaws - foam at mouth.

Mouth: Strong metallic copper slimy taste with flow of saliva - constant protrution and retraction of the tongue like a snake - when drinking the fluid, the fluid descends with gurgling sound abdomen contracted, colic, violent and intermittent, intussusception.

Stool: Cholera, with cramps in abdomen and calves.

Respiratory: suffocative attacks worse 3 a.m. (Am-c.), spasm and constriction of chest. Spasmodic asthma alternating with spasmodic vomiting, whooping cough, better, swallowing water - cramps in calves and soles.

Epilepsy: Epilepsy, aura begins in knees. Clenched thumbs.

Skin: Skin blush chronic psoriasis and lepra *(Hughes)*

Modalities: *Worse* before menses; from vomiting, contact. Better during perspiration, drinking cold water.

Relationship: Copper is found in Dulcamara, Cuprum sulph in 1-3% Sol. in inoperable Sarcoma - Cuprum cyanatum. (meningitis basilaris); Cholas terrapina (cramps in calves and feet; rheumatism, with cramp-like pains); Plumb.; Nux; Veratr. Cuprum oxydatum nigrum 1x (all kinds of worms, including tape-worms and trichinosis according to Zopfy's 60 years' experience).

Dose: 6-30c *(Boericke)*

It is this power to relieve internal spasm which renders it appropriate to the collapse stage of cholera, of which it is also like Sulphur, a prophylactic either when worn next to the skin or taken internally.

Mossa regards Cupr. as one of the remedies for the effects of fright and relates the case of a girl, who after a fright was affected by involuntary motions of left arm and leg developing into pronounced general chorea.

'Schwencke' cured a case of epilepsy of forty years standing with Cupr. after Bell. and Hyo. had done some little good. The patient was aged 45. The fits began suddenly towards morning with chewing motion of lower jaw, gnashing of teeth, becomes upright and rigid in bed; shrieks, attacks become more severe, arms and legs were thrown outwards and trunk arched upwards. Cupr. was now given. For a time the attacks continued severely, but gradually improvement set in and in less than three months they ceased altogether. The anger in this case and the ill-humour in Mossa's are noteworthy.

Is antidoted by sugar or white of egg mixed with milk and given freely. Hepar or Potash soap may be used after poisoning from food prepared in copper vessels.

Causation: Suppression or fright.

(JHC)

239. *Curare*

(Woorari-Arrow poison)

Muscular paralysis without impairing sensation and consciousness. Paralysis of respiratory muscles. Reflex action diminished. Debility of the aged (Baryta) and from loss of fluids. Catalepsy. Nervous debility Trismus (Tetanic spasm of jaw muscle) Glycosuria with motor Paralysis.

Curare decreases the output of Adrenalin. Vomiting of bile in cirrhosis of liver. Diabetes Mellitus 4th dilution (Dr. Burkhard.)

Head: Ptosis of right side.

Ears: Swelling of lobes of ear.

Face: Facial and buccal paralysis. Tongue and mouth drawn to right. Red face.

Respiratory: Threatened paralysis of respiration on falling asleep.

Short breath, short dry cough, provokes vomiting, followed by fainting. Chest sore to pressure. Very distressing dyspnoea.

Arms: Weak, heavy, cannot lift the fingers. Weakness of hands and fingers in pianists - favours development of Corns.

Relations: Curare antidotes strychnin.

Dose: 6-30 *(Boericke)*

A condition resembling catalepsy has been induced by it, immobility with fixed gaze on waking - Two cases of diabetes in middle aged men have been cured by 'Burkhard' with Cur. 4. Its relation to hydrophobia and Tetanus is probably antipathic - if the poisoning is due to punctured wound rubbing in tobacco or salt will neutralise it. In yellow-brown spots on skin. (Sep., Lyc., Nux-v., Sul.) *(JHC)*

An arrow poison prepared by the savages of South America and is of indefinite origin.

This remedy is indicated when there is depression of the motor nervous structures. In the nervous debility of the aged, numbness of the arms as if a weight was hung to them. It is of service in the paralysis of respiration, the breath stopping on falling asleep.

Paralytic dyspnoea and pulmonary emphysema are also benefitted by its use. It has rendered some service in leprosy when the skin presents a dirty appearance. The blood oozes from the skin.

There are tubercles on the nose, with loss of hair and teeth and swelling of the lobes of the ear with discharges of pus.

Compare: Conium, Gelsemium, Causticum. (Blackwood)

240. *Cyclamen*

(Sor bread)

Large doses produce violent purging and vomiting. Disturbed digestion with very salty saliva. Anaemic and chlorotic conditions. Affections of Uterus. Gastro-intestinal and genito-urinary tracts affected, including secondary anaemia and various reflexes, sleepiness, moroseness and lassitude, cough at night while asleep, without waking especially in children. (Cham., Nit. ac.)

Grives over duty neglected, depression with weeping, desire to be alone - flickering before eyes. Sneezing with itching in ears, dim vision, worse on waking with spots before eyes - flickering of various colors. Sees countless stars. Disturbance of vision associated with gastric disturbances - Salty taste - Worse fat food - Diarrhoea after every cup of coffee - Hiccough. Satiety after a few mouthfuls - Disgust to meat especially pork - desire for lemonade - no thirst all day - Pain about anus and perineum as if a spot were suppurating when walking or sitting - Menses profuse, black, membranous, clotted, too early, with labor like pains from back to pubes - flow less when moving about. Menstrual irregularities with megrim and blindness or fiery spots before eyes. Hiccough during pregnancy - after menses swelling of breasts with milky secretion. Pain in parts where bones lie near surface - burning, sore-pain heels. Cramp like contraction of right thumb and index finger - Acne in young women, pruritus better scratching and appearance of menses.

Worse: Open air, evening, sitting, standing and cold water.

Better: During menstrual flow, by moving about, rubbing parts in warm room, lemonade.

Dose: 3rd attenuation. *(Boericke)*

Cyclamen has a traditional reputation as a remedy for affections of the uterus and appendages - It is in many ways analogous to Pulsatilla from which it differs mainly in having no amel from open air, and in not having thirstlessness as so frequent an accompaniment of other conditions.

It is suited to the phlegmatic temperament, blonde, leucophlegmatic subjects with chlorotic conditions, disinclined for labour and easily fatigued; special senses enfeebled or their functions suspended. Debility, torpidity of mind and body - Squint especially in connection with menstrual irregularities or fevers, after convulsions, convergent squint, left eye drawn inwards - Suppressed skin eruption causing to amenorrhoea and partial blindness. *(JHC)*

241. Cypripedium

(Yellow lady's slipper)

The skin symptoms correspond to those of poisoning by Rhus for which it has been found an efficient antidote. Nervousness in children from teething and intestinal trouble. Debility after gout - Hydrocephaloid symptoms, result of long exhausting diarrhoea, sleeplessness. Cerebral hyperaesthesia in young children often the result of overstimulation of brain.

Child cries out at night, is wakeful and begins to laugh and play.

Dose: Tr. to 6c. *(Boericke)*

Cupr. has great repute as a nervine among eclectics and in domestic practice, it ranks with Scutellaria and Valerian. A strong infusion causes exhilaration followed by calmness and is much resorted to by women whose nerves are shattered by long illness or excessive indulgence in tea or coffee. *(JHC)*

Mother tincture of the fresh root, and dilutions.

This remedy is indicated in despondency, in mild cases of delirium tremens, debility, sleepiness, reflex epilepsy, and in cases of spermatorrhoea. When this mental condition is present there is profound indifference to everything, even to his studies, duties and common courtesies of life, inability to study, think or listen to lectures.

It is used in reflex convulsions occurring in children of an excitable, nervous temperament, or where there is functional irritation of the brain, which renders the child sleepless, even at night. The child's disposition is very changeable, being playful at one moment and irritable and fretful the next. It should be thought of in cases of teething or of intestinal irritation.

There is sleeplessness. With restlessness of the body and twitching of the limbs; she desires to talk, pleasant ideas constantly crowding on the mind.

Compare: Scutellaria, Valeriana, Ignatia)

(Blackwood)

242. *Daphne Indica*

(Spurgelaurel)

Acts on lower tissues, muscles, bones and skin, sudden lightening jerks in different parts of the body - craving for tobacco. Burning in stomach, parts of the body feel separated (Bapt). Fetid breath, urine, sweat.

Head: Feels as if skull would burst - as if head were separated from body -

Mouth: Tongue coated on one side only (Rhus).

Urine: urine thick, turbid, yellowish, like rotten eggs.

Sleep: Absolute inability to sleep, some times caused by aching of bones. Dreams with nightmare - Dreams of cats, black cats.

Dose: 1 to 6c. *(Boericke)*

Its pains are erratic and electric-like. It is like 'FAMBOS' in the craving for tobacco - Swaying sensation in the head when walking - Sensation as if the vertex were screwed up in a vice - Sensation as if the arms were detached from the body, yet they are under complete control of the will.

Agg: From tobacco. *(JHC)*

This remedy is indicated in cases of mercurio - syphilitica affections where the muscles, bones, and skin are involved. The head feels distended as if it would burst, or as if it were separated from the body. There are rheumatic pains in the feet, thighs, and knees which shift from place to place.

Compare: Mezereum, Aurum metallicum.

(Blackwood)

243. *Digitalis*

(Fox glove)

Comes into play in all diseases, where the heart is primarily involved, where the pulse is weak, irregular, intermittent, abnormally slow and dropsy of external and internal parts. Weakness and dilatation of the myocardium. It greatest indication is in failure of compensation and especially when auricular fibrillation has set in. Slow pulse in recumbent posture, but irregular and dicrotic on sitting up. Auricular flutter and fibrillation especially when subsequent to rheumatic fever. Heart block, very slow pulse. Other symptoms of organic heart disease, such as great weakness and sinking of strength, faintness, coldness of skin, and irregular respiration; cardiac irritability and occular troubles after tobacco; jaundice from induration and hypertrophy of the liver frequently calls for digitalis. Jaundice with heart disease; faint as if dying, bluish appearance of face. Cardiac muscular failure when a systole is present, stimulates the heart muscles, increases force of systole, increases length. Prostration from slight exertion, collapse.

Mind: Anxious, Melancholic, dull, lethargic with slow pulse.

Eyes: Changes in acuteness of perception of shades of green.

Stomach: Excessive nausea, great weakness in stomach, faintness, tenderness of epigastrium, copious salivation, neuralgic pain in stomach, enlarged sore painful liver.

Stool: White chalk like, ashy pasty stools.

Urine: As if a straw was being thrust back and forth - urethritis.

Male: Nightly emission, with great weakness of genitals after coitus, hydrocele, scrotum enlarged like a bladder, gonorrhoea, balanitis (Merc), dropsical swelling of genitals.

Respiratory: Desire to take a deep breath, breathing irregular, difficult, deep sighing, cough with raw, sore feeling in chest. Expectoration sweetish. Senile pneumonia. Great weakness in chest. Dyspnoea, constant desire to breathe freely; lungs feel compressed; chronic bronchitis, passive congestion of the lungs, giving bloody sputum due to failing myocardium. Cannot bear to talk. Haemoptysis with weak heart.

Heart: Irregular heart especially of mitral disease. Very slow pulse. Intermits, weak, cyanosis. Inequality of pulse, it varies, sudden sensation as if heart stood still. Pulse weak and quickened by least movement.

Extremities: Swelling of the feet. Fingers go to sleep easily. Sensation in legs as if a red hot wire suddenly darted through them. *(Dudgeon)*

Sleep: Starts from sleep in alarm, that he is falling from a height.

Skin: Blue distended veins on lids ears, lips, and tongue. Dropsical itching and jaundice.

Modalities: Worse when sitting erect, after measles and music.

Better When stomach is empty in open air.

Relation: *Adonis, Crataegus (a true heart tonic), Kalmia, Spigel, Liatris - Convallaria* (Heart disease with vertigo and digestive disturbances.)

Dose: 3-30 will bring about reaction, when the drug is homoeopathically indicated, but for palliative purposes the physiological dosage is required. (For this purpose the tincture made from the fresh plant in doses of 5-20 drops, when the cardiac stimulation is desired) (The infusion of 1½% dose ½ to 1 oz if the diuretic action is wanted). The tincture may be given on sugar or bread and nothing liquid be taken for 20 minutes before or after its administration of the powdered leaves 1½ to 2 grains in capsules Digitoxin 1-250 grain. No matter what form of Digitalin is given, the dose should be reduced as soon as the pulse rate has been lowered to 80 beats in minute and the normal rhythm has been partially or completely restored. Under such conditions a good rule is to cut the dose in ½ and still more, if there be sudden falling of the urinary output. *(Boericke)*

Sensation as if heart would stop beating if she moved (Cocaine - fears that unless constantly on the move heart will cease beating).

Pulse full, irregular, very slow and weak, intermitting every third, fifth or seventh beat.

Aggravation: When sitting, especially when sitting erect, motion. *(HC. Allen)*

Heart stimulant - Pulse is slow or irregular - There may be a condition of cyanosis present - Cold, clammy sweat - Heart is dilated - tired heart - pulse is slow and feeble - cardiac dropsy - anasarca -

patient cannot lie down and is obliged to sit up. The jugular veins are distended - urine is scanty. Mitral regurgitation - aortic valve - pneumonia and chronic bronchitis in the aged - blueness of the skin - eye lids, lips and tongue - renal congestion, nephritis and post scarlatinal dropsy - jaundice - passive congestion of the liver - nocturnal emissions - great weakness of the genital organs. Compare - Strophanthus, Kalmia latifolia, Arsenicum album, Sparteine. *(Blackwood)*

244. *Dioscorea Villosa*

(Wild yam)

As a remedy for many kinds of pain especially colic and in severe, painful affections of abdominal and pelvic visera; it ranks with the polychrests of the Materia Medica. Persons of feeble digestive powers, tea drinkers with much flatulence - Gall stone colic.

Sinking at the pit of the stomach - pain along sternum and extending into arms - hiccough - relieved by standing erect.

Abdomen: Pains suddenly shift to different parts, appear in remote localities as fingers and toes. Sharp pains from liver, shooting upward to right nipple - feeble action of heart.

Male: Relaxation and coldness of organs - strong smelling sweat - emission in sleep - with weak knees.

Modalities: *Worse* evening and night, lying down and doubling up - *Better* standing erect, motion, in open air, pressure.

Dose: Tr. to 3rd pot. *(Boericke)*

'Burt', who made a heroic proving of this remedy says the grand sphere for the use of Dioscorea is among neurosis of the bowels and stomach, where the coeliac and umbilical plexuses are in a state of great hyperaesthesia. The pain and spasm being unbearable. 'Hale' considers as characteristic a constant pain aggravated at regular intervals by paroxysms of intense suffering Any kind of colic or neuralgia with these characteristics may indicate Dioscor. Dioscor causes pain in the bowels, spasmodic twisting, writhing, drawing, lancinating, pulsating, burning, pains radiate upward and downward - frequent, sharp, darting pains from one part to another. *(JHC)*

Flatulence after meals, after eating, especially tea-drinkers are often subject to violent colic. *(HC Allen)*

Bilious colic, gall stones, the pain is made worse by bending forward and lying down, and is relieved by standing up and bending backward. Cholera morbus, cholera infantum, neuralgic dysmenorrhoea, and ovarian neuralgia - seminal emissions, lustful dreams of women. *(Blackwood)*

245. *Diphtherinum*

(Potentized Diphtheritic virus)

Adapted to patients prone to catarrhal affections of respiratory organs, scrofulous individuals. Diphtheria, laryngeal diphtheria, post-diphtheritic paralysis. Malignancy from the start, glands swollen, tongue red, swollen; breath and discharge very offensive. Diphtheritic membrane thick, dark. Epistaxis, profound prostration, swallows without pain, but fluids are vomited or returned by the nose.

Dose: 30-200 or C.M. Potency. Must not be repeated too frequently.

(Boericke)

The well known features of the disease of which this nosode is a product must be the guide to its use. It should be more efficacious in the potencies against diphtheria, both as prophylactic and cure, than the serum injections. In all probability, it will be found useful in the paralysis of diphtheria and other like kinds of spinal affections. It needs clinical development and a proving in the potencies. *(JHC)*

246. *Dolichos Pruriens*

(Cowhage)

A right sided medicine, with pronounced liver and skin symptoms. A general intense itching without eruption. Exalted nervous sensibility, senile pruritus. Haemorrhoidal diathesis.

Pain in throat, worse swallowing, below right angle of jaw, as if splinter were imbedded vertically. Pains in gums prevents sleep.

Colic from getting feet wet. Constipation with intense itching, bloated abdomen white stools. Swelling of liver - haemorrhoids with burning sensation.

Intense itching with no swelling or rash, worse across shoulders, also about elbows and knees and hairy parts. Jaundice. Yellow in spots; itching excessively at night. Herpes zoster (Ars.).

Modalities: Worse at night, scratching, right side.

Relation: Rhus t., Bell., Hep., Nit ac., Fagopyr.

Dose: 6th potency, Tincture drop doses in Haemorrhoids. *(Boericke)*

The most characteristic symptoms of Dolichos are - a general intense itching without eruption *agg:* by scratching and a pain in the throat on right side below angle of jaw as if a splinter were embedded vertically in it. Cold water burns on the itching skin. *(JHC)*

This remedy is indicated when there is an intense itching over the body without any visible eruption - it relieves the itching that attends jaundice. It is of service in constipation when there is an intense itching of the skin, a distended abdomen and dark coloured stools. *(Blackwood)*

247. *Doryphora*

(Colorado Potato - Bug)

The centre of this drug's action seems to be in the urinary organs and hence its employment in gonorrhoea and gleet. Urethritis in children from local irritation and gleet. Great trembling in extremities. Prostration, swelling of body. Burning sensation. Urinary difficult micturition. Urethra inflamed with excruciating pain when urinating. Pain in back and loins severe trembling in limbs.

Relation: Antidote - Stram.

Dose: 6-30. *(Boericke)*

Doryphora in its general effects bears a strong resemblance to Cantharis. An extensive proving has been made and to this have been added the effects of poisoning from handling the insects, and from inhaling the vapour, when they have been burned or scalded. Like Canth, Doryphoa produces burning in mouth, throat, gullet, stomach, abdomen, rectum, and urinary passages, strangury, urethritis and itching, burning, and inflammation of glans penis. *(JHC)*

This remedy is indicated in urethritis. There is difficult micturition, the urethra is inflamed and the passage of the urine is painful; there is pain in the lumbar region, trembling of the extremities and great prostration.

Compare: Cantharis, Apis mel.

(Blackwood)

248. *Drosera*

(Sundew)

Affects markedly the respiratory organs and was pointed out by Hahnemann as the principal remedy for whooping cough. Drosera can break down resistance to tubercle and should therefore be capable of raising it (Dr. Tyler). Laryngeal phthisis is benefitted by it. Phthisis pulmonum, vomiting of food from coughing with gastric irritation and profuse expectoration. Pains about the hip joint. Tubercular glands.

Respiratory organs: Spasmodic, dry irritative cough, like whooping cough, the paroxysms follow each other very rapidly; can scarcely breathe; chokes. Cough very deep and hoarse, worse after midnight; yellow expectoration with bleeding from nose and mouth, retching, deep hoarse voice, hoarseness.

Harassing and titillating cough in children - not all through the day, but commences as soon as the head touches the pillow at night.

Asthma when talking, with contraction of throat at every word uttered.

Modalities: *Worse* after midnight, lying down, on getting warm in bed, drinking, singing, laughing.

Compare: Chelid., Corall., Cupr., Causanea, Argent., Meny.

Dose: First to 12th attenuation.

(Boericke)

Teste who places Drosera in his Zincum group of medicines, mentions that it grows in damp priaries, along the border of marshes and is avoided by animals. Barrish states that when eaten by sheep it gives them a cough, which is fatal to them. Teste refers to the fact sheep eating Drosera leaves acquire a nocturnal cough and die and that the pleurae of cats to which Drosera had been administered were found studded with tubercles.

"Buchmann of Alvensleben" agrees with Hahnemann that "Dros" in high attenuation should not be repeated. *(JHC)*

This agent is an antispasmodic, sedative and expectorant. Its action is upon the respiratory organs, where it produces a dry, irritating, spasmodic cough.

Spasmodic, explosive cough, with dryness of the air passages - Pertussis - the cough is deep, hoarse and worse after midnight.

Irritating cough of children beginning as soon as their head reaches the pillow, sore throat of clergymen. Laryngeal phthisis.

Compare: Naphthalin, Mephitis.

(Blackwood)

249. *Duboisia*

(Cork wood Elm)

Acts chiefly on the nervous system, eyes, upper respiratory tract. Recommended in pharyngitis sicca, with black, stringy mucus. It dilates the pupils, dries the mouth, checks perspiration, causes headache and drowsiness. On the eyes it acts more promptly than atropia, much stronger as a Mydriatic. Red spot floats in the field of vision. Sensation as if stepping on empty space. Vertigo with pale face, not gastric in origin. Scarlet fever, locomotor ataxia, palliative in exophthalmic goitre.

Mind: Silly and nonsensical.

Eyes: Conjunctivitis, Mydriasis, pain over eyes.

Dose: 3 to 12 potency. *(Boericke)*

Duboisia belongs to the same order as Belladonna and its alkaloid. Sulphate of Duboisia has been used as a substiture for Atropine. Its application to the eye has caused marked constitutional symptoms of fever, delirium, stupor and dry mouth. A symptom which may prove a key note is red spot floating in the field of vision. Dryness of mucous membranes is very characteristic - cold feeling in the eyes. Sensation as if stepping on empty space. Anhalonium. (Coloured vision) *(JHC)*

250. Dulcamara

(Bitter sweet)

Hot days and cold nights, towards the close of summer are especially favourable to the action of Dulcamara and is one of the remedies that correspond to their symptoms to the conditions found as effects of damp weather, colds after exposure to wet, especially diarrhoea. It has a specific relation also to the skin, glands and digestive organs, mucus membranes secreting more profusely while the skin is inactive. The rheumatic trouble induced by damp cold are aggravated by every cold change and some what relieved by moving about. Results from sitting on cold, damp ground. Icy coldness. One sided spasms, with sleeplessness. Paralysis of single parts. Congestive headache with neuralgia and dry nose. Patients living or working in damp, cold basements (Nat. sulph.) Eruption on hands, arms or face around the menstrual period.

Head: Scald head, thick brown crusts.

Nose: Stuff up when there is a cold rain.

Face: Tearing in cheek extending to ear, orbit and jaw, preceded by coldness of parts and attended by canine hunger. Humid eruption on cheeks and face generally.

Mouth: Facial neuralgia, worse slightest exposure to cold.

Stomach: Aversion to food, burning thirst for cold drinks.

Abdomen: Cutting pain about navel, swelling of inguinal glands.

Stool: Green, watery, slimy, bloody, mucus from damp cold weather.

Urine: Must urinate when getting chilled - urine has thick mucus, purulent sediment.

Female: Before appearance of menses a rash appears on skin or sexual excitement.

Respiratory: Cough after physical exertion.

Back: Stiff neck, pain in small of back as after long stooping, stiffness and lameness across the neck and shoulders after getting cold and wet.

Extremities: Feet icy cold, warts on hands. Perspiration on palms of hands. Rheumatic symptoms after acute skin eruptions.

Skin: Adenitis, Pruritis, always worse in cold wet weather, urticaria, brought on by exposure or sour stomach - warts large, smooth, on face and palmar surface of hands.

Modalities: Worse at night, from cold in general, damp rainy weather.

Better from moving about external warmth.

Dose: 2-30 *(Boericke)*

This feature among others renders them all good antidotes to mercurius - Baryta carb is the complement of Dulcamara.

(JHC)

251. *Echinacea*

(Purple Gone - Flower)

We are indebted to the Eclectic school for this remarkable medicine as a Corrector of blood dyscrasia'. Acute auto infection. Symptoms of blood poisoning, septic conditions generally. Diarrhoea in typhoid. Gonorrhoea, boils, erysipelas and foul ulcers. Gangrane goitre with exophthalmic symptoms, full doses, also injecting 5-10 drops into Thyroid gland. Tendency to malignancy in acute and subacute disorders. Last stages of cancer to ease pain. Venom infections. Cerebro-spinal meningitis. Puerperal infection. Tired feeling. Piles. Pustules. Acts on vermiform appendix thus has been used for appendicitis, but it promotes suppuration and a neglected appendicitis with pus formation would probably rupture sooner under its use. Lymphatic inflammation, crushing injuries, snake bites and stings generally. Foul discharges with emaciation and great debility.

Dose: Tr 1 to 10 drops every two hours and larger doses. *(Boericke)*

The closest analogue of Ech. is Baptisia. In snake bites it compares with Lobelia purpurascens. In boils with Anthracin.

(JHC)

This agent poduces warmth and tingling of the parts over which it passes. The flow of saliva is augmented, and the secretions from the glands in general are stimulated, and digestion is improved, defective metabolism is corrected and nutrition is improved under its influence. Larger doses produce a drowsiness with mental dullness, and severe headache. The tongue is coated white, the desire for food is lessened. There is a general lassitude with aching, alternate chills and flashes of heat over the body. The skin takes on an unhealthy condition.

This remedy is indicated in cases of blood poisoning and septic conditions. They may be the result of an auto-infection, defective elimination or from poisons introduced from without.

It is indicated in typhoid, septic, and puerperal fevers, when there are flashes of heat and chilliness over the back. The patient is profoundly prostrated. There is headache with periodical flushing of the face.

It is useful in uraemic poisoning, the urine is scanty, contains albumin, and all the symptoms of uraemic poisoning are present.

In diphtheria, stomatitis materna, ulcerated sore throat and post-nasal catarrhs, it is used both locally and internally.

In bed sores, chronic ulcerations, glandular indurations, furuncles and carbuncles, it is of service both locally and internally.

Compare: Baptisia, Arsenicum, Rhus-t., Hepar., Calcarea sulphurica. (Blackwood)

252. *Elaps Corallinus*

(Coral - Snake)

Similar to snake poisons generally. Has a very marked black discharge. Cold things disagree. Desire for sweetened butter milk. Nausea and vomiting. Prostrating diarrhoea of consumption. Acidity of stomach with faint feeling. Sudden pain in stomach. Spasm of oesophagus. Pharynx constricted; food and liquids suddenly arrested and then fall heavily into stomach. Spasms followed by paresis. Cold feeling in stomach, fruits and ice water lie very cold. Right sided paralysis. Must have oscillatory motion. Rheumatic constitutions. Ear, nose and throat symptoms important.

Mind: Fear of rain; can speak but cannot understand speech.

Ears: Cerumen black and hard with difficult hearing or serous greenish discharge, offensive, buzzing and illusion of hearing.

Nose: Chronic nasal catarrh with fetid odor and greenish crusts, nostrils stopped up.

Chest: Coldness in chest after drinking - stitches in apex of right lung.

Stomach: Feels cold.

Modalities: *Worse* eating fruit, cold drinks, wet weather.

Dose: 6-30. *(Boericke)*

Elaps is distinguished from the other serpent venoms, by the prominent blackness of its discharges and haemorrhages, black ear wax - I cured with Elaps 200 very old standing case of irritating rash in axilla (right) with recurrent suppuration of axillary glands - dreams of dead person. *(JHC)*

A snake found in Brazil, of the family Ophidia. This remedy is indicated in violent headaches which are felt first in the left, then in the right eye, and extend fiom the forehead to the occiput. Also when there are pains in the ears with sudden deafness, with roaring and cracking in the ears at night.

It is useful in nasal catarrh and ozaena when there are dry plugs and mucus in the nose. There is cough and haemoptysis. The blood is black and there are severe pains through the lungs, and a sensation of coldness of the chest.

Compare: Lachesis, Colchicum.

(Blackwood)

253. *Elaterium*

(Squirting cucumber)

This is an invaluable remedy in violent vomiting and purging especially if the evacuations are copious and watery. It is a very efficient remedy in certain forms of dropsy. Much yawning and stretching, ("Beriberi"), choleraic conditions, urticaria and mental disorders coming on as a consequence of suppressed malaria. Irresistable desire to wander from home at night. Effects of damp weather.

Stool: Watery, copious, forceful squirting diarrhoea, frothing, olive green, with cutting in abdomen.

Fever: Chill comes on with much yawning and stretching, lasting all through chill. Pain in extremities, darting into fingers and toes. Chills and fever with spurting diarrhoea.

Modalities: *Worse* from exposure on damp ground.

Compare: Bry., Croton., Gambogia.

Dose: 3-30.

As a hydragogue cathartic to produce free discharges in dropsies - Elaterin - 1-20, grain (palliative only.) *(Boericke)*

The signature of Elat. is too obvious to be missed. Profuse watery stools, coming out with a gush, which is the main characteristic of the drug is plainly typified in the explosion, by means of which the ripe fruit scatters its seeds. The property of Elat to cause draining of the tissues of their water contents has been used to cause the absorption of dropsical fluids. Minute doses will often effect this. Elat promotes the opening of abscesses and boils. *(JHC)*

254. *Epigea Repens*

(Trailing Arbutus)

Chronic cystitis with dysuria, tenesmus after micturition, muco-pus and uric acid deposit, gravel, renal calculi. Fine sand in urine of a brown color. Burning in neck of bladder whilst urinating and tenesmus afterward. Pyelitis, incontinence of urine, croaking noise and rumbling in bowels.

Dose: Tr. in 5 drop doses every 3 hours. *(Boericke)*

Hale mentions Epigea as having been a popular remedy in renal calculi throughout the United States ever since the settlement. It has been successful in removing dysuria and strangury as well as urinary tenesmus.

Hale once gave to a patient who had a bloody muco purulent sediment in the urine with intense dysuria. 10 drops of the tincture 6 times a day. A copious deposit of fine brown sand was observed and all symptoms were relieved.

255. *Epihysterinum*

(A nosode)

This is one of Dr. Burnett's nosodes, used by him in cases of haemorrhage and obtained as I conclude, from a case of haemorrhage in a patient suffering from fibrous tumour, possibly with malignant elements. At any rate, I have found it of great value in controlling uterine haemorrhage, whether connected with fibrous growth or not. I have used it in the 30th upwards giving one or two doses weekly.

Compare: In fibrous tumours and uterine haemorrhages - Thlaspi Bursa Pastoris, Fraxinus. A, Hydrastis and its alkaloids. *(JHC).*

A nosode from the tissues of fibroid tumor of uterus, possibly with malignant elements.

Symptoms: Uterine haemorrhage, whether connected with fibrous growth or not. *(B. K. Sarkar) Calcutta*

256. *Epiphegus*

(Beech drop)

A remedy for sick, neurasthenic and nervous headaches, especially in women brought on or made worse by exertion, shopping etc. Tongue coated yellow, bitter taste. Drowsy after meals. Loose stools. Subinvolution, with painful menstruation and congestion.

Head: Pressing pain in temples from within outwards, worse left side.

Viscid salivation, constant inclination to spit. Sick headache coming on when deviating from ordinary pursuits. Headaches from nerve tire caused by mental or physical exhaustion preceeded by hunger.

Modalities: Worse from working in open air. Better from sleep.

Dose: 1-30c. *(Boericke)*

A slender branching herb without leaves, of a dull purple or yellow brown colour, growing as a parasite on the roots of beech-trees. Tincture of whole fresh plant in full flower.

A very characteristic symptom is, constantly want to spit, saliva viscid when this symptom occurs in connection with a headache Epiphegus will almost certainly cure.

I have cured with it many cases of headache, some of them desperately severe. The conditions are *agg:* from working in open air; from rising up in bed amel: from a good sleep. *(JHC)*

257. *Equisetum*

(Scouring rush)

Principal action on the bladder. A remedy for enuresis and dysuria.

Frequent urging with severe pain at the close of urination. Urine flows only drop by drop, sharp burning, cutting pain in urethra while urinating.

Relation: *Hydrangea, Ferrum phos, Apis, Canth., Linaria, Chimaph.* Equisetum contains Silica in appreciable quantity.

Dose: Tr. to 6th potency. A decoction, teaspoonful doses or the tincture in hot water is found useful to allay irritability of urinary tract, calculus, dysuria, etc., also for pleuritic effusion and dropsy. (Boericke)

Enuresis-wets bed at night, when he dreams he always sees a crowd of people. Linaria has enuresis with frequent painful urging to urinate, causing the patient to rise at night. (Farrington) *(JHC)*

Enuresis, diurnaet. Nocturna, profuse watery urine, where habit is the only ascertainable cause. *(HCA)*

258. *Erechthites*

(Fireweed)

Haemorrhages are caused and cured by this remedy. Persistent haemorrhage from the bladder. Haemorrhage from any part especially lungs, always attended by excitement of the circulation. Flashes of heat and coldness. Scanty urine. Oedema of extremities.

Skin: Symptoms like Rhus poisoning.

Relation: Erig, Millef., Ham., Rhus t.

Dose: Tincture - Locally for poison oak.

(Boericke)

Fire weed so called, because it grows abundantly in clearing which have been burnt out and has been used empirically in haemorrhages; especially, metrorrhagia, and as a local application in skin affections, herpes, eczema, psoriasis, and indolent ulcers. Another marked feature is increased appetite and also increased feeling of strength and desire for exercise. According to "Hale" oil of fire weed is also extracted from `Erigeron' and is said by chemists to be identical with Turpentine. All three cause active and passive haemorrhages, the former being the primary and the latter the secondary action.

259. *Erigeron*
(Fleabane)

Haemorrhages are caused and cured by this remedy. Persistent haemorrhage from the bladder. Haemorrhage from the uterus with painful micturition. Profuse bright red blood. Pain in left ovary and hip. Chronic gonorrhoea, with burning micturition, continual dribbling.

Dysentery, with soreness and burning in bladder. Tympanites.

Female: Metrorrhagia with violent irritation of rectum and bladder and prolapsus uteri. Bright red flow. Menorrhagia, profuse Leucorrhoea; bloody lochia returns after least motion, comes in gushes, between periods. leucorrhoea with urinary irritation, pregnant women with weak uterus, a bloody discharge with slight exertion. Bleeding haemorrhoids, nose bleed instead of menses. (Bry)

Modalities: Worse left side.

Relation: Terebinthina.

Dose: Tr. to 3rd potency. Oil of Erigeron 1x internally for tympanitis. An enema of one dram of the oil with the yolk of an egg and pint of milk will reduce the most enormous tympanities. *(Boericke)*

260. *Eriodictyon*
(Yerba Santa)

A remedy for asthmatic and bronchial affections. Bronchial phthisis, with night sweats and emaciation. Asthma relieved by expectoration. Cough after influenza. Further absorption of effusion in pleural cavity. Appetite poor and impaired digestion Whooping cough.

Respiratory: Wheezing asthma with coryza and mucus secretions. Dull pain in right lung. Burning in fauces. Chronic bronchitis, bronchial tuberculosis with profuse easily raised, bronchial secretion giving relief.

Relation. Grind Aral, Eucalyptus, Ipec.

Dose: Tr. In doses 2 to 20 drops and attenuation. *(Boericke)*

Eriodictyon, says Allen, has a strong Terebenthine taste and abounds in a Resinon matter which sometimes exudes so copiously that in drying the specimens stick firmly together and to the paper. "Yerba Santa" (Holy plant) is a popular expectorant remedy in Mexico and California. By Homoeopaths it has been chiefly used in pthisical condition especially bronchial phthisis. Asthmatic breathing with accumulation of mucus, the asthma being relieved when the mucus is got rid of. *(JHC)*

This remedy is indicated in chronic bronchitis, bronchial tuberculosis and asthma, when these are attended with a profuse, easily raised bronchial secretion which brings relief. It has relieved the cough that remained as a sequela of influenza. There is usually a thickening of the bronchial mucous membrane. The appetite is poor and the digestion is impaired.

Compare: Eucalyptus, Grindelia robusta. *(Blackwood)*

261. *Eryngium Aquaticum*
(Button Snake Root)

A remedy for urinary disorders. Strangury etc. with nervous erethism. Thick yellow mucus discharges. Influenza, uridrosis, sweat of urinous odor in evening.

Dose: Tr. to 3rd potency.

(Boericke)

Eryngium acts on the mucus membranes producing thick yellow mucous discharges from eyes, ears, nose, mouth, bowels, urethra and vagina. Haemorrhage from stomach and bowels. *(JHC)*

It is of service in urethritis, when there is a thick, yellow discharge, with difficult urination, and spasmodic stricture, and pain behind the pubes, and in cases where there is an escape of the prostatic fluid from the slightest provocation.

Compare: Conium, Cannabis sativa, Clematis. *(Blackwood)*

262. *Eschscholtzia Californica*

(California poppy)

Experiments upon animals showed it to act more powerfully than morphine which is contained in the plant. It causes general weakness, torpor, accelerated respiration, complete paralysis of the limbs. Slowing of circulation.

A soporific remedy which is harmless.

Use the tincture. *(Boericke)*

263. *Eucalyptus Globulus*

(Blue gum tree)

Eucalyptus is a powerful antiseptic and destructive to low forms of life, a stimulating expectorant and an efficient diaphoretic. Atonic dyspepsia, gastric and intestinal catarrh. A remedy with marked effects on catarrhal processes, malaria and intestinal disturbance. Influenza. Fever of relapsing character. Produces diuresis and great increase of urea. Haemorrhages internally and locally (Hamam). Typhoid. Symptoms of exhaustion and toxaemia. Conditions of the mucous surfaces of the air passages, genito-urinary organs and gastro-intestinal tract. A gastro intestinal irritant with pain in stomach and upper intestines, several hours after eating.

Head: Coryza.

Nose: Stuffed up sensation, then watery coryza. Nose does not stop running. Tightness across bridge, chronic catarrhal purulent and fetid discharge.

Throat: Enlarged, ulcerated tonsils and inflamed throat - use tincture locally.

Stomach: Slow digestion, much fetid gas.

Abdomen: Acute diarrhoea, dysentery.

Urine: Acute nephritis, complicating influenza, catarrh of bladder, urethral carbuncle.

Respiratory: Asthma with great dyspnoea and palpitation, moist asthma, expectoration white, thick mucus, bronchitis in the aged, bronchorrhoea. (Bal. peru). Profuse expectoration of offensive mucopus. Irritative cough. Whooping cough in rachitic children. Fetid form of bronchitis, bronchial dilatation and emphysema.

Extremities: Pricking sensation, followed by painful aching. Nodular swellings over metacarpal and metatarsal joints.

Fever: Elevation of temperature. Continued and typhoid fevers, scarlet fever (protective and curative) show a tendency to foulness, high temperature, accelerated but not strong pulse. Use the tincture.

Oil of Eucalyptus. The volatile oil possesses in common with other terpenes, the property of converting water, in presence of air and sunlight into hydrogen peroxide or to convert oxygen into ozone which is the explanation usually given of its deodorizing and antiseptic properties.

Dose: Tr. 1 to 20 drop doses and lower potencies.

Also oil of Eucalyptus in 5 drops doses.

(Boericke)

The gum tree is a native of Australia and is transplanted to marshy districts in mild climates on account of its capability of absorbing water and its alleged power of destroying malarial poisons. It has been familiarised to everybody during the influenza epidemic as a prophylactic and disinfectant. The provings show that it causes most of the ordinary influenzal symptoms. It is therefore homoeopathic to the disorder. C.E. Fischer has cured with it many cases of dysentery. Dr. Arthur Dalzell related two striking cases of bronchial asthma promptly relieved with 5 drop doses of oil of Eucalyptus given in a table spoonful of water. The dose was given last thing at night. It follows Arsenic in relapsing fevers. *(JHC)*

This agent is a disinfectant, antispasmodic, expectorant and an antipyretic. When the oil is applied to the skin it acts as an irritant and increases the local blood supply and produces systemic effects. When the vapour is inhaled it has a local effect upon the mucous surfaces as well as a general effect. In the mouth it leaves a pungent, aromatic or camphor-like impression. It excites a flow of saliva and leaves an astringent flavor in the mouth, The appetite and digestion are improved; the secretion of the gastric intestinal fluid is increased. Medium doses produce a sensation of buoyancy, whilc large doses produce drowsiness, depression and paresis of the limbs. The skin is pale and cold; the pulse is small and compressible; the pupils are contracted, the breathing is short and irregular; the urine and urea are increased; the heart's action is increased; the arterial tension is first increased and later lowered. It is eliminated by the kidneys and through the skin and bronchial mucous membranes.

Therapeutics

This remedy is indicated in subacute and chronic malarial infectious cases, in which large quantities of quinine have been employed. There is frequently a drain upon the system, as from a diarrhoea or dysentery. There may be an atonic dyspepsia present which is dependent upon a gastric catarrh. It meets many of these cases, when it acts as a reconstructive, assisting assimilation and hastening convalescence. It is also indicated in typhoid, typho-malarial and other septic fevers when there is a dull, congestive headache and a diarrhoea of a thin, watery, offensive character. It is useful in catarrhal affections of the bronchial mucous membranes, bronchorrhoea, and other chronic conditions that are accompanied by free muco-purulent expectoration. It is useful in tubercular and hectic fevers with profuse, exhaustive sweats, and in asthma of debilitated anaemia subjects with great dyspnoea and palpitation of the heart. Inhalation of the fumes from the drug is of service in these cases.

It should be remembered in atonic dyspepsia, chronic, gastric and intestinal catarrh. The digestion is slow, and there is a burning, hot sensation in the stomach.

It is beneficial in chronic catarrh of the bladder, in chronic nephritis, granular degeneration of the kidneys, pyonephrosis, and in hydronephrosis.

It should be studied in diseases of women at the climacteric period in those who are distressed with flatulence, palpitation of the heart, sudden flushing of the face; also in leucorrhoea, when it may be employed both locally and internally.

Compare: Baptisia, Arsenicum album, Cinchona, Balsam peru, Copaiva.

(Blackwood)

264. *Eugenia Jambos*
(Rose Apple)

Eugenia produces a state of intoxication like alcohol. Everything appears beautiful and larger; excitement soon changing to depression. Acne simple and indurated. The pimples are painful to some distance around. Acne Rosacea. Nausea better smoking. Comedones.

Head: Headache as if a board were lying on right side. Talkative. Hot lachrymation.

Extremities: Nightly Cramp in soles of feet (Cupr., Zinc).

Skin: Cracks about toes, fissures between toes, skin recedes from the nails, forming pus. *(Boericke)*

Malabar plum tree - Rose apple - like Eucalyptus, Eugenia causes a condition of drunkenness. It makes the prover very talkative and indolent.

Amel: After urination, sky and trees more joyous and clear but after a quarter of an hour everything became gloomy again. *(JHC)*

Mother tincture of the fresh seeds; and dilutions. Of the tincture, 1 to 3 drops. Homoeo, 3x. This remedy is indicated in comedones, simple acne, and acne rosacea, when there is an inflamed area about the pimple. There are fissures of the skin, especially between the toes.

Compare: Beriberi, Aqua. (Blackwood)

265. *Euonymus Atropurpurea*
(Wahoo-burning bush)

Brunettes more easily affected, producing headache, mental disturbances and much distress in hepatic and renal region. Albuminuria, Migraine, passive congestion and torpor of liver. Chronic catarrhal affections of stomach and intestines. Weak heart. Chronic rheumatism and gout.

Dose: Tr. and lower attenuation.

(Boericke)

Euonymus Atropurpurea like Eonimin and Euon. Europ, is a favourite liver remedy among Eclectics. A lady who tasted the juice of the bark related her experience to Hale: I felt immediately a sick weakening feeling all through the nervous system, dull heavy pain through upper portion of head together with enlarged blurred feeling and I seemed so drawn up from the floor, that it seemed difficult to place my foot down, when walking with sufficient firmness to stand up; a tipping over sensation when sitting and walking, a deathly sickness at stomach, with perspiration and heat in face, in alternation with chills in the back and back parts of the arms. Some of the symptoms returned next day, but were dissipated by vinegar which must be looked upon as its antidote. *(JHC)*

266. *Eupatorium Aromaticum*

(Pool Root)

Nervous erethism, restlessness and morbid watchfulness, hysteria and chorea. Low fevers and extreme restlessness. Aphthous disease. Sore nipples; sore mouth in infants, vomiting of bile, pain in stomach, headache and fever.

Dose: Tr. to 3rd potency. *(Boericke)*

E. aromat, when chewed, produces in the mouth a warm aromatic pungent sensation as is regarded as a "warm stimulating tonic". Hale quotes eclectic authorities as commending this plant in "aphthous stomatitis". In women and children also for burning in the stomach with nursing sore mouth before and after confinement. Like E, Purpur, it has been used for gravel and the Indians use it as a cure for Ague. *(JHC)*

Common name, white snake root. This remedy is indicated in hysteria, nervous irritability, restlessness and flatulence. It is of service in Aphthae, nursing sore mouth and sore nipple. In these cases it should be applied locally. *(Blackwood)*

267. *Eupatorium perfoliatum*

(Thorough wort)

Known as Bone set from the prompt manner in which it relieves pain in limbs and muscles that accompanies some form of febrile diseases, like malaria and influenza. Eupatorium acts principally upon the gastro-hepatic organs and bronchial mucous membranes. It is a boon in miasmatic districts, along rivers, marshes etc. and in all conditions, where there is a great deal of bone pain. Cachexia from old chronic bilious intermittents. Worn out constitutions from inebriety. Sluggishness of all organs and functions. Bone pains, general and severe. Soreness. Marked periodicity. (Ars., China, Cedron)

Head: Soreness of eyeballs. Occipital pain after lying down with sense of weight.

Respiratory: Coryza with sneezing. Hoarseness and cough with soreness in chest. Influenza, chronic loose cough, worse at night.

Fever: Chill between 7 and 9 a.m. preceded by thirst with great soreness and aching of bones.

Extremities: Aching pain in back. Aching in bones of extremities with soreness of flesh. Aching in arms and wrists.

Modalities: *Worse* periodically. Better by conversation.

Relation: Bry., Sep., Nat m., Chel., Nyct., Arbon tristis.

Dose: Tr. to 3rd attenuation. *(Boericke)*

Eupat. Perfol. is an old world remedy having been recommended by Dioscorides for ill conditioned ulcers, dysentery, stings of reptiles, chronic fevers, obstructed liver. The leading characteristic for its homoeopathic use is the distressing bone pain it causes, such as are found in connection with malarial fevers and influenza. I have found Eup. perf. most useful in influenza. Bryonia is the closest analogue, but Bryonia has free sweat and the pains make the patient keep still. Eup. perfol. has scanty sweat and its pains cause restlessness. *(JHC)*

Insatiable thirst before and during chill and fever. Knows chill is coming because he cannot drink enough. *(HC Allen)*

This remedy is indicated in bilious and intermittent fevers, dengue and influenza, when there are severe pains in the back and legs, as though the bones were broken, with soreness of the eyeballs and yellowness of the conjuctivae and face.

It is of service in bilious fevers when there is an excruciating headache, with soreness of the scalp and eyeballs, redness of the face, nausea, bilious vomiting and prostration, soreness in the hepatic region, with constipation and high colored urine.

It is useful in intermittent fever, when the chill appearing from 7 to 9 a.m. one day, and at noon the next. There is thirst before and during the chill and fever, there are severe bone pains and bilious vomiting. It is to be studied in dengue, when the bone pains are severe; also in influenza when there is great soreness over the body, with pains as though the bones would break. There is hoarseness and a cough, with soreness of the larynx and chest; he must support the chest with his hands during coughing. The pulse is weak; there is coryza, thirst and bilious derangement.

Compare - Bryonia alba, Chelidonium. (Blackwood)

268. *Eupatorium purpureum*

(Queen of meadow)
(Gravel root)

Albuminuria, diabetic, strangury, irritable bladder, enlarged prostate are a special field for this remedy. Excellent in renal dropsy. Chills and pains run upwards. Impotency and sterility. Home sickness.

Head: left sided headache with vertigo.

Urinary: Deep dull pain in kidneys, burning in bladder and urethra on urinating. Insufficient flow, milky strangury, haematuria, constant desire, bladder feels dull, dysuria. Vesical irritability in women. Diabetes insipidus.

Compare: Sensecio, Cannab sat., Helon., Phos. ac., Triticum, Epigea. (Boericke)

Potency: 1st potency.

The common name 'Gravel Root' Indicates the traditional use of the drug and in the hands of eclectics, it has done good work in case of irritable bladder, diabetes insipidus incontinence of urine and calculus affections. E. Perf., Colch (Compare for nausea at smell of food) *(JHC)*

269. *Euphorbia lathyrus*

(Gopher plant Caper spurge)

The fresh milk juice is exceedingly acrid, when applied to the skin and the fruit is highly purgative and poisonous. The juice causes redness, itching pimples, some- times gangrene. The symptoms point to its use in Erysipelas, Poison Oak etc. Rheumatic pains during rest. Paralytic weakness in joints.

Dose: 3-30. *(Boericke)*

The chief symptom of E. lathy. are - Retching, and vomiting and bloody stools with brilliant eyes, flushed face, the abdomen is drawn inward. The whole body is stiff and icy cold. Uneasiness. *(JHC)*

270. *Euphorbium*

(Spurge)

(The resinous juice of Euphorbia Resinifera)

An irritant to the skin and mucous membranes. Burning pain in bones. Pains in limbs and paralytic weakness in the joints. Important respiratory and skin symptoms. Terrible burning pains. Pains of cancer. Everything appears larger than it really is.

Skin: Vesicular erysipelas.

Dose: 3-6 Potency. *(Boericke)*

Euphorbium officinarum. Gum Euphorbium. The respifera exudation or juice of Euphorbia resnified exported from Morocco. Euphorbia resinifera is a Cactus like plant of the Euphorbiaceae.

Gum Euphorbium is one of the group of Euphorbian drugs and should be studied with Croton tig. and Ricinus. Like these it produces gastro-intestinal irritation and all degrees of irritation of the skin.

It also affects the eyes, teeth and bones. Burning pains in the bones is an indication and along with Euphorb Helerodoxa, it is a remedy for the pains of cancer. (In a desperate case of Sarcoma of the pelvic bones under my care nothing gave greater relief to the pains than repeated doses of Euphorb. 6c. *(JHC)*

271. Euphrasia
(Eye Bright)

Manifests itself in inflaming the conjuctival membrane, especially producing profuse lachrymation. Patient is better in open air. Catarrhal affections of mucous membranes, especially of eyes and nose.

Profuse acrid lachrymation and bland coryza, worse evening. Hawking up of offensive mucus.

Head: Catarrhal headache.

Nose: Profuse fluent coryza.

Eyes: Catarrhal conjunctivities, discharge of acrid matter. The eyes water all the time, acrid lachrymation, bland coryza. (Opp. Cepa). Discharge thick and excoriating (mercur-thin and acrid) Burning and swelling of the lids. Frequent inclination to blink. Free discharge of acrid matter. Sticky mucous on cornea, must wink to remove it. Pressure in eyes. Little blisters on cornea. Opacities, Rheumatic iritis. Ptosis (Gels., Caust.).

Rectum: Constipation.

Female: Menses painful, flow lasts only an hour or day. Amenorrhoea with ophthalmia.

Male: prostatitis.

Modalities: Worse in evening, indoors, warmth, south winds, from light. Better from coffee. In dark. *(Boericke)*

According to Grauvogl, the 'Signature' of a black spot in the Corolla which looks like the pupil marked Euphrasia as an eye medicine to the ancients and homoeopathic experiments have fully confirmed its old time reputation. Eye symptoms appear in great variety and the irritation extends to the skin around the eye and to the nose, producing nasal catarrh and affection of external nose.

Sensation, as if dust or sand in eyes, as if a hair hung over eyes, as if upper lips were made of wood, stiffness of left cheek or tongue. 'Ames' of Rickland, Ohio has recorded the case of an old man of 79 to whom he gave Euphras 3x for lachrymation and sneezing, with the result that it relieved him, in addition of a prostatic trouble, he had for some years, compelling him to rise frequently in the night to urinate. This led 'Ames' to give Euphr. in other case of prostatic trouble with good results. As an eye lotion Euphr. has great value. I have seen corneal opacities removed by its prolonged use. *(JHC)*

Pertussis, excessive lachrymation during cough, cough only in day time. *(HCA)*

272. *Eupion*

(Wood tar distillation)

Marked female symptoms and backache. A remedy for uterine displacements. Pain in back, followed by a bland leucorrhoea. Menses too early and copious, flow thin. Intense sweat from slightest. exertion. Disgusting dreams. Sensation as if whole body were made of jelly.

Female: Burning in right ovary, Gushing in leucorrhoea, chronic tubal disease. Uterine flexion. Menses too early and copious. During menses, irritable and disinclined to talk, burning and stitches in chest and heart. After menses yellow leucorrhoea with severe backache. When pain in back ceases, the discharge gushes out. Sore pain between labia during urination, pruritus pudendi, labia swollen.

Extremities: Cramps in the calves worse at night.

Relationship: Kreosot, Graph., Lach.

Dose: 3rd potency. *(Boericke)*

On distilling wood tar, a volatile oil is obtained, which separates into a lighter and heavier oil, the heavier oil is Kreosote, the lighter is Eupion.

The effects of Eupion, which was proved by "Wahle' in Rome, who also proved paraffin, bear a close resemblance to those of Kreosote, but are by no means, identical with them. A large number of the symptoms centre in the female sexual organs. Some of them being very characteristic - Nose bleed occurs, when menstrual flow intermits. Lachesis. (Pain ceases when discharge appear).

(JHC)

273. *Fabina Imbricata*

(Pichi)

A South American shrub cultivated in southern california. It is a Terebinthine diuretic. It has also tonic and Cholagogue properties, used in the treatment of nasal catarrh, jaundice, dyspepsia and to increase the secretion of bile. (Albert Schneider). Useful in the Uric acid diathesis, cystitis, gonorrhoea, prostatitis, dysuria, vesical catarrh with suppurative prostatic conditions, post gonorrhoeal urinary conditions, cholelithiasis and liver affections, vesical tenesmus and burning after urination. Excoriating urine and calculi.

Dose: Ten and twenty drops of Tr.

(Boericke)

274. *Fagopyrum*

(Buck wheat)

Its action on the skin producing pruritus is very marked. Viscible pulsation of arteries. Fluent coryza. Offensive excretions. Itching Erythema. Pruritus Senilis. Post nasal catarrh, dry crusts, granular appearance of posterior nares with itching.

Head: Itching in and around eyes and ears.

Nose: Fluent coryza with sneezing, followed by dryness and crust formation.

Stomach: Eructations of scalding, hot, acid watery substance, better coffee. Bad taste in the morning. Persistent morning nausea, drooling.

Heart: Throbbing in all arteries after retiring, palpitation with oppression. Pulse irregular. Intermittent, rapid, light feeling in chest.

Female: Pruritus vulvae with yellow leucorrhoea, worse rest. Burning in right ovary.

Extremities: Vehement itching in arms and legs, worse towards evening. Feet numb and pricking.

Skin: Itching, better by bathing in cold water, worse scratching, touch and retiring, sore red blotches, blind boils. Itching of knees and elbows and hairy portions. Itching of hands, deep in, vesicular, pustular, phlegmonous dermatitis. Skin hot swollen.

Modalities: Better cold water, coffee, worse in afternoon from sunlight, scratching.

Relationship: Compare - Dolichos, Bovista, urtica.

Dose: 3rd potency and 12x. *(Boericke)*

275. *Fel Tauri*

(Ox-gall)

Increases the duodenal secretion, emulsifies fats and increases the peristaltic action of the intestines. Liquefies bile and acts as a purgative and cholagogue. Disordered digestion, diarrhoea and pain in nape of neck are among its chief symptoms. Obstruction of gall ducts. Biliary calculi, jaundice.

Stomach: Tendency to sleep after eating.

Relationship: Merc., Dulc., Cholesterin, in biliary lithiasis, China. Calculobili—Triturate Gall stones - 10 to 12x (Gall Stones).

Dose: Lower triturations. Purified Ox gall 1 to 10 gr. *(Boericke)*

Inspissated gall triturated with sugar of milk; or dilutions may be made with water. Ox gall is a remedy of very ancient use. It is used in the old school, mostly as a purgative, for preventing putrefacting peristalsis. It is sometimes given along with Opium to prevent the constipating effect of that drug. In the stomach bile is a foreign body precipitating Pepsin and causing irritation of the stomach. It does not aid the digestion either of albumin or of farinaceous substances; Fel. T. has been proved homoeopathically by Buchner and has produced a few characteristic symptoms, disordered digestion, diarrhoea, headache, pains in joints and cramps. It removes a tendency to sleep after eating. Several symptoms were noticed in nape of neck.

Relations: compare - Cholesterinum, Merc., Dulc. (JHC)

This agent increases the duodenal secretions, emulsifies fats, and increases the peristaltic action of the intestines. It liquifies the bile and acts as a purgative and cholagogue.

It is of service in cases of jaundice due to obstruction, when the stools are very offensive, of a light, clay color. It is also employed as an intestinal antiseptic.

(Blackwood)

276. *Ferrum Met*

(Iron)

Best adapted to young weakly persons anaemic and chlorotic, with pseudoplethora, who flush easily, cold extremities, over - sensitiveness, worse after any active effort, weakness from mere speaking or walking though looking strong. Pallor of the skin, mucous membranes, face, alternating with flushes, orgams of blood to face, chest, head, lungs etc. Irregular distribution of blood. Pseudo plethora. Muscles flabby and relaxed.

Mind: Slight noises unbearable, excited from slightest opposition. Sanguine temperament.

Head: Hammering, pulsating, congestive pain in back of head.

Face: Flushed from least pain, emotion or exertion, red parts become white.

Mouth: Pain in teeth, relieved by icy cold water.

Stomach: Voracious appetite or absolute loss of appetite. Loathing of sour things. Spits up food by the mouthful, vomiting immediately after eating. Vomiting after midnight. Intolerance of eggs.

Stool: Cramping pain in rectum, prolapsus recti, itching of anus, especially young children.

Female: Women who are weak, delicate, chlorotic yet have a fiery red face, menses too early, too profuse, last too long, pale watery sensitive vagina, prolapse of vagina.

Pulse: Full but soft and yielding, also small and weak. Heart suddenly bleeds into the blood vessels.

Fever: General coldness of extremities, head and face hot, chill at 4 a.m. Heat in palms and soles. Profuse debilitating sweat.

Modalities: Better walking slowly about. Better after rising.

Worse: While sweating, while sitting still, after cold washing and over heating - midnight aggravation.

Antidotes: Ars., Hep.

Complementary: Chin., Alum., Ham.

Dose: States of debility, where the blood is poor in Hematin, require material doses. Plethoric, haemorrhagic conditions, call for small doses, from second to sixth potency. *(Boericke)*

Ferrum, the Mars of alchemists is one of the prominent constituents of the animal body, being present in considerable quantity in the blood. It is present in many articles of daily food and when given in excess to men or animals its first effect is to increase the amount of iron in blood, stimulate the appetite, augment the heart beats and the bodily vigour. The cheeks are flushed as if in blooming health, but in spite of the bloom in appearance, there is pallor of hips and mucous membranes, great fatigue and breathlessness and any motion will set up the symptoms. Delicate girls, fearfully constipated with low spirits. Feet swell - intolerance of eggs. Diarrhoea coming on when the patient begins to eat. Many remedies have it immediately after eating. *(JHC)*

Persons of sanguine temperament, pettish, quarrelsome, disputative, easily excited, least contradiction angers. *Amel:* from mental exertion.

Vertigo with balancing sensation, as if on water, on seeing flowing water, when walking over water or when crossing a bridge.

Cinchona. The vegetable analogue follows well in nearly all diseases, acute or chronic.

Aggravation: At night, at rest, especially while sitting still. *(JHC)*

This agent when taken internally blackens the teeth and the tongue. In small doses it acts as a stomach tonic, if not continued too long. Should large doses of a preparation showing an acid reaction be administered for a prolonged period, anorexia, nausea, and indigestion result. In the stomach the various preparations are changed into a chloride. It combines with the red blood corpuscles and brings the haemoglobin up to the normal standard. Under its influence the muscular power of the heart is increased, the arteries are contracted and the blood pressure is increased. The urea is increased, and micturition is rendered more frequent. It is eliminated by the faeces, bile, urine, skin, mucous, and serous surfaces. The stools are dark.

Should its use be continued over a prolonged period the digestion is impaired. There is thirst, gastric oppression, nausea, vomiting, with pain or a sense of fullness in the head and dizziness and increased heat in the body. The breathing is labored; acne appears upon the face, breast and back. There are haemorrhages from the mucous surfaces, with plethora, and other indications of vascular changes.

This remedy is indicated in cases of anaemia, with debility, when the face and lips are of a pale bluish colour. The face becomes red and flushed from the least pain, emotion, or exertion, there is profound muscular relaxation and prostration.

The anaemia may appear under the mask of plethora or congestion; at times the face presents an ash pale or greenish color; with pain or exertion, it becomes a fiery red; at which time there is vertigo, ringing in the ears, palpitation of the heart and dyspnoea. Accompanying these symptoms of anaemia and chlorosis there is weakness and relaxation of the whole muscular system, together with emaciation and coldness of the extremities. The patient finds a degree of relief from walking about slowly inspite of the great exhaustion. On account of the pronounced anaemia, the stomach is unable to perform its function, and there is vomiting of food after eating, or coughing. The ejected material is acid and sour. The stools are apt to consist of undigested food.

The diarrhoea is painless, and is worse during the morning and may be involuntary, watery and slimy. It may excoriate the anus, and be attended with a fiery red face.

This type of a chronic diarrhoea is frequently seen in anaemic children. It usually appears soon after eating or drinking, there is no pain or effort, and it contains much undigested substance. At times the bowels are constipated. There is ineffectual urging to stool, the hands and feet are cold , while the pale, anaemic face become fiery red on the least effort.

In nocturnal enuresis it is of service when the urine is of a dark, red color. There is an irritability of the urethra and neck of the bladder, and a degree of anaemia. It is of service in cases of chronic vesical catarrh and gleet. In the management of chronic degeneration of the kidneys with albuminuria it is efficacious the anaemia and prostration are pronounced, and anasarca is usually present.

It is useful in the females who are anaemic and weakly. There is profuse menstruation, the menses are too frequent and last too long. Before the period there is stinging headache with ringing in the ears; during the period she must keep quiet as the least exertion renders the flow more profuse. The menses intermit for a few days. There may be much itching, pruritus of the vulva in delicate, weakly women, who suffer from a leucorrhoea, which is watery and milky in character, and is smarting and corroding.

It is indicated in tuberculosis of the young, florid subjects, when there is a tendency to congestion of the blood to the lungs and haemoptysis, with palpitation of the heart and flying pains through the chest. The patient is anaemic, becomes flushed easily and suffers from dyspnoea.

In intermittent fever, when quinine has been abused and there is a high degree of anaemia, which is marked by a pseudo-plethora, it is indicated. The spleen is enlarged, there is congestion to the head and a tendency to vomit all foods taken. The patient sweats easily, especially at night during sleep or on being covered.

Rheumatism of the left deltoid muscle is relieved by the remedy. It is tearing in character, is worse at night, driving him out of bed, and motion diminishes the pain.

Compare: Graphites, Natrum mur., Arsenic. *(Blackwood)*

277. *Ferrum Magneticum*

(Load stone)

Marked symptoms in intestinal tract. Pain in nape of neck. Paralytic weakness, small warts on hands.

Dose: 3rd potency.

As with Ferrum there is agg. during a meal, flatulence, grumblings, movements in abdomen, with urgent diarrhoea after a meal. The appearance of warts may indicate that Fer. Mag. is related to the sycotic constitution. *(JHC)*

278. *Ferrum Phos*

(Phosphate of Iron)

In the early stages of febrile condition, it stands midway between sthenic activity of Aconite and Bell and the asthenic sluggishness and torpidity of Gel. The typical Ferr. Phos subject is not full blooded and robust, but nervous, sensitive, anaemic with the false plethora and easy flushing of Ferrum. Prostration marked; face more active than Gels. The superficial redness never assumes the dusky hue of Gels. Pulse soft and flowing, no anxious restlessness of Acon. Susceptibility to chest troubles. Bronchitis of young children. In acute exacerbation of tuberculosis, a fine palliative of wonderful power. Corresponds to Grauvogls oxygenoid constitution, the inflammatory, febrile, emaciating, wasting consumptive.

The remedy for first stage of all febrile disturbances and inflammations, before exudation sets in, especially for catarrhal affections of the respiratory tract. Ferr. phos 3x increases haemoglobin. In pale anaemic subjects with violent local congestions. Haemorrhages bright from any orifice.

Head: Headache better cold applications.

Nose: First stage of cold in the head, epistaxis.

Throat: Mouth hot, fauces red, inflamed. Ulcerated sore throat. Tonsils red and swollen. Eustachian tube inflamed. Sore throat of singers, subacute laryngitis with fauces inflamed and red (2x). After operation on throat and nose to control bleeding and relieve soreness. First stage of diphtheria. Ranula in vascular, sanguine constitutions.

Stomach: Aversion to Meat and Milk, vomiting of undigested food, sour eructations.

Urine: Diurnal enuresis.

Respiratory: First stage of all inflammatory affections. Expectoration of pure blood in pneumonia.

Heart: Short, quick, soft pulse.

Extremities: Stiff neck, articular rheumatism, crick in back, rheumatic pain in shoulder, whitlow.

Modalities: *Worse* at night and 4 to 6 a.m., touch, jar, motion, right side.

Better: Cold applications.

Dose: 3-12 potency. *(Boericke)*

Schussler deduces the following indications for iron when the muscular cells which have grown flaccid through loss of iron receive a compensation for their loss, the normal tensional relation is restored; the annular fibres of the blood vessels are shortened to their proper measure, the capacity of these vessels again becomes normal and the hyperaemia disappears and in consequence the inflammatory fever ceases.

Iron will cure:-

1. The first stage of all inflammations, caused by hyperaemia.
2. Pains.
3. Haemorrhages.
4. Fresh wounds, contusions, spasms, as it removes hyperaemia.

Schussler generally used the 12x trituration. Aversion to meat and milk.

(JHC)

It is a white or bluish, almost tasteless powder. This remedy is indicated during the first stages of catarrhal and febrile disturbances and inflammation before exudation has taken place; also as a reconstructive in those who are anaemic, children who are weakly, with a failing appetite, and who lose weight and strength.

It is useful in acute bronchitis and hyperaemia of the lungs when the sputum is free; there is no restlessness and irritability that characterize Aconite. In capillary bronchitis and broncho-pneumonia it meets the febrile and general condition, but it is useless when cyanosis has once taken place.

It should be remembered in haemoptysis when there is a slight, bright haemorrhage. The patient is frequently overgrown, has a tendency to phthisis and suffers from bronchial catarrh, headache an epistaxis. In entero-colitis and cholera infantum it is indicated when the child is quiet and inclined to be drowsy, there is tenesmus, the stools are slimy and contain streaks of blood.

It is also of service when there is a tendency to rickets; the limbs are tender and motion is painful. It should be studied in acute tuberculosis and for the acute attacks of chronic tuberculosis.

It should be remembered in diurnal enuresis that is dependant upon irritation of the trigone of the bladder. There is pain in the neck of the bladder; he must urinate at once. The pain is worse while standing, and is relieved while lying down. Compare: Gel., China., Acon., Kali m. *(Blackwood)*

279. *Ferrum Picricum*

(Picrate of Iron)

Is considered a great remedy to complete the action of other medicines. The symptom that specially calls for it is failure of the function of an organ under exertion, e.g., the voice fails after public speaking. Acts best in dark haired patients, plethoric with sensitive livers. Warts and epithelial growths, corns with yellowish discoloration. Senile hypertrophy of the prostate. Epistaxis, chronic deafness and tinnitus due to gout. Meatus dry. Pseudoleucaemia.

Urinary: Frequent micturition at night with full feeling and pressure in rectum. Smarting at neck of bladder and penis.

Extremities: Hands covered with warts.

Dose: Second and third trituritition.

(Boericke)

It has cured many cases of warts and corns as I have repeatedly verified. He (Dr. Cooper) considers it specially indicated for warts on the hand, when they are multiple. Cooper has observed that warts, especially old pedunculated warts frequently accompany chronic deafness. P.C. Majumdar (Indian Hom. Review oct. 1899) cured a student suffering from anaemia and malarious fever off and on for a year, who had these symptoms among others, impaired hearing of both ears, buzzing, hissing, vertigo, indigestion, headache, and tired feeling after bodily or mental exertion. He considers Ferr. pic. suited to the results of malarious fever, sexual excesses and loss of blood. Ferr. pic. is apt to aggravate if given too low. *(JHC)*

It is almost a specific in nose bleed.

(HC Allen)

280. Ficus Religiosa

(Ashwathya)

This east Indian drug causes and cures haemorrhages of many kinds; Haematemesis, menorrhagia, haemoptysis etc. Bloody urine.

Stomach: nausea, vomiting of bright red blood, pain and sick feeling in stomach.

Relation: Acalypha, Millefol., Thlaspi., Ipecac.

Dose: First potency. *(Boericke)*

We owe this remedy to Dr. Sarat Chandra Ghose of Midnapore, who made the first proving and thereby discovered its power to cause and cure haemorrhages of many kinds. *(JHC)*

281. Filix mas - Aspidium

(Male fern)

A remedy for worm symptoms, especially with constipation. Tape worm, soporific conditions. Torpid inflammations of lymphatic glands. (maceration of fresh root). Pulmonary tuberculosis in young patients, no fever, with limited ulcerated lesions, formerly classified as scrofula.

Abdomen: Bloated, gnawing pain, worse eating sweets, diarrhoea and vomiting, worm colic with itching of nose, pale face, blue rings around eyes. Painless hiccough.

Dose: First to third potency. For expulsion of tape worm a full dose of ½ to 1 dram of the oleoresin; fasting.

(Boericke)

Tincture of fresh root or fresh root grated - male fern has been recognised as a vermifuge from the time of Galen and Dioscorides credits it with the power of causing sterility and abortion.

A fragmentary proving in Allen's appendix records a case in which 15 to 20 drops of the tincture given 3 times a day to a women suffering from bloated abdomen with more or less pain caused diminution of the bloating but also, severe prolapse of vagina, pain and tenesmus of bladder with copious and frequent emission of urine with intense pain, Filix was discontinued and then Chimaphila relieved. *(JHC)*

Tincture of the fresh rhizome; and dilutions. U.S.P. Aspidium, Oleoresina Aspidii.

The great use of this remedy has been in the removal of Tape worms.

(Blackwood)

282. *Fluoricum Acidum*

(Hydro-fluoric acid)

Especially adapted to chronic diseases with syphilitic and mercurial history. Glabella region bloated. Acts especially upon lower tissues and indicated in deep destructive processes; bedsores, ulcerations, varicose veins and ulcers. Patient is compelled to move about energetically. Complaints of old age or the prematurely aged, with weak, distended blood vessels. Hobnailed liver of alcoholics. Goitre (Dr. Woakes) (Kali fluroide produced bronchocele in dogs). Early decay of tooth. Old cases of nightly fevers coming on periodically.

Mind: Indifference towards those loved best, inability to realise responsibility, buoyancy, mentally elated and gay.

Eyes: Sensation as of wind blowing through eyes.

Male: Swollen scrotum.

Skin: Varicose veins, itching especially of orifices, dropsy of limbs.

Relationship: Calc. fluor., Silica.

Dose: sixth to thirtieth potency.

(Boericke)

T.F. Allen has recorded an experience showing the applicability of Fl. ac. in Whitlow. Amel from cold washing distinguishes it from Silic. A constant irresistable desire to walk in the open air. It does not fatigue is characteristic of Fl. ac. *(JHC)*

In persons who have worked, who have been working day and night to establish a business, or to keep it up, and when there has been constant use of the brain it is suitable. In mental depression and melancholy, with great sadness, in young men who have destroyed the nervous system by vicious practices, by secret vice. It is particularly suitable for that disorder of the human economy where men have continuously changed their mistresses. There is a state in which a man is never satisfied with one woman, but continually changes, and goes from bad to worse until he is a debauche. If a young man cannot keep away from women, he is not so bad off if he will only keep to one, but he goes from one to many, until he stands upon the street corners and, in his lust, craves the innocent women that go along the street.

To him there is no place like home. Now, when man arrives at the state when he wants to go somewhere else, that he wants to go away from home, that he is disturbed at home, that everything annoys him at home, that he no longer loves his children as he once did, he needs fluoric acid.

He wants to bathe the face and head in cold water; such bathing is grateful. The feet burn and are put out of bed in the night; he hunts around in bed for a cool place for the feet and hands. The soles perspire, and the palms perspire and the sweat is acrid, making the parts sore; excoriation from the sweat between the toes. Worse from drinking tea and coffee. Warm drinks bring on a diarrhoea, or flatulence, or disturbance in the stomach, and cause indigestion to manifest itself in various ways. The symptoms are worse standing and sitting and better in the open air.

It is a remedy of great depth of action. It so disturbs the functions that there are peculiar outward signs in the nails, in the hair, in the skin, they are all imperfectly developed.

The nails are crippled, likewise corrugations in the nails; the nails grow too fast and grow awkwardly; that is, they are deformed and crippled, too thick in some places.

It is very analogous to Sil., and it is one of the natural followers of Sil. where 'Sil' has been too frequently repeated by persons who do not know that Silicea does its best in a single dose and that it is a long acting and slow medicine.

Think of the remedy, in fistula leading to the teeth, fistula lachrymalis and fistula in Ano.

Intense uncontrollable sexual desire. Mental exhaustion from overwork or from vices.

Dry scales, itches very much, bald places - Exostoses - Nasal bones all destroyed, and the nose becomes flat, the teeth decay or break off or ulcerate at the roots - craves cold water and is continually hungry. Often that all gone sensation in the stomach. Is always eating and is relieved from eating - Chronic ulcers of the throat not necessarily syphilitic. This patient craves pungent, spicy, highly seasoned things. The most vicious kind of chronic diarrhoea - Morning diarrhoea - protrusion of the anus during defaecation. Itching around and in anus in perineum - itching violent. Squamous eruptions upon the body, dry cutaneous eruptions upon the body, very scaly. *(Kent)*

283. *Formalin*

(Aqueous solution 35% of Formaldehyde gas)

Is a powerful disinfectant and deodorant, a potent poison. Prevents growth and kills almost any pathogenic micro-organism. It seems to have the peculiar property of eating into malignant tumors, leaving the surrounding healthy tissue uncharred and unchanged. A plug of cotton wool soaked in a 20% solution of formaldehyde and applied for a few hours will produce a necrotic slough, which must be scraped away before the next application, otherwise it hardens.

Formalin in hot water as vapor is the most valuable therapeutic agent in pertussis, phthisis, in catarrhal affections of upper air-passages.

Mind: Forgetfulness.

Head: Vertigo.

Respiratory: Dyspnoea, laryngismus stridulus, whooping cough.

Skin: Puckers skin like leather, wrinkles, scales off. Eczema in neighbourhood of wound. Damp sweat most marked on right upper extremity.

Dose: A vapour in hot water in respiratory affections. (1% spray) otherwise 3x potency. *(Boericke)*

284. *Formica Rufa*

(Myrmexine)

(Tr. from crushed live Ants)

An arthritic medicine. Gout and articular rheumatism, pains worse motion, better pressure. Right side most affected. Chronic gout and stiffness in joints. Acute outburst of gouty poisons, especially when assuming the neuralgic forms.

Tuberculosis, carcinoma, and Lupus, chronic Nephritis. Complaints from over lifting. Apopletic diseases. Has a marked deterrent influence on the formation of polypi.

Head: Nasal polypi.

Extremities: Rheumatic pains; stiff and contracted joints, weakness of lower extremities. Rheumatism comes on with suddenness and restlessness. Sweat does not relieve. Relief after midnight and rubbing.

Skin: Red, itching and burning.

Modalities: *Worse* cold, and cold washing, dampness before a snowstorm.

Better: Warmth, pressure, rubbing, combing hair.

Dose: 6-30.

Compare: Formic acid: Chronic myalgia. Muscular pains and soreness. Gout and articular rheumatism, which appear suddenly. Pains usually worse on right side, motion, and better from pressure. Failing vision. Increases muscular strength and resistance to fatigue. Feels stronger and more fit in ordinary walking. Marked diuretic effect, greater elimination of products of disassimilation, particularly urea. Tremor. Tuberculosis, chronic nephritis and carcinoma, Lupus, etc., have been treated successfully with injections of Formic acid of a dilution corresponding to the 3rd and 4th centesimal.

In prescribing it for varicose veins, polypi, catarrh, Dr. J.H. Clarke orders an ounce or two of a solution of Formic acid in the proportion of one part of the acid to eleven of distilled water. Of this one teaspoonful is taken in a tablespoonful of water after food once or twice daily. Pain in aponeurosis and muscles of head, neck, and shoulders before a snowstorm. Rhus-t., Dulc., Urt., and Juniperus contain Formic acid; wood alcohol, when taken as a constituent of a beverage so common in these prohibition days, is not eliminated easily and is slowly converted into Formic acid, attacking the brain and causing death or blindness.

Dr. Sylwestrowica of the Hering Research Laboratory of Hahnemann College. Philadelphia contributed his experience with Formic acid, as follows:

The best field for the formic acid treatment are cases of a typical gout. Under this classification are to be mentioned disturbances in the muscles, such as myositis, periostitic proceses of the bones in form of doughy swellings, changes of the fascias such as Dupyutren's contraction, skin troubles such as chronic eczema, psoriasis and loss of hair, kidney disturbances such as subacute and chronic nephritis. In these cases formic acid in 12x and 30x hypodermically 1 cc. is indicated at intervals of 2-4 weeks. Eight to twelve days after the first injection an aggravation is often noticed.

In acute rheumatic fever and acute gonorrhoeic arthritis Formic acid 6x every six days 1 cc., sometimes 12x in sensitive patients shows often splendid results abolishing the pains and preventing reccurrence.

Chronic arthritis needs a special discussion. Clinical experiments of the Hering Research laboratory of the Hahnemann Medical College of Philadelphia on a great number of cases of arthritis with formic acid showed that it preferably acts on the ligaments, capsule and bursa of the joints. Such kind of cases respond very readily to treatment.

The prognosis depends to a large extent upon the etiology of the case. The most satisfactory cases are chronic arthritis in connection with gouty diathesis. Chronic arthritis following an attack of acute rheumatic fever shows also remarkable results although often pains of a neuralgic character persisting in certain spots are very stubborn. Finally chronic arthritis of traumatic nature can be cured by formic acid. In the later case formic acid 6x showed quicker and better results than 12x or 30x which are indicated in the previous cases. In general the disappearance of the stiffness of the joint is the first sign of improvement. Then the pain and swelling cease gradually in 1-6 months time.

The prognosis of the formic acid treatment is not so favourable in chronic arthritis in which deformans processes have already taken place on the articular surfaces. Such process in the beginning can be checked completely, advanced cases frequently show an improvement. But there is always the possibility that this improvement is only temporary, This is particularly to be expected in the cases of the so called arthritis deformans in which even the inflammations on the ligaments and capsula are of a very progressive character.

Dose: Sixth to thirtieth attenuation.
(Boericke)

Formica rufa - It is of use in all kinds of apoplectic diseases. It strengthens the brain (Hering) - Causation - checked foot sweat.

285. Fragaria

(Wood - strawberry)

Acts on digestion and mesenteric glands, prevents formation of calculi, removes tartar from teeth and prevents attacks of gout. The fruit has refrigerant properties. Strawberries produce symptoms of poisoning in certain susceptible individuals, such as urticarial rashes (strawberry anaphylaxis). Here give Fragaria High potency.
(Boericke)

General anasarca and especially swollen tongue - The well known 'strawberry tongue' is an indication for its use. An infusion of the root is used for drying up the breasts in women who wish to wean their children. It diminishes the size of the breasts and dries up the milk. *(JHC)*

This agent when used freely prevents the formation of calculi, and removes the tartar from the teeth, and prevents attacks of gout. It is of service in urticarious, petechial and erysipelatous eruptions.
(Blackwood)

286. Franciscea

(Manaca)

Chronic stiffness of muscles. Gonorrhoeal rheumatism. Syphilis and rheumatism, great heat over body, much aching, better sweat. Pain in back of head and spine, band like feeling around head, pericarditis with rheumatism. Rheumatic pain in feet and lower parts of legs. Urine contains Uric acid.

Dose: Tincture or fluid extract 10-60 minims.
(Boericke)

Franciscea is a Brazilian remedy of great local repute as an antisyphilitic and anti-rheumatic. It is a poison causing violent purgation and emesis. Many cases of acute, sub-acute and chronic cases of rheumatism have been reputed cured with the tincture by homoeopaths, also pericarditis complicating rheumatism. *(JHC)*

287. *Fraxinus Americana*

(White ash)

Enlargement of Uterus - Fibrous growth, sub-involution, and prolapse. Uterine tumors, with bearing down sensations. Fever, sores on lips. Cramps in feet. Cold creeping and hot flashes. Infantile eczema.

Female: Uterus enlarged and patulous. Watery, unirritating, leucorrhoea. Fibroids with bearing down sensation, cramps in feet, worse in afternoon and night. Dysmenorrhoea.

Relationship: Epiphegus, Sepia, Lillium.

Dose: 10-15 drops of Tr. 3 times a day. *(Boericke)*

Fraxinus has had a fragmentary proving, but the chief clinical authority for its use is Dr. Burnett, who regards it as a uterine tonic in all heavy states of the uterus with prolapse, bearing down and relaxed ligaments. He calls it "The medicinal Pessary" I have repeatedly verified his indications. It is an organ remedy of the first hand. It is also indicated in uterine tumours, especially fibroids with bearing down sensations. *(JHC)*

The remedy is indicated in enlargement and subinvolution of the uterus, when attended with prolapsus and a bearing down sensation. *(Blackwood)*

288. *Fuligo Ligina*

(Soot)

Acts on glandular system, mucous membranes and obstinate ulcers, epidermis, tetters, eczema, chronic irritation of mucus membranes of mouth, pruritus vulvae, uterine haemorrhage, cancer, especially of scrotum - chimney sweeper's cancer, epithelial cancers, cancer of womb with metrorrhagia. Sadness, thoughts of suicide.

Compare: Kreosot.

Dose: 6th trituration *(Boericke)*

289. *Fucus vesiculosis*

(Sea Kelp)

A remedy for obesity and non-toxic goitre, also exophthalmic. Digestion is furthered and flatulence diminished. Obstinate constipation. Forehead feels as if compressed by an iron ring. Thyroid enlargement in obese subjects.

Relation: Phytol, Thyroidine, Badiaga, Iodum.

Dose: Tr. 5 to 60 drops 3 times a day before meals. *(Boericke)*

Fucus is a tissue remedy of great power and must be compared with Iodine of which it contains a large proportion. The symptoms have been obtained from patients taking the medicine for the reduction of obesity. The rapidity of digestion is increased and flatulence diminished. Goitre has been cured with it in teaspoonful doses of tincture given 2-3 times a day. *(JHC)*

290. *Fuchsina - Magneta*

(A coloring substance used in adulteration of wine)

Produces redness of ears, deep red discolouration of mouth, swollen gums, with burning and tendency to salivation, deep red urine, albuminous and light red, profuse diarrhoea, with abdominal pains, cortical substances of kidneys degenerated, useful in cortical nephritis with albuminuria.

Dose: 6x to 30th potency.

(Boericke)

291. *Galium Aparine*

(Goose Grass)

Galium acts on the urinary organs, is a diuretic and of use in dropses, gravel and calculi. Dysuria and cystitis. Has power of suspending or modifying cancerous action. Has clinical confirmation of its use in cancerous ulcers and nodulated tumors of the tongue. Inveterate skin affections and scurvy. Favours healthy granulations and ulcerated surfaces.

Dose: Fluid extract, half dram doses, in cup of water or milk. Three times a day.

(Boericke)

It is a popular remedy for cancer, given internally and used externally as a solvent for gravel and stone-nodulated tumour of tongue diagnosed to be cancer (See Hale). - Psoriasis of the hand. *(JHC)*

Galium Aparine - Cleavers - This remedy is indicated in dysuria, cystitis with much burning upon urinating. It is also of service in nodular tumors of the skin and tongue, and in severe types of skin diseases.

Compare - Cannabis sativa, Cantharis, Copaiva, Berberis vul. *(Blackwood)*

292. *Gallium acidum*

(Gallic acid)

Should be remembered as a remedy in phthisis. It checks the morbid secretions, gives tone to the stomach and increases the appetite. Passive haemorrhages when pulse is feeble and capillaries relaxed. Cold skin. Haematuria, Haemophilia, itching of skin. Pyrosis.

Dose: First trituration, and pure acid 2 to 5 grain doses. *(Boericke)*

Gallic acid the well known astringent derivative of Tannic acid, obtained from galls or oak apples. It is used in old school practice as a local application to arrest haemorrhages. In pulmonary haemorrhage and in the excessive expectoration and the night sweats of pthisis it has been found of a special service. Bayles said it rapidly checks secretions, gives general tone to the stomach, increases appetite and removes constipation. Gall-ac. is used in popular practice to check excessive menstruation. *(JHC)*

293. *Gambogia*

(Gummi Gutti)

The use of this drug in homoeopathy has been confined to its action on the alimentary tract. It produces a diarrhoea very similar to croton. From its pathogenesis, it is very evident that it has very intense and definite action especially on the gastro-enteric tract.

Gastro-enteric symptoms: Feeling of coldness at edge of teeth. Great irritability of the stomach, burning, smarting and dryness of the tongue and throat. Pain in the stomach after food. Tenderness in epigastrium. Pain and distention of abdomen from flatulence after stool. Rumbling and rolling. Dysentery with retained scybala with pain in sacral region. Diarrhoea with sudden and forcible ejection of bilious stool. Tenesmus after, burning at Anus.

Modalities: *Worse* towards evening and at night.

Dose: 3-30 *(Boericke)*

The chief reputation of gamboge among homeopaths is as remedy for diarrhoea - profuse watery diarrhoea, particularly with old people is characteristic. Stool preceded by excessive cutting in navel, stool expelled all atonce after urging and is followed by a feeling of great relief. Stools yellow (colour of the drug, green) bloody, lienteric. Burning in anus after stool, anus sore and excoriated, frightful vomiting and purging with fainting. Burning in the liver - like many other yellow bile like drugs, Gamboge acts markedly on the liver. Agg: towards evening or at night. There is periodicity in symptoms. *(JHC)*

294. Gaultheria

(Wintergreen)

Inflammatory rheumatism, pleurodynia, sciatica and other neuralgias, come within the sphere of this remedy. Cystic and prostatic irritation, undue sexual excitement and renal inflammation.

Stomach: Acute gastritis, severe pain in the epigastrium - prolonged vomiting. Uncontrollable appetite - notwithstanding irritable stomach gastralgia from nervous depression. (give 5 drop of 1x of oil)

Dose: Tr. and lower potencies. *(Boericke)*

Tincture of fresh leaves - oil obtained from leaves. An evergreen trailing vine found in cool damp woods. The oil contains methyl salicylate and is one of the sources of salicin. *(JHC)*

295. Gelsemium

(Yellow Jasmin)

Centers it action upon the nervous system, causing various degrees of Motor paralysis. General prostration. Dizziness, drowsiness, dullness and trembling. Slow pulse, tired feeling, mental apathy, paralysis of various groups of muscles about the eyes, throat, chest, larynx, sphincter, extremities, etc. Post-diphtheritic paralysis. Muscular weakness. Complete relaxation and prostration. Lack of muscular co-ordination. General depression from heat of sun, sensitive to a falling barometer, cold and dampness brings on many complaints. Children fear falling, grab nurse or crib. Sluggish circulation. Nervous affections of cigar makers. Influenza. Measles. Pellagra.

Mind: Dullness, languor, listless, apathy regarding his illness.

Head: Vertigo, band feeling, occipital, headache. Dull, heavy ache, with heviness of eyelids, pain in temple extending into ear.

Eyes: Ptosis; eyelids heavy, dim sighted, orbital neuralgia with contraction and twitching of muscles, serous inflammation, hysterical amblyopia.

Face: Hot, heavy, flushed, besotted looking.

Mouth: Tongue Trembles.

Throat: Post-diphtheritic paralysis, feeling of lump in throat, pain from throat to ear.

Stomach: Gelsemium patient has no thirst.

Stool: Diarrhoea from emotional excitement, cream coloured, tea green.

Urine: Profuse, clear watery partial paralysis of bladder, retention.

Female: Dysmenorrhoea.

Male: Spermatorrhoea without erections, scrotum continually sweating.

Respiratory: Dry cough, with sore chest and fluent coryza, spasm of the glottis, acute bronchitis.

Heart: A feeling as if it were necessary to keep in motion or else hearts action would cease, weak slow pulse of old age.

Back: Dull, heavy pain, pain in neck, especially upper sterno cleido muscles. Dull aching in lumbar and sacral regions.

Extremities: Loss of power of muscular control, cramp in muscles of forearm, writer's cramp, trembling.

Sleep: Sleepless from nervous irritation (Coffea)

Fever: Wants to be held, because he shakes so. Pulse slow, full soft, chilliness up and down back, Heat and sweat stages, long and exhausting. Dumb ague with much muscular soreness, nervous chills, bilious remittent fever, chill without thirst along spine.

Skin: Hot dry, itching measle like eruptions, measles, catarrhal symptoms, aids in bringing out eruptions.

Modalities: *Worse* - very damp weather, fog, before a thunderstorm, emotion or excitement, bad news, tobacco smoking, when thinking of his ailments, at 10 a.m.

Better: Bending forward, by profuse urination, open air, continued motion, stimulants.

Relation: Ignatia (gastric affections of cigar makers); Baptisia, Ipecac, Acon., Bell., Cimic., Mag. phos. Gelsemium contains Mag phos.

Alcoholic stimulants relieve all complaints; where Gels in useful.

Dose: Tr. to 30th attenuation, 1 to 3rd most often used. *(Boericke)*

Gelsemium, which belongs to the same order of plants as Nux vomica and Curare is not only one of the most important additions to the Materia Medica for whose introduction we are mainly indebted to Hale, but it is also in the first rank of importance among the vegetable polychrests. A drug is of importance in homoeopathy not so much by reason of the great number of the symptoms it causes, as by possessing a number of well marked and clearly characterised symptoms which correspond to symptoms constantly met with in everyday practice. It was this which at once gave Gels., a place among the polychrests of homoeopathy. Like its botanical relatives, Gels. is a great paralyser. It produces a general state of paresis, mental and bodily.

Gels. is adapted to children and young people, to persons of a nervous, hysterical temperament, to irritable, sensitive, excitable people. The following provings related by Dr. George Logan of Ottawa (Med, adv, xxiii 125) show the power Gels has over the mental sphere. The subject was Mrs. Logan who describes her experience thus. It increases the power of recollection of memories. It appears to me that I can remember almost anything I love to recall. Now this is my invariable experience, whenever I take Gels., no matter whether in the 3rd or 1000th potency - and I have been in the habit of using it for twenty years. I am writing this under the influence of the drug.

In coryza and hay fever, Gels. has an important place. Early morning sneezing and streaming colds are a strong indication. Chill beginning in hands, or feet, running up back - itching of skin eruption like measles.

The stools of Gels whether loose or constipated are mostly yellow like the flower. The colour comes out also in the colour of the tongue and bilious symptoms generally - (J.G. Blackley pointed out the suitability of Gels to writers cramp and professional paralysis. Complaints from sudden change from hot or dry to damp air. Agg: damp weather, cold damp atmosphere. Causation: Depressing emotions, fright, anger, bad news, sun, heat, damp weather, warm or cold, thunder storms, alcohol, self abuse. *(JHC)*

This agent in toxic doses produces paralysis of the roots of the motor cerebral nerves and the motor area of the spinal cord and as a result paralysis of all muscles of the body. This is followed by a cutaneous anaesthesia. Convulsions in animals and at times in man. The breathing is rendered slower and shallower and is frequently irregular, death results from asphyxia due to depression and ultimately paralysis of the respiratory center. The heart's action is reduced, the pulse is slower, weaker than normal, while the arterial tension is lowered. The temperature is reduced.

Through its action on the third cranial nerve, mydriasis and ptosis results. The sixth nerve may be affected when a convergent strabismus may result with diplopia and dimness of vision. There is extreme muscular weakness and prostration while the patient is drowsy, but the mind is not affected till carbonic acid narcosis takes place. *(Blackwood)*

296. Gentiana Lutea

(Yellow Gentian)

Stomach symptoms marked. Acts as a tonic, increasing appetite.

Head: Vertigo, worse rising or motion, better open air, frontal headache.

Better-eating and open air, brain feels loose, head tender. Aching in eyes.

Throat: Dry, thick saliva.

Stomach: Acid risings, ravenous hunger, nausea, weight and aching in stomach, inflation and tension of stomach and abdomen (Pothos). Colic, umbilical region sensitive to touch, flatulence.

Dose: First to 3rd attenuation. *(Boericke)*

The yellow Gentian is the source of the well known 'tonic' of allopathic practice. In the homoeopathic provings, (by Watzke, Buchner and others), the chief symptoms have been noted in the alimentary sphere and among them 'ravenous hunger' is marked. It has thus some claim to be a positive tonic as it may cause increased appetite in health. It has dry mouth, bitter or earthling taste, nausea, vomiting, colic, diarrhoea with yellow stools (it is the yellow Gentian), rheumatic pains, sensations of constriction are marked and common, weakness, dull feeling, morose mood, febrile condition. *(JHC)*

297. Geum Rivale

(Water avens)

Water avens N.O. Rosacea - Tr. of plant in flower. Hering is the authority for this medicine. Only one symptom has been recorded but it is very definite. Tearing jerking pains which instantly unfit him for everything, seem to shoot from deep within the abdomen, below the umbilicus to the end of urethra. As soon as he eats anything they return, then he is obliged to lie down. They are like electric shocks, excessively severe and always occur twice in succession. *(JHC)*

298. *Ginseng*

(Aralia Quinquefolia - Wild Ginseng - Panax)

Said to be a stimulant to the secretory glands, especially, salivary. Acts on the lower part of the spinal cord. Lumbago, sciatica and rheumatism. Paralytic weakness. Hiccough. Skin symptoms. Itching pimples on neck and chest.

Male: Rheumatic pains after frequent emissions. Weakness of genital organs, voluptuous tickling at the end of urethra, sexual excitement. Pressure in testicles.

Extremities: Hands feel swollen, skin feels tight. Contraction - coldness in back and spine. Bruised pain in small of back and thighs, nightly digging in right lower limb to toes. Burning heat in tips of fingers. Eruptions on upper inner thighs. Stiff contracted joints, heaviness of lower limbs. Crackling in joints. Stiffness in back.

Dose: Tincture to 3rd potency.

(Boericke)

The symptoms of the Chinese and the American Ginseng are taken together, as the two are probably identical. The name is said to signify the resemblance of man or man's thigh. The root is forked like that of a mandrake. Fabulous prices are given for it in Manchuria, as much as p. 40 per pound being paid for certain qualities of it. The wild Ginseng of Siberia is said to be the best. The natives along the Ussuri river use it boiled for headaches, colds, fevers, stomach pains. In America it is a domestic remedy for the after pains of labour. The shape of the root might indicate an action on the pelvis and lower limbs and J.H. Henry (H.R. XI 493) says it acts on the lower part of the spinal marrow; is indicated by bruised pains in small of back and thighs (on rising from bed) and great languor, with paralytic rheumatic pains in lower limbs, arthritic swelling of the foot, which had been exerted a long time, violent pain in big toe. He mentions also Nightly digging in right lower limb from hip to big toe, cramp pains from right hip to toes, lancinating tearing in right tarsal joint. He considers it specific in lumbago, sciatica and chronic rheumatism, with frequent desire to urinate and sexual excitement. *(JHC)*

299. *Glonoine*

(Nitroglycerine)

Recent German provings of Glonoine confirm the original American provings and clinical indications and bring out very marked nerve disturbances. Great lassitude, no inclination to work, extreme irritability, easily excited by the slightest opposition ending in congestive head symptoms. The sixth potency alone produced itching all over body with later, acne and furuncle formation, also bulimy.

Great remedy for congestive headaches, hyperaemia of the brain from excess of heat or cold. Excellent for the intercranial, climacteric disturbances, or due to menstrual suppression. Children get sick when sitting before an open fire. Surging of blood to head and heart. Tendency to sudden and violent irregularities of the circulation, violent convulsions associated with cerebral congestion. Sensation of pulsation through- out body, pulsating pains. Cannot recognize localities.

Head: Confusion. Effects of sunstroke, heat on head. Head heavy, but cannot lay it on pillow. Cannot bear any heat about head. Throbbing headache. Head feels enormously large, as if skull were too small for brain - increases and decreases with the sun.

Ears: Each beat of heart is heard in ears, full feeling.

Dose: 6-30. Potency. *(Boericke)*

lon. is one of the many monuments of Hering's therapeutic genius. The note of the action of Lon is a tendency to sudden and violent irregularities of the circulation. It acts very quickly and very violently. The signature of this potent explosive may be said to be bursting and expansion. Amel: Cold application and cold air. Belladonna has *Amel:* bending head back and covering head - where as Glon. *amel:* uncovered.

Causation: Sun, Bright show, Fire heat. Hair cut. *(JHC)*

This agent increases the pulse rate and produces a general throbbing of the vessels. The throbbing is most marked in the head and gradually becomes worse till there is a violent, bursting frontal headache with giddiness, fullness of the head, flushed face and sensation of constriction of the throat, accompanied by vomiting, faintness and complete insensibility. Large doses occasion heart failure in diastole.

Increases the pulse rate - general throbbing of the vessels - throbbing is most marked in the head-congestion and hyperaemia of the brain - violent and appear suddenly - sunstroke - congestive throbbing headaches - puerperal convulsions - cerebral congestion of children when Belladonna does not afford desired relief - tinnitus aurium. It should be remembered in acute and chronic interstitial nephritis when the arterial tension is high. Also in cases of increased vascular tension of the aged. In angina pectoris, asthma and heart failure it is of service when the pulse is small, wiry and there is pallor, anaemia of the brain and collapse. Use the physiological dose in these cases. *(Blackwood)*

300. Glycerinum

(Glycerine)

Glycerinum is used homoeopathically, dynamized glycerine. Seems to act deep and long, building up tissue, hence of great use in marasmus, debility - mental and physical, diabetes etc. It disturbs nutrition in its primary action and secondarily, seems to improve the general state of nutrition (Dr. Wm. B. Griggs).

Urinary: Profuse and frequent urination - increased specific gravity and sugar - Diabetes.

Dose: 30th and higher potencies. Pure Glycerine in teaspoonful doses T.I.D. with lemon juice for pernicious anaemia.

(Boericke)

301. Gnaphalium

(Cut weed - old Balsam)

A remedy of unquestioned benefit in Sciatica, when pain is associated with numbness of the part affected. Rheumatism and morning diarrhoea. Polyuria.

Female: Weight and fullness in pelvis, dysmenorrhoea with scanty and painful menses.

Back: Chronic backache, in lumbar region, better resting on back, lumbago with numbness in lower part of back and weight in pelvis.

Extremities: Cramps in calves of legs and feet when in bed, rheumatic pains in ankle joints and legs, intense pain along the sciatic nerve, numbness alternates with pain. Better drawing limbs up, flexing thigh on abdomen. Gouty concretions. Pain in joints as if they lacked oil. Chronic muscular rheumatism of back and neck.

Relation: Xanthoxyl, Cham., Puls.

Dose: 3-30th potency. *(Boericke)*

Gnaphal has been used mainly in affections of sciatic nerve. But it has also an action on the abdominal organs. The special indication for its use in sciatica and lumbago is, numbness alternating with pain. There is also sexual excitement in male provers, pain and irritation in the prostate gland. A very important observation made by MC. George is on the value of Gnaph in dysmenorrhoea - weight and fullness in pelvis. Flexing the thigh on abdomen may possibly be a key note. *(JHC)*

It has relieved flatulent colic, when the pains are in various parts of the abdomen, which is sensitive to pressure; also cholera morbus, when with the colic there is vomiting and purging *(Blackwood)*

302. *Gossypium*
(Cotton plant)

A powerful emmenagogue used in physiological doses. Homoeopathically, it corresponds to many reflex conditions depending on disturbed uterine function and pregnancy. Gossypium will relieve tardy menses, especially with sensation that the flow is about to start and yet does not do so. Tall bloodless patients with nervous chills.

Stomach: Nausea with inclination to vomit before breakfast.

Female: Intermittent pains in ovaries, tumour of breast with swelling of auxiliary glands, morning sickness.

Dose: Tr. to 6th attenuation. *(Boericke)*

Gossyp. has been mainly used in affections of the female generative organs. It has been taken in the form of the extract to procure abortion. The symptoms of the external organs are strongly marked and the ovaries are the seat of pains which come and go and in the uterus there are bearing down pains. Intermittent pains in the ovaries is characteristic. The morning nausea and salivation indicate the remedy for morning sickness of pregnancy. *(JHC)*

It is useful in uterine subinvolution and fibroids, when the patient is anaemic, complains of gastric pain and debility. *(Blackwood)*

303. *Granatum*
(Pomegranate)

As a vermifuge for the expulsion of Tapeworm, and homoeopathically for the following symptomatic indications. Salivation with nausea and vertigo, spasm of the glottis.

Head: Vertigo very persistent.

Stomach: Constant hunger.

Abdomen: Pain worse about umbilicus.

Skin: Itching of palms.

Dose: 1-3 potency. *(Boericke)*

Pomegranate is a well known vermifuge especially used for the expulsion of taenia. For this a decoction of the rind of the fruit is used. Swelling of navel - protrusion in inguinal rings. *(JHC)*

It contains an alkaloid called Pelletierine. This remedy is employed as a taenicide and taeniafuge of the tape worm. All the symptoms ascribed to it are but those that result from the taenia. *(Blackwood)*

304. *Graphites*

(Black lead - Plumbago)

Like all the carbons this remedy is an anti-psoric of great power and especially active in patients who are rather stout, of fair complexion, with tendency to skin affections and constipation, fat, chilly and costive, with delayed menstrual history, take cold easily. Children, impudent, teasing, laugh at reprimands. Has a particular tendency to develop the skin phase of internal disorders. Eradicates tendency to erysipelas. Anaemia with redness of face. Tendency to obesity. Swollen genitals. Gushing leucorrhoea. Aids absorption of cicatrical tissue. Induration of tissue. Cancer of pylorus. Duodenal ulcer.

Mind: Music makes her weep.

Head: Burning on vertex.

Eyes: Eyelids red and swollen. Eczema of the lids, fissured.

Ears: Dryness of inner ear. Moisture and eruptions behind the ears. Hears better in noise.

Nose: Smell abnormally acute, cannot tolerate flowers.

Stomach: Aversion to meat, sweets nauseate. Hot drinks disagree. Constrictive pain in stomach. Stomach pain *Amel.:* eating, hot milk and lying down.

Abdomen: Must loosen clothing.

Female: Leucorrhoea, pale, thin, profuse, white, excoriating.

Nails: Thick, black and rough. Matrix inflamed.

Skin: Eruptions oozing out a sticky exudation. Unhealthy, every little injury suppurates.

Modalities: *Worse* warmth, at night, during and after menstruation.

Better: In the dark, from wrapping up.

Dose: 6-30 potency. *(Boericke)*

Suited to women inclined to obesity who suffer from habitual constipation with a history of delayed menstruation. What Pulsatilla is at puberty, Graphites is at the climacteric. Leucorrhoea acrid, excoriating, occurs in gushes day and night. Stool intolerable odour. Decided aversion to coition (both sexes). After calcarea in obesity of young women with large amount of unhealthy adipose tissue. *(H.C. Allen)*

Degenerative changes in the skin, hair, nails, and glands. Inclined to obesity. Fair complexion, subject to constipation, climacteric period. Eczema, rhagades, excoriations, ulcers, skin may be dry. Constipation. Gastric catarrh, intestinal fermentation, abdomen distended with gas, putrid. Cramping pains in the stomach, relieved by eating, disgust for meats and sweets. Diarrhoea - stools are brown, fluid, offensive. Menses are scanty. Leucorrhoea acrid, excoriating. Mastitis, cracks in the nipples. Compare - Pulsatilla, sepia. *(Blackwood)*

Plumbago. Black lead. An allotropic modification of Carbon. The finest specimens contain traces of iron 0.4 to 0.6 percent; poor qualities as much as 4 percent. Trituration of prepared black lead from finest English drawing pencils.

Graphites is suited to persons who have a tendency to put on unhealthy fat. There is clean tongue. Milk agrees well, especially hot milk. Salivation.

The male sexual organs are affected as well as the female; uncontrollable sexual excitement with violent erections.

The skin of Graphites is rough, hard and dry. Eczematous and herpetic eruptions predominate. Cracks and fissures. Offensive discharges and secretions. Sweat stains yellow; sour, offensive.

Warmth of bed agg: itching and amel: crampy pain in stomach.

Head: Humid scabs on the head. After scratching more sore and humid; later drying up to a white scurf. Abundant desquamation of the scalp. Perspiration smelling acid or very offensive, colouring the linen yellow. The hair turns grey.

Ears: Fetid smell and discharge of blood and of pus from the ears.

Appetite: Immoderate hunger with acidity of the stomach.

Stool and Anus: Obstinate constipation, with hard faeces, knotty and scanty. Stools of a putrid, sour smell with burning at the rectum or of sanguinous mucus - Mucous diarrhoea - Diarrhoea, with tightness of the abdomen Faeces of a very small size, like a worm. Lumbrici and ascarides, Taenia. Itching, sensation of excoriation, and swelling of the anus. Prolapsus recti with the varices, as if the rectum were paralysed.

Sexual organs: Eruption of pimples on the prepuce, and on the penis. Leucorrhoea, white and liquid, like water, with tension of the abdomen, and weakness in the back.

Neck and back: Stiffness in the nape of the neck. Violent pain in the nape of the neck and the shoulders, on stooping the head and on raising the arms, like a tearing incision.

Upper limbs: Tearing and lancinating in the shoulders. Sensation of contraction in the joint of the elbow, on extending the arms - Cramp and tearing in the hands.

Mouth: Pain, as from excoriation, vesicles and ulcers on the tongue - Bitter taste in the mouth, the tongue being much coated - profuse salivation - speech impeded by paralysis of the muscles.

Lower limbs: Arthritic tearing in the hip joint, the feet and the toes. Stiffness of the instep - shooting pain, like that of an ulcer, in the heel and in the soles of the feet on rising from the sitting posture - cold feet even in the evening in bed feet burning - fetid sweat on the feet - contraction of the toes-swelling and distortion of the toes - corn.

Obstinate dryness of the skin and absence of perspiration - Encysted tumours - unrefreshing sleep at night, followed in the morning by a comatose sleep. *(JHC)*

305. Gratiola

(Hedge Hyssop)

Acts especially on gastro-intestinal tract, chronic catarrhal conditions, leucorrhoea and gonorrhoea. Obstinate ulcers. Useful in mental troubles from overweening pride especially useful in females. Nux-v. symptoms in females often met by Gratiola.

Head: Rush of blood.

Stool: Green frothy water, forcibly evacuated without pain. Constipation.

Female: Nymphomania, Menses too profuse, premature and too long. Leucorrhoea.

Dose: 2nd to 3rd potency. (Boericke)

Cooper regards it as the vegetable Antacid. Buvier says, Teste saw four cases of nymphomania in females to whom herb doctors had given injections of decoctions of freshly gathered Gratiola. Causation - Abuse of coffee. *(JHC)*

This agent is an emetic, diuretic, cathartic, and in toxic doses is an active poison.

This remedy is indicated in cholera infantum and diarrhoea when there is nausea and vomiting of a yellow, bitter, sour tasting fluid, which comes up without any special exertion. The passage from the bowels consists of green frothy water, which is forcibly evacuated. Following the passage there is burning in the rectum and anus. It is frequently the remedy to relieve the bowels and stomach troubles that appear as a result of taking large quantities of ice water. *Compare:* Croton tiglium, Veratrum album. *(Blackwood)*

306. Grindelia

(Rosin wood)

Both Grindelia Robusta and Grindelia Squarrosa have been used for the symptoms here recorded. There is practically no difference in their action, although G. Squarrosa is credited with more splenic symptoms. Dull pain and fullness in left hypochondrium, chronic malaria, gastric pains associated with splenic congestion induces paralysis, beginning in extremities, its action is shown on the heart first, quickening, then retarding it.

Acts on the cardio - pulmonary distribution of the pneumogastric in dry catarrh (Tart. emetic in muco-purulent). Produces a paresis of the pneumogastric interfering with respiration. Smoothering after falling asleep. Asthmatic conditions, chronic bronchitis. Bronchorrhoea with tough mucus difficult to detach.. Raises the blood pressure. Nausea and retching of gastric ulcer. Sugar in urine. An effective dose to Rhus poisoning locally and internally. Also for burns, blisters, vaginal catarrh and herpes zoster. Hyperchlorhydria, when attended with asthmatic and other neurotic symptoms. Hyperaemia of gastric mucous membrane with difficult respiration.

Head: Pain in eye balls.

Respiratory: Stops breathing when falling asleep, wakes with a start and gasps for breath. Must sit up to breathe, cannot breathe when lying down. Pertussis with profuse mucous secretion.

Dose: Tr. in 1-15 drops doses and lower potencies. *(Boericke)*

The Grindeliae are a genus of asteroid composites growing on the pacific coast and inland on the mountains. The terminal heads of yellow flowers and the leaves are usually covered with a viscid balsamic secretion, from which they have been called Gum plants. A tincture is made of the leaves and unexpanded flowers. Bundys proving of G. squarrosa was made with a tincture of the dried plant.

There was a kind of paralysis of the vagus nerve, on falling asleep the respiratory movement would cease and would not be resumed until he wakes up from the resulting suffocation. One writer obtained excellent results from Grindelia in a number of cases of asthma and emphysema with dilated heart. Dr. Foster's patient was awakened by asthmatic attacks, the room seeming too small. After getting quiet, just as he would commence to lose himself in sleep he would suddenly awaken again because he seemed to have forgotten to breathe, Grind. R. 30 relieved. It removed aversion to darkness in one patient, who wanted a light in the room all night. Symptoms are Amel: by movement, Agg: in the dark, and on falling asleep. *(JHC)*

This remedy is indicated in chronic bronchial asthma and chronic spasmodic bronchial cough, when they are attended with profuse, tenacious expectoration, which gives relief. The breath stops when the patient goes to sleep and awakes with a start, gasping for breath. It is useful in irregular heart action and in hay-fever when associated with difficult breathing it is used locally and internally as an antidote for Rhus toxicodendron poisoning.

Compare: Sanguinaria, Eriodictyon. *(Blackwood)*

307. *Guaco*

(Mikania, Climbing Hemp Weed)

Acts on nervous system and female organs. Antidotes to bites of scorpions and serpents. Cholera. Bulbar paralysis. Syphilis. Cancer. Deafness. Tongue heavy and difficult to move. Spinal irritation, spinal symptoms most marked and verified. Beer drinkers threatened with apoplexy. Diarrhoea and dysentery with aching in sacrum and loins.

Back: Pain along spine.

Extremities: paralysis of extremities.

Dose: 3-6 potency. *(Boericke)*

Guaco has a local repute as a remedy for the bites of serpents, for hydrophobia cholera and cancer. In the homoeopathic provings rice water stools occurred and difficulty in swallowing as in hydrophobia. *(JHC)*

308. *Guaiacum*

(Resin of Lignum Vitae)

Chief action on fibrous tissue and is especially adapted to the arthritic diathesis. Rheumatism, and tonsillitis. Secondary syphilis. Very valuable in acute rheumatism. Free foul secretions. Unclean odor from whole body. Promotes suppuration of abscesses. Sensitiveness and aggravation from local heat. Contraction of limbs, stiffness and immobility. Feeling that he must stretch.

Head: Gouty and rheumatic pain in head and face, extending to neck. Worse cold wet weather. Pain often ends in a stitch.

Throat: Acute tonsillitis.

Stomach: Desire for apples and other fruits. Aversion to milk.

Respiratory: Feels suffocated - Pleuritic stitches.

Back: Aching in nape. Stiff neck and sore shoulders.

Extremities: Rheumatic pain in shoulders, arms and hands. Growing pains. Sciatica and lumbago. Gouty tearing with contractions. Immovable stiffness. Ankle pain extending up the leg, causing lameness. Joints swollen, painful and intolerant of pressure, can bear no heat. Stinging pain in limbs. Arthritic lancinations followed by contraction of limbs. A feeling of heat in the affected limbs.

Modalities: Worse from motion, heat, cold wet weather, pressure, touch, from 6 p.m. to 4 a.m.

Better: External pressure. Follows Sepia.

Dose: Tr-6c. *(Boericke)*

It is a remedy in gout and rheumatism and a diuretic but lately it has also taken a place in old school therapeutics as a remedy for consumption.

It acts on mucous membranes, muscles, joints and bones, and causes contraction of tendons with resulting deformity. Gouty nodosities on joints. Verwey (H.R. ix, 627) treated a lady who for several years had a frequently recurring gouty inflammation of the knees. Guai. 30 was given (after Chi. 30 had failed to relieve) without obvious benefit. Guai. 1 was now given and after a few hours the swelling broke and the pains quickly subsided. A short time after, the same patient accidentally injured the same knee. Under Guai. 1 the swelling soon broke and the pain was relieved.

Rheumatism in syphilitic and mercurial patients. Acute tonsillitis, simple or rheumatic. Syphilitic sore throat. Burning in the throat.

Guaiac., says Ozanam, seems to combine the properties of Bell, Apis, and Bar c. It has the erythematous or inflammatory angina with bright redness of Bell, the oedema of Apis, and the phlegm with tendency to suppuration of tonsils of Bar. c and Apis (H.R. ii 217). Proell records the cure of a case of secondary syphilis in a gentleman.

Guaiac is better than Caust, which it follows well when either gout or rheumatism causes distortion of limbs. *(JHC)*

It is useful in chronic rheumatism of the upper extremities and in Lumbago when there is a stiffness of the parts. The joints are swollen, tender, and cannot bear pressure or heat. It has been employed in the treatment of secondary syphilis. Compare - Mezereum, Mercurius, Rhus tox. *(Blackwood)*

309. Gun powder

(Carbon - Sulph - Kali - Nit)

There is no proving of Gun - powder, but I made an experiment on myself with the 2X, as I have mentioned in my article on Kali - Nit in my Dictionary of Materia Medica.

The indications for the remedy are broad and clear, so that no fine differentiation of symptoms is required. The list of diseases named under 'Clinical' will be a sufficient guide, coupled with the broad indication, blood poisoning. Gun powder corresponds to suppuration in a great number of forms - many of them septic. I have not found it disagree with any other remedy, so that there need be no fear of alternating it with some other remedy, if particularly indicated.

In some country districts a decoction of gun powder is given increase its effects.

Relation: Calendula externally is also complementary. Also - Thuja, Silica, Baryta Carb (Septic tonsils) agree very well.

Nitre with sulphur and charcoal forms Gun Powder. A teaspoonful of this in hot water was a favorite remedy for gonorrhoea among soldiers in days when black powder was used. In the triturations, Gun powder has cured ascarides in adults. In some experiments made by myself with Gun power 2x, severe Herpes facialis involving right eyebrow and right side of nose developed. *(JHC)*

310. Hamamelis Virginica

(Witch Hazel)

Venous congestion, haemorrhages, varicose veins and haemorrhoids, with bruised soreness of affected parts seem to be the special sphere of this remedy. Acts upon the coats of the veins causing relaxation with consequent engorgement. Passive venous haemorrhages from any part. Great value in open, painful wounds with weakness from loss of blood. After operations, supersedes the use of morphia.

Head: Wants 'the respect due to me' shown.

Stool: Haemorrhoids, bleeding profusely with soreness - Dysentery - pulsation in rectum.

Female: Vicarious menstruation, uterine haemorrhage, bearing down pain in back. Menses dark profuse with soreness in abdomen. Metrorrhagia occurring midway between menstrual periods. Vagina very tender. Profuse leucorrhoea. Vulva itches - Milk-leg, haemorrhoids. Metrorrhagia, passive flow - vaginismus - ovaritis - phlegmasia alba.

Male: Varicocele, pain in testicles, orchitis, testicles enlarged, hot and painful, Epididymitis.

Respiratory: Haemoptysis.

Skin: Bluish chilblains, phlebitis, purpura, varicose veins and ulcers.

Modality: *Worse* warm moist air.

Dose: Tr-6c. Distilled extract locally.
(Boericke)

The deep red colour of the tincture of Hamamelis may be taken as the signature of its therapeutic action. No remedy has a wider sphere of usefulness in cases of haemorrhage and disordered blood vessels. A number of interesting superstitions are associated with the Shrub - and shoots of it are used as divining rods, for discovering water and metals. Hamamelis is called for in cases of varicose angina where the veins of the pharynx are large and blue. The parts from which the flow of blood proceeds feels sore and bruised. It relieves the excessive thirst, that most patients with heart troubles complain of - complementary to Ferrum in Haemorrhages. *(JHC)*

This agent is an astringent, styptic, sedative and tonic. It acts upon the veins much as Aconite does upon the arteries, and results in venous congestions, and haemorrhages. Full doses produce a throbbing in the head.

In varicose veins of the legs it is of service both locally and internally. Also in varicose veins of the throat, when the veins are distended and the parts are of a bluish color, there is more or less soreness of parts and pain upon swallowing, with hawking and raising of mucus and blood. The patient takes cold easily, especially in a warm, moist or a relaxing air, that favors venous stasis. Haemorrhoids, that bleed profusely, are sore and painful, and attended with burning, fullness and heaviness, as if the back would break. The anus feels sore and raw and there is an urging as for stool, while the haemorrhoids is of a bluish color.

In phlebitis, with soreness, it is of great service and may be applied locally in the form of a wet dressing, and given internally.

It is met with in lacerated and contused wounds, where it not only controls the haemorrhage, but removes the pain and soreness, also cases of epistaxis. It is also indicated in these cases when the flow is profuse from the nose, but is venous in character, relieving a distressing headache.

It should be remembered in haemoptysis, when the blood is venous. There may be a slight tickling that induces a cough, or it may come up without effort, or coughing.

The menses are profuse and dark and are attended with soreness in the abdomen. Following any traumatism of these parts, the menstruation is attended with great pain, uterine haemorrhage that appears as the result of riding in a carriage over rough ground or from severe jolting of the body. It relieves vaginismus, with intense soreness of the parts, also prurigo of the vulva, when the parts are of a dark purplish color.

Haematuria, haematemesis and chilblains, when the parts are of bluish color, have been relieved by this remedy.

Subacute ovaritis incident to pregnancy and menstruation, and gonorrhoeal infection, when the organ is greatly inflamed, and extremely tender to touch, it should be employed both locally and internally.

Compare: Melilotus, Ipecacuanha, Millefolium. *(Blackwood)*

311. Hekla Lava

(Lava Scoriae from Mt. Hecla)

Marked action upon the jaws. Of great use in exostosis, gum abscess, difficult teething, nodosities, caries of bone etc. Osteitis, periostitis, osteosarcoma, rachitis. Tumours in general. Bone necrosis. Necrosis and sinus after mastoid operation.

Face: Facial neuralgia from carious teeth and after extraction. Toothache with swelling about jaws. Enlargement of maxillary bone.

Dose: Lower trituration. *(Boericke)*

I have chosen the single word Hecla in preference to Hecla Lava, as being simpler and more convenient. The ash and scoriae of this volcano contain Silica, Alumina, Lime, Magnesia, with some oxide of Iron. When travelling in Iceland, Garth Wilkinson noticed that the sheep in the vicinity of Hecla had immense exostoses on the jaws. Another effect noticed was the drying up of the milk both in sheep and cows. The finer ash which fell on pastures at a distance, was the most deleterious, the gross ash near the mountain was inert. In cows, post-mortem examination showed the intestines filled with ashes, hardened to a mass, and stomach coated over with a pitch-black membrane spotted with brown, and difficult to remove by washing, the jaw teeth were covered with a shining metallic crust. Several young horses died from lumps on the jaw-bones, so large as to cause dislocation. Sheep when slaughtered, were found to be of bluish hue internally, and the intestines were friable. In many cases worms from two to three inches long, with pale grey bodies and brown heads, and a little thicker than a horse hair, were found in the bronchia. In sheep the osseous and dental systems were much affected. The head-bones, and especially the jaw-bones, swelled and became so friable that when boiled they fell to pieces. The thigh, and especially the shin bones, swelled and bulged. The jaws, were sometimes covered with large swellings which spread and were looser of texture and darker in colour than the bone; these could be separated from the bone without injuring it; but in some fatal cases a hole going down to the marrow was discovered under the swelling. Garh Wilkinson adds to the above that he has used Hecla with excellent effect in toothache, gum abscess, swellings about the jaws and in difficult dentition. Clinical experience has shown the power of Hecla to arrest many forms of bone disease, including osteosarcoma, scrofulous and syphilitic osteitis and exostoses. The swellings amenable to it are painful and sensitive to touch; Agg; from touch and pressure. The glands are affected almost as much as the bones: "induration and infiltration of cervical glands, studding neck like a row of pearls." The right side has been more predominantly affected. The subjoined schema is compiled mainly from cured symptoms.

Compare: Conchiol, Silic., Calc., Slag., Phos., Stilling, Sulph., Kali-iod., Amphisb., Symphyt, Ruta. *(HCA)*

312. *Helleborus*

(Snow Rose)

Produces a condition of sensorial depressions. Sees, hears, tastes imperfectly and general muscular weakness which may go on to complete paralysis, accompanied by dropsical effusions. Hence a remedy in low states of vitality and serous disease. Characteristic aggravation from 4 to 8 p.m. (Lycop). Sinking sensation. State of effusion in hydrocephalus. Mania of melancholy type.

Mind: Involuntary sighing. Complete unconsciousness. Picks lips and clothes.

Head: Rolls head. Bores head into pillow.

Mouth: Horrible smell from the mouth, Falling of lower jaw. Meaningless picking of lips - Grinding of teeth - Chewing motion - greedily swallows water.

Extremities: Automatic motion of one arm and leg.

Sleep: Cri-encephalique.

Skin: Pale, dropsical.

Dose: Tr. to 3 potency.

Compare: Hedera Helex for Hydrocephalus. *(Boericke)*

Helleborus Niger or Black Hellebore was one of the drugs used to produce the "Helleborism, of the ancients" the subject of Hahnemann's famous essay; but the drug most commonly employed was the white hellebore, or Veratrum album, which belongs to another family, the Melanthaceae. "Black Hellebore receives its name from the external colour of its root; the root of Ver. alb. is extremely white. Teste quotes Hahnemann as saying: I conclude from various observations that one of the first effects of Black Hellebore is a kind of stupor, a dullness of the sensorium commune, a condition where, with sight unimpaired, nothing is seen very fully, and the patient does not pay any attention to anything; with the hearing perfectly sound, nothing is heard distinctly; with perfectly constituted gustatory organs, everything seems to have lost its taste; where the mind is often or always without ideas; where the past is forgotten or little remembered; where nothing gives one any pleasure; where one's sleep is very light, and a really sound, refreshing sleep is not to be had; and where one desires to work without having the necessary strength or attention required for it. Teste groups Hell. n. in the Chamomilla class, with Gratiola and Viola Tric, all of which cause a particular derangement of the cerebral functions and even of the whole nervous system; a painful increase of the sentient action, followed by a considerable depression of the vital forces, and a certain disorder of the mental faculties. He cured with Hell. n. a case of epilepsy in a little girl five weeks old after the failure of Cann. Cham. was given to the nurse. Hell. n. directly to the patient. *(JHC)*

Physiological action: this agent produces salivation and stimulates the secretions of the liver and pancreas; it also increases the peristaltic action of the intestines. There is hyperaemia of the kidneys, while the urine is scanty. The uterine mucous membrane is congested. The brain cord and serous surfaces show a general hyperaemia and anasarca. Toxic doses cause paralysis, with a rapid pulse and sudden arrest of the heart. With the paralysis there is a tremor, followed by violent convulsions.

This agent contains two active medicinal principals, Helleborein and Helleborin; the former is an active cardiac poison and drastic purgative; the latter acts as a narcotic producing in animals at first inquietude, which is soon followed by paresis, both of motion and sensation. *(Blackwood)*

313. *Heloderma*

(Gila Monster)

The results of the bites is a benumbing paralysis like paralysis agitans or locomotor ataxia. There is no tetanic phase - a condition almost reverse in objective symptoms to Hydrocy - acid or strychnia. The most unusual action of the drug is noted upon the eye of the mouse. The eyeball becomes more prominent and the cornea shows opacities. The exophthalmus is due to the pressure of the blood behind the eye ball (Boyd). Homoeopathically, it is indicated in many forms of diseases characterised by great coldness - 'arctic coldness'. Cold waves from occiput to feet or ascending.

Extremities: Numbness and trembling, cyanosis of hands. Coldness Sensation as if walking on sponge and as if feet were swollen. Staggering gait. Cock's gait. When walking lifts feet higher than usual and puts down heel hard. Feel cold as ice, or burn. Stretching relieves pains in muscles and limbs. Fever: Internal coldness, as if frozen to death. Cold rings around body, cold waves. Cold spots. 'Arctic' coldness temperature sub-normal 96° (Camph).

Dose: 30 potency. *(Boericke)*

At any rate it is agreed that there is one lizard that is a Heloderma and our remedy is the poison obtained therefrom. An ugly disagreeable looking creature the head long and blunt, eyes black and bead like, tail half the length of the body thick set and club like. The entire body cased in a thinly coated armour, marked curiously with yellow and black. It is sluggish and slow of movement when kept in the dark but may develop great activity when brought into the sunlight. It is most tenacious of life, the only vulnerable part seems to be at the junction of the head with the spine a blow on which will kill it. *(JHC)*

Synonyms, Heloderma Horridus, Gila Monster. A large Lizard of the Order Saurii. Prep: Triturations of the virus, and dilutions.

Dose: Dilutions from the 6th up.

Physiological action - This poison when introduced into the human system produces a sensation of coldness and a paralysis that simulates paralysis agitans or locomotor ataxia.

This remedy is to be studied in all conditions when there is a sensation of coldness of the body, internal coldness as if frozen, together with a staggering, ataxic gait.

Compare: Camphora, Argentum nitricum. *(Blackwood)*

314. *Helonias*

(Unicorn root)

Sensation of weakness, dragging and weight in the sacrum and pelvis, with great languor and prostration, are excellent indications for this remedy.

There is a sensitiveness expressed as a consciousness of womb. Tired, back ache in females. The weakness shows itself also in a tendency to prolapse and other malposition of the womb. The menses are often suppressed and the kidneys congested. It seems as if the monthly congestion instead of venting itself as it should through the uterine vessels, had extended to the kidneys. With it all there is a profound melancholia. Patient must be doing something to engage the mind. Remember it for women with prolapsus from atony, enervated by indolence and luxury (better when attention is engaged - hence when the doctor comes), or for those worn out with hard work, tired strained muscles, burn and ache, sleepless, diabetes mellitus and insipidus. Constant aching and tenderness over kidneys.

Mind: Patient is better when kept busy.

Back: Pain and weight in back, tired and weak. Aching and burning across the lumbar region extending down the legs. Great languor, better exercising.

Female: Dragging in sacral region with prolapse especially after a miscarriage. Pruritus Vulvae. Conscious of womb. Menses too frequent, too profuse.

Urine: Albuminous.

Dose: Tr. to 6c. *(Boericke)*

It is a uterine remedy of great power. Uterine tonic, consciousness of the womb and relaxation of uterine ligaments, misplacements and prolapse have been removed. Has prolapse of uterus, ulceration of cervix, dark offensive leucorrhoea. Is irritable, finds fault with everyone and cannot bear contradiction. Severe backache - Helon 30. Easily fatigued by any work, who complain of a tired backache, a tired feeling extending into the limbs. Some of this passes off after commencing work. Intense pruritus, vulvar and vaginal for several weeks. She could tear the flesh out. It was so intense. Thin albuminous leucorrhoea evidently the cause of pruritus - In general it is a close analogue of Puls. - in its local and general symptoms - Compare also Sep., Pic. ac., (tired aching and some burning in back and legs)

(JHC)

This agent in large doses is a cardiac poison. Cattle die as the result of eating it. In medicinal doses it is an emetic, tonic, diuretic and vermifuge.

While these complaints may be general, and the remedy indicated in both sexes, they are frequently associated with diseases of the kidneys and generative organs of the female. An examination of the mucous surfaces and of the blood shows that a condition of anaemia is present.

The leucorrhoeal discharge has an offensive odour, and there is a persistent itching of the genitals. Following confinement, it is useful when there is a tendency to prolapsus and other malposition of the uterus. She complains of heaviness and dragging of the pelvic organs.

It is of service in prolapsus of the uterus, which is either the result of indolence and luxury or of hard work, either mental or physical. The patient is conscious of a womb.

It prevents abortions which occur as the result of the slightest over exertion or irritating emotions.

It should be remembered as a possible remedy in cases of salivation, and in nervous dyspepsia, and chronic gastritis when debility is a pronounced symptom. The patient's ailments are ameliorated while she is doing something.

Compare: Aletris farinosa, Lilium tigrinum, Phosphoric acid, Murex.

(Blackwood)

315. Hepar sulph calcareum

(Hahnemann's Calcium Sulphate)

Suits especially scrofulous and lymphatic constitutions, who are inclined to have eruptions and glandular swellings. Unhealthy skin. Blondes with sluggish character and weak muscles. Great sensitiveness to all impressions. Sweating Patient pulling blanket around him. Locally it has a special affinity the respiratory mucous membrane, producing croupous catarrhal inflammation, profuse secretion and also easy perspiration. After abuse of mercury, infected sinus with pus formation. The tendency to suppuration is most marked and has been a strong guiding symptom in practice. The lesions spread by the formation of small papules around the side of the old lesions. Chilliness, hypersensitiveness, splinter like pains, craving for sour and strong things are very characteristic. Feeling as if wind were blowing on some part. The side of the body on which he lies at night becomes gradually insufferably painful, he must turn. Pellagra (material doses required), syphilis after anti specific gross medication.

Mind: The slightest cause irritates him, dejected and sad. Ferocious. Hasty speech.

Eyes: Ulcers on cornea, iritis, with pus in anterior chamber, purulent conjunctivitis.

Ears: Discharge of fetid flow from ears whizzing and throbbing in ears with hardness of hearing. Pustules in auditory canal and auricle. Mastoiditis.

Nose: Sore, ulcerated. Sneezes every time he goes into a cold dry wind with running of nose, later thick offensive discharge. Smell like old cheese, hay fever.

Face: Yellowish complexion. Middle of lower lip cracked, ulcers in corners of mouth.

Mouth: Ptyalism Gums and mouth painful to touch and bleed readily.

Throat: When swallowing, sensation as of a plug and of a splinter in throat, quinsy with impending suppuration.

Stomach: Longing for acids. Aversion to fat food. Heaviness and pressure in stomach after a slight meal.

Abdomen: Hepatitis, Hepatic abscess.

Stool: Clay coloured and soft, sour, white, undigested, loss of power to expel even a soft stool.

Urine: Voided slowly, without force, drops vertically.

Male: Herpes, itching of glans, franeum and scrotum. Suppurating inguinal glands.

Humid soreness on genitals and between scrotum and thigh.

Female: Itching of pudenda. Abscesses of labia with great sensitiveness. Extremely offensive leucorrhoea.

Respiratory: Loses voice and coughs when exposed to dry cold wind. Hoarseness with loss of voice. Dry hoarse cough excited, whenever any part of the body gets cold or uncovered or from eating anything cold - choking cough.

Extremities: Finger joints swollen - Nail of great toe painful on slight pressure.

Skin: Abscesses - suppurating glands - Acne in youth. Unhealthy skin, every little injury suppurates - skin with deep cracks on hands and feet. Ulcers very sensitive. Sweats day and night without relief - wants to be wrapped up warmly. Chronic and recurring urticaria. Herpes circinatus.

Fever: Dry heat at night. Profuse sweat, sour sticky offensive.

Modalities: Worse from dry cold winds.

Better: In damp weather, from wrapping head, from warmth, after eating. Hepar antidotes bad effects from mercury.

Dose: 1-200c. The higher potencies may abort suppuration, the lower promote it.

If it is necessary to hasten it, give 2x.

(Boericke)

"Liver of Sulphur" is a name which was given by the old chemists to several sulphur compounds whose colour was supposed to resemble that of liver - neither it is not identical in composition or properties with calcium sulphate (Gypsum) of Schussler. Being a chemical combination of Calc. carb. and sulph., it has some of the properties of both, but is very different from either. It is useful to compare them. Sensitiveness to noise - to odours - dissatisfaction with oneself and others - dreamy - atra-bilious mood. A sort of ferocious spleen as though one could murder a man in cold blood (and benevolent disposition). Silicea and merc: are inimical - but if hepar is given as an intermediary no unpleasant effects will occur. There is a semi-paralytic condition of rectum and bladder somewhat like that of Alumina. The stools are passed with great difficulty even when clay like and soft. Micturition is impeded, obliged to walk a while before the urine passes. Teste puts Hep. in his Pulsatilla group with Sil., Calc., Graph., and Phos.

The slightest injury causes suppuration - oversensitive, physically and mentally - quick, hasty speech and hasty drinking - extremely sensitive to cold air - urine voided slowly, without force, drops vertically - cough when any part of the body is uncovered, croupy, choking, strangling, from exposure to dry west wind - sensation of a splinter, fish bone or plug in the throat. Middle lower lip cracked - diarrhoea of children with sour smell. Sweats profusely day and night without relief Amel: warmth in general, wrapping up warmly especially of the head, in damp wet weather.

(H.C. Allen)

316. Hippomanes

(A meconium deposit of the Amniotic fluid taken from the colt)

The old famous Aphrodisiacum of the greek authors.

Stomach: Icy coldness.

Male: Sexual desire increased, prostatitis, drawing pain in testicles.

Extremities: Sprained sensation in wrist. Great weakness of hands and fingers. Chorea.

Dose: 6-30. *(Boericke)*

A normally white, usually dark olive green, soft, glutinous mucous substance, of a urinous odour, which floats in the allantois fluid, or is attached to the allantois membrane, of the mare or cow, chiefly during the last months of pregnancy. Trituration of the dried substance taken from the tongue of a newly-born filly.

The clinical experience with this remedy has been so limited, that but few characteristic indications have been made out. These, however, are peculiar. Icy coldness in stomach. Violent pain in wrists. Paralysis of wrist in morning in bed. Weakness of hands and fingers so that he cannot hold anything. A case of chorea was cured on these last symptoms. There is weakness, restlessness, melancholy. The headache is *Amel.* lying on painful side, *Agg:* walking in sun. Chilliness, *Amel.:* from being covered. A peculiar sensation is as if the head would fall forward on walking; as of a plug in the throat; as if a swelling retarded the flow of the urine. There is desire to lie down, but no relief on doing so.

Relations: Antidoted by Coffee; Caust. relieved the paralysis of wrist.

Compare Anac. (Plug sensation) (JHC)

317. Hippozaenium

(Glanderine-mallein Farcine)

This powerful nosode introduced by Dr. J.J. Garth Wilkinson, covers symptoms which suggest integral parts of consumption, Cancer, Syphilis etc. and promotes useful service in the treatment of Ozaena, Scrofulous, swellings, pyaemia, erysipelas, chronic rhinitis, saneous secretion.

Nose: Catarrh, ozaena.

Face: All glands swollen, painful, from abscesses.

Respiratory: Bronchitis in the aged.

Dose: 30 potency. *(Boericke)*

Mallein, Glanderin, Farcin. The nosode of glanders or farcy. The disease is called Glanders when the catarrhal symptoms are pronounced; Farcy when these are not noticeable, the skin being chiefly affected, with deposits in the lungs. Homoeopathic preparations of both have been made. Triturations of sugar of milk saturated with the virus.

I have used it with excellent effect in cases of inveterate nasal catarrh and glandular enlargement. The nasal affection may go on to Ozaena, ulceration of nasal cartilages and bones. It has cured papules and ulcerations in frontal sinuses, pharynx and trachea, hoarseness, old cases of bronchitis especially in old persons, where suffocation from excessive secretion seemed imminent. Bronchial asthma, whooping cough. A cough commencing at Christmas and lasting till June has been cured by it. *(JHC)*

318. Hoang Nan

(Strychnos - Gaultheriana. Tropical Bind Weed)

Exhaustion with vertigo, numbness and tingling in hands and feet, involuntary action of lower jaw. Pustules and boils; tertiary syphilis and paralysis. Eczema, prurigo and ulcers, leprosy, cancer, of glandular structures and bites of serpents. Removes fetor and haemorrhage in cancer relieves the healing process. Follows Arsenic.

Dose: Five drops of Tincture may be increased to twenty. *(Boericke)*

Hoang - Nan is a plant indigenous to Tonquin, where it has a great reputation as a remedy for leprosy, hydrophobia, snake bites and diseases of the skin - The red dust of the bark contains the most active properties. The native method of preparing the medicine is by moistening the mixture of three powders with a little vinegar and forming the paste into pills of about a centimeter in diameter - According to Hansen, prurigo, pustular eczema, in parts well supplied with sebaceous glands (face, neck, genitals) boils, carbuncles, constitutional syphilis, cancer of the glands and general malnutrition were also met by the remedy the dose of which is 5-30 drops of the tincture three times a day -

Compare: Nux-v., Curare, Angustura, Brucea antidys, Hydrocotyle. (JHC)

A tincture is prepared of the bark. This remedy is indicated in diseases of the skin, such as eczema, prurigo, old ulcers, secondary syphilis, cancer, leprosy and serpent bites.

It should be remembered in pustular eczema, and in prurigo in parts that are well supplied with sebaceous glands. It is useful in leprosy, as under its action the patient improves, the anaesthesia disappears and sensibility returns. *(Blackwood)*

319. Homarus

(Digestive juice of live Lobster)

Dyspepsia, sore throat and headache seems to be a combination that may be controlled by the remedy. Frontal and temporal pain chiefly with soreness in eyes. Throat sore, raw, burns, with tough mucous. Pain in stomach and abdomen better after eating. Belching. Chilliness and pain all over. Itching of skin.

Modalities: *Worse* from milk, after sleep.

Better: From motion, after eating.

Relationship: Compare - Sepia, Asterias, Astacus, Aethusa.

Dose: 6th potency. *(Boericke)*

The effects of Lobster on some persons and under some conditions are well known. Persons have been known to die after eating lobster and thereafter drinking milk. Cushing put a little of the poison into warm milk and in 10 mts. it was a hard mass. Agg. from milk should be a strong indication for its use. For patients who are awakened in the night by the necessity to pass wind Homarus should be the remedy. The symptoms generally are Agg. after sleep, in the morning on waking, at night, on drawing a long breath, from drinking milk. Amel. from inhaling cold air. L.H. Hallock relates small amount of Lobster salad had been eaten, an hour later general pruritus commenced, worse in lower extremities especially in the calves. The itching was of a biting, burning character. No amel. by rubbing or scratching, almost unendurable - it lasted two hours inspite of bathing with hot and cold water, fresh and salt. No sooner had the itching abated than lips, nose, eyes began to swell, till the eyes were closed and lips almost completely inverted.

Causation: Milk - effects of. *(JHC)*

The digestive fluid found just behind the mouth of the live lobster. This remedy is useful in dyspepsia with pain in the stomach and abdomen that is relieved after eating. It is of service in pharyngitis when the throat is raw, and burns and in headache that is worse in the temples. *(Blackwood)*

320. Hydrangea

(Seven Barks)

A remedy for gravel, profuse deposit of white amorphous salts in urine. Calculus, renal colic, bloody urine. Acts on ureter. Pain in lumbar region. Dizziness. Oppression of chest.

Urine: Burning in urethra and frequent desire. Urine hard to start. Heavy deposit of mucus. Sharp pain in loins, especially left. Great thirst, with abdominal symptoms and enlarged prostate. (Ferr. pic., Sabal.). Gravelly deposits. Spasmodic stricture. Profuse deposit of white amorphous salts.

Relationship: Compare: Lycop.; Chimaphil., Berberis, Pareira; Uva, Sabal., Oxydendron; Geum - Water-Avens. (Severe jerking pains from deep in the abdomen to end of urethra; affections of bladder, with pains in penis; worse, eating; relaxed mucous membranes, with excessive and deprived secretions; imperfect digestion and assimilation.) Polyctrichum - Haircap moss (according to Dr. A.M. Cushing in mother tincture or infusion for enlarged prostate - prostatitis.)

Dose: Tincture. *(Boericke)*

Like some other members of the Saxifragaceae, Hydrang. has a traditional reputation as a stone breaking remedy having been used in calculus diseases for many years. Dr. Nottingham, of Lansing, says (Ame. Hom., November 15, 1899) that in physiological doses it produces giddiness, oppression of the chest, and acts as a cathartic, diuretic, sialogogue, and narcotic. He used it with brilliant results in the following case: Mr. B., 71, tall slender, dark, was exceedingly irritable and frequently subject to violent paroxysms of anger. For many years he had been accustomed to make the most reckless use of drugs, and was always requesting his homoeopathic doctor to give him something stronger. For eight years he had suffered from vesical sphincter irritation, with dribbling of urine, severe spasms of prostate, renal catarrh, yellow sand in urine, and even small calculi. After persistent use of best indicated remedies with no effect, the fluid extract of Hydrang. was given, a teaspoonful every three or four hours, and the symptoms disappeared in a remarkably short time. Cooper has also used this remedy (which, he says, is the thirstiest plant known) with good effect in diabetes, in cases presenting with great thirst, with abdominal symptoms and in enlarged prostate. It appears to act strongly on the neck of the bladder. Hansen adds that it is particularly useful for profuse deposits of white amorphous salts in the urine; and has arrested the tendency to formation of calculi; relieves distress from renal calculus, with soreness over region of kidneys and bloody urine.

Relations: Compare - Berb., Sabal s., Solidago. v., Uva ursi, Thlaspi. b., Ocim. c. *(JHC)*

This remedy is indicated when there is frequent urination with burning and acute, sharp, quick pain in the urethra. There may be a partial suppuration of the urine with general irritation and aching pain in the back. This may be dependent upon the passage of gravel, uric acid, or amorphous salts.

It should always be remembered in these cases as a sedative for the pain in the bladder, ureters or kidneys. It is useful in Uric acidaemia, when there are severe pains in the back and the urine contains an excess of solids. Also an irritation of the bladder of an acute character, as is observed following confinement. *(Blackwood)*

321. *Hydrastis*

(Golden Seal)

Acts especially on mucus membranes relaxing them and producing a thick yellowish ropy secretion. The catarrh may be anywhere - throat, stomach, uterus, urethra. It is always characterised by this peculiar mucous discharge. Hydrastis is especially active in old easily tired people, cachetic individuals with great debility, cerebral effects prominent, feels his wits sharpened, head cleared, facile expression. Weak muscular power, poor digestion and obstinate constipation. Lumbago, emaciation and prostration. Its action on the liver is marked. Cancer and cancerous state, before ulceration when pain is the principal symptom. Goitre of puberty and pregnancy. Small pox internally and locally. The power of Hydrastis over smallpox, seen in modifying the disease, abolishing its distressing symptoms, shortening its course, lessening its danger and greatly mitigating its consequences.

Nose: Sinusitis; thick tenacious secretion from posterior nares, excoriating discharge. Ozaena with ulceration of septum. Tends to blow nose all the time.

Ears: Eustachian catarrh.

Mouth: Shows imprint of teeth, stomatitis, ulceration of tongue, fissures towards the edges.

Stomach: Weak digestion. Bitter taste.

Back: Dull, heavy, dragging pain and stiffness, particularly across lumbar region, must use arms in raising himself from seat.

Rectum: Constipation.

Urine: Gleety discharge.

Female: Menorrhagia, pruritus vulvae with profuse leucorrhoea.

Respiratory: Expectoration, thick yellow, tenacious expectoration.

Skin: Eruptions like variola, ulcers.

Dose: Tr. to 30th attenuation.

(Boericke)

The so called root of Hydrastis from which the Tr. is made is really a perennial underground stem, thick, knotty and yellow. The yellow colour is very intense and it has been used by Indians as a dye. For though by no means a specific in all cases of cancer, it is in cancer cases that Hydrastis has won its chief fame, and I think it may fairly be said that more cases of cancer have been cured with it than with any other single remedy. Appetite bad, the power of digesting bread and vegetables, especially weak and causing eructations. The action of the bowel is either infrequent and constipated or frequent with loose, soft, light coloured stools - The female genital organs are very much affected, metrorrhagia, leucorrhoea, pruritus vulvae, scirrhus of uterus, of breasts, sore mouth of nursing women, sore nipples. Like many other yellow medicines it has a marked action on the liver, causing jaundice and liver enlargement. It is worthy of note that most remedies which powerfully act on the skin will also cause an asthmatic state.

(JHC)

This agent is a stomach and intestinal tonic, increasing the secretion of the gastric and intestinal juices and promoting the appetite, it increases the peristaltic action of the stomach and intestinal walls, increasing their muscular tone and favours a more normal evacuation of the bowels. It has a stimulating influence upon the respiration and circulation, increasing the arterial tension, as a result of its action upon the myocardium, which is more permanent than that imparted by many other agents; a similar action is observed upon the muscles in general. It is mildly antiperiodic. If continued over a long period it will derange the digestion and constipation results. It is also a protoplasmic poison, arresting the movements of the white blood corpuscles. It contains two alkaloids,

Hydrasting which is considered identical with Berberin, and acts as a tonic, antiperiodic and causes ringing in the ears; and Hydrastine, which affects the mucous membrane. These alkaloids while not toxic in medicinal doses, have produced death in the larger animals. There were convulsions, decreased blood pressure and failure of the heart in diastole. The elimination of this agent is largely through the kidneys.

It should be remembered in catarrhal conditions of the gall ducts, and catarrhal jaundice when there is no pain, as well as cholelithiasis. The tongue is coated yellow and slimy, there are eructations of a sour, putrid nature. The patient complains of an atonic dyspepsia. The stools are pale and scanty. There is palpitation of the heart, and a sensation of faintness and a gone feeling referred to the epigastrium.

The bowels are usually constipated and the stools often mixed with mucus. In these cases from three to ten drops of reliable tincture should be given before each meal and on retiring, in a cup of hot water.

It is useful both locally and internally in cases of stomatitis of nursing women, aphthous sore mouth in delicate children. The gums may be loosened from the teeth and spongy, and bleed easily. The tongue is large and shows the imprint of the teeth. It is to be especially remembered if mercury and chlorate of potash have been extensively employed without results.

It has been employed in ulceration of the skin and fissured nipples, indolent ulcers, lupus, eczema and leprosy during the ulcerative stage, when it meets the secondary symptoms, the lowered vitality and impaired constitutional effects.

In those suffering from cancer it has given a degree of relief, and has improved the general health, and while it may have no influence over the cancerous dyscrasia and but little over carcinoma, it has favourable influence over scirrhous tumors developing in glandular tissue, and especially if there is a history of atonic dyspepsia, gastric catarrh, a constipated state of the bowels and liver, with a broad indented tongue and distress after meals. It is reputed to have cured cancer of the mammary gland when the tumor was hard and painful and the general indication for the remedy was present. However this may be, it is of great service in non-malignant mammary gland tumors during the menstrual period, and in those local circumscribed enlargements that occur in the gland more or less suddenly.

It is a valuable remedy in leucorrhoea, which may be uterine or vaginal. It is profuse, yellow, tenacious and the patient complains of great prostration, sensitiveness in the hepatic region, constipation and haemorrhoids.

It should be remembered in pruritus vulvae, with superficial ulcerations and fungoid developments. There may be bleeding associated with the profuse leucorrhoea and many of the constitutional symptoms of the remedy. In these cases it should be used locally as well as internally.

It has been employed in gonorrhoea when the discharge is yellow and thick.

(Blackwood)

322. *Hydrocotyle*

(Indian Penny wort)

Curative in disorders that exhibit interstitial inflammation and cellular proliferation in any part. Hypertrophy and induration of connective tissue. Has considerable reputation in Leprosy and Lupus, when there is no ulceration. The skin symptoms are very important. Of great use in ulceration of womb.

Difficulty in maintaining the upright posture. Very copious perspiration. Pains of cervical cancer.

Female: Pruritus of vagina, heat within vagina, granular ulceration of womb.

Skin: Great thickening of epidermoid layer and exfoliation of scales. Intolerable itching, especially of soles, elephantiasis.

(Boericke)

Hydrocot. has been long known as an Indian remedy. Boilean was the first to use it as a remedy in leprosy. It has been tested pathogenetically and clinically and its place has been fairly well defined. The skin and the female generative organs are the chief seats of the drug's action. A great variety of skin affections have been cured with it, Acne, eczema Pemphigus, Lupus, Copper coloured eruption, papular eruption on face, intolerable itching in various places - Hydrocotyle acts on the male sexual organs also causing weight in the male uterus, the prostate gland - A patient of mine, who was taking Hydroc, for Eczema, with advantage complained of persistent dreaming all the time he was asleep and an unpleasant mouth on waking in the morning.

Dose: Tr. to 6th potency.

Tr. 5 drops dose. *(JHC)*

323. *Hydrocyanic Acid*

(Prussic acid)

One of the most toxic agents known. Convulsions and paralysis express the action of this remedy. Spasmodic constriction in larynx, feeling of suffocation, pain and tightness in chest, palpitation, pulse weak, irregular. Sinking sensation at the epigastrium. Hysterical and epileptic convulsions. Cyanosis. Collapse due to some pulmonary condition, not a cardiac collapse. Catalepsy. Cholera. State of collapse. (Ars. Verat). Coldness. Tetanus. Narcolepsy.

Mind: Fears everything, horses, wagons, houses, falling, etc.

Stomach: Drink rumbles through throat and stomach. Great sinking at pit of stomach.

Heart: Violent palpitation. Pulse weak, irregular.

Dose: 6 and higher potencies.

(Boericke)

HCN. is one of the deadliest and most rapidly acting of poisons. Hence its applicability in cases of critical intensity such as the collapse stage of cholera. Sudden cessation of all discharges, convulsions during severe attack of illness. It acts powerfully on the coeliac ganglia, causing intestinal cramps and colics - face flushed, bluish tint - the characteristic blue tint of HCN is apparent after death in some poisoning cases - coldness is a great feature with the remedy marble coldness within and without. Blue tinge of the skin is also characteristic.

(JHC)

324. *Hydrophobinum*

(Lyssin-saliva of rabid dog)

Affects principally the nervous system, aching in bones. Complaints from abnormal sexual desire. Convulsions brought on by dazzling light or sight of running water.

Stool: Desire for stool on hearing or seeing running water.

Urine: Constant desire to urinate on seeing running water.

Worse: Sight or sound of running water or pouring water or even thinking of fluids, dazzling or reflected light, heat of sun, stooping.

Compare: Xanthium spinosum - Cockle - said to be specific for hydrophobia and is recommended for chronic cystitis in women.

Dose: 30th potency. *(Boericke)*

Lyssin: The nosode of rabies. Trituration of sugar of milk saturated with the saliva of a rabid dog. Trituration might also be made of Pasteurs strongest virus. This remedy has been pretty extensively used in practice, not only in cases of Hydrophobia, but in many disorders in which the key note symptoms have been present. These are exquisite: sensitiveness to breath of air, to bright objects, especially the surface of water, to sounds, and most of all to the sound of running water. Even the thought of it is enough to bring on an aggravation or a convulsion. Cases of dysentery with pain and tenesmus on hearing water running from a tap have been cured with Hydrop. Cannot bear heat of sun. Thirst with inability to swallow. Copious viscid saliva. Causation - dog bite. *(JHC)*

325. *Hyoscyamus*
(Henbane)

Disturbs the nervous system profoundly. It is as if some diabolical force took possession of the brain and prevented its function. It causes a perfect picture of mania of a quarrelsome and obscene character. Inclined to be unseemly and immodest in acts, gestures and expressions. Very talkative and persists in stripping herself, or uncovering genitals. Is jealous. Afraid of being poisoned etc. Its symptoms also point to weakness and nervous agitation, hence typhoid and other infections with coma vigil. Tremulous weakness and twitching of tendons. Subsultus tendinum. Muscular twitchings, spasmodic affections, generally with delirium. Non inflammatory cerebral activity. Toxic gastritis.

Mind: Very suspicious, talkative, obscene, lascivious mania, uncovers body, jealous, foolish, great hilarity, inclined to laugh at everything. Delirium with attempt to run away - low muttering speech - constant carphologia - Deep stupor.

Throat: Stinging dryness - Uvula elongated.

Male: Impotence, lascivious, exposes his person, plays with genitals during fever.

Chest: Dry spasmodic cough at night, (Worse lying down, better sitting up) from itching in the throat as if uvula were too long.

Extremities: Picking at bed clothes.

Sleep: Starts up frightened.

Nerves: Great restlessness, every muscle twitches. Will not covered.

Modalities: *Worse* - at night, during menses, after eating, when lying down. Better - stooping.

Dose: 6-200. *(Boericke)*

Hyoscyamus (Hog-bean) is allied to Belladonna botanically, and in pathogenetic action the two drugs are much alike in their main features. But when examined closely their differences are sufficiently well marked to render their distinction easy. Though sometimes growing near rivers, Bell. flourishes best in a chalky soil. Hyos. is found growing on old rubbish heaps near ruins, on roadsides and sometimes by the seashore. The flower of Bell. is of a dull, purplish brown; of Hyos. a dirty yellow with claret coloured streaks. Bell is a smooth plant, whilst Hyos. is densely covered with thickly woven hairs, and by a sticky, heavy smelling exudation.

A patient had objected to the taste of water in which Hyo-ϕ had been mixed so Dr. Mills took a teaspoonful just to taste it. A few moments later I found that it produced a queer feeling throughout the body. I felt as though without weight, as though I walked through and on air. My head felt light. I had an insane desire to laugh and shout. It was only by the utmost use of my will power that I could keep myself from doing something ridiculous. I can liken the condition only to one of mild hilarious intoxication - a funny drunk. I knew I was silly, but I could not help it. To keep myself from losing my dignity before the nurses and the family, I locked myself in the bathroom for a few minutes and made faces at myself in the mirror. The condition passed off in half an hour. These two experiences, brief as they were, cover a large share of the ground occupied by Hyo. The delirium of Hyo. is more of the low, muttering type, whilst that of Bell. tends to be violent and furious. Hyo. also has fits of ungovernable rage, but the violence is not so sustained as that of Bell. The face of Bell. is red, of Hyo. pale or bluish. Hyo. corresponds to a greater variety of cases of melancholia than Bell., and here one great characteristic is suspicion so frequently met with in cases of insanity or of those on the borderland.

Twitching is one of the grand characteristics of Hyo. Another feature of the Hyo. insanity is uncovering. Nymphomania, lascivious mania, lies naked in bed and chatters. Hyo. corresponds to the typhoid state; tongue dry and unwildy, sees things too large or too near and grasps at them; picks the bed-clothes and mutters. Hyo. is one of our best remedies in toothache, having well defined symptoms. Hyos. 30 is one of the most useful remedies in restlessness and sleeplessness. *(JHC)*

While in its action this agent has many points in common with Belladonna and Stramonium, yet each has an individuality of its own.

It is serviceable in the insomnia of childhood, when there is more or less twitching of the muscles; they scream out during sleep, as though frightened. In the adult it is of service when the insomnia is dependent upon nervous excitement.

It is frequently useful in cases of an incessant, dry, spasmodic cough, with tickling in the throat, which is aggravated from lying down and is relieved by sitting up. There is an elongated uvula in many of these cases. *(Blackwood)*

326. Hypericum

(St. John's wort)

The great remedy for injuries to nerves, toes and nails. Crushed fingers especially tips, excessive pain, fullness is a guiding symptom to its use. Prevents lock jaw. Punctured wounds. Relieves pain after operation. Quite supersedes the use of morphia after operations. (Helmuth). Spasms after every injury. Has an important action on the rectum, haemorrhoids. Coccydynia. Spasmodic asthmatic attacks with changes of weather or before storms, better by copious expectoration. Injured nerves from bites of animals. Tetanus, Neuritis, tingling burning and numbness. Constant drowsiness.

Mind: Feels as if lifted high in air or anxiety, lest he fall from heights.

Head: As if touched by an icy cold hand. Throbbing in vertex. Head feels longer elongated to a point.

Rectum: Haemorrhoids with pain, bleeding and tenderness.

Back: Pressure over sacrum.

Extremities: Crawling in hand and feet. Neuritis.

Respiratory: Asthma worse foggy weather and relieved by profuse perspiration.

Modalities: (Worse) in cold, dampness, in a fog, in close room, least exposure, touch. (Better) bending head backward.

Compare: Ledum for punctured wounds and bites of animals.

Dose: Tr to 3rd potency. *(Boericke)*

The leaves of various species of hypericum are sprinkled with pellucid dots and black glands, which contain an essential oil. These which are most conspicuous in H. perforatum have evidently given the signature which has lead to the chief use of the plant in medicine namely as a remedy for wounds or perforations of the integuments. The leaves more over are lance shaped. The particular kinds of wounds for which Hyp. has been found of signal service are wounds of parts rich in nerves, brain, spine (spinal irritation from falls) coccyx, finger ends, wounds from stepping on nails or any punctured wounds. The characteristic of the Hyp. wounds is that they are very sensitive to touch (Ledum punctures are not particularly sensitive to touch). Roehrig (H.R. XII. 40) considers Hyp. externally and internally the nearest thing to a specific in bleeding piles. *(JHC)*

327. Iberis

(Bitter Candy Tuft)

State of nervous excitement. Has marked action upon the heart. Possesses great efficacy in cardiac diseases. Controls vascular excitement in hypertrophy with thickening of the heart's walls. Cardiac debility after influenza. Liver region full and painful. White stools.

Head: Conscious of heart's action.

Heart: Palpitation with vertigo and choking in throat. Pulse full, irregular, intermittent. Worse least motion and in warm room, dropsy and enlarged heart. Violent palpitation induced by slightest exertion or by laughing or coughing, darting pain through heart, cardiac dyspnoea - wakes with palpitation about 2 a.m. Throat and trachea fills up with mucus. Cough causes redness of face. Tachycardia.

Extremities: Numbness and tingling in left hand and arm.

Modalities: *Worse* lying down on left side, motion, exertion, warm room.

Dose: Tr. to 1st potency. *(Boericke)*

Old school authorities had mentioned Iberis as useful in the treatment of Hypertrophy of the heart. This lead Hale to have the remedy proved. Sylvester had observed that Iberis controlled the violence and sharp action of the heart and softened the pulse, hence its great service in hypertrophy. The cardiac symptoms of the drug are very pronounced and well marked, consisting of pains, dull or stitching, with palpitation and breathlessness on slightest exertion, pains down the left arm and numbness, intermittent pulse. Choking sensation in throat was also marked. The stools were white as those of Digit. On turning on left side a sharp sticking pain is felt as if a needle were present crosswise in the ventricles and pricked at each contraction - Iberis ϕ one drop in a powder on the tongue 2 or 3 times a day - After about 10 days, the heart felt almost suddenly into its perfect regular unconscious beat and retired at once and finally from further observation. Proctor has repeatedly given Iberis since then in similar cases, with the same success 'Conscious of heart's action' may possibly prove a key note for its use. *(JHC)*

These symptoms may be associated with pericarditis, myocarditis and nervous derangement of the heart when its action is characterized by violence and irritability. There are severe stitching pains in the cardiac region, the pulse is full but irregular, and all the symptoms are aggravated by motion.

Compare: Cactus grand., Crataegus., Amyl-nit. *(Blackwood)*

328. Ichthyolum

(A combination of sulphonated hydrocarbons; a fossil product of complex structure found in Tyrol, supposed to be fish deposits, contains 10% sulphur.)

Its action on skin, mucous membranes and kidneys is prompt and useful. It is strongly anti-parasitic. Redness, pain and inflammation; decreases tension. Excellent in winter coughs of old people. Polyarthritis. Chronic rheumatism - Uric acid diathesis. Hay fever, chronic hives, tuberculosis, aids nutrition. Alcoholism when nothing will stay on stomach.

Face: Skin feels dry and itches. Acne on chin.

Nose: Bland coryza, stuffed feeling, feels sore inside. Irresistible desire to sneeze.

Stomach: Nausea, increased appetite.

Urine: Increased in quantity and frequency, burning pain in meatus - Uric acid deposits.

Respiratory: Coryza, dry tasting cough, bronchiectasis and pthisis. Bronchitis especially in the aged.

Skin: Heat and irritation, itching, scaly and itching eczema, crops of boils. Pruritus of pregnancy, Psoriasis, Acne rosacea, erysipelas.

Dose: Lower potencies - Externally, it is used as an ointment with Lanoline 20% to 50% for chronic eczema and psoriasis. Also acne rosacea and gouty joints. Chilblains, scabies, rectal suppositories for senile prostate. *(Boericke)*

This is an unproved remedy which has been used in old-school therapeutics as external application, and internally in skin affections, rheumatism, scrofula, nephritis, and gonorrhoea. It is a powerful antiseptic. As an external application to rheumatic joints it has achieved marked results. A solution of equal parts of Ichthyol and water is warmed and applied to the affected joint on calico and covered with heated cloths, outside of which is an impervious fabric to prevent evaporation. Pure Ichthyol or an ointment of Lanoline and Ichthyol may be used instead. Gouty joints have also been benefited. Ichthyol appears to act by virtue of its power of allaying pain and inflammation but there can be no doubt that a thorough proving would bring out a specific relationship to the maladies in which it has been used with success. "Scarpa" claims to have used it with excellent effect in a large number of cases of pthisis.

Relationship: Ichth. belongs to the Petroleum class of remedies. *(JHC)*

329. *Ignatia*

(St. Ignatius bean)

Produces a marked hyperaesthesia of all the senses, and a tendency to clonic spasms. Mentally the emotional element is uppermost and co-ordination of function is interfered with. Hence it is one of the chief remedies for hysteria. It is especially adapted to the nervous temperament. Women of sensitive, easily excited nature dark, mild disposition, quick to perceive, rapid in execution. Rapid change of mental and physical condition opposite to each other. Great contradictions, alert, nervous, apprehensive, rigid, trembling patients who suffer acutely in mind or body, at the same time made worse by drinking coffee. The superficial and erratic character of its symptoms is most characteristic. Effects of grief and worry. Cannot bear tobacco. Pain in small circumscribed spots (Oxal ac.). The plague. Hiccough and hysterical vomiting.

Mind: Changeable mood, introspective, silently brooding, melancholic, sad, tearful, not communicative, sighing and sobbing, after shocks, grief, disappointment.

Head: Feels hollow, worse stooping, headache as if a nail were driven out through the side, congestive headaches following anger or grief. Worse smoking or smelling tobacco, inclines head forward.

Face: Twitching of muscles of face and lips.

Mouth: Sour taste, toothache, worse after drinking coffee and smoking.

Throat: Feeling of a lump in throat that cannot be swallowed - better eating something solid, Tonsils inflamed, swollen with small ulcers. Follicular tonsillitis.

Stomach: All gone feeling in stomach, much flatulence, hiccough, sinking in stomach, relieved by taking a deep breath.

Rectum: Itching and stitching up the rectum, prolapse, painful constriction of anus after stool - haemorrhage and pain. Pressure as of a sharp instrument from within outward.

Respiratory: Dry spasmodic cough in quick successive shocks. Coughing increases the desire to cough. Much sighing, worse in the evening, little expectoration leaving pain in trachea.

Female: Menses black, too early, too profuse or scanty, feminine sexual frigidity.

Extremities: Ulceration, pain in soles.

Sleep: Jerking of limbs on getting to sleep, insomnia from grief, cares, with itching of arms and violent yawning.

Fever: Chill with thirst, during fever. Itching, nettle rash all over body.

Skin: Itching, nettle rash, very sensitive to draught of air. Excoriation, especially around vagina and mouth.

Modalities: *Worse* in the morning, open air, after meals, coffee, smoking, liquids, external warmth.

Better: While eating, change of position.

Dose: 6-200 potency. *(Boericke)*

One minor inconvenience attending these notions is that patients have become very shy of the drug and resent having it prescribed for them thinking that their doctor deems them hysterical if he does prescribe it - In intermittent fever it is the only remedy that will cure certain cases. The seeds of Ignatia contains a larger proportion of strychnia than those of Nux vomica and the great difference in the characteristic features of the two medicines prove the wisdom of considering medicines apart from their so called active principles. There are many activities in plants besides the alkaloids they may contain and these are often the determining factors of the drugs' specific action. Ign. is not suitable for persons or patients in whom anger, eagerness or violence is predominant, but for those who are subject to rapid alternations of gaiety and disposition to weep or other characteristic emotional states. The consequences of worry no less than grief call for Ign. Special action of Ign. in cases of moods. Globus hystericus. It must be borne in mind, that the absence of any particular characterisic of a drug is no contra-indication to its provided other indications are sufficiently pronounced, Ign. will cure many painful conditions of the anus and rectum, including piles and prolapse when characterised by sharp stitching pain shooting up the rectum. Headaches terminate with a profuse flow of urine. The characteristic cough of Ignatia is an irritable and irritating cough, the longer the cough lasts the more the irritation to cough increases. Kent describe it as 'the longer the cough lasts the more the irritation to cough increases'. Kent describes it as Hack, Hack-ety-hack ending in sobbing. Chill *agg:* by external heat (wraps, stove) - External chilliness and internal heat. Ign. is one of the chilly medicines, like - Nux-v., Caps., and Ars. - There is great aversion to tobacco, which agg. many symptoms. Aversion to warm food, meat, alcohol, desire for sour things, for bread, especially rye bread agg: from emotion, from sweets, coffee, strong smells, from ascarides, when yawning. It is best administered in the morning if there is no hurry - Ign. hides her grief. Puls. shows it - Prolapsus ani. Causation, grief, fright, worry, disappointed love, jealousy, old spinal injuries. *(JHC)*

Habitat, Philippine Islands. Physiological action: Though chemically and botanically similar to Nux vomica, these two remedies are not interchangeable but each has a therapeutic individuality of its own. Ignatia is primarily a spinal remedy, producing a hyperaesthesia of the senses with a tendency to hysterical spasms and a loss of harmony in the co-ordination of the various portions of the body. When the excitability is exhibited by anger, vehemence and irascibility is exhibited by anger, Nux vomica is indicated. In ignatia there is a rapid alternation of gaiety and a disposition of weep. There are symptoms of neuralgia.

This remedy is indicated in those of a nervous temperament who are sensitive and easily excited. They have dark hair and skin and a mild disposition, and a contradiction of the symptoms which are continually changing; there is a fever with no thirst, the sore throat is relieved by swallowing. There is a sensitiveness that is relieved by pressure. The chill is relieved by uncovering and the headache is relieved by stooping. There is a marked sensitiveness to pain and suffering from hysterical weakness, nervous exhaustion and faintness.

It is of service in those suffering from the effects of chagrin, grief, loss of friends, bad news and misfortunes, when the patient broods over her troubles in concealment rather than in public. She is introspective, silent and given to sighing and weeping.

It is an important remedy in hysteria when there is extreme sensitiveness to all external impressions, she laughs and cries alternately, she suffers from globus hystericus, passes large quantities of pale limpid urine. She cannot share her sorrow or anger with anyone, she does not or cannot cry, weeps inwardly, and cannot become reconciled to what has occurred.

It is indicated in many cases of melancholia when the general symptoms of the remedy are present.

It is of service in cases of anger and ill humor, when she resents the slightest suggestion of a blame or contradiction, and retains these in her mind and is continually irritated from thinking of them.

These patients are subject to neuralgias about the head; it is described as a pressing, boring, localized pain confined to one spot. The pain is aggravated from talking, listening or paying close attention; is ameliorated by stooping forward. The attack terminates in vomiting and in the passages of large quantities of urine.

It should be remembered in ciliary and facial neuralgias when emotional excitement and twitching of the muscles of the face and eyelids ae present. There may be spasmodic closure of the jaws and biting of the side of the cheek and tongue.

It has been employed in epilepsy and eclampsia when the attack is precipitated by some sudden emotion or when dependent upon a reflex irritation.

It should be remembered in indigestion when this is dependent upon depressing emotions. There is marked distension of the stomach and abdomen with but little eructation of gas, but there is an excessive discharge of flatulence, which is offensive but is passed without any exertion of the abdominal muscles.

It should be studied in chronic gastritis when there is empty retching and at times vomiting of mucus and food, a heavily coated tongue, foul breath, constipation and morning aggravation in neurotic, hysterical women.

It should be remembered in hyperchlorhydria, and gastralgia when there is hiccough, empty retching which is relieved by eating, salivation and an empty or gone sensation referred to the epigastrium.

It should always be remembered in functional nervous states in those of the peculiar temperament of Ignatia; there is usually a history of fright or violent emotion.

It is to be borne in mind in prolapse of the rectum. This may occur with slight exertion at stool or without any movement. It may be associated with constipation which is very similar to that of Nux vomica, with the constant ineffectual urging to stool that results only in prolapsus of the rectum.

It is indicated in a diarrhoea that is painless and is characterized by a sudden urging. Often tenesmus, rumbling and emissions of flatus.

It should be thought of during menstruation when this is irregular, too early or profuse, and even suppressed from the effects of grief; a suppressed sorrow.

It has a place in the management of ovarian neuralgia when the mental symptoms of the remedy are present and she declares she cannot and will not stand this suffering.

It should be remembered in sexual frigidity and sterility when the patient is sensitive and easily irritated but hides her grief and nurses her sorrow.

It is of service in sciatica in nervous, hysterical subjects. It is worse during cold weather; at night the pain is intermittent, boring and tearing in character. The pain is such that the patient must move about.

There is a nervous reflex cough; it is constant and the patient claims it is due to tickling in the pharymx, larynx or trachea, but in reality is reflex from a remote organs as the ovaries, uterus, or due to worms. It is worse while lying down and is in no way relieved, but on the contrary aggravated, by coughing, but can be controlled by the will.

Compare - Chamomilla, Coffea cruda, Nux vomica. *(Blackwood)*

330. *Ilex Aquifolium*

(American Holly)

Intermittent fever, marked eye symptoms. Spleen pain. All symptoms better in winter.

Eye: Infiltration of cornea, staphyloma, nightly burning in orbits, rheumatic inflammation of eye. *(Boericke)*

With 5 drop doses of the 1x given 4 times a day Dr. Hendricks cured several cases of rheumatic inflamation of the eye, with periostitis of the frontal bone which almost always leads to staphylomatous degeneration of the cornea. *(JHC)*

331. *Indigo*

(Dye stuff)

Marked action on the nervous system and of undoubted benefit in the treatment of Epilepsy with great sadness. Excited mood and desire to be busy. Neuraesthenia and hysteria. Pure powdered Indigo placed on the wound cures snake and spider poison (Kali permang, Golondrina, Cedron. Stricture of oesophagus, blue colour (Cupr.)

Head: Vertigo with nausea. Convulsions.

Stomach: Eructations.

Rectum: Prolapse of rectum, with horrible itching at anus.

Urinary: Constant desire to urinate.

Nervous: Hysterical symptoms, where pain predominates. Excessive nervous irritation. Epilepsy, flashes of heat from abdomen to head, fit begins with dizziness. Aura from a painful spot between shoulders - reflex spasms from worms.

Compare: Oestrus cameli, an Indian medicine for epilepsy. *(Boericke)*

Dose: 3-30 potency.

Indigo was introduced into medicine as a remedy for epilepsy. It has been extensively proved by homoeopaths and observations have also been made of its effects on epileptic patients who were receiving large doses from old school practitioners - Indigo in cases of epilepsy but with little success except in cases arising from the presence of worms (Teste). E.P. Colby gave it in all cases of epilepsy coming under his care during 12 years with the result that he apparently cured 10% and reduced the frequency of attacks in many more. The dosage is not mentioned but was probably crude. In the dynamic cures of epilepsy effected by indigo, there has been great melancholy, which the patient has sought to hide, spending many nights crying alone. Or a furious excitable disposition before the attacks and mild and timid later.

For epilepsy - Compare - Sulphur with sinking sensation, hot flushes, worm fever, *Kali-brom.* - with acne.

Act. R. with waving sensation in brain.

Bufa - with vehement or excitable temperament. *(JHC)*

332. *Indium*

(Metal Indium)

Headache and migraine. Seminal emissions. Backache.

Head: Pain in head when straining at stool, with nausea. Sleepiness.

Male: Horribly offensive smell of urine after standing a short time. Emissions too frequent, diminished power. Testicles tender. Drawing pain in spermatic cord.

Dose: 6-200

Compare: Selenium, Titanium. (Male sexual organs). (Boericke)

It has been proved under the direction of Bell, mostly in the potencies and the symptoms mark it out as allied in action to Selenium and Titanium in its general action and particularly in the male sexual sphere. There is diminished power and control, frequency of nocturnal emissions, sexual dreams of perversion, which should render it of service in some cases of sexual psychopathy - Violent pain in the head when straining at stool. This is not infrequently met within the practice and I have given great relief with Ind. 200 to a patient who had this symptom. *(JHC)*

333. *Indol*

(A crystalline compound derivable from Indigo, but also a product of putrefaction of Proteids)

Primary action is to increase the elimination of indican - Auto intoxication.

Compare - Skatol. Persistent desire to sleep, dull, discontented mental state, hideous, delusions and nervousness, constant motion of fingers and feet. Intestinal putrefaction.

Dose: 6th attenuation. *(Boericke)*

334. *Influenzinum*

(The nosode of Influenza)

The nosode of influenza has with many practioners taken the place of Baptisia as the routine in epidemics. It may be given in 12th or 30th potency, either in the forms of tincture, pilules of discs, or 10 globules may be dissolved in six ounces of water and of this a dessert spoonsful may be given for a dose. It may be repeated every 2 hours. This will be found sufficient to control a large proportion of the cases. The general directions I give to my patients are these - when colds appear in a family, let all those who are unaffected take Ars. 3 TDS and let the patient take Influ-30 every hour or two. This generally prevents the spread of the trouble and clears up the colds, whether they are of the influenza type or not. Influenza has the property of developing old troubles, and thus it takes an infinite variety of forms in different persons, so that influenza, need not be expected to cure all cases unaided, or indeed, to be appropriate to every case.

Compatible : Act. r., Ars., Bel., Hep., Merc., and many others. (JHC)

335. *Insulin*

(An active principle from the pancreas which affects sugar metabolism)

Besides the use of Insulin in the treatment of diabetes, restoring the lost ability to oxidize carbohydrate and again storing glycogen in the liver, some use of it homoeopathically has been made by Dr. Wm. F. Bakery, showing its applicability in acne, carbuncles, erythema with itching eczema. In the gouty transitory glycosuria, when skin manifestations are persistent give three times daily after eating. Given a persistent case of skin irritation, boils or varicose ulceration with polyuria, it is indicated.

Dose: 3x to 30x. *(Boericke)*

336. *Inula*

(Seawort)

A mucous membrane medicine. Bearing down sensations in pelvic organs and bronchial symptoms are most marked. Substernal pain. Diabetes.

Respiratory: Dry cough, worse at night and lying down, larynx painful, chronic bronchitis, cough with much thick expectoration, with languor and weak digestion. stitches behind sternum. Teasing cough with much and free expectoration. Palliative in tubercular laryngitis.

Dose: 1-3 potency. *(Boericke)*

A very pronounced effect was observed in the pelvic organs, pressing and dragging towards the rectum and genitals, headache and labour-like pains. Inula is one of the remedies, which has sensation as of something alive, moving about internally, also twisting as of a ball in umbilical region, as if a substance would come out of rectum and genitals. Another peculiar sensation is, as though someone was poking him with a finger in various parts of the body, especially in diaphragm, so painful he awoke with clenched teeth. *(JHC)*

This agent is an expectorant, diuretic, diaphoretic an emmenagogue.

This remedy is indicated in a teasing, persistent cough with profuse expectoration and substernal pain.

It is of service in chronic metritis. The menses are too early and painful; there is a violent backache, with labor like pains and a dragging sensation in the pelvic organs, which are engorged and relaxed.

Compare: Corallium, Viburnum opulus.
(Blackwood)

337. *Iodoformum*

(Iodoform)

Should not be forgotten in the treatment of tubercular meningitis both as a local application to the head and internally (Bacil). Tuberculous conditions. Subacute and chronic diarrhoea of children.

Head: Meningitis.

Eyes: Dilated.

Abdomen: Cholera infantum, chronic diarrhoea, stools greenish, watery, undigested, with irritable temper.

Dose: Second trituration. Three grains on the back of the tongue will relieve attack of asthmatic breathing. *(Boericke)*

All the symptoms of acute meningitis have been produced in some instances and this fact has been turned into good account by homoeopathists - The external use of it has set up eczema. In one case, that of a soldier who had had iodoform applied to his arm, a scarlatina like rash appeared, spreading from the arm over the body and ending in desquamation. Scarlatina was actually diagonised but some doubt was raised and suspicion being thrown on the idf; a piece of silver was placed in the mouth. Immediately a garlic taste was experienced showing the presence of 'Idf'; which other tests confirmed. 'Idf' imparts a garlic odour to silver. *(JHC)*

338. Iodum

(Iodine)

Rapid metabolism. Loss of flesh with great appetite. Hungry with much thirst. Better after eating. Great debility, the slightest effort induces perspiration. Iod. individual is exceedingly thin, dark complexioned with enlarged lymphatic glands, has voracious appetite but gets thin. Tubercular type. All glandular structures, respiratory organs, circulatory system are especially affected; they atrophy. Iodine arouses the defensive apparatus of the system by assembling the mono-nuclear leucocytes whose phagocytic action is marked at a given point. Lead poisoning. Tremor. Iodine craves cold air.

Acute exacerbation of chronic inflammation. Arthritis deformans. Acts prominently on connective tissue. The plague, goitre. Abnormal vaso-constriction, capillary congestion followed by oedema, ecchymosis, haemorrhages, and nutritive disturbances are the pathological conditions at the basis of its symptomatology. Sluggish vital reaction, hence chronicity in many of its aspects. Acute catarrh of all mucous membranes. Rapid emaciation, not with standing good appetite and glandular atrophy call for this remedy, in numerous wasting diseases and in scrofulous patient. Acute affections of the respiratory organs. Pneumonia, rapid extension. Iodine is warm and wants cool surroundings. Weakness and loss of breath going upstairs. Adenoid vegetations. Tincture internally and locally to swollen glands and rattle snake bites.

Mind: Anxiety when quiet.

Head: Rush of blood and feeling of a tight band.

Eyes: Acute dacryocystitis.

Nose: Sneezing, sudden violent influenza, dry coryza becomes fluent in open air; fluent hot coryza. Acute nasal engorgement associated with high blood pressure.

Throat: Eustachian deafness, thyroid enlarged, goitre.

Stomach: Ravenous hunger.

Urine: Dark, yellow green.

Female: Ovaritis, wedge like pain from ovary to uterus, swindling of mammary glands, wedge like pain in the right ovarian region.

Respiratory: Pain in larynx, croupy cough, cold extends downwards.

Extremities: Joints inflamed and painful, pains in bones at night, white swelling, gonorrhoeal rheumatism. Rheumatism of nape and upper extremities, cold hands and feet. Acrid sweat of feet. Pulsation in large arterial trunks. Rheumatic pains; nightly pain in joints, constrictive sensations.

Skin: Hot, dry, yellow and withered, glands enlarged, nodosities.

Modalities: (Worse) when quiet, in warm room, (Better) walking about, in open air.

Complementary: Lycopod, Badiaga.

Dose: 3-30. Large dose expels tape worms, locally microbicide. *(Boericke)*

The most prominent feature of the action of Iodium is its power of causing absorption. I have seen it given with excellent effect in the lower attenuations, when swollen and deformed joints have been left behind after an attack of acute rheumatism.

Goitres are equally amebable to ·its resolvent action - Eats ravenously yet emaciates is a key note. It seems as if the waste of tissue set up the desire for absorbing great quantities of food. Absence of appetite is also among the effects of iodum and either condition may indicate it - I gave 5 drops of Iod 3x in a wine glass of water half an hour before meal times and her appetite returned with such vigour, she could not choose but to eat and was soon restored to a normal mental and bodily state - Iod is especially suited to persons of dark hair and complexion, dark yellow tawny skin. There is increased erethism, patient very excitable and restless, moving about from place to place. It is indicated by induration or atrophy of testes, ovaries and uterus. The salivary glands and pancreas are especially affected by Iod and a diarrhoea of milky like whey stools often indicative of pancreatic disease is especially amenable to its action. Nash thinks Iod is one of the remedies affected by the moons changes. In case of goitre, where it is indicated, he gives a powder of Iod. C.M. every night for four nights after the moon has passed the full.

Causation: Nervous shock and disappointed love. *(JHC)*

This agent when applied externally and locally is a disinfectant and rubefacient, parasiticide, antiseptic vesicant and caustic. When applied to the skin it produces a yellow, brown or black stain and is an irritant and caustic in proportion to its strength and frequency of its application. The discoloration may be removed by sodium hyposulphite of ammonia. In combination with the albumin it prevents putrefaction. When large amounts are frequently applied desquamation of the skin is produced, at times rapid vesication and possibly sloughing. It reflexly dilates the blood vessels of the organs subjacent to the area to which it is applied and thus it is a counter irritant. When its vapor is inhaled it produces irritation of the mucous membrane of the respiratory passages and cough, sneezing, increased secretion of mucus, dyspnoea and more or less pain is felt in the chest. Inhalation of a small amount acts as an antiseptic and prevents decomposition of the secretions.

When taken in small doses it is a gastric tonic and in very small doses it is a gastric sedative allaying nausea. From large doses their is salivation, general discomfort and colicky pains. Excessive dose have resulted in death due to severe gastro - enteritis.

Through its action on the nervous system it produces depression of the spirits, mental distress and apathy. He complains of lassitude, muscular debility, increased feebleness with a lowering of the heart's action.

When its use is protracted there is a metallic taste in the mouth with increased salivation, tendernes of the teeth and gums, nausea and coryza with gastric irritation, acneiform eruptions, which may be vesicular, or of a purpuric variety. As its use is continued the coryza becomes more pronounced and oedema of the eyelid, lachrymation and occular pains develop.

There is atrophy of the mammae, testicles and ovaries. This condition of absorption extends in a degree to all tissues normal and pathological. Small doses of Iodine and of the iodide have changed a latent hyperthyroidism to an active form.

This remedy is indicated in those with dark hair and eyes who are scrofulous. The lymphatic glands are large, hard and usually painless. A condition of torpidity glands are large, hard and usually painless, and condition of torpidity and sluggishness is present. They have great appetite but gradually become emaciated. They are weak, get out of breath easily when climbing stairs or an ascent. There is a constant formation of gas in the stomach. The patient is usually irritable and sensitive to the slightest wrong, is despondent, given to fears, is restless, frequently irritable and sensitive to real or fanciful wrongs.

It is of service in colloid goitre and scrofulous enlargement, and indurations of other glands when the general characteristics of this remedy are present.

It is useful in croup that is the attended with wheezing and a sawing respiration, the face is pale and cold and the child grasps the larynx. In these cases the inhalation of the vapor often acts well.

It should be remembered in croupous pneumonia of scrofulous subjects with a tendency to tuberculosis. It is during the second state that it is usually indicated, when hepatization is extending. There is great dyspnoea, the fever is high, the sputum contains much blood, and the skin is dry. The pneumonic process often involves the apex of the lung.

It is of benefit in chronic bronchitis, when there is a tendency to tuberculosis. The cough is dry, hacking and fatiguing and is attended with but little expectoration; there is a sensation of itching behind the sternum; there is great debility, emaciation, even while living well. The glandular system often shows involvement.

This is one of the remedies that has shown some results in fibrinous bronchitis. It is of value during the last stages of tuberculosis when the voice is rough and coarse, the skin is dry, there is emaciation and night sweats.

The various combinations of Iodine have been extensively employed as Iodide of Stannum, Iodide of Antimony and Iodide of Arsenic.

It is occasionally indicated in the pericarditis that attends pneumonia and rheumatism, also in cardiac hypertrophy when there is a sensation as though the heart was squeezed.

It has been employed in articular rheumatism when the parts are hot and swollen, the skin shiny, the pains are severe, shift and wander from the joints to the meninges of the brain and heart, also in gonorrhoeal arthritis, house maids's knee joint, especially in the syphilitic, and following excessive use of mercury.

In acute chronic pancreatitis this was Rademacher's great remedy, when there is an increased flow of saliva, with violent vomiting of a sour, watery substance, with a diarrhoea of a soft, watery, foamy stool. In acute conditions there is fatty diarrhoea. There is a voracious appetite and yet there is a gradual emaciation going on. There is a soapy taste in the mouth. Rademacher gave a tablespoonful every hour of a solution consisting of thirty drops of the tincture in eight ounces of water.

It has been of service in cancerous degeneration of the cervix of the uterus when there are cutting pains in the abdomen with haemorrhages at every stool. There may be an acrid corroding leucorrhoea that stains and corrodes the linen. This is aggravated at the menstrual period.

It has been employed in atrophy of the ovaries and mammary glands. There may be amenorrhoea or an excessive menstruation and the patient may complain of a wedge like pressing pain from the right ovary downward.

It should be thought of in aged men when there is incontinence of the urine with hypertrophy of the prostrate, with atrophy or enlarged hardened testicles that are free from pain.

It should be remembered in the salivation of mercury and that of pregnancy. It is of service in syphilitic conditions such as iritis and syphilitic ulcer of the nose and throat and when there are coryzas that are fluent, profuse, hot and attended with sneezing. There is headache over the frontal sinuses.

It is of service in chronic deafness with adhesions of the middle ear and glandular enlargement and catarrh of the Eustachian tube.

It has been found curative in persistent headache with vertigo, dizziness and hypertension of the aged.

Compare: Spongia tosta, Bromine, Mercurius. *(Blackwood)*

339. Ipecacuanha

(Ipecac-root)

The chief action is on the ramifications of the pneumogastric nerve, producing spasmodic irritation in chest and stomach. Morphic habit. The principal feature of Ipecacuanha is its persistent nausea and vomiting, which form the chief guiding symptoms. Indicated after indigestible food, raisins, cakes etc. Especially indicated in fat children and adults who are feeble and catch cold in relaxing atmosphere, warm moist weather, spasmodic affections. Haemorrhages, bright red and profuse.

Stomach: Tongue usually clean, mouth moist, much saliva, constant nausea, vomits food, bile, blood, mucus.

Abdomen: Amebic dysentery, with tenesmus, little thirst. Cutting, clutching, worse around the navel.

Stool: Like frothy molasses, griping at navel, dysenteric, slimy.

Female: Uterine haemorrhage, profuse bright, gushing, with nausea, vomiting during pregnancy. Pain from navel to uterus - menses too early and too profuse. Respiratory constriction in chest, cough incessant and violent with every breath; Bleeding from lungs with nausea; Hoarseness.

Fever: Intermittent fever, after quinine, slightest chill, nausea.

Compare: In Asthma - Blata orientalis.

Dose: 3-200. *(Boericke)*

Constant nausea Ipe. is very likely to be of use. With this there is a clean or not very dirty tongue - profuse salivation with nausea - perhaps the relationship of Ipe. to China may have something to do with its large sphere of usefullness in intermittent fever. Jahr recommended that in all cases of intermittents, in which no other remedy is particularly indicated Ipc. should be given with. The cough of Ipe. is dry, spasmodic, constricted, asthmatic - threatened suffocation from accumulation of mucus. In whooping cough, a characteristic is the spasmodic rigidity of the patient. Child loses breath, turns pale, stiff and blue, strangling with gagging and vomiting of mucus, bleeding from nose or mouth - Ipe. is a medicine of great importance in haemorrhages. The blood is bright red and the flow steady. A great keynote for Ipe. in haemorrhage (whether of lungs, bowels, uterus or other parts) is nausea with haemorrhage - threatened abortion, with internal heat. The symptoms of Ipe. develop in this order -

1.Gastric. 2. Respiratory 3. Spinal. 4. Genito-urinary, 5. Cutaneous. *(JHC)*

There is a sense of fulness in the stomach, cutting pains in the stomach and below the stomach, going from left to right. The cutting pain in colic goes from left to right. The patient is unable to stir or breathe until that pain passes off. It holds him transfixed in one position, coming like the stabbing of a knife in the region of the stomach, or above the navel, going from left to right, and is attended with prostration and nausea. Though there is sometimes thirst, it is usually absent. When Ipecac does its best work, there is thirstlessness.

You will see Ipecac patients tossing over the bed as much as they do when they need Rhus, turning and tossing, and moving the hands and feet, with restlessness. This is especially the case when the spine is somewhat involved. Ipecac has symptoms that look like tetanus; it has opisthotonous.

Inflammation of the lower portion of the bowel, the rectum and the colon. The tenesmus is awful, burning and continuous urging with the passage of only a little mcuus and blood.

The chest complaints of Ipecac are interesting. Ipecac is especially tne infants' friend and is commonly indicated in the bronchitis of infancy. The usual bad cold that ends in chest trouble in infants is a bronchitis. It is very seldom that an infant gets a true pneumonia, is generally bronchitis with coarse rattling which can be head throughout the room, and the trouble has come on pretty rapidly.

You can readily see the value of Ipecac in whooping cough. It has the paroxysmal character, the red face, vomiting and gagging with the cough. The red face, thirstlessness, violent whoopig, with convulsions, with gagging and vomiting of all that he eats are the symptoms that you will generally find.

It is useful in cases of humid asthma, in cases of asthmatic bronchitis, when they suffer from the damp weather and from sudden weather changes; every little cold rouses up this bronchial attack; and he suffocates and gags when he coughs, or spits up a little blood. He has to sit up nights to breathe, and the attacks are common and frequent. *(Kent)*

340. Iridium

(Metal)

Intestinal putrefaction and septicaemia, anaemia, increases red corpuscles, epilepsy, lupus, rheumatism and gout. Uterine tumors, spinal paresis, exhaustion after disease. Children who are puny, weak limbed, and grow too fast. Nephritis of pregnancy.

Head: Wooden feeling in right side of head.

Dose: 6 and higher. *(Boericke)*

Indium is a rare metal of the platinum group found in platinum ore. A feeling as of a triangle on face, the base formed by the two malar bones, the apex in the vertex. Laboucher says it is admirable in all cases of anaemia, is better than China for the aged and persons exhausted by disease for puny, weak limbed children and those who grow too fast. *(JHC)*

A metallic element, ductile, silvery, and softer than lead.

This remedy is useful in megrim. The pain is in the temples and forehead, and is associated with sleeplessness, nausea, weakness and a feeling of emptiness in the stomach at 11 a.m.

It is of service in seminal emissions when there is diminished sexual power. The testicles are tender, and there are pains along the spermatic cord.

Compare: Anacardium, Selenium.
(Blackwood)

341. *Iris Tenax*

(Iris minor)

Iris Tenax - dry mouth, deadly sensation at point of stomach, pain in Ileo-caecal region, appendicitis, pain from adhesions after. *(Boericke)*

Grows very luxuriantly in the clay ground and on the hill sides of Oregon. The fibre of the plant is so strong, that it is used by Indians for making cord, and weaving into bags. The most remarkable symptoms were, no doubt the fearful pain in the Ileo-caecal region and the hard chill at 2 p.m. *(JHC)*

342. *Iris Versicolor*

(Blue flag)

Thyroid, Pancreas, Salivary, Intestinal glands and gastro intestinal mucous membranes, are especially affected. Increases the flow of bile. Sick headaches and cholera morbus are a special therapeutic field for its action.

Stomach: Burning of whole alimentary canal, vomiting sour, bloody, biliary nausea. Profuse flow of saliva, deficient appetite - constipation - give 30th.

Modalities. *Worse* in evening and at night from rest. *Better* from continued motion. *(Boericke)*

The blue flag is in great repute as a remedy among the Indians of North America - The action on the salivary glands and pancreas was very much marked and Iris has proved an excellent remedy in affections of these organs.

'Kitchen' found Iris the most effective all round remedy in cases of vomiting of all kinds. It is a great remedy in bilious sick headache. C.C. Conant said he had repeatedly verified right sided headache, beginning with a blue and very severe in front of head - In pancreatic diabetes Iris v. Should have a very important place. It has cured cases of herpes zoster (right side) eczema capitis, impetigo figurata and Psoriasis. Amel: by moderate motion and it should not be forgotten that constipation as well as diarrhoea may be a strong indication - Iris has thick ropy saliva (Ipecac saliva is thin), Iris agg: 2-3 a.m., Iris. v. is temporarily amel.: by drinking cold water. *(JHC)*

This is the vegetable mercury. The chemical constituents are an acrid resin, camphoraceous body, fat, sugar, gum tannin and possibly an alkaloid. This agent has a profound action upon the gastric intestinal tract, the glandular and nervous system. It produces acidity of the gastrointestinal secretion, acid diathesis and acidity. There is a sensation as though the contents of the stomach had turned to vinegar. This acidity is the central feature in the action of the drug. Disturbances of the functions of the pancreas, lymphatic glands and skin, as shown by the abnormal secretions from the bowels, condition of the urine, the violent pains in the various parts of the body, and great mental irritability and depression. The headaches are frequently produced by eating sweets. In hemicrania it is of service. Hyperchlorhydria, vomiting of food, especially following the taking of rich or fat foods. Pancreatitis, glycosuria, intolerable itching which is worse at night, psoriasis.

In those cases of eczema it will be found most useful if given in the tincture or one of the lower potencies every three hours. It should be remembered in enlarged thyroid of recent date. Compare - Ipecacuanha, Podophyllum, Sanguinaria. *(Blackwood)*

343. *Jacaranda*
(Brazilian Caroba tree)

Has reputation as a remedy in venereal diseases and rheumatism. Morning sickness. The urinary and sexual symptoms are important. Rheumatic symptoms.

Urinary: Urethra inflamed, discharge of yellow matter.

Male: Heat and pain in penis, painful erections, phimosis, prepuce painful and swollen. Chancroid. Chordee. Itching pimples on gland and prepuce.

Extremities: Gonorrhoeal rheumatism and syphilitic arthritis.

Dose: Tr. to 3rd potency. *(Boericke)*

Contact of urine with chancre causes tearing pains which affect whole organism. Prepuce much swollen, could not be drawn over glans, on attempting to do so, copious discharge of yellow green pus. *(JHC)*

This remedy is indicated in feeble minded masturbators in whom there are irritations and pain about the prepuce, and glans of the penis, also in rheumatic pains and syphilitic arthritis.

It should be remembered in cystitis and gonorrhoea, when there is much inflammation and pricking pains in the prepuce. The lips of the urethra are inflamed and there is a yellow-white discharge.

Compare: Thuja *(Blackwood)*

344. *Jalapa*
(Jalap)

Causes and cures colic and diarrhoea. The child is good all day, but screams and is restless and troublesome at night.

Dose: 3-12 potency.

Compare: Colocynth. *(Boericke)*

The characteristic stool of Jalap is watery, sour smelling and bloody. There is cutting colic before and during the stool. The most marked agg. is at night. A child may be quite all day but screams and tosses about all night. In such a case Jalap is very likely to be the remedy, whether the child is suffering from diarrhoea or other complaint. The abdominal pain is very severe as if the abdomen would be cut to pieces. *(JHC)*

This remedy is indicated when there is diarrhoea with pain and gripping in the bowels with flatulence. The stools are watery, sour smelling and at times bloody. There may be colic before and during the stool. This is worse at night. The child is good all day but screams and tosses about all night.

It should be remembered in the entero-colitis of adults with cutting pains, especially in the sigmoid. There is a general coldness and blueness of the face. Prostration and fainting.

Compare:- Camphor, Colocynthis.
(Blackwood)

345. *Jatropha*
(Purging nut)

Of value in cholera and diarrhoea. The abdominal symptoms are most important. Suppressed measles.

Stomach: Very easy vomiting.

Stool: Diarrhoea, forced discharge, loud noise in abdomen like gurgling of water, coming out of a bung hole.

Extremities: Coldness of whole body.

Dose: 3 to 30th potency. *(Boericke)*

Jatropha is one of the most active of the euphorbeans and strongly resembles Croton in its action, especially in the urgent gushing stools and the irritation and pimples of the skin. One of the most notable characteristics of Jatropha is the very marked and peculiar gurgling it causes. Much noise in abdomen as if a bottle was being emptied followed later by a thin stool. At times the purging is accompanied by copious vomiting of watery albuminous ropy liquid. Sudden desire for stool is marked. Water is almost immediately vomited. It corresponds more to the earlier than the collapse stage of cholera.

Cramps are predominant. The patient writhes in bed with pain. The characteristic is a rice water discharge, it has vomiting and purging; more or less sweat, more or less cramps. Suppression of urine, the great prostration, syncope and rapid onset peculiar to cholera and it has this to differentiate it from all other remedies - the vomit and purging and evacuations are thick, albuminous, lumpy, instead of thin and watery - Patient seeks to cool himself by throwing off covers and lying on ground, summer diarrhoea occurring suddenly, Veratrum has more pain and more pronounced collapse - It has not the albuminous vomiting of Jatr. - not so much rumbling as Ars. (Vomits water as soon as drunk), Elat. (Gushing noisy stools)*(JHC)*

346. *Jequirity*
(Crab's eye vine)

Epithelioma, lupus, ulcers, granular lids.

Eyes: Purulent conjunctivitis, inflammation spreads to face and neck. Granular ophthalmia, Keratitis.

Dose: Mother tincture diluted locally and 3x internally. *(Boericke)*

Arbus precatorius (Jequirity) is a climbing plant, a native of India, but has been introduced to the western tropics and its use as an eye remedy was discovered by the natives of Brazil, who gave it the name Jequirity. It has small nearly globose seeds which are of a brilliant scarlet colour with a black scar, indicating where they were attached to the pods. These are used for necklaces and as a standard of weight under the name of Ratti - Thirty grains of powdered seeds are allowed to soak for 24 hours in 1000 grammes of water - the patient with granular ophthalmia bathes his eye, with the filtered product thrice daily for 3 days, at the end of which time he has become the subject of a severe conjunctivitis, which may be either purulent and more allied to the diphtheritic form. By the 15th day the inflammation ceases and the granulations are found to be much diminished in size or even destroyed. The intensity of inflammation may be regulated by the strength of the solution. Sometimes the inflammation does not confine itself to the eyes but effects the lids with an intense inflammation which spreads to the face, neck and chest. *(JHC)*

347. *Jonosia Asoka*

(Bark of an Indian tree introduced by Dr. D.N. Ray, Calcutta)

Has extensive sphere of action on female organs. Amenorrhoea and metrorrhagia.

Gastric - Desire for sweets, also acid things, thirst, excessive nausea, obstinate constipation, haemorrhoids.

Dose: Tincture. *(Boericke)*

Saraca Indica or Jonosia Asoka - In an ordinary leucorrhoea or leucorrhoea mixed with blood or bloody discharge, the physicians have uniformly and universally found it to be a sovereign remedy - from my own personal knowledge, I can vouch for the authenticity of those brilliant cures and nobody can doubt its efficacy as a splendid uterine remedy. (Dr. Gosh). It has obstinate constipation, protrusion of haemorrhoids. Amenorrhoea.

Personal observations of Dr. Gosh.

Asoka is a noted plant in our country and its therapeutic properties in curing and alleviating all sorts of menstrual troubles and uterine disorders date long back. In the cure of leucorrhoea its action can never be questioned and upon bloody leucorrhoea whether acute or chronic, it exerts an exhilarating and permanent curative action, which sometimes appears to be a miracle. It is said to posses a stimulating effect on the endometrium and on the ovarian tissue. It is extensively employed in uterine ailments, especially menorrhagia, which is the outcome of utreine fibroids and other causes.

It has been found to be an excellent medicine for the complaints appearing at the time of menopause. For barrenness it is generally used with success.

In bleeding piles, its efficacy has been verified by us. In bleeding piles the colour of the blood is red, the patient experiences severe pain and stiff feeling in the back and suffers from constipation, there is burning sensation from passing urine and there is also burning of the hands, feet and eyes in the evening. The patients of Asoka are generally affectionate, nervous, sentimental, gloomy and religious.

Dose: Dil - ϕ and 3x and 2x are generally used. (Dr. S.C. Gosh - Book - Drug of Hindoosthan)

Asoka Janosia has gained universal reputation as a great saviour of women from all ailments peculiar to the fair sex. Why should any woman suffer so long as this great saviour survives on earth - Asoka. Q-5 drops TDS - It may be used as an intercurrent remedy and complementary to Abroma Augusta, Xanthoxyllum, Aletris Farinosa, Viburnum Opulus, Viburnum Prunifolia, Ova toasta, Pulsatilla,

Sepia, Cimicifuga, Caulophyllum etc. with great success. *(Dr. Yudhbir Sinha)*

348. *Juglans Cinerea*

(Butter nut)

A faulty elimination that produces jaundice and various skin eruptions is pictured by this drug. The sharp occipital headache usually associated with liver disturbances is very characteristic. Pain in chest, axilla and scapula with suffocative sensation. Feeling as if all internal organs were too large, especially those of left side. Cholelithiasis.

Head: Sharp occipital headache.

Skin: Red, like flush of scarlatina, jaundice with pain about liver and right scapula. Itching and pricking when heated. Pustules, eczema, especially on lower extremities, sacrum and hands, erythema and erysipelatous redness.

Dose: Tr. to 3rd potency. *(Boericke)*

The green rind rubbed on tetters and ringworms dispels them - One patient who was taking 'Jug. c' for acne developed all the symptoms of angina pectoris. But the skin is the organ most of all affected by the drug. All kinds of eruptions have been caused or cured by it, including scarlatina and rodent ulcer. *(JHC)*

This agent acts upon the liver, duodenum, small intestines and colon. Producing an increased activity of the bile forming function of the liver, and increasing the secretions from the glands of the intestinal tract. Large doses produce large bilious evacuations from the bowels with severe intestinal pain and colic, similar to those produced by Iris versicolor. These evacuations from the bowels are attended by a sensation of burning and are followed with tenesmus, the odor of the stools is similar to that of onions. It produces pain in both hypochondriac regions, with stitching pain in the region of the liver that extends to the right shoulder and under the right scapula. The hepatic area is sensitive under palpation. Under its action the blood becomes darker in character and more fluid than is normal.

It also produces occipital headache in which the pains are sharp and shooting in character, and are associated with tenderness of the liver, and a catarrhal condition of the duodenum and jaundice. There are sharp pains under the right shoulder blade which might remind one of Chelidonium or Bryonia. The patient often awakes about 3 a.m. with a severe occipital headache. There are bilious stools of a yellow-greenish color, their passage is attended with a sensation of burning in the anus and is followed by tenesmus.

It should be remembered in cases of occipital headaches when the pain appears during the early morning, is severe and cutting in character. It is partially relieved after arising. It is most frequent in those with enlarged sensitive livers. The pain may be present during the forenoon, when it is usually referred to the right side of the head and the right temple.

There may be a sensation as though the head was enlarged. The headache may be accompanied with frequent urination. The passing of the urine is attended by a sensation of burning in the urethra. Occasionally there is a sensation as of sinking in the stomach complained of, attending the headache. The tongue has a yellow coating.

It should be studied in cases of retrosternal pain when there is a sensation as of suffocation. This is observed when exercising and compels the patient to stand still. It is associated with gastric and hepatic symptoms and led to its use in a case of angina pectoris, which it speedily relieved.

It is of service in cholangitis and in cholecystitis and the attending jaundice when there are sharp cutting pains in the region of the gall bladder that appear independent of movements. This pain extends and is felt under the right scapula. In these cases there is frequently a morning occipital headache. The patient is obliged to get out of bed and move about to find relief from the pain.

It is an important remedy in diseases of the skin which vary in character from scaly to pustular and from papules to bulla. Associated with the skin lesion there is usually a toxic condition of the intestine, the urine showing an excess of indican.

It should be remembered in erythema nodosa when there are extensive patches of eruptions on the body and extremities that are attended with general constitutional disturnbances.

It should be remembered in chronic eczema when it is of an impetiginous variety. The secretions are semipurulent, ichorous in character and there is soreness and an intolerable itching and smarting. When this remedy is indicated there is an unhealthy condition of the intestinal tract.

Compare - Iris ver., Bryonia, Chelidonium. *(Blackwood)*

349. *Juglans Regia*

(Walnut)

Skin eruptions are prominent.

Head: Confused, feels as if head were floating in air, occipital sharp pain, styes.

Skin: Comedones and acne of the face, crusta lactea with soreness around ears. Itching and eruptions of small red pustules. Scalp red and itches violently at night. Chancre - like ulcer. Auxcillary glands suppurate.

Dose: Tr. and lower potencies.

(Boericke)

It was said that in the golden age, when men lived on Acorns, the gods lived on the Walnuts and hence the name Juglans, (Jovel's Glans or Jupiters Nuts) - The remarkably brain-like appearance of the nut has given rise to the notion that it is a brain food. Remarkable symptoms of inflammation and ulceration appeared in the male sexual organs. This to a large extent belongs to the general integumatory action of the remedy. Farrington says 'Jug. r.' is one of the best remedies in Tinea Favosa especially in the scalp behind the ears, itching is intense at night, so that the patient has difficulty in sleeping. One of the provers was cured of an itching eruption of the legs from which he had suffered in winter for four years, the itching commencing as soon as he began to undress. The itching is agg. at night, warmth of bed. It removed a winter rash *agg:* by undressing. *(JHC)*

350. *Justicia Adhatoda - Basaka*

(An Indian shrub., Singhee)

Highly efficacious medicine for acute catarrhal conditions of the respiratory tract (used in the beginning).

Respiratory: Dry cough from sternal region all over chest. Hoarseness, larynx painful, paroxysmal cough, with suffocative obstruction of respiration. Cough with sneezing, severe dyspnoea with cough. Tightness across chest. Asthmatic attacks, cannot endure a close warm room, whooping cough.

Dose: 3 and higher - severe aggravation have been noticed from lower potencies.

(Boericke)

Allopathic use and opinions.

Expectorant, anti-spasmoic and alteratively, the flowers and roots with ginger and (SITAB) are given in ague, rheumatism, constipation, asthma, chronic bronchitis and other chest affections. Leaves are smoked in Asthma.

Dr. Watt has also brought to notice the use of Adhatoda leaves in rice cultivation in Sutlej valley. The fresh leaves are scattered over recently flooded fields prepared for the rice crop and the native cultivators say that they not only act as a manure but also a poison to kill the aquatic weeds that otherwise would injure rice.

In acute bronchitis it was found always to afford relief, especially where the sputum was thick and tenacious, acting in very much the same way as Ipecac.

There is no doubt however that it relieves the irritable cough by its soothing action on the nerves and by liquifying the sputum which makes expectoration easy.

It is not effective in relieving attack of bronchial asthma. In pulmonary tuberculosis, it has no action whatever.

Personal observation of Dr. S.C. Ghose.

In coryza it is highly curative where sneezing troubles the patient. In whooping cough, I have the greatest confidence in it as long as or whenever catarrhal symptoms are noticed. The cough of Justicia is incessant and severe. The chest seems pregnant with phlegm and there is audible rattling of mucus but very little is expectorated or it is loosened only with repeated hawking.

It has also great loss of appetite and there is also obstinate constipation.

(Dr. S.C. Ghose)

Dose: Give 3 drops of ϕ or 1 drop of 1X ϕ ID *(Dr. Yadubir Sinha)*

351. *Kali Arsenicum*

(Fowlers solution)

The Kali Ars. patient tends towards malignancy and inveterate skin diseases. He is restless, nervous and anaemic.

Skin: Intolerable itching worse undressing. Dry, scaly, wilted acne, pustules worse during menses. Chronic eczema, itching worse from warmth, walking, undressing, psoriasis, lichen, phagedenic ulcers, fissures in bends of arms and knees. Gouty nodosities, worse change of weather. Skin cancer, where suddenly an alarming malignancy without any external signs sets in. Numerous small nodules under skin.

Dose: 3-30c. *(Boericke)*

Kali ars. has been tested, consists of Arsenious acid 1 part, Carbonate of potash 1 part, compound tincture of lavender 3 parts, distilled water 95 parts. Dilutions should be made from this.

It is not possible to separate entirely the Pathogenesis of Ars. alb. and Kali ars. Kali ars. is the favourite form in which Arsenic is prescribed by the allopaths, consequently the bulk of observations from over dosing are due to this preparation; and as it is named Liquor arsenicalis it is considered as Arsenic and nothing else.

Skin: Dry, wilted skin; emaciated to a skeleton - On three different occasions, swelling of face and eyelids, then erysipelas invading whole face ending in desquamation in a week - Acne, appearance like that in early stage of variola. Miliary eruption - Herpes zoster behind right ear, rt. side of neck, rt. shoulder, rt. upper arm, rt. chest, a few isolated vesicles Lt. side of neck, severe attack of shingles rt. side of chest - Eruption covering entire body except scalp, comes out in red papulae, varying in diamater from size of pin's head to that of a three cent piece; vesicles form on summit, suppurate, crusts form and fall off, leaving a sore which heals; the places occupied by these sores are marked by a dark - coloured cicatrix, and the skin generally has dusky look, intolerable itching, stinging, and burning, especially on undressing at night; it is agg; on trunk, legs and forearms; mind much depressed - Lichen confluens over whole body except face, palms, and soles, and part of chest; the rest studded with papulae, particularly distinct about outer sides of thighs, arms, and back; they are covered with very minute, flimsy, whitish scabs, causing a powdery appearance of skin; head very scurfy; hair crisp and dry; often irritation in skin, which becomes reddened and cracked, particularly about bend of arms and knees - one of the earlier signs is a minute papular rash, which by and by assumes the form of delicate, brownish scales giving the skin an unwashed appearance; esp. observed on parts protected from light by clothing. After taking it for three weeks, suddenly, after feeling ill for a few hours, a copious rash made its appearance on face, hands, and chest, like measles; accompanied by catarrhal symptoms, swelling of face, lips, eyelids, yellow — furred tongue, gastro-intestinal irritation, intense lameness of feet, standing giving great pain; complete aphonia followed in a few days, desquamation commenced on tenth day; redness lasted some weeks - Epithelial cancer supervened after prolonged medication with Kali ars. Psoriasis - A clerk had taken arsenic for a long time for psoriasis, palms and soles became spreckled over with corns, finally epithelial cancer of scrotum appeared (Hutchinson) - dry chronic eczema; skin of arms thicker and rougher than natural, covered with flimsy exfoliations of epidermis; very irritable itching and tingling when she gets warm; intensely fissured about bends of elbows and wrists occasional exacerbation, with eruption of distinct vesicles: languor and lassitude; pale, sallow complexion, catamenia irregular - Patches of psoriasis on back, arms, and spreading from elbows, and anteriorly on legs, size of crown piece, and indolent - Psoriasis; scaly itchings, causing him to scratch till an ichorous fluid discharges, forming a hard cake - discolouration of skin after psoriasis and lepra - Psoriasis in numerous patches, with great itching; the patches becoming more active, scale off, and are replaced by smaller patches that leave behind them a red skin - Jaundice.

(JHC)

352. *Kali Bichromicum*

(Bichromate of potash)

The special affinities of this drug are the mucous membranes of stomach and air passages, bones and fibrous tissues. Kidneys, heart and liver are also affected. Incipient parenchymatous nephritis. Nephritis and gastric disturbances. Cirrhosis of liver. Anaemia and absence of fever are characteristics. General weakness bordering on paralysis. It is especially indicated for fleshy, fat, light complexioned persons subject to catarrhs or with syphilitic or scrofulous history. Symptoms are worse in the morning; pains migrate quickly; rheumatic and gastric symptoms alternate. Moré adapted to subacute rather than the violent acute state. Mucous membranes everywhere are affected, catarrh of pharynx, larynx, bronchi and nose, and a tough stringy, viscid secretion is produced, which is a very strong guiding symptom for this drug. Perforation of the septum. Chronic atonic catarrh. polypus. Dilatation of stomach and the heart.

Head: Aching and fullness in glabella bones and scalp feels sore.

Eyes: Discharge ropy and yellow. Descemetitis.

Nose: Snuffles of children, especially fat, chubby babies. Pressure and pain root of nose, septum ulcerated, fetid smell, discharge thick, ropy, greenish yellow, tough elastic plugs, loss of smell, coryza with obstruction of nose, violent sneezing. Inflammation of frontal sinus with stopped up sensation.

Mouth: Dry, tongue red shining smooth and dry, broad, flat, indented, thickly, coated, feeling of hair on tongue.

Throat: Uvula relaxed, oedematous, bladder-like. Pseudo membranous deposit on tongue and soft palate.

Stomach: Round ulcer of stomach, dislike water, cannot digest meat.

Desire for beer and acids, gastric symptoms are relieved after eating.

Stool: Jelly like, gelatinous, worse morning.

Urinary: Burning in urethra. After urinating a drop seems to remain, which cannot be expelled, ropy mucus in urine. Pyelitis, urine mixed with epithelial cells, mucus, pus or blood, haematochyluria.

Male: Itching and pain of penis with pustules. Agg: at night, constriction at root of penis, at night on awakening; syphilitic ulcers, with cheesy tenacious exudation. Erections.

Female: Yellow, tenacious leucorrhoea, pruritus of vulva with great burning and excitement, prolapsus uteri, worse in hot weather.

Respiratory: Profuse yellow expectoration, very glutinous and sticky, coming out in long stringy and very tenacious mass, worse when undressing.

Back: Cutting through loins.

Extremities: Pains fly rapidly from one place to another, soreness of heels when walking. Tendo-achilles swollen and painful.

Skin: Ulcer with punched out edges.

Dose: 3x and 30c and higher - the lower preparation of this salt should not be kept too long. *(Boericke)*

1. Discharge from mucous membranes of tough stringy mucus or muco pus which adheres to the part and can be drawn out in strings.
2. The occurrence of pain in small spots.
3. Punched out perforating ulcers occurring on skin, mucous membranes and affecting bones.
4. Pains wander from part to part, rheumatic pains alternate with gastric symptoms.

Hair sensation is marked, chiefly on the posterior part of the tongue and in the left nostril - one of its effects is odourless stools. Asthma always followed coitus, agg. from coitus and also from emission. Blindness followed by headache, the sight improves as the pain becomes worse. *(JHC)*

It is an important remedy in spasmodic croup, when the dry, ringing cough has given way to a barking, hoarse cough and a tenacious expectoration.

It should be studied in chronic bronchitis, when the cough is hoarse and croupy. There is hoarseness and tightness complained of, and the expectoration is tenacious and viscid. The cough is worse after arising; if the patient has had his meal there may be vomiting.

It has been employed in gastric ulcer, when the severe localized symptoms and mucous secretions have been the guiding indications. *(Blackwood)*

353. *Kali Bromatum*

(Bromide of Potash)

Like all potash salts, this weaks the heart and lowers temperature. Rheumatism is caused by it. General failure of mental power, loss of memory, melancholia, anaesthesia of the mucus membrane especially of eyes, throat and skin, acne, loss of sexual desire, paralysis. Leading remedy in psoriasis. Nodular form of chronic gout. Symptoms of apoplectic attacks. Uraemic or other wise, Somnolence and stertor, convulsions, aphasia, albuminuria. Epilepsy (with salt free-diet).

Mind: Imagines he is singled out as an object of divine wrath, night terrors.

Head: Numb fielding in head.

Throat: Anaesthesia of fauces, pharynx and larynx.

Stomach: Intense thirst, persistent hiccough.

Abdomen: Cholera infantum, internal coldness.

Male: Debility and impotence, effects of sexual excesses.

Female: Exaggerated sexual desire.

Extremities: Fidgety hands, busy twitching of fingers.

Skin: Acne of face, pustules, itching, worse on chest, shoulders, Anaesthesia of skin. Psoriasis.

Sleep: Restless sleep, night terrors, Horrible dreams, somnambulism.

Modalities: Better, when occupied mentally or physically.

Dose: A few grains of the crude salt to the 3rd Trituration. Said to be much more active, if salt is eliminated from the diet.

(Boericke)

At the same time K. Brom. has a very profound action on the generative organs and the mental side of the generative sphere. Sensual, lascivious fancies, Satyriasis and nymphomania and finally impotence and wasting of the sexual organs. The cases of epilepsy, in which it is curative, are chiefly those associated with sexual excess or abuse in men and those in which the fits occur during or near the menstrual period in women - It is indicated also in cases of epilepsy occurring at the new moon and when headache follows the fit. One of the most troublesome accidents of the allopathic use of K. Brom. is the production of eruptions of many kinds but most notably acne.

Acne has a very definite relation to the sexual organs, being especially noticeable at puberty and in women at the menstrual period. I know of no remedy of such universal usefulness in case of simple Acne as K. Brom - 30. The memory is lost, forgets how to talk - drowsiness is one of the key notes of the drug, drops asleep in his chair and if aroused falls asleep again immediately. 'Flooding especially in young women'. A number of cases of ovarian cyst have disappeared under its action, also fibroids and fatty tumours. Kali. brom. is more particularly adapted to persons inclined to obesity, to children, to nervous women.

Compare: Eug. Jambos in acne; K. Brom. fidgety hands; Zincum fidgety feet.

Causation: Emotional disturbance sexual excess. *(JHC)*

This agent acts as a depressant of the motor and sensory nerves, which terminates in paralysis if it is continued. The gait becomes trembling, uncertain, and there is a lack of co-ordination. The capillaries are so contracted, metabolism is interfered with and anaemia results, the breath is offensive, and there is an eruption on the skin which at first is papular, but in time becomes pustular and furuncular in character.

It is useful in cerebral irritation, with congestion during dentition and acute diseases, also in nervous restlessness, when the patient cannot keep still, but must move, keeps the hands and fingers moving - "Fidgety hands".

It is indicated in Spermatorrhoea from excessive sexual desire, amorous dreams and nocturnal emissions. It is employed in somnambulism and the night tremors of children; also for restlessness and sleeplessness, due to worry and grief of any form. It has relieved spasmodic dry, croupy, nervous, hysterical cough, when the result of a neurosis or reflex irritation. It should be remembered in young, fleshy people with acne of a bluish-red color, and pustular, leaving bluish-red scars. *(Blackwood)*

354. *Kali Carbonicum*

(Carbonate of potassium)

The 'weakness' characteristic of all potassium salts is seen especially in this, with soft pulse, coldness, general depression, and very characteristic stitches, which may be felt in any part of the body or in connection with any affection. All Kali pains are sharp and cutting, nearly all better by motion. Never use any salts of Potash, where there is fever (T.F. Allen). Sensitive to every atmospheric change and intolerance of cold weather. One of the best remedies following labor. Miscarriage, for consequent debilitated states. Early morning aggravation is very characteristic. Fleshy aged people in dropsical and paretic tendencies. Sweat, backache and weakness. Throbbing pains. Tendency to dropsy. Tubercular diathesis. Pains from within out and of stinging character. Giving out sensation. Fatty degenerations. Stinging pains in muscles and internal parts. Twitching of muscles. Pain in small spot on left side, Hypothyroidism. Coxitis.

Mind: Very irritable, hypersensitive to pain, noise, touch.

Head: Headache from riding in cold wind. Great dryness of hair, falls out.

Eyes: Swelling over upper lid, like little bags.

Nose: Stuffs up in warm room, ulcerated nostrils.

Mouth: Gums separate from teeth, pus oozes out, pyorrhoea, Aphthae.

Stomach: Flatulence, desire for sweets, sour eructations, nausea, constant feeling as if stomach were full of water. Anxiety felt in stomach.

Rectum: Large, difficult stools. Haemorrhoids large, swollen painful. Itching ulcerated pimples around anus. Large discharge of blood with natural stool. Easy prolapsus.

Urine: Obliged to rise several times at night to urinate. Involuntary urination when coughing, sneezing etc.

Male: Deficient sexual instinct. Excessive emissions followed by weakness.

Female: Menses early, profuse or too late, pale and scanty; complaints after parturition.

Respiratory: Dry hard cough about 3 a. m. with stitching pains and dryness of pharynx. Bronchitis. Whole chest is very sensitive, expectoration scanty and tenacious but increased in morning and after eating. Hydrothorax, coldness of chest, wheezing, cough with relaxed uvula, better in warm climate.

Heart: Burning in heart region. Weak, rapid, intermittent pulse.

Back: Small of back feels weak. Severe backache during pregnancy and after miscarriage. Hip disease. Pain in nates and thighs and hip joint. Lumbago with sudden sharp pains extending up and down back and to thighs.

Extremities: Backs and legs give out, tearing pains in limbs with swelling. White swelling of knee, tearing in arms from shoulder to wrist. Limbs go to sleep easily. Soles very sensitive. Pain from hip to knee, pain in knees.

Skin: Burning as from a mustard plaster.

Sleep: Drowsy after eating - wakes about 2'o clock and cannot sleep again.

Modalities: Worse after coition, cold weather, from soup and coffee, in morning and 3 o' clock.

Better: Warm weather, though moist, during day, while moving about.

Antidote: Camph and coffea.

Dose: 30th and higher. Do not repeat too often. Use cautiously in old gouty cases, advanced Bright's and tuberculosis.

(Boericke)

Potassium carbonate sometimes called vegetable alkali exists in all plants and was originally obtained from the ashes left after burning wood and vegetable structures. It corresponds to conditions in which these tissues are relaxed. Joints give way, the back feels as if broken, the patient feels compelled to lie down in the street. The climactering flushings of K. Carb. are associated with disturbances of the heart. Palpitations are most violent. He places it in the front rank as a knee remedy. Among the grand characteristics (1) stitching lancinating pains, also called jerking pains agg: during rest, lying on affected side. (2) Early morning *agg:* 2-4 a. m. (3) The occurrences of bag like swellings over the eye, between the eye brows and the upper lids.

It is suited to persons of soft tissues with tendency to be fat. Easy sweating may be placed in the same category, combination of "Sweat, backache and weakness." The backaches of K. Carb are very important. The pain often extends downwards to the buttock and even to the knee waking at 2 a.m.-K. Carb. 30 cured but meantime he developed this symptom. Great weakness of right thigh, as if it would give out when walking. This giving out feeling is very characteristic of the remedy. Complaints after coition in males. Cannot bear to be touched, starts when touched ever so lightly, especially on the feet, when eating she was so weary, she fell asleep and could not finish her meal. K. carb. is suited to the aged; rather obese, lax fibre; to dark haired persons; and inclined to be fat - Apis and Ars. (Puffing of face and eyes) K-Carb will bring on the menses, when Nat. m., though apparently indicated fails. *(JHC)*

355. *Kali Chloricum*

(Chlorate of Potassium)

Acts very destructively upon the kidneys producing a croupous nephritis, haemoglobinuria etc. Parenchymatous nephritis with stomatitis. Produces most acute ulcerative and follicular stomatitis. Coma, toxaemic condition of pregnancy, urinary symptoms, chronic nephritis, hepatitis, septicaemia, anaemia.

Mouth: Mucous surface red tumid, with grey based ulcers.

Stool: Diarrhoea profuse, greenish mucus.

Dose: 2-6 potency. Use cautiously locally as it is poisonous. *(Boericke)*

Most acute ulceration and follicular stomatitis. The whole mucous surface was red and timid and in the cheeks, lips, etc. were numerous grey-based ulcers.

(JHC)

This is the most poisonous of all the salts of potash, and its indiscriminate use in physiological doses should be discouraged.

This remedy is indicated when there is acute ulcerative process, with septic discharge and decay of animal tissue going on.

It is useful in follicular and ulcerative stomatitis, the nursing sore mouths of mothers and infants, and gangrene of the mouth of children, cancrum oris. The mouth and gums are tender and may be gangrenous; the saliva is foetid and purulent; the tongue is coated and there are ulcers with gray bases over the mucous surfaces. The urine may contain blood and albumin. This same process may involve the stomach, when there is a sensation of weight and of burning in the epigastrium. *(Blackwood)*

356. *Kali Cyanatum*

(Potassium cyanide)

Sudden sinking sensation. Cancer of tongue and agonizing neuralgia have been benefited by this drug. Sick headache, sciatica, epilepsy.

Tongue: Power of speech lost but intelligence intact.

Dose: 6-200 potency. *(Boericke)*

Strong tetanic convulsions, slow breathing, loss of consciousness. A woman had cancerous ulcer of right side of tongue involving the root. With a view of relieving the woman's sufferings "Petroz" gave her

Gr. 1/100 of K. Cy. once in 4 days. In a fortnight the suffering was diminished, the tongue appeared less thick and speech easier. The case went on to complete and permanent cure. *(JHC)*

357. *Kali Hydriodicum*

(Iodine of Potassium)

The profuse watery acrid coryza that the drug produces services as sure guiding symptom, especially when associated with pain in frontal sinus. It acts prominently on fibrous and connective tissues producing infiltration, oedema etc., glandular swellings. Purpura and haemorrhagic diathesis. Syphilis may be indicated in all stages. In acute form with evening remitting fever, going off in nightly perspiration. (2) Second stage, mucous membranes and skin ulcerations. (3) Tertiary symptoms, nodes. Give material doses. Diffused sensitiveness (glands, scalp, etc). Rheumatism in neck, back, feet, especially heels and soles, worse cold and wet. Iodide of potash. In material doses acts in the different forms of fungoid disease (Thrush, ring worm etc). Often simulating syphilis and bacterial diseases like tuberculosis, symptoms like loss of, weight, spitting of blood etc. Tea tasters cough due to inhaling the fungus, also brings about often favourable reaction in many chronic ailments even when not clearly symptomatically indicated.

Head: Pain intense over eyes and root of nose. Facial neuralgia.

Nose: Profuse, acrid, hot, watery, thin discharge, ozaena with perforated septum.

Eyes: Syphilitic Iritis.

Respiratory: Larynx feels raw, expectoration like soap-suds, greenish, pneumococcic meningitis. Pleuritic effusion, cold travels downward to chest.

Extremities: Rheumatism of knees with effusion, sciatica.

Skin: Glands enlarged, rough nodules.

Dose: We use as a rule, the first dilution from 6-20 drops a day. If after a week no decided progress is visible one drop of the Tr. Iodine is added to each hundred of the first dilution.

30th potency *(Boericke)*

I rarely find occasion to use it in lower attenuation than the 30th, Agg. at the Sea side-enlarged lymphatic glands, syphilitic nodes, condylomata, and tumours of the breast and uterus have been removed by it. The solvent action of the drug is most powerfully excited on the more lowly organised tissues. Womb packed with fibroids, pain in right inguinal region. It acts on the tissues, much in the same way as syphilis does, dissolving them-glands atrophy, tissues especially connective tissues and ligaments, inflame and ulcerate - hard lumps like nodes on the scalp which pain excessively. All symptoms agg. by drinking cold milk - But perhaps the most satisfactory action of K. Iod. in the 30th is in rickets and rickety conditions, along with its many attendant symptoms. It gives a better chance of removal of that very obstinate symptom, tinnitus aurium, a single dose of K. Iod. 30 to be given.

Causation: Drinking cold milk. *(JHC)*

It is useful in coryza and lachrymation, when there is a violent sneezing, with acrid water running from the nose, and great redness of the nose, throat and pharynx. There are throbbing and burning pains in the nasal and frontal bones, with ulcerations of the cartilages, and, as a result, there is a foul, sickening smell and a discharge of green plugs or yellow pus. The gums recede from the teeth, which are loose, the breath is offensive, and there is a bloody saliva. It should be remembered in all glandular enlargements when dependent upon syphilis.

It acts as an antidote in lead poisoning. *(Blackwood)*

358. Kali Mur

(Chloride of Potassium KCl)

Although not proven this remedy has a wide clinical use through its introduction by Schussler. It certainly is of great value in catarrhal affections, in sub acute inflammatory states, fibrinous exudations and glandular swellings. White or gray coating of base of tongue and expectoration of thick white phlegm seem to be a special guiding symptom. Bursitis, Praepatellaris.

Head: Crusta lactea, Dandruff.

Ears: Chronic, catarrhal conditions of the middle ear, snapping and noises in the ear.

Mouth: Coating of tongue, grayish white, dry or slimy.

Throat: Follicular tonsillitis, tonsils inflamed, enlarged, so much, can hardly breath, grayish patches of spots in the throat and tonsils. Adherent crusts in vault of pharynx. Hospital sore throat. Eustachian catarrh.

Stomach: Fatty or rich food causes indigestion.

Stool: Constipation, high coloured stools, diarrhoea, after fatty food. Clay coloured, white or slimy stools, dysentery, purging with slimy stools. Haemorrhoids bleeding, blood dark and thick, fibrinous, clotted.

Female: Menstruation irregular, scanty or excessive, dark clotted like tar, Leucorrhoea non irritating, bland.

Back and Extremities: Rheumatic fever, exudation and swelling around the joints, nightly rheumatic pain, worse from warmth of bed, hands get stiff while waiting.

Respiratory: Loss of voice, hoarseness, asthma with gastric derangements, mucus white and hard to cough up - loud noisy stomach cough, cough short, acute and spasmodic like whooping cough, expectoration thick and white, rattling sounds of air passing through thick tenacious mucus in the bronchi, difficult to cough up.

Skin: Acne, erythema and eczema with vesicles containing thick white contents.

Dry flour-like scales on the skin.

Modalities: Worse rich food, fat.

Dose: 3-12 Potency. *(Boericke)*

It is to Schussler that we owe the introduction of this salt into homoeopathy. His account of it is this - It is contained in nearly all the cells and is chemically related to fibrin. It will dissolve white or greyish - white secretions of the mucous membrane and plastic exudations. This gives the indication for it in catarrhs in croupous and diphtheritic exudations and in the second stage of inflammation of serous membranes when the exudation is plastic. When the cells of the epidermis lose molecules of K. mur in consequence of a morbid irritation, then the fibrin comes to the surface as a white or whitish gray mass, when dried this forms a mealy covering. If the irritation has seized upon the tissues under the epidermis, then fibrin and serum are exuded, causing the affected spot on the epidermis to raise the blisters. Similar process may take place in and below epithelial cells. Chronic catarrhal condition of middle ear. Closed Eustachian tubes. Snapping and noises in the ear. Greyish white dry or slimy tongue. Haemorrhoids bleeding, blood dark, fibrous, clotted. Diphtheria. Rheumatic fever with exudation and swelling around the joints. The symptoms are agg: by motion, by any fatty or rich food or pastry. It is said to have cured cataract after Calc. fl. had helped. I have cured with it rheumatism affecting most left shoulder and elbow. Agg: in morning on rising. The great key note of K. mur is whiteness, whiteness of secretions exudations, eruptions, of tissues. There are next-to-tough fibrinous exudations and discharges, too readily clotting blood, hence embolism, induration and hard swellings.

Causation: Vaccination, sprains, burns, blows, cuts, rich food. *(JHC)*

Cataract, Mumps-swelling of the parotid gland. Epilepsy after suppression of skin eruptions, in growing nails, warts on hands.

Potency: 6X, 12X, 30, 200. *(H.C.Allen)*

359. Kali Nitricum

(Nitrate of Potassium-saltpeter)

Often indicated in asthma, also valuable in cardiac asthma. Of great value in sudden dropsical swelling over the whole body. Gastro intestinal inflammation, with much debility and relapse in phthisis, call for this remedy. Suppurative nephritis.

Nose: Swollen feeling, worse right nostril, polypus.

Stool: Diarrhoea from eating veal (Calf's flesh).

Respiratory: Bronchitis with sharp short, dry hacking cough, asthma with excessive dyspnoea, oppression worse in the morning, congestion of lungs, spasmodic croup.

Heart: Pulse weak, small, thready.

Compare: Gunpowder (Nitre with sulphur and charcoal - 2x trit.) "Blood poisoning", septic suppuration, protective against wound infection. Herpes facialis crops of boils, carbuncles, osteo-myeletis - Cannab. sat., contains a large amount of Kali nit.

Dose: 3, 30. *(Boericke)*

K.N. is known in old school practice principally as a "refrigerant diuretic" and as the active agent in the well known "Nitre papers" which are burnt for producing fumes to allay attacks of asthma. It has also been used in rheumatism, and for incontinence of urine in children. That its antiasthmatic properties are homoeopathic is abundantly shown in the respiratory symptoms it produces. Its diuretic properties are utilised homoeopathically in Diabetes insipidus and its use in enuresis, must come in the same category. K.N. acts with great intensity on the abdominal and pelvic organs producing most painful colics, diarrhoea and dysentery; in the male sexual sphere, excitement and pain in testes and cords; in the female, menorrhagia with flow of ink-like blackness. Agg: from eating veal-easy intoxication by wine or beer was noted by several provers. A peculiar symptom is a sour taste in the throat. Another peculiar symptom is in connection with the asthmatic state. The breathlessness is so great, that the patient though thirsty can only drink a sip at a time between the breaths. Allen thus defines the asthma of K.N.; Asthma with excessive dyspnoea, faintness and nausea, with dull stitches or with burning pain in chest, rather free expectoration - Nitre with sulphur and charcoal forms gun powder.

A teaspoonful of this in hot water was a favourite remedy for gonorrhoea among soldiers in the days when black powder was used. In the trituration, gun powder has cured ascarides in adults. In some experiments made by myself with Gun powder 2x, severe herpes facialis involving right eye brow and right side of nose was developed, agg from veal, wine or beer, 3 a.m. cough, in morning, by coffee - suited to asthmatic constitutions and chest complaints. *(JHC)*

This remedy is of service in rheumatism, myalgia and lumbago, when the urine is strongly acid and the solids are greatly increased.

It is useful in the relief of asthma, when a blotting paper should be saturated with a solution of the salt in the proportion of one drachm to the ounce of hot water. The paper should be dried and burned in a pitcher or narrow mouth jar and the fumes inhaled. *(Blackwood)*

360. Kali Permanganicum

(Permanganate of Potassium)

Intense irritation of nose, throat and larynx. Diphtheria. Dysmenorrhoea. Bites of serpents and for other animal poisons. Septic conditions; tissues infiltrated with tendency to sloughing.

Locally, 1 dram to a quart of water, to correct fetor in cancer, ulcer, ozaena, and other foul odors. Also as an injection in leucorrhoea and gonorrhoea. Internally, 2X dilution in water. Saturated solution locally in eruption of smallpox.

Pottassium permanganate for Morphine poisoning: Potassium permanganate is recognized as being the most effective chemical antidote in cases of morphine or opium poisoning, acting directly on the morphine and oxidizing it to less toxic substances. To be effective the permanganate must come in direct contact with the opium or morphine in the stomach; hypodermic or intravenous injections are absolutely useless, as the salt would be decomposed by the blood serum at once. The proved treatment is administration of two to five grains of potassium permanganate in dilute aqueous solution as soon as possible after the poison is taken, this amount to be increased if very large doses of the poison have been taken. Washing out the stomach with a quantity of 1 to 500 solution of permanganate is as recommended, using at least a pint of this solution either by a stomach pump or by enforced vomiting. Permang. of potash counteracts effects of alkaloids of many poisonous plants, owing to its oxidizing powers if given before the alkaloid has been absorbed. (Dr. Chestnut in Dept. of Agriculture). *(Boericke)*

K. Pm. is the well known disinfectant and has been chiefly used in medicine for local application in diphtheria and other conditions where there are fetid discharges. A proving by H.C. Allen has brought out the fact that the medicine is homoeopathic to both. There was intense irritation of nose, throat and larynx, with sanious and bloody discharges and constant inclination to swallow although swallowing gave great pain. Profuse salivation and constant flow of ropy mucus from the stomach were among the noted effects. The uvula was swollen and red. Extreme fetor of breath and sanious discharges call for it in diphtheria Kraft, who has used it largely in diphtheria gives it in this way: A few grains are dissolved in a tumbler of water sufficient to make it very red. A teaspoonful of this is put into another tumbler of water, and a teaspoonful out of the second tumbler is given every hour or two. The swollen uvula is also noteworthy. The exterior of the throat is very sensitive. A patient of mine made a curious use of K. pm. externally. He had wart on the tip of his nose, for which I had given him thuja internally and externally in vain, and later causticum internally with no better success. He on his own account applied a strong solution of K.pm. in the form of condy's fluid and it disappeared in a week-Kali pm. antidotes opium. *(JHC)*

361. Kali Phos

(Phosphate of potassium)

One of the greatest nerve remedies. Prostration. Weak and tired. Especially adapted to the young. Marked disturbance of the sympathetic nervous system conditions arising from want of nerve power, neurasthenia, mental and physical depression are wonderfully improved by this remedy. The causes are usually excitement, overwork and worry. Besides it corresponds to states of adynamia and decay, gangrenous conditions. In these two directions, it has won many clinical laurels. Remember it in the treatment of suspected malignant tumors. After removal of cancer, when in healing process skin is drawn tight over the wound. Delayed labor.

Mind: Anxiety, nervous dread, lethargy, indisposition to meet people. Extreme lassitude and depression. Very nervous, starts easily, irritable, brain fag, hysteria, night terrors, somnambulance, loss of memory, slightest labour seems a heavy task. Great despondency about business, shyness, disinclined to converse.

Head: Cerebral anaemia - Headache of students and those worn out by fatigue.

Ears. Humming and buzzing in the ears.

Mouth: Breath offensive, fetid.

Tongue: Coated brownish like mustard. Excessively dry. Toothache with easily bleeding gums. Gums spongy and receding.

Throat: Gangrenous sore throat.

Abdomen: Diarrhoea, foul putrid odor occasioned by fright with depression and exhaustion, prolapsus recti.

Female: Menstruation too late or too scanty in pale irritable sensitive, lachrymose females. Too profuse discharge, deep red or blackish red, thin and not coagulating, sometimes with offensive odor. Feeble and ineffectual labour pains.

Urinary organs: Enuresis, very yellow urine.

Respiratory: Asthma. Least food aggravates. Short breath on going upstairs.

Modalities: *Worse* excitement, worry, mental and physical exertion, eating, cold, early morning.

Dose: 3rd to 12th trituration. The highest potencies seem to be indicated in certain cases. *(Boericke)*

According to Schussler, K. Phos. is contained in the cells of the brain, nerves, muscles, blood (corpuscles and plasma) and intercellular fluids and a disturbance in the motions of its molecules produces; (1) In thought cells, despondency, anxiety, fearfulness, homesickness, suspiciousness, agoraphobia (morbid fear of open spaces and crowds), weak memory. (2) In vaso-motor nerves, first small and frequent pulse, later, retarded (3) in sensory nerves, pains with sensation of paralysis. (4) In motor nerves, weakness of muscles and nerves even to paralysis. (5) In trophic fibres of sympathetic nerves: retarded nutrition. Alopecia areata (Schussler). Excretion of golden or orange yellow. The urine is very yellow, tongue with brownish mustard like coat. Has cured impotence and seminal losses on these indications (J.C. Nottingham), frequent micturition agg: when menses come on. It is suited to pale, sensitive, irritable persons - Herring says Mushroom contain K. Ph. and hence are useful after weakening illness to restore muscle and nerve.

(JHC)

This remedy is indicated in derangements of the nervous system such as neurasthenia, prostration, insomnia, loss of mental vigor, and muscular debility following acute diseases. The patient is gloomy, depressed, with a loss of memory and a tendency to look on the dark side of things; it is of service in melancholia and mania that arise as a result of overstrain of the mind or from an exhausting drainage that affects the nerve centers, also homesickness, when haunted by visions of the past.

It is useful in enuresis, when dependent upon paralysis of the sphincter and a general weakness in the aged.

It should be remembered in low typhoid conditions when there is mental depression and delirium. The tongue is dry, brown, and there are sordes upon the teeth. The breath is offensive; there is a putrid diarrhoea and the patient is prostrated. It is indicated in the headache of those who are exhausted, students who have overstudied. The pain is relieved by gentle motion and is attended with a weary, empty, gone feeling in the region of the stomach.

Compare: Gel., Zincum, Muriatic acid.
(Blackwood)

362. Kali Sulph

(Potassium sulphate)

Ailments accompanied by profuse desquamation. Applicable to the later stages of inflammation. Yellow mucus and serous discharges, profuse and intermittent. Has been found of much use in oxaluria.

Head: Rheumatic headache, beginning in evening. Bald spots. Dandruff and scald head.

Nose: Cold with yellow slimy expectoration. Enlargement of the nasal pharyngeal mucous membrane.

Stomach: Tongue coated yellow and slimy, dread of hot drinks.

Respiratory: Rattling of mucus in chest, Bronchial asthma, and yellow expectoration - cough worse in evening and in hot atmosphere.

Extremities: Pain in nape, back and limbs, worse in warm room, shifting wandering pains.

Fever: Rise of temp at night, intermittent fever with yellow slimy tongue.

Skin: Psoriasis (Ars., Thyroid), eczema, burning, itching papular eruption, nettle rash, polypi, ring worm of scalp or beard with abundant scales.

Modalities: *Worse* in evening, heated room, better: Cool open air.

Dose: 3-12 potency. *(Boericke)*

K.S. in reciprocal action with iron effects the transfer of the inhaled oxygen to all the cells, containing iron. K.S. answers to the process of desquamation, which takes place after scarlatina, measles, erysipelas of the face etc. when a sulphate and any oxide of iron comes in contact, they surrender their oxygen and form sulphurate of iron. By more oxygen this may be further decomposed into sulphuric acid and an oxide of iron. K.S. is Schusslers Pulsatilla - The leading indications are those given by Schussler. The yellow colour of the discharges, the skin and mucous membrane appearances.

Agg: warmth - Amel: in open air - M.E. Douglas reports a case of Asthma, with thick yellow expectoration, much rattling in chest, laboured breathing, talking almost impossible cured with K. Sul. 3x, five grains every hour in the attack - "Hansen" cured with K. Sul. 3x a case of Psoriasis beginning on right leg, later attacking left leg and left elbow. The guiding symptom was "great desquamation of the epidermis." *(JHC)*

This remedy is indicated during the third stage of inflammation, when the discharge is yellow. There is an evening rise of temperature. The patient feels better while in the cool air. It is of service in conjunctivitis, when the discharge from the eyes is yellow.

It is useful during the last stages of bronchitis and broncho-pneumonia, when there is rattling of mucus in the chest. The cough is worse during the evening, and in a warm atmosphere. The sputum is yellow. It should be remembered in rheumatism, when the pains are worse from warmth, and wander and shift about.

Compare - Pulsatilla, Kali bichromicum.

(Blackwood)

363. Kalmia Latifolia

(Mountain Laurel)

A rheumatic remedy, pain shift rapidly, nausea and slow pulse frequently accompanying. Also has a prominent action on the heart. In small doses it accelerates the heart action, in larger it moderates it greatly. Neuralgia, pains shoot downwards with numbness. Fulgurating pains of locomotor ataxia. Protracted and continuous fevers with tympanities. Paralytic sensations, pains and aching in limbs, accompany nearly every group of symptoms. Albuminuria.

Head: Vertigo.

Eyes: Stiff drawing sensation when moving eyes, scleritis, pain increased by moving eyes.

Face: Worse right side.

Stomach: Nausea, pain in pit of stomach, worse by bending forward, relieved by sitting erect.

Urinary: Frequent, with sharp pains in lumbar region.

Heart: Weak slow pulse, palpitation, worse leaning forward, gouty and rheumatic metastasis of heart. Sharp pains take away the breath.

Back: Lumbar pain of nervous origin.

Extremities: Deltoid rheumatism especially right. Pains affect a large part of limb or several joints and pass through quickly, pains along ulnar nerve.

Sleep: Sleepless, wakes very early in morning.

Modalities: Worse leaning forward.

Compare: Spigelia, Pulsatilla.

Dose: Tr. to 6 potency. *(Boericke)*

Kalmia Latifolia, which has large and showy flowers is found in the northern parts of United states. Its flowers yield a honey said to be deleterious and its leaves and shoots certainly are so to cattle. K. Angustofolia, probably for the same reason has received the name of lamb kill. The powder leaves of some are used as a local remedy in some skin diseases. The hard wood of K. Latifolia is used in the manufacture of various useful articles. The Canadian patridge is said to become poisonous as human food after feeding on "Kalmia berries". Stiffness of the skin (especially of the eyelids) is most remarkable. Tobacco heart. The rheumatic pains proceed from above downwards, but some of the sensations ascend. Kalmia has a sun headache. Agg: and Amel: with the sun, beginning in occiput, going over forehead, comes on at sunrise gets Agg: towards noon and declines as sun sets. Insufficiency of the mitral valve - Led: pains shoot up, Kalm. Pains shoot down - Kalm is more suited to gout or rheumatism shifting from joints to heart.
(JHC)

Adapted to acute neuralgia, rheumatism, gouty complaints, especially when heart is involved as a sequel of rheumatism or gout. Rheumatism; pains intense, change place suddenly, going from joint to joint, hot, red, swollen, worse from least movement. Pulse slow, scarcely perceptible (35 or 40 per minute). Pale face and cold extremities. It follows Spig. well in heart disease. *(H.C. Allen)*

364. Kaolin

(Bolus alba. China clay - Alumina silicate)

A remedy for croup and bronchitis.

Nose: Yellow, sore, scabby.

Respiratory: Soreness of chest, along trachea, cannot stand percussion, gray sputa, capillary bronchitis, larynx and chest sore - membranous croup - extends down trachea.

Dose: Lower triturations. *(Boericke)*

365. Kousso Brayera

(Hagenia Abyssinica)

A vermifuge - Nausea and vomiting, vertigo, precordial anxiety, slowing and irregular pulse, subdelirium and collapse rapid and extreme prostration - to expel Tape worm.

Dose: 1/3 oz - mix with warm water and let stand 15 mts. - stir well and administer. May be preceded by a little lemon juice. (Merrel)

Relation: Mallotus - Kamala - An efficient remedy for Tape worm in 30-60 Minims of Tr. taken in cinnamon water.
(Boericke)

The flowers of Kousso are a favourite remedy for Tapeworm with the natives of Abyssinia, and the use of them in European practice for that purpose has led to the observation of the few symptoms recorded, among which thirst, nausea and vomiting are prominent. In one case miscarriage was caused. The mode of administration as a taenifuge is as follows: Take a quarter of an ounce of the dried flowers, boiling distilled water four ounces. Infuse fifteen minutes without straining. The powder is to be taken with the infusion, in the morning, fasting. Two such draughts may be given. It is best to give a purgative before and an hour or two after the draught. A remark by Alexander Milne is significant to homoeopaths: Though Kousso leads to the expulsion of the worm, it does not seem to improve the morbid condition which favours its production. (Living taenia placed in an infusion of Kousso mixed with milk were killed in about half an hour). The prostration caused by the treatment is so great that Milme advises a course of Cinchona and Iron to follow.

Relations: Compare: Cucurb., Granat., Filix. m. *(JHC)*

366. Kreosotum

(Beech wood Kreosote)

Kreosotum is a mixture of phenols obtained from the distillation. Pulsation all over the body and profuse bleeding from small wounds. Very severe old neuralgic affections, pains rather aggravated by rest. Excoriating burning and offensive discharges. Haemorrhages, Ulcerations, cancerous affections, rapid decomposition of fluids and secretions and burning pains, over grown, poorly developed children. Post - Climacteric diseases, tumefaction, puffiness, gangrene, ailing of teething children.

Mouth: very painful dentition, child will not sleep, very rapid decay of teeth, with spongy bleeding gums, teeth dark and crumbly.

Throat: Putrid odor.

Abdomen: Cholera infantum in connection with painful dentition, green stools, nausea, dry skin, exhaustion etc.

Urine: Offensive, violent itching of vulva and vagina, worse when urinating. Enuresis in the first part of night, must hurry when desire comes to urinate.

Female: Corrosive itching within vulva, burning and swelling of labia, violent itching between labia and thighs. During menses, difficult hearing. Leucorrhoea, yellow acrid, odor of green corn, worse between periods, menstruation flow intermits, ceases on sitting or waking, reappears on lying down.

Respiratory: Hoarse with pain in larynx-winter coughs of old people with heavy pressure on sternum, copious purulent expectoration.

Modalities: Worse in open air, cold, rest, when lying, after menstruation.

Better: From warmth, motion, warm diet.

Dose: 3-30c. The 200c to sensitive patients. *(Boericke)*

A product of distillation of wood tar. Its name derived from the Greek means 'flesh preserver'. Teste observed that it acted particularly well on infants in the cradle and congenital syphilis was a very strong indication for it. The marked action of "Kre" on the dentition confirms this - The teeth decay almost as soon as they appear. Kreo is one of the most important remedies in enuresis. The chief urinary features are (1) copious pale urine. (2) sudden great urging, the patient cannot go quick enough. (3) The child wets the bed during the first sleep which is very profound. In my own experience Kreo 3 and 30 meets a very large proportion of toothache cases where the teeth are decayed, especially if the gums are scorbutic. Vomiting of pregnancy. leucorrhoea putrid. Annoying itching at genitals at times, music makes him weep. Kreo retains food several hours and vomits it undigested. *(JHC)*

367. *Lac Caninum*

(Dog's milk)

This remedy is of undoubted value in certain forms of sore throat and diphtheria and rheumatism. Corresponds to a low-vitiated, non-feverish type of sickness. The keynote symptom is erratic pains alternating sides. Feels as if walking on air or not touching the bed when lying down. Great lassitude, ozaena. Decided effect in drying up milk in women who cannot nurse the baby. Great weakness and prostration. Sinking spells every morning. Mastitis.

Mind: Despondent, visions of snakes.

Head: Sensation of walking or floating in the air.

Mouth: Profuse salivation, cracking of jaw while eating.

Throat: Tonsillitis and diphtheria symptoms change repeatedly from side to side, shining glazed appearance of deposit, pearly white or like pure white porcelain, stiffness of neck and tongue.

Female: Flow in gushes, breasts swollen, painful before and better on appearance of menses - Worse least jar-helps to dry up milk. Galactorrhoea.

Extremities: Sciatica-right side, legs feel numb and stiff, cramps in feet.

Rheumatic pains in extremities and back, from one side to other, pain in arms to fingers. Burning in palms and soles.

Sleep: Dreams of snake.

Modalities: Worse morning of one day and in the evening of next. Better - cold, cold drinks.

Relation: Lac felinum (Cat's milk) - Ciliary neuralgia, eye symptoms, photophobia, asthenopia, dysmenorrhoea.

Lac vaccinum: (Cows milk) Headache, rheumatic pain, constipation.

Lac vaccinum coagulatum (Curds) nausea of pregnancy.

Lac Deflor.: - dreams of going on a journey. (Cow's Skimmed milk)

Lactis vaccini floc. (Cream) - Diphtheria, leucorrhoea, menorrhagia, dysphagia.

Dose: 30 and the highest. *(Boericke)*

Lac. can., the bitch's milk is not a novelty in remedies. Successful in the treatment of diphtheria - a large number of the symptoms were manifested in the region of the throat. Curative and prophylactic in diphtheria. An alternation of sides. Rheumatic and other affections having this peculiarity of changing from side to side are very likely to be benefited by lac. can. Corners of mouth and alae nasi cracked. One prover had delusions about snakes, imagined she was surrounded by them, was afraid to close her eyes at night for fear of being bitten by a large snake which she Imagined was beside the bed-imagines he wears someone else's nose. Sensation of lightness and levitation. Cannot bear one part of her body to touch another, must keep even her fingers apart.

Relations: According to Nichols, Lac. can. acts best in single dose, if repeated should be given at exact intervals. Spreads fingers apart. Cannot bear one finger to touch the other (Lac. felin - cannot bear one foot to touch the other.) *(JHC)*

For nervous, restless, highly sensitive organisms. Very forgetful, absent minded. Make purchases and walks away without them - In writing uses too many words.

Nothing worth living for, could weep at any moment - Chronic blue condition, every thing seems so dark that it can grow no darker. Serviceable in almost all cases when it is required to dry up milk (Asaf. to bring back or increase it - Lac. d) - Probably no remedy in the materia medica presents a more valuable pathogenesis in symptoms of the throat or one that will better repay a careful study. *(H.C. Allen)*

368. *Lac Defloratum*

(Skimmed milk)

A remedy for diseases with faulty nutrition. Sick headaches with profuse flow of urine during pain. Car sickness.

Head: Pain begins in forehead to occiput, in morning on rising. Intense throbbing with nausea, vomiting, blindness and obstinate constipation, worse noise, light motion, during menses with great prostration and better by pressure and bandaging head tightly.

Stool: Constipation - Stools hard, large with great straining. Painful lacerating anus.

Dose: 6-30 c. and higher. *(Boericke)*

The idea of potentising skimmed milk originated with Swan upon reading Donkins `Skim Milk' treatment for Diabetes and Bright's disease - violent headache and the constipation - As milk contains within it an epitome of all the tissues and salts of the animal which secreted it, it is natural to expect of it a wide range of action in the attenuations. Thirst for large quantities. Often depression with crying and palpitation. The symptoms which specially indicate it in diabetes are, intense thirst, wasting - menses suppressed suddenly from putting hands into cold water - loss of weight or else obesity - Burnett maintains that excess of milk in the diet of children after they have cut their first teeth renders them susceptible to colds. Most symptoms occur in the morning. *(JHC)*

Vomiting incessant, no relation to eating: first of undigested food, intensely acid, then of bitter water; of pregnancy. Constipation-faeces dry and hard. A woman who had taken 10 or 12 enemas daily often passed 4 or 6 weeks without an evacuation - constipation of 15 years standing. Feels completely exhausted. *(H.C. Allen)*

369. *Lachesis*

(Bush master and surucucu)

Like all snake poisons, Lachesis decomposes the blood rendering it more fluid hence a haemorrhagic tendency is marked. Purpura, septic states. Diphtheria and other low forms of disease, when the system is thoroughly poisoned and the prostration is profound. The modalities are most important in guiding to the remedy. Delirium tremens with much trembling and confusion. Very important during the climacteric and for patients of a melancholic disposition. Ill effects of suppressed discharges. Diphtheria carriers. Sensation of tension in various parts. Cannot bear anything tight anywhere.

Mind: Loquacity - Derangement of the time sense.

Head: Sun headaches - relieved by onset of discharge (menses or nasal catarrh)

Ears: Wax dry hard.

Mouth: Gums swollen, spongy, bleed.

Tongue: Swollen, burns, trembles, red, dry and cracked at tip, catches on teeth - toothache, pain extends to ears.

Throat: Worse left side, swallowing liquids, quinsy, septic parotiditis. Pain aggravated by hot drinks, chronic sore throat, with much hawking. Mucus sticks and cannot be forced up or down, very painful, worse slightest pressure, touch is even more annoying - Worse swallowing saliva or liquids, pain into ear. Collar and neck band must be very loose.

Stomach: Made better by eating. Empty swallowing more painful than swallowing solids.

Abdomen: Cannot bear anything around waist.

Stool: Constipated, offensive, anus feels tight. Haemorrhages from bowels like charred straw, black particles. Haemorrhoids protrude, become constricted, purplish, stitches in them on sneezing or coughing. Constant urging in rectum, not for stool.

Female: Pain relieved by the flow (Eupion), left ovary very painful and swollen - Mammae inflamed bluish - Acts especially well at beginning and close of menstruation.

Male: Intense excitement of sexual organs.

Respiratory: Suffocation on lying down, when anything is around throat, compels patient to spring from bed and rush for open window. Feels he must take a deep breath. Cough dry, suffocative, worse pressure on larynx, after sleep, breathing almost stops on falling asleep.

Back: Worse rising from sitting posture.

Extremities: Pain in tibia (may follow sore throat).

Sleep: Patient sleeps into an aggravation, sudden starting when falling asleep. Sleepiness, yet cannot sleep, wide awake in evening.

Skin: Bluish, purplish appearance, boils, carbuncles, ulcers, senile erysipelas, wens, cellulitis, varicose ulcers.

Modalities: (Worse) after sleep, lachesis sleeps into aggravation, ailments that come on during sleep, left side, in the spring, warm bath, pressure or constriction, hot drinks, closing eyes - (better) appearance of discharges, warm applications.

Dose: 8-200. Doses ought not to be repeated too frequently. If well indicated, a single dose should be allowed to exhaust its action. *(Boericke)*

The effect of handling the virus and preparing the lower attenuations was to throw Herring into a fever with tossing delirium and mania much to his wife's dismay.

The four grand characteristics of lachesis are (1) Agg: Sleep (2) Excessive sensitiveness of the surface with intolerance of touch or constriction. (3) Left sideness and the direction left to right, symptoms begin on the left side and either remain there or proceed to the right. (4) Amel: from the onset of discharge. Wherever one or more of these features is prominent in any case Lach. will most likely prove the remedy. Agg: By closing the eyes (vertigo) is allied to this - *Lach* especially suits cholereic women with freckles and red hair. Women who have never been well since the change of life - Thin rather than fat persons. Persons who cannot stand the sun and who are agg: in summer weather. Tremor of tongue is a leading feature of many Lach. states. Frantic loquacity, jumps from one subject to another - talks, sings, or whistles constantly - insane jealousy. Patient is always making mistakes in the time of day. The throat is especially the seat of Lach. Lach is also one of the most prominent remedies in appendicitis. Cancer of the breast, when assuming a bluish appearance will be helped by Lach. Sleeps into an attack of asthma. *(JHC)*

This agent produces irritation of the larynx, trachea and heart. The blood is decomposed and haemorrhages result. A low asthenic condition is developed, which is followed by convulsions and unconsciousness.

This remedy is indicated when there is hypersensitiveness of the body, and especially to the clothing about the neck. The patient feels worse after a sleep. The complaints are mostly upon the left side of the body, and many of them appear at the climacteric period. It should be studied in mania, when there is great loquacity, the patient is restless and wants to be on the move; is jealous, suspicious of being poisoned; refuses the medicine, and believes she is under a super human power.

It is of service in headache that occurs from the heat of the sun. They are attended with a very pale face, also headaches and coryza that are the result of a cold and are relieved as soon as the discharge is established.

It is indicated in facial erysipelas upon the left side: at first it is bright red, but later it becomes dark bluish, or purplish. The cellular tissue is infiltrated. The patient is weak, drowsy, and may be delirious.

It should be remembered in chronic pharyngitis and laryngitis, when there is much hawking of mucus which cannot be forced up or down. There is a sensation of a lump in the left side of the throat which seems to go up and down when swallowing. The throat is sensitive to touch, the distress is worse after sleep. It is also of service in diphtheria when there is great difficulty in swallowing, great foetor, and the parts are purple and livid.

It is useful when there is congestion of the left ovary. It is swollen and indurated. The distress is relieved by a discharge of blood from the uterus. The menses are scanty, black and offensive and the pains are relieved as the flow starts. It benefits those suffering from climacteric troubles when there is palpitation of the heart, flushes of heart, haemorrhages, vertex headache and fainting. All the complaints are worse after sleep and she cannot endure anything tight about the throat or waist.

It relieves diarrhoea when the stools are offensive and there is a constant urging and hammering in the rectum. It is also of use in constipation when the anus is sensitive and feels constricted.

It should be remembered in pneumonia when a septic condition is threatened. The expectoration consists of pus and blood, and there is a profuse perspiration over the body, also in all forms of septic inflammations when the parts are sensitive, of a bluish appearance and there is an offensive odor from the surface.

Compare: Acid Nitricum, Crotalus hor., Natrum mur. *(Blackwood.)*

370. Lachnantes

(Spirit weed)

Head, chest and circulation are affected. Bridge of nose as if pinched. A remedy for Torticollis, rheumatic symptoms about neck. Tuberculosis. Light complexioned people, disposed to talk, a flow of language and the courage to make a speech.

Head: Feels enlarged; bridges of nose feels as if pinched.

Back: Chilliness between the shoulder blades, pain and stiffness in back.

Neck: Drawn over to one side in sore throat. Rheumatism of the neck, stiffness of neck. Pain in nape as if dislocated.

Relationship - Fel. Tauri, nape of neck pains and great tension there.

Dose: 3rd potency. Tincture in Phthisis, unit doses once or twice a week or 3 drops every four hours. *(Boericke)*

Lachnan. is a herb, growing in sandy swamps near the coast. The root is red and fibrous, leaves sword - shaped, stem hairy, flowers yellow, wooly. The head, the chest and the circulation seem most prominently affected by Lachn. - Icy coldness of body - The loquacity of Lachn. is remarkable. Herring said the Indians chew the plant when they meet the white man to give them a flow of language. The white pigs and sheeps of Virginia lose their hoofs, if they feed on Lachnan while the black varieties eat it without inconvenience. *(JHC)*

It is indicated in severe headaches, migraine, the pain is intense, upon the right side of the head. There is a sensation as though the head was split open with a wedge. The pain is such that she must cry. The whole body is cold, moist and clammy, vomiting aggravates. The painful parts feel enlarged and are made worse from the least noise.

(Blackwood)

371. Lacticum Acidum

(Milk acid)

Morning sickness, diabetes and rheumatism offer a field for this remedy, troubles in the breasts. Locally in the tuberculous ulceration of vocal cords.

Stomach: Tongue dry parched, thirst, voracious hunger, copious salivation, water brash, nausea, especially in pale anemic women, nausea better eating. Worse smoking.

Chest: Pain in breasts, with enlargement of axillary glands and pain extends into hand.

Extremities: Rheumatic pain in joints and shoulders, wrists, knees, with much weakness. Trembling of whole body while walking, limbs feels chilly.

Urine: Large quantities passed frequently - saccharine.

Relation: Sarcolactic acid, Lithia, Phos. ac.

Dose: 3rd - 30c. (6-10 drops in a small glass of water in acute gastro enteritis) (Cartier) *(Boericke)*

Lactic acid was discovered by `Scheele' in sour milk, the result of spontaneous fermentation of sugar of milk under the influence of Casein. It is also met with in many vegetable products, which have turned sour. Many valuable observations have been made on patients taking substantial doses for diabetes - Pain, swelling and stiffness and tenderness of joints agg: by motion. Diabetes is the affection for which it has been most given in old school practice, but it has also proved of great power in the homoeopathic attenuations. Nash regards the concomitance of rheumatic pains as the chief guiding symptoms here. He records a case of diabetes with rheumatic fever supervening, cured with lact. ac. 200. Copious night sweat is a feature of Lact. ac., but sweat is not offensive.

Compatible: Meat diet in diabetes.

Incompatible: Coffee. Agg: symptoms. *(JHC)*

372. *Lactica Virosa*

(Acid Lettuce)

The remedy acts principally upon the brain and circulatory system. Delirium tremens with sleeplessness, coldness, and tremor. Hydrothorax and ascites. Impotence, sense of lightness and tightness affecting whole body, especially chest. Seems to be a true galactogogue. Marked action on extremities.

Female: Increase of milk in breasts.

Compare: Spiranthes (Galactogogue)

Dose: Tincture. *(Boericke)*

Poisonous Lettuce. The sleep provoking powers of Lactica are recognised by sensitive persons who eat ordinary garden lettuce in salad. Fatigue during stool and also sleepiness during stool; are peculiar and may prove characteristic. *(JHC)*

373. *Lapis Albus*

(Silico-fluoride of calcium)

Affections of glands, goitre, pre-ulcerative stage of Carcinoma, burning stinging pain in breast, stomach and uterus, connective tissue about glands specially affected. Fat anaemic babies with iodine appetite. Ravenous appetite. Remarkably successful in scrofulous affections, except in malarial cases. Uterine carcinoma. Fibroid tumors with intense burning, pains through the part with profuse haemorrhage. Glands have a certain elasticity and pliability about them rather than the stony hardness of Calc. fluor. and Cistus.

Ears: Otitis media suppurative.

Skin: Scrofulous abscesses, and sores, enlargement and induration of glands especially cervical, lipoma, sarcoma, carcinoma, pruritus.

Relation: Silica, Badiaga, Ars. iod., Calc. iod., Con., Kali iod., Asterias. *(Boericke)*

Silico-fluoride of calcium. A species of genesis found by Grauvogal in the mineral springs of Gastein. These waters flow over Gneiss formations into the valley of Achen where goitre and cretinism abound. Grauvogl, who introduced this remedy, cured with it a case of carcinoma and he and others have cured cases of goitre and scrofulous glands. It has shown great power over new growths of many kinds.

In two cases of cervical glands cured by L. alb. 6, Dewey relates that a ravenous appetite developed while the remedy was being taken. The swelling of the glands was elastic rather than stony hard. In one of the patients the swelling was as large as a goose egg in the right sterno-clavicular region. The 30th and 200th caused such intense pruritus that the patient refused to take any more medicine of any kind. Since then "Whiting" has cured many cases of pruritus and also of dysmenorrhoea with Lap. alb. Miss `X', 34, normal till she had measles at 20, since then pain at commencement of menstruation, so severe as to cause fainting. This severe pain would continue for a day or until the flow was established.

Lapis alb. 200 cured in six months. Dr. Gregory cured a young man of a tumour of the lip with Lap. a. 30. *(JHC)*

Silico fluoride of Calcium. A mineral substance found floating in the spring of Gastein, Germany. This remedy is indicated in enlargement of the lymphatic glands when they have a soft and doughy feel and are movable. It is useful in non-encapsulated goitre.

Comp.: Calc. iod., Con., Badiage. *(Blackwood)*

374. *Lappa-arcticum*

(Burdock)

Very important in skin therapeutics. Eruptions on the head, face and neck, pimples, acne, styes and ulceration on the edge of the eyelids, profuse and frequent urination. Crops of boils and styes (Anthracin).

Female: Uterine displacements: An exceedingly sore bruise feeling in uterus with great relaxation of the vaginal tissues. Apparently entire lack of tonicity of pelvic contents. These symptoms are aggravated by standing, walking, a mis step or sudden jar.

Dose: Tr. to 3rd potency. *(Boericke)*

It has been given from the earliest times for prolapsus uteri, sterility, milky urine and sores about joints. A large number of symptoms were observed in the skin (Acne, eczema, especially scalp) and mucous membranes, eruptions and discharges. It is one of the remedies which have been successful in curing uterine prolapse. *(JHC)*

375. *Lathyrus*

(Chick pea)

Affects the lateral and anterior column of the cord. Does not produce pain. Reflexes always increased. Paralytic affections of lower extremities, spastic paralysis, lateral sclerosis, Beriberi, Athetosis, infantile paralysis. After influenza and wasting, exhaustive diseases, where there is much weakness and heaviness, slow recovery of nerve power. Sleepy, constant yawning.

Mouth: Burning pain in tip of tongue.

Extremities: Tips of fingers numb, tremulous, tottering gait, excessive rigidity of legs, spastic gait, knees knock against each other when walking. Cramps in legs worse cold and cold feet. Cannot extend or cross legs when sitting. Myelitis with marked spastic symptoms. Rheumatic paralysis. Gluteal muscles and lower limbs emaciated. Legs blue, swollen if hanging down. Stiffness and lameness of ankles and knees, toes do not leave the floor, heels do not touch floor. Muscles of calves very tense. Patient sits bent forward, straightens up with difficulty.

Urine: Increased bladder reflex. Frequent, must hurry.

Dose: 3rd potency. *(Boericke)*

These are the symptoms:-

1. Lumbago, incontinence of urine, complete loss of sexual power, pains in lower and sometimes upper limbs, tremors, invasion of disease is sudden, often coming on after a damp, cold night.
2. The lower limbs are affected with anaesthesia and motor paralysis. In the cases of horses as well as in human beings, the symptoms often remained

in abeyance until cold damp weather set in. Men are more sensitive to it than women. It should be like Nux a Mans medicine.

Causation: Cold damp weather.
(JHC)

This agent produces symptoms that simulate paraplegia, which is worse during damp and wet weather. The leg becomes stiff, the gait is unsteady, and there is aching of the parts, without severe pain. These symptoms have been attributed to a transverse myelitis with degeneration of the cord, as sclerosis of the pyramidal tract.

This remedy should be studied in cases of spastic paraplegia, in chronic myelitis with marked spastic symptoms, in cases where there is an excessive knee - jerk with rigidity of the parts, also in cases of spinal anaemia and in multiple sclerosis.

The cardinal indications for this remedy are the sudden loss of power in the lower extremities, with rigidity of the legs, spastic gait, which is often tremulous. The onset of the disease is sudden and it is aggravated by coldness and damp weather.

Compare: Zincum pic., Argentum nit.
(Blackwood)

376. Latrodectus Mactans

(Spider)

The bite produces tetanic effects that last several days. A picture of Angina pectoris is presented by the action of the drug. The praecordial region seems to be the centre of the attack. Constriction of chest muscles with radiation to shoulders and back. Lowered coagulability of blood.

Skin: Coldness of whole surface. Skin cold as marble.

Dose: 6th potency. *(Boericke)*

Tincture of living spider - skin cold as marble, countenance expressive of deep anxiety - in 36 hours from the time he was bitten he took 3 1/2 quart bottles of the best rectified whisky without showing the least symptom of intoxication. *(JHC)*

377. Laurocerasus

(Cherry Laurel)

Spasmodic tickling cough, especially in cardiac patients is often magically influenced by this drug. Lack of reaction especially in chest and heart affections. Drink rolls audibly through oesophagus and intestines. General coldness, not ameliorated by warmth. Violent pain in stomach with loss of speech, spasms of facial muscles and oesophagus. Asphyxia neonatorum.

Respiratory: Cyanosis and dyspnoea, worse sitting up. Patient puts hands on heart. Cough with valvular disease. Exercise causes pain around heart. Tickling dry cough, dyspnoea, constriction of chest, cough with copious, jelly like, or bloody expectoration. Small and feeble pulse. Threatening paralysis of lungs. Gasping for breath, clutches at heart.

Heart: Mitral regurgitation, clutching at heart and palpitation. Cyanosis neonatorum.

Dose: Tr. to 3rd potency. Cherry laurel water, 2-5 drop doses. *(Boericke)*

Laurocerasus the so called 'Laurel' of our gardens. `Lauro' has cyanosis both of newborn infant and of heart disease. If fluids are forced down the throat they roll audibly into stomach. There are suffocative spells about the heart agg: by sitting up, the patient is compelled to lie down (as with Psor) though some heart symptoms have the opposite condition and compel the patient to sit up. Inclined to loss of flesh and haemorrhages, that are small in quantity and bright in colour. In nervous affections constant jerks, cannot keep still and the characteristic gasping are leading indications - cough with valvular heart disease. *(JHC)*

378. Lecithin

(A Phosphorus containing complex organic body prepared from the yolk of egg and animal brains).

Lecithin is important in the vital processes of plant and animal organisms. Lecithin has a favourable influence upon the nutritive condition and especially upon the blood hence its use in anaemia and convalescence, neurasthenia and insomnia. Increasing the number of red corpuscles and amount of hemoglobin. Excellent galactogogue, renders milk more nourishing and increases quantity. Causes an immediate decrease in the excretion of the phosphates. Mental exhaustion and impotence. Tuberculosis causing marked improvement in nutrition and general improvement. Tired, weak, short breath, loss of flesh, symptoms of general breakdown, sexually weak.

Dose: 1/2 to 2 grains of crude and potencies - 12th potency. *(Boericke)*

379. Ledum

(Marsh Tea)

Affects especially, the rheumatic diathesis going through all the changes from functional pain to altered secretions and deposits of solid earthy matter in the tissues. The Ledum rheumatism begins in feet and travels upward. It affects also the skin, producing an eruption like poison oak, and is antidoted thereto, as well as to stings of insects. There is a general lack of animal heat and yet heat of bed is intolerable. For punctured wounds, produced by sharp pointed instruments or bites, particularly if the wounded parts are cold, this is the remedy. Tetanus with twitching of muscles near wound.

Face: Red pimples on forehead and cheeks.

Rectum: Anal fissures, Haemorrhoidal pain.

Extremities: Gouty pains shoot all through the foot and limb and in joints, but especially small joints. Swollen, hot, pale. Throbbing, in right shoulder. Pressure in shoulder, worse motion, cracking in joints, worse warmth of bed. Gouty nodosities, ball of great toe swollen (Bothrops), rheumatism begins in lower limbs and ascends (Kalmia opposite). Ankles swollen, soles painful, can hardly step on them. Easy spraining of ankle.

Skin: Itching and warmth of bed. Antidote to Rhus poisoning.

Modalities: Better from cold, putting feet in cold water, worse at night and from heat of bed.

Relationship: Ledum antidotes spider poisons.

Compare: Ruta, Ham., Bellis., Arnica.

Dose: 3-30 potency. *(Boericke)*

It is a native to damp regions of North of Europe and that no animal except the goat eats it on account of the strong resinous smell of its leaves, which keeps off lice and prevents flour from getting mouldy.

Redness, swelling and throbbing in point of index finger from prick of a needle - Ledum aborted a felon in a few days. (Ten years ago I stepped on a nail and ever since then have had a pain running up to the thigh) - "Nash says" Led. 200 is unequalled as a remedy for black eye from a blow. Ledum has often been given to horses when they go lame and draw up their legs. Constitutions abused by alcohol. Ruta for periosteum, symphytum for bone, Hypericum for nerve, Staphisagria for pediculosis. Causation: Abuse of alcohol, hair cutting, suppressed discharges, wounds, bruise bites, punctured wounds, Stings. *(JHC)*

This agent retards the capillary circulation, especially of the extremities and external surfaces of the body, and there is coldness of extremities. The articulations of the small joints are enlarged and there are deposits and nodosities. Eczema develops.

This remedy is indicated in those of a rheumatic diathesis, when the disturbance begins in the feet and extends to the body. The secretions are altered and deposits take place about the joints; the muscles are sore and there are sticking, tearing pains in various parts of the body. The pains change their location suddenly and are worse at night and from warmth, although the patient is chilly.

It is not to be thought of only in acute rheumatic conditions, but also in chronic gouty nodes and concretions where the same group of symptoms are present; the process extends upwards.

It is of service in ecchymosis from slight injuries, especially in gouty and intemperate subjects.

It is an important remedy for the soreness of the soles of the feet and heels that is observed following exposure to colds and getting wet.

It should be remembered locally for the injuries and wounds made by pointed instruments; also as a local application for stings of mosquitoes and wasps.

It should be remembered in wounds of the eye, for ecchymosis of the conjunctiva and intra-ocular haemorrhages.

It should be studied in chronic eczemas and papular eruptions on the forehead and face that is observed in habitual drunkards.

It has been employed locally as an antidote to Rhus poisoning.

Compare - Rhus tox, Hamamelis, Arnica, Bellis per. *(Blackwood)*

380. Lemna Minor

(Buckweed)

A catarrhal remedy. Acts especially upon the nostrils. Nasal polypi, swollen turbinates. Atrophic rhinites. Asthma from nasal obstruction, worse in wet weather.

Nose: Putrid smell.

Mouth: Putrid taste.

Modalities: *Worse* in damp, rainy weather, especially heavy pains.

Dose: 3-30 Potency. *(Boericke)*

In a man I cured with Lemna 3x given three times a day an aggravated nasal catarrh. In the morning he filled two pocket hand-kerchiefs with yellow defluxion before he could feel his nose clear. *(JHC)*

This remedy should be studied in cases of nasal catarrh, when the nares are obstructed. There is a foul smell from the nose and an offensive taste when awaking in the morning. These conditions are worse in damp weather; and especially during heavy rains.

It has benefited cases of polypi and hypertrophy of the turbinates, with post nasal catarrh and atrophic rhinitis.

Compare: Teucrim, Sanguinaria.

(Blackwood)

381. Leptandra

(Culvers Root)

A liver remedy, with jaundice and black tarry stools. Bilious states. Enfeebled portal circulation, malarial conditions.

Dose: Tr. to 3rd potency. *(Boericke)*

As one of the grand characteristics of its relatives digitalis is white stools, the grand characteristic of lept is black stools. *(JHC)*

382.Liatris Spicata Serratula

(Colic Root)

A vascular stimulant, increases functional activity of the skin, mucous membranes. Of use in dropsy due to liver and spleen diseases, also renal dropsy. Here the suppressed urination is most favourably influenced. General anasarca due to heart and kidney disease. Diarrhoea with violent urging and pain in lower part of back, colic. Locally applied to ulcers and unhealthy wounds. A prompt diuretic.

Dose: 1 to 4 drams of Tr. of infusion. *(Boericke)*

1. Dropsy from material enlargement of liver and spleen.
2. Dropsy with almost total suppression of urine. After other remedies had failed, `Liatris' was given and on the second day, the patient passed a gallon and half of urine. It has a popular repute as a specific in chronic diarrhoea - it acts better if Sul. or Merc. cor. is given first. *(JHC)*

This agent is employed in gonorrhoea, gleet, and nephritis with dropsy. *(Blackwood)*

383. Lilium Tigrinum

(Tiger Lily)

Manifests powerful influence over the pelvic organs, and is adapted to many reflex states dependent on some pathological conditions of uterus and ovaries. More often indicated in unmarried women. The action of heart is very marked. Pain in small spots. Rheumatic arthritis.

Mind: Profound depression of spirits, fears some organic and incurable disease, aimless hurried manner.

Eyes: Myopic astigmia.

Stool: Constant desire to defaecate from pressure in rectum. Early morning urgent stool.

Female: Menses early, scanty, dark, clotted, offensive, flow only when moving about. Bearing down sensation with urgent desire for stool, as though all organs would escape. Ceases when resting. (Sep., Lac. c., Bell.). Congestion of uterus, prolapse and anteversion, acrid brown leucorrhoea.

Extremities: Cannot walk on uneven ground. Pain in back and spine.

Relationship: Cact., Helon., Murex., Sep., Platina., Pallad.

Dose: The middle and higher potencies seem to have done best. Its curative action sometimes is slow in developing itself.
(Boericke)

A patient to whom I have given Lil. tig. 30 said, it caused a sensation in the abdomen as if the contents were tied up in knots. C. Sigmund Raue has observed, excellent results from Lil. tig. 3x and 30 in cases of uterine fibroid presenting the characteristic symptoms of the remedy. I never obtained good results from Lil. tig., until I gave it in the 30th attenuation
(JHC)

Affects principally, the left side of the body - Tormented about her salvation with ovarian or uterine complaints. Consolation agg. Profound depression of spirits, can hardly avoid weeping, is very timid, fearful, and weeps much. Indifferent about what is being done for her - must keep busy to repress sexual desire - aimless hurried motion. Rapid heart beat 150 to 170 per minute. *(HC Allen)*

This agent acts upon the uterus and ovaries, producing irritation and congestion and subacute inflammation. Reflexly it affects the heart and nearly all the other organs of the body.

This remedy is indicated in nervous hysterical women when the uterus and ovaries are engorged with blood; there may be uterine displacement and subinvolution. These conditions may be the result of getting up too soon following confinement.

It should be remembered in melancholia and the mental disturbance that are dependent upon the uterine and ovarian irritation. She can hardly avoid weeping, is very timid, anxious about her present and future welfare, believes her disease cannot be cured. She is always in a hurry but accomplishes nothing, she fears being alone or that she will become insane. In other cases there is mania when she curses, strikes and has obscene thoughts, is wild and crazy.

It is an important remedy in uterine, ovarian and mammary neuralgia, especially if there is uterine displacement, chronic metritis with acrid leucorrhoea that excoriates the vagina. There is tenderness over the uterine region. In some cases there is a sensation of weight and pressure downward of the abdominal and pelvic contents as is observed in enteroptosis. This is attended by the mental symptoms of the remedy and is relieved by sitting supporting the abdominal walls or pressing upward on the vulva. In these cases the menses appear too early, are scanty, dark and offensive. Flow only when moving about, it ceases when she is quiet.

It is of survive in disturbances of the heart that are reflex to some uterine disturbance, there may be a sensation as though the heart contained too much blood or as if it were grasped by a hand and squeezed, and relaxed gradually, so called false angina. Some of these patients complain of a severe headache.

Compare - Cimicifuga racemosa, Cactus grand., Helonias. (Blackwood)

384. *Lithium Carbonicum*

(Carbonate of Lithium)

Chronic rheumatism connected with heart lesions and asthenopia, offer a field for this remedy. Rheumatic nodes. Uric acid diathesis, whole body is sore. Gout and tophi.

Head: Headache ceases while eating.

Stomach: Gnawing relieved by eating.

Respiratory: Pain in mammary glands which extend into the arms and fingers.

Extremities: Rheumatic pains throughout shoulder - joint, arm and fingers and small joints generally.

Skin: Barber's itch (Use high).

Modalities: (Worse) in morning, right side, (Better) rising and moving about.

Relationship: *Lithium lacticum,* rheumatism of shoulders and small joints relieved by moving about, worse-resting.

Dose: 1-3rd trituration. *(Boericke)*

The skin of Lithium carb patient is dry and harsh like a nutmeg-grater. According to Allen the Lactate of Lithia has been found valuable for subacute rheumatism of the shoulder joint. *(JHC)*

This remedy should be studied in rheumatic, gouty subjects who suffer from cardiac, renal or eye lesions; it is indicated in chronic rheumatic endocarditis when there is soreness about the heart. There is throbbing with dull stitches in the cardiac region, and a sensation of trembling or fluttering of the heart. It is of survice in soreness of the bladder with sharp sticking pains extending to the neck of the bladder in rheumatic subjects.

It is also useful in rheumatic affections of the eyes with hemiopia, the right half of objects is invisible. In many of these cases there is an acidity and gnawing of the stomach, which is relieved by eating.

Compare: Lycopodium, Benzoic acid. *(Blackwood)*

385. Lobelia Inflata

(Indian tobacco)

It is a vasomotor stimulant, increases the activity of all vegetative processes, spends its force mainly upon the pneumogastric nerve, producing a depressed relaxed condition with oppression of the chest and epigastrium, impeded respiration, nausea and vomiting.

Languor, relaxation of muscles, nausea, vomiting and dyspepsia are the general indications that point to the use of this remedy in asthma and gastric affections. Best adapted to light complexioned, fleshy people. Bad effects of drunkenness. Suppressed discharges. Diphtheria, catarrhal jaundice.

Ears: Deafness due to suppressed discharges.

Mouth: Mercurial taste.

Stomach: Extreme nausea and vomiting, faintness and weakness at epigastrium. Profuse salivation with good appetite.

Respiratory: Dyspnoea from constriction of chest. Better by rapid walking.

Modalities: (Worse) tobacco, afternoon, slightest motion, cold, especially cold washing, (Better) By rapid walking (Chest pain), toward evening and from warmth.

Dose: Tincture to thirtieth potency. *(Boericke)*

According to Hale, this plant was used by the Indian as an emetic detergent, in the same way as Verat. alb. was used by the ancients to produce Helleborism. But the chief modern exponent of Lobelia, is Samuel Thompson, of New Hampshire, who founded the modern Botanic School. His chief remedies were, besides Lobelia, Cayenne pepper and the vapour bath. There can be little doubt that he accomplished much with these, but his unbounded faith in Lobelia, led, in some instances, to fatal poisoning.

It was a true instinct on the part of Teste that led him to class Lob. i. with Sul. though the provings and clinical experience do not fully bear out what he says about its skin action.

A woman got a piece of mutton bone down her windpipe and into one of the bronchia. She was taken to the London Hospital, but the idea of operation was abandoned as hopeless and she was sent out. Lob. I. ac. was given five drops three times a day. Soon a most violent cough was set up, in the course of which the patient coughed up a large quantity of fetid pus and finally the bone.

Lob. i. may cause a rash which exfoliates, and it has cured many cases of psoriasis. *(JHC)*

386. *Lolium Temulentum*

(Darnel)

Has been made use of in cephalalgia, sciatica, paralysis, prostration and restlessness.

Extremities: Gait unsteady, trembling of all limbs, loss of power in extremities. Violent pain in calves as if bound with cords. Cold extremities, spasmodic motions of arm and legs. Cannot write, cannot hold a glass of water. Trembling of hands as in paralysis.

Dose: 6th potency. *(Boericke)*

The name Darnel means stupefied and the plant's evil reputation is of very ancient date. The symptoms are the result of observations made on persons poisoned by eating meal containing an admixture of Lol. tem. Allen mentions an assertion that Lolium is much infested with ergot, and that it is to this that the poisoning symptoms are due, the unaffected grain being inert; and Allen notes in support of this that the poisonings have been most frequently observed in low, wet districts, and during wet seasons, provings are needed to decide this. The chief symptoms are: Confusion of mind, at times delirium;' very great depression. Nausea and vomiting of the bread containing it and mucus with it. Paralysis, tremors and convulsions. Cold rigors, internal chilliness; cold sweat. A very characteristic symptom is: Tightness in the calves; violent pain in the calves as if bound with cords. This tightness affects the rest of the legs in less degree. "Bonino" has cured a carpenter, 29, who had had trembling of the hands eleven years, agg: morning. Later the legs also began to tremble. His father and brother were similarly affected. Merc. v. and Agar. only relieved temporarily. Lol. tem. cured. *(JHC)*

This remedy is useful in paralysis, and trembling of the extremities, with prostration and restlessness.

Compare - lathyrus. *(Blackwood)*

387. *Lycopodium*

(Club Moss)

This drug is inert until the spores are crushed. Its wonderful medicinal properties are only disclosed by trituration and succussions. In nearly all cases where lycopodium is the remedy, some evidence of urinary or digestive disturbance will be found. Corresponds to Grauvogle's Carbonitrogenoid constitution, the non-eliminative lithaemic Lycopodium is adapted more especially to ailments gradually developing, functional power weakening, with failures of digestive powers, where the function of the liver is seriously disturbed. Atony, malnutrition, mild temperaments of lymphatic constitution, with catarrhal tendencies, older persons where the skin shows yellowish spots, earthy complexion, uric acid diathesis etc. Also precocious, weak children, symptoms characteristically run from right to left, act especially on right side of body and are worse from about 4-8 p.m. In kidney affections, red sand in urine, backache, in renal region, worse before urination. Intolerant of cold drinks, craves everything warm. Best adapted to persons intellectually keen, but of weak muscular power. Deep seated, progressive chronic diseases. Carcinoma. Emaciation. Debility in morning. Marked regulating influence upon the glandular (Sebaceous) secretions. Pre-senility. Ascites in liver disease. Lycop. patient is thin, withered, full of gas and dry. Lacks vital heat, has poor circulation, cold extremities, pain come and go suddenly. Sensitive to noise and odors.

Mind: Melancholy, afraid to be alone, Hurried when eating, apprehensive, spells and writes wrong words.

Head: Shakes head without apparent cause. Pressing headache on vertex, worse from 4 to 8 p.m. Great falling out of hair. Eczema, moist oozing behind ears, premature baldness and gray hair.

Eyes: Styes in lids near internal canthus. Eyes half open during sleep.

Ears: Humming and roaring with hardness of hearing.

Nose: Sense of smell very acute, nose stopped up, snuffles, fanlike motion of alae nasi.

Face: Blue circles around eyes, copper coloured eruption. Itching scaly herpes in face and corners of mouth.

Mouth: Blisters on tongue. Bad odor from mouth.

Throat: Stitches on swallowing, better warm drinks, ulceration on tonsils, beginning on right side, diphtheria, deposits. Spread from right to left, worse cold drinks.

Stomach: Desire for sweet things, food tastes sour, great weakness of digestion. Eating over so little creates fullness, incomplete burning eructations, rise only to pharynx, there burn for hours, likes to taste food and drink hot.

Abdomen: Hernia, right side, liver sensitive.

Stool: Stool hard difficult small, haemorrhoids very painful to touch, aching.

Urine: Slow in coming, polyuria during the night, heavy red sediment, child cries before urinating.

Male: No erectile power, impotence, premature emission. (Cal., Sel., Agn.)

Female: menses too late, last too long, vagina dry, coition painful, varicose veins of pudenda, leucorrhoea.

Respiratory: Expectorations gray, thick, bloody, purulent, salty.

Heart: Aneurism. (Baryta carb)

Extremities: One foot hot, the other cold. Chronic gout with chalky deposits in joints. Profuse sweat of the feet, pain in heel on treading on a pebble. Painful callosities of soles. Toes and fingers contracted. Sciatica worse right side. Cannot lie on painful side, cramps in calves and toes at night in bed. Limbs go to sleep - twitching and jerking.

Fever: Chill between 3-4 p.m., followed by sweat.

Skin: Chronic eczema associated with urinary, gastric and hepatic disorders, skin becomes thick and indurated, varicose veins. Dry shrunken skin, especially palms. Hair become prematurely gray. Viscid and offensive perspiration, especially of feet and axilla. Psoriasis.

Mod: Worse right side, from above downward, 4 to 8 p.m., from heat of warm room, hot air, bed, warm applications, except throat and stomach which are better from warm drinks, better by motion, after midnight, from warm food and drink, on getting cold, from being uncovered.

Relationship: Lycop. acts with special benefit after Calcarea, and sulph, Iod., Graphites, Lach., Cheledon - Lycop. is the only vegetable that takes up Aluminium. (T.F. Allen). Hydrastis follows Lycopod. in indigestion.

Dose: 6-200c. *(Boericke)*

Lycopodium is one of the pivotal remedies of the materia medica and an intimate acquaintance with its properties and relations is essential to a proper understanding of the materia medica as a whole. Lyco ranks with sulphur and calcarea in the central trio around which all the rest of the materia medica can be grouped - practice on keynote symptoms alone is an absurdity, but the right use of key note symptoms is an immense saving of labor (1) Agg. from 4 to 8 p.m. (2) Any affection commencing on the Rt. side and spreading to left. (3) Agg. from uncovering (Sil. must wrap up the head) (4) Amel: from warm drinks Agg: from cold food and drink. (5) Fan like movement of Alae nasi. (6) Half open condition of the eyes during sleep. (7) Spasmodic asthma always ushered in by unusual excitement and attended by peculiar mental depression. (8) Right foot hot, left foot cold.

Fear of being alone, of men, of his own shadow. Lyco is a remedy for misers - Lyco has cured many cases of right inguinal hernia, especially in children. Lyco is one of the great remedies for constipation where purgatives have been abused. Lyco has a very large range in respiratory affections. Salt sputa, milky. Cannot endure noise. For warts, 2 grain tablet of Lyco. 6 was given at bed time the warts soon began to shrivel - in 6 weeks all gone. Agg: from eating cabbage, vegetables, beans, and peas, with husks, bread especially rye bread and pastry. Agg: Cold food and drink, wet weather, Wine, milk, before menstruation, suppressed menstruation. I have known some very good prescribers almost abandon this remedy on account of unexpected aggravation. Inguinal hernia (Nux vomica more on left-Lyco right). *(JHC)*

For persons intellectually keen but physically weak, upper part of body emaciated, lower part semi-dropsical, predisposed to lung and hepatic affection, especially the extremes of life, children and old people. Baby cries all day, sleeps all night (rev-Jalap and Psorinum) - Ailments from fright, anger, mortification or vexation with reserved despleasure. (Staph.)

Red sand in urine on child's diaper (phos) - child cries before urinating. Bad effects of: onions, bread, wine, spirituous liquors, tobacco smoking and chewing;
(H.C. Allen)

This agent in the powder or pollen form is employed as a dusting powder for chaffing. When triturated and the spores with their dense cellulose covering rupture, the oil within them is liberated and an agent of great therapeutic value is liberated, which acts upon the digestive organs, retarding their action; there is flatulence, constipation and congestion of the liver. There is pain under the ribs and around the waist, shooting pains under the shoulder blades. Pain in the gastric region. Haemorrhoids; veins are distended and may bleed, the extremities are cold. The skin presents a dirty appearance and the complexion is pale, jaundiced, or there are liver spots. The mucous membranes take on an atonic condition; congestion, catarrhal inflammation results with flatulence and distension of the intestines, urination is painful, the urine contains a brick dust sediment, and an excess of uric acid.

This remedy is indicated in those whose intellectual development over balances the physical. The complaints are deep-seated and develop gradually. The gastro-intestinal and urinary symptoms are prominent in many cases. The complaints start on the right side and go to the left, are worse from 4 to 8 p.m. The patient finds relief in the open air, the urine contains a heavy, red sediment of uric acid and there are pains in the region of the kidneys and bladder, in the limbs and joints.

It is of service in various derangements of the digestive organs when there are large accumulations of flatulence; he may feel hungry but a few mouthfuls fill him, and he feels distended, but belching does not bring any relief.

It is an important remedy during the acid stage of chronic gastritis when there is a sensation of burning in the stomach, with sour acid eructations; the epigastric region is distended and sensitive to touch. The patient feels sleepy after eating. There is mental depression, the bowels are usually constipated.

It should be remembered later in the history of the case when there is a chronic atonic indigestion, solid food causes great pain, there is slowness of digestion, great accumulation of flatus and at times vomiting of undigested food long after it has been eaten.

It is indicated in hyperchlorhydria when there is a large amount of flatulence and constipation. The appetite may appear excessive but while eating there is a feeling of fullness and distension when he has eaten little. There are acid eructations and the urine contains uric acid deposits. In some of these cases there is hiccough after meals.

It is indicated in chronic congestion of the liver when there is pain and distress and heaviness in the hepatic region. There is fermentation and rumbling of gas. The complexion is jaundiced, yellowish gray or of a dingy yellow hue. It will at times relieve symptoms that are dependent upon chronic congestion of the liver.

It is of service in haemorrhoids; these may bleed, they are painful when the patient is sitting, intestinal fermentation and mental despondency are present.

There is usually a condition of constipation, the stools hard and dry and there is but little desire for stool and a spasmodic stricture appears whenever there is such a desire.

It is indicated in the uric acid diathesis when there are deposits of uric acid crystals in the urine, which is scanty, cloudy, has a foul odor and causes a burning sensation when it passes.

It should be remembered in the dysuria of children when they cry before urinating, the diaper is stained yellow and the urine flows in fits and starts.

It is an important remedy early in the case to prevent the formation of renal calculi, also in interstitial nephritis when the gastric, hepatic and urinary symptoms correspond.

It is a useful remedy in coryza and nasal catarrh when the nose is stopped, especially at night; the discharge is often purulent and consists of crusts and plugs. There may be a tendency to recurrent polypi of the nose.

It is of survive in tonsillitis and diphtheria, especially when the disease starts on the right side and extends to the left. There is a fan-like motion of the alae nasi; a 4 p.m. aggravation and renal symptoms are present.

It is a valuable remedy in the bronchial catarrh of the aged when there is dyspnoea on least exertion, and violent attacks of coughing from least provocation or inhalation of anything that is irritating. The symptoms are worse later in the afternoon and are usually attended with renal and gastric symptoms of the remedy.

It is an important remedy in chronic pneumonia or cases of delayed resolution when there is a muco-serous or muco purulent expectoration; there is difficult breathing, fan-like motion of the alae nasi, the condition is worse during the late afternoon; the intestinal distension and urinary finding indicate this remedy.

It has been of great service in chronic rheumatism and gout when the afternoon aggravation, gastric and urinary findings are present.

It has yielded fine service in gouty and uric acid conditions when the eyes are involved.

Compare: Nux vom, Ant. crud., Nat. mur. *(Blackwood)*

388.Lycopus Virginicus

(Bugle-weed)

Lowers the blood pressure, reduces the rate of the heart and increases the length of systole to a great degree. Passive haemorrhages. (Adrenalin 6x)

A heart remedy, and of use in exophthalmic goitre and haemorrhoidal bleeding indicated in diseases with tumultuous action of the heart and more or less pain, haemoptysis due to valvular heart disease. Beneficial in toxic goitre used in the pre-operative stage. Dose: 5 drops of Tr. *(Beebe)*

Heart: Rapid heart action of smokers, pre-cordial pain, constriction, tenderness pulse weak, irregular, intermittent tremulous, rapid, cyanosis, heart's action tumultuous and forcible. Palpitation from nervous irritation, with oppression around heart, rheumatoid, flying pains, associated with heart disease. Cardiac Asthma (Sumbul).

Respiratory: Wheezing cough, with haemoptysis, bleeding small but frequent.

Urine: Pain in testicles.

Relationship: Ephedra — Teamsters tea (in exophthalmic goitre), Fucus, Spartein, Crataegus, Adrenalin 6x.

Dose: 1-30. *(Boericke)*

Briggs of Fot Lovell (St' Louis Periscope IX-329) relates the cure of a patient of Tarentula bite by application of a liquid made by Lycopus. He says the Cherokee Indians allow themselves to be bitten by Rattle snakes, Centipedes and Tarentula, chewing as an antidote large quantities of Lycopus and swallowing the juices.

(JHC)

389. Magnesia Carb

(Carbonate of Magnesia)

Gastro-intestinal catarrh, with marked acidity. Often used with advantage for complaints arising in people who have been taking this drug to sweeten the stomach. Is frequently indicated in children. Whole body smells sour. Disposed to boils. Broken down `worn out' women, with uterine and climacteric disorders. With numbness and distension in various parts and nerve prostration. Sensitive to the least noise, touch, etc. Affections of the antrum of Highmore. Effects of shock, blows, mental distress. Sense of numbness, nerve prostration, tendency to constipation after nervous Strain, sensitive to least touch-it causes starting, or cold winds or weather or from excess of care and worry with constipation and heaviness, intense neuralgic pains.

Face: Toothache, especially during pregnancy, worse at night, ailments from cutting wisdom teeth.

Stomach: Desire for fruit, acids, and vegetables. Eructations sour and vomiting of bitter water. Craving for meat.

Stool: Green watery, frothy like a frog-ponds's scum, milk passes undigested and sour in nursing children.

Female: Sore throat before menses appear, late and scanty.

Respiratory: Salty bloody expectoration.

Extremities: Tearing in shoulders as if dislocated, right shoulder painful, cannot raise it-whole body feels tired and painful, especially legs and feet.

Modalities: Worse warmth of bed, change of temperature, cold wind or weather every three weeks, rest. Better - warm air.

Dose: 3-30 potency. *(Boericke)*

The state of nervousness indeed by excess of cares and worries of life. Mag. c 200 repeated 3-4 times a day has given untold relief to many a patient of this kind. One leading note of Mag. c is sensitiveness. The least touch causes starting-Cooper mentions it as a possible remedy in pyorrhoea alveolaris. For children who are puny and sickly, who refuse their milk and get pain in the stomach, if they take it, diarrhoea, colic, stools green, like a scum of a frog pond - jellylike lumps, aphthae, marasmus. Mag. c is a sovereign remedy.

Caution: Cutting wisdom teeth, injudicious feeding, milk. *(JHC)*

This agent produces irritation and catarrh of the mucous membrane of the alimentary tract, with acid and sour eructations, sour smelling, flatulent stools and sour perspiration.

It also acts upon the genital organs of the female, disturbing menstruation.

This remedy is indicated in catarrhal enteritis when the passage resembles the green scum seen upon the frog pond. At times there are white particles in the stool. The stool is sour, the odor from the body is sour, the eructations are sour. The child looks pale, sickly, and is disturbed by cold.

It should be remembered in acid dyspepsia with heartburn, when there is marked acidity of the gastric and intestinal secretions, with a constant sour taste in the mouth - Starchy foods disagree, as does milk.

It is beneficial in sick headaches when there is a persistent nausea and vomiting of extremely acid material; at times this may take the form of a supra orbital or infra orbital neuralgia. The pains are sharp and shooting in character, are worse at night, during rest, so that the patient gets up and walks about. The pains are also worse from a draft of air, change of the temperature to cold, and from touch.

It should be remembered in marasmus of children; they are puny and sickly; milk causes pain when taken into the stomach. There are colicky pains; the stools are green and sour.

It is of service in delayed and scanty menstruation; also in menorrhagia when the flow is thick and dark like pitch and is worse at night.

Compare - Aloe s, Rheum.(Blackwood)

390. Magnesia Mur

(Murate of magnesia)

A liver remedy with pronounced characteristic constipation. Chronic liver affections with tenderness and pain, extending to spine and epigastrium, worse after food, especially adapted to diseases of women, with a long history of indigestion and uterine disease, children who cannot digest milk. Evil effects of sea bathing.

Dose: 5 drops of Tincture. 3-200.
(Boericke)

Mag. m. is one of the leading remedies in foot sweat. The characteristic stool is knotty and conglomerate like sheep's.
(JHC)

Children during difficult dentition are unable to digest milk. Constipation, stool hard, scanty, large, knotty, like sheep's dung, difficult to pass, crumbling at verge of anus. *(HCA)*

391. Magnesia Phos

(Phosphate of Magnesia)

The great anti-spasmodic remedy. Cramping of muscles with radiating pains. Neuralgic pains relieved by warmth. Especially suited to tired, languid, exhausted subjects, indisposition for mental exertion. Goitre.

Ears: Severe neuralgic pain, worse washing face and neck with cold water.

Mouth: Toothache, better by heat and hot liquids. Complaints of teething children.

Abdomen: Enteralgia, flatulent colic, forcing patient to bend double, relieved by rubbing, warmth, pressure, accompanied by belching of gas, which gives no relief. Bloated full sensation in abdomen, must loosen clothing, walk about and constantly pass flatus.

Female: Menstrual colic, membranous dysmenorrhoea, menses too early, dark, stringy.

Respiratory: Spasmodic cough, whooping cough. Intercostal neuralgia.

Heart: Angina pectoris.

Fever: Chills run up and down the back with shivering.

Extremities: Involuntary shaking of hands; paralysis agitans, cramps in calves, twitchings, chorea, writers' and players' cramp, tetanic spasms, weakness in arms and hands, finger tips stiff and numb. General muscular weakness.

Mod: Worse right side, cold touch, night, Better - Warmth, bending double, pressure, friction.

Dose: 1-12 potency. Sometimes the highest potencies are preferable. Acts especially well, given in hot water.

(Boericke)

Mag. phos. is one of the most important of Schusslers original additions to the materia medica. It is contained in blood corpuscles, muscles, brain, spinal marrow, nerves, teeth. Disturbance of its molecules results in - pains, cramps, paralysis. The pains are shooting like lightning or boring, often combines with or alternating with a sensation of constriction, at times wandering, amel: by warmth, by pressure, agg: by light touch. Nash says - all kinds of pain (though cramping pain is the most characteristic - burning pain - Ars) H.C. Allen says Amel: by hot, warmth, pressure, bending double.

(JHC)

This remedy is indicated in tired, exhausted, neurotic subjects, when suffering from darting, spasmodic pains, which are relieved by pressure and warmth.

It is of service in enteralgia and flatulent colic. The pains are spasmodic, forcing the patient to bend double. There is a belching of gas, but it brings no relief. The pains are relieved by pressure, friction, and the application of heat.

It is also of benefit in menstrual colic and membranous dysmenorrhoea when the troubles are purely spasmodic. It should be remembered in spasmodic twitching of muscles and the spasms of teething children.

It is useful in spasmodic cough, and whooping cough when the spasms come in paroxysms without expectoration.

It should be remembered in chorea, and contractions of a single muscle, and cramps, such as writers' pains and violin players' cramps.

Compare: Colocynth, Kali phos., Dioscorea *(Blackwood)*

392. Magnesia Sulph

(Epsom Salt)

The skin, urinary and female symptoms are most marked. The purgative action of sulphate of magnesia is not a quality of the drug, but a quality of its physical state, which renders its absorption impossible. The properties inherent in the substance itself can only be discovered by attenuation.

Physiologic Dosage. Mag. sulph is of diagnostic and therapeutic value in Gall stone colic. From 2-4 teaspoonfuls in glass hot water taken at onset of a colicky attack may abort or stop the colic.

Epsom salt is one of the most active saline cathartics, operating with little pain or nausea, especially if pure. It has but little if any effect on intestinal paralysis, its action causing a rush of fluid into the intestine, which by producing a distention of the bowel produces evacuation. It causes little or no irritation in the intestine. In common with the other salines, it is the classical evacuant to be employed in connection with mercurials and anthelmintics and in cases of poisoning. Epsom salt usually acts with in one to two hours, more quickly if taken in hot water, and in the morning before breakfast. The ordinary dose as a mild laxative is a heaping teaspoonful, as a cathartic two to four teaspoonfuls. The taste may be improved if necessary by the addition of a little lemon juice and sugar. Besides its chief use as a saline cathartic, Mag. sulph is used to a considerable extent, externally in saturated solution as an antiphlogistic and as antipruritic in erysipelas, ivy poisoning, cellulitis and other local inflammations. Use on compresses, saturated with solutions.

Dose: The pure salt to the 3rd potency. Locally 1:4 in water in septic conditions, erysipelas, orchitis, boils, etc. (Boericke)

Recently old school authorities have discovered in this cathartic a remedy for dysentery. The diuretic action of the drug with great thirst has led to its successful use in diabetes. The diarrhoea is accompanied with great thirst - Warts are allied to epithelioma and H.T. Webster has cured many causes of warts of children - giving as much of the salts as would lie on a dime (six penny) TDS. *(JHC)*

This remedy is indicated in profuse leucorrhoea that renders the patient weak and exhausted, with pain in the small of the back. The urine is turbid and deposits a copious red sediment, its passage being attended with stitching pains in the urethra.

There are small pimples all over the body which itch violently. In physiological doses it is useful in dropsy when the skin is cool. In such cases it causes active elimination by both the kidneys and intestinal tract.

In small doses it is of service in dysentery, also in constipation. It is highly beneficial in reducing pelvic infiltration following acute inflammation. In these cases it should be incorporated into a vaginal suppository and inserted in the vagina. *(Blackwood)*

393. Magnetis Poli Ambo

(The magnet)

Hahnemann is his preface says that he does not expect ordinary mechanical, materialistic and atomistic heads to be able to regard diseases as immaterial alterations of the vitality, or pure dynamic derangements of our state of health, and medicinal powers as merely virtual almost spiritual forces. He asks how they can reconcile with their materialistic notions the fact that a single imponderable spark from a Leyden Jar gives a shock to the strongest man and yet no ascertainable ponderable substance is communicated to his body.

Although each of the poles presents something peculiar in its power of altering the human health, yet each of them seems, when applied twice or more often, to produce alternating action which resemble those of the opposite pole.

My own experience with the magnetism is confined to Mgt. P Aust. 2M, but that is sufficient to give me confidence in prescribing attenuations of these remedies when their indications arise. The leading symptoms of Mag. are, burning lancinating pains throughout the body, pains as if broken in joints, where cartilages of two bones touch, shooting and jerking, disturbed sleep, headache as if a nail is driven in. Agg: by motion; toothache agg: from cold and on contact with cold. Boericke has added tendency of old wounds to bleed a fresh. *(JHC)*

394. Magnetis Polus Arcticus

(North pole of the magnet)

The symptoms of M. P. arct. were obtained by applying it on the region of the 4th and 6th dorsal vertebrae at a distance of four or five fingers breadth from the body. A number of well characterised symptoms were experienced in the teeth and jaws. There was swelling, heat and redness of one cheek. Sensations of coldness are marked. There is coldness where the magnet is applied. The eyeballs feel cold as if it were a lump of ice in the socket. On the other hand there is a sensation as if blood was rushing towards the point touched by the Magnet. Somnambulism. Sensation as if scalp adhered to skull. Tooth ache agg: breathing through mouth. *(JHC)*

Disturbed sleep. Somnambulism. Cracking in cervical vertebrae. Sensation of coldness. Toothache. *(Boericke)*

395.Magnetis Polus Australis

(South Pole of the Magnet)

I have cured so many cases of in growing toe nail with M. P. Aust. 2M, that I invariably give it in the first place, when there are no symptoms plainly indicating another remedy. Hahnemann has seen the following symptoms. Sore pain on the inner side of the nail of the big toe, when walking, as if the nail had grown into the flesh on the side, very painful on being slightly touched and the shoe pressing on the toes and on the nail of the big toe when walking as from corns. Varicose veins, left lower leg. Aching when standing or when the leg is hanging down, removed by placing it horizontally. Frequent feeling of hot water, running hanging affected part, but only when leg is down, at times throbbing there when leg hangs down. M. P. Aust. C.M. one dose - Agg: hanging down.

Compare: Toe nails - Graph, Sil, Nit. ac, Thuja. (JHC)

Severe pain in inner side of nail of the big toe (Ingrowing nail), easy dislocation of joints of foot, feet are painful when letting them hang down. *(Boericke*

396. Malandrinum

(Grease in Horses)

A very effectual protection against small pox (Thuja, Silica). Efficacious in clearing of the remnants of cancerous deposits.

Skin: Scab on upper lip, with stinging pain when torn off, aching in forehead, dry, scaly, itching, rhagades of hands and feet in cold weather and from washing. Toes feel scalded and itch terribly. Bone like protuberances.

Dose: 30 and highest. *(Boericke)*

According to Jenner, the origin of Cow-pox is infection of the udders of cows by contact with grass on which a horse infected with `Grease' has trodden. This assertion is to some extent confirmed by the experiences of homoeopaths, who have found in Maland, a very effectual protection against infection with small pox and against vaccination. I have cured with it cases of unhealthy, dry, rough skin, remaining for years after vaccination. Burnett has cured with it a case of knock-knee in a child who was constantly handling his penis - In bad effects of vaccination. In general, children handling genitals. *(JHC)*

397. Mancinella

(Hippoman-Manganeal apple)

Skin symptoms most marked. Dermatitis with excessive vesiculation, oozing of sticky serum and formation of crusts. To be remembered in mental depressed states at puberty and at climacteric with exalted sexuality. (Loss of vision. Pain in the thumb.

Mind: Sudden vanishing of thoughts. Fear of becoming insane.

Skin: Vesicles, large blisters as from scalds, pemphigus.

Dose: 6-30 potency. *(Boericke)*

It is one of the trees around which the Upas legends have clustered. It is certain that the juice, which resembles pure white milk does possess a considerable amount of acridity and that some persons suffer great pain from incautiously handling it. Perhaps its most dangerous property is that of causing blindness, if by chance the least drop of the milk or smoke of the burning wood comes in contact with the eyes. Fixed idea that she would become insane. Fear of getting crazy *(JHC)*

398. Manganum Aceticum

(Manganese Acetate)

Manganum causes anaemia with destruction of the red corpuscles. Jaundice, nephritis with albuminuria. Fatty degeneration of liver. Paralysis agitans, cellulitis, subacute stage, promotes suppuration and hastens regeneration.

Symptoms of chronic poisoning, according to Professor Von Jaksch, were involuntary laughter and involuntary weeping and walking backwards. Strongly exaggerated reflexes and physical disturbances evidenced by men making fun of each other's gait. Paraplegia progressive, wasting, feeble and staggering gait.

Inflammation of bones or joints with nightly digging pains. Asthmatic persons who cannot lie on feather pillow. Syphilitic and chlorotic patients with general anaemia and paralytic symptoms often are benefited by this drug. Gout, chronic arthritis. For speakers and singers. Great accumulation of mucus. Growing pains and weak ankles. General soreness and aching; every part of the body feels sore, when touched, early tuberculosis.

Head: Anxiety and fear, better lying down.

Ears: Feel stopped, cracking on blowing nose, pain from other parts extends to ears. Deafness in damp weather. Whistling tinnitus.

Respiratory: Chronic hoarseness, every cold rouses up a bronchitis.

Female: Flushes of heat at climacteric.

Extremities: Every part of body feels sore when touched, tending to fall forward. Walks stooping forward, paralysis agitans.

Skin: Chronic eczema associated with amenorrhoea, worse at menstrual period or at menopause.

Dose: 3-30. *(Boericke)*

Its medicinal as well as its physical relationship with iron is very close. There is one curious symptom they have in common, cough amel: by lying down.

Blood: Destroys red corpuscles and causes anaemia. *(JHC)*

Relation: Am. m. in rheumatism of heels, Cupr. in Psoriasis.

This remedy should be remembered in cases of general anaemia when the menses are early, scanty or there are menstrual discharges between the periods. These patients are prone to catarrhal disturbances such as laryngeal catarrh and hoarseness and aphonia or laryngo tracheitis especially in those who are using the voice constantly.

It is indicated in laryngeal phthisis as a palliative when there is rawness and great soreness. It is useful in boys whose voices are changing and who are troubled with catarrh and an effort to clear the throat.

It should be studied in periostitis and articular rheumatism when the pains shift from joint to joint. The pain is worse at night.

It produces symptoms of paraplegia, progressive wasting, feebleness and staggering gait, and paralysis.

In certain skin diseases it has afforded great relief in anaemic patients with delayed menstruation and aggravation about this period.

Compare: Conium, Ferrum.

(Blackwood)

399. Mangifera Indica

(Mango Tree)

One of the best general remedies for passive haemorrhages, uterine, renal, gastric, pulmonary and intestinal. Rhinitis, sneezing, pharyngitis and other acute throat troubles, suffocative sensation, as if throat would close, relaxation of mucous membrane of alimentary canal. Catarrhal and serous discharges, chronic intestinal irritation. Varicose Veins, drowsiness, Atonic conditions, poor circulation, relaxed muscles.

Skin: Itching of palms, skin as if sun burnt, swollen, white spots, intense itching. Lobes of ears and lips swollen.

Relation: Compare - Erigeron, Epilobium.

Dose: Tincture. *(Boericke)*

400. Medorrhinum

(The gonorrhoeal virus)

A powerful and deep acting medicine, often indicated for chronic ailments due to suppressed gonorrhoea. For women with chronic pelvic disorders. Chronic rheumatism. Great disturbance and irritability of nervous system. Pains intolerable, tensive, nerves quiver and tingle, child dwarfed and stunted. Chronic catarrhal conditions in children. Nose dirty, tonsils enlarged, thick yellow mucus from nostrils, lips thickened from mouth breathing. State of collapse and trembling all over. History of sycosis. Often restores a gonorrhoeal discharge. Intensity of all sensations. Oedema of limbs, dropsy of serous sacs. Disseminated sclerosis.

Mind: Weak memory, cannot speak without weeping, time passes too slowly, is in a great hurry, fear in the dark and of some one behind her, melancholy with suicidal thoughts, hair dry, crispy, itching of scalp, dandruff.

Face: Small boils break out during menses.

Stomach: Very thirsty, craving for liquor, salt, sweets etc, warm drinks. Pernicious vomiting of pregnancy.

Abdomen: Rests more comfortably lying on abdomen.

Stool: Intense itching of anus.

Urine: Nocturnal enuresis.

Female: Intense pruritus, sensitive spot near os uteri, leucorrhoea thin, acrid, excoriating, fishy odor, sterility, metrorrhagia.

Male: Nocturnal emissions.

Respiratory: Incessant, dry night cough, better lying on stomach.

Extremities: Legs heavy, cannot keep them still, ankles easily turn when walking. Burning of hands and feet, finger joints enlarged, puffy, gouty concretions. Heels and balls of feet tender. Soreness of soles.

Skin: Incessant itching, worse night and when thinking of it. Fiery red rash about anus in babies, copper colored spots, favus, tumours and abnormal growth.

Fever: Wants to be fanned all the time, chills up and down back, coldness of legs, hands and forearms, flashes of heat in face and neck. Night sweat and hectic.

Sleep: Dreams she is drinking - sleeps in knee chest position.

Mod: (Worse) when thinking of ailment, from daylight to sunset, heat, inland - (Better) at the sea shore, lying on stomach, damp weather (Caust).

Dose: The very highest potencies only of service, must not be repeated often. *(Boericke)*

She could not read in the evening and in the morning, the lids would be closed and she suffered much on getting them separated. Many cases of stunted growth and arrested development in children are due to latent gonorrhoea and syphilis. Syphillinum has agg: from sunset to sunrise as also have all the great anti-syphilitic remedies. Medorrh. has Agg: from sunrise to sunset, always brighter in evening. Agg: in early morning hours. There is a state of collapse and a desire to be fanned - There is scarcely a spot on the body that is not full of pain - obstinate rheumatism. Burnett regards Medorrh. as the mother of pus and catarrh - sycotic asthma agg 2 to 4 a.m. amel: at sea side. Fiery red rash developing about the anus in babies a few days old. Constipation with hard dry stools. Medorr. is the remedy used in single doses, but is rarely, if ever, to be given in the acute stages of a disease. Leaning far back amel: constipation, can only pass stool so. Chronic rheumatism of joints, agg: inland, amel: near sea. *(JHC)*

This remedy is indicated in chronic diseases and constitutional dyscrasias dependent upon a latent gonorrhoea.

It should be remembered in chronic arthritis, gout, rheumatism, neuralgia and diseases of the spinal cord that can be traced to this as its origin. It bears the same relation to spinal nervous diseases that Psorinum does to those of the skin and mucous membranes.

It is of servive in the chronic pelvic diseases of women that date from a gonorrhoeal infection.

It is beneficial in those who are dwarfed and stunted both physically and mentally; children that are pale and rachitic, dull and weak.

It is often curative in gleet, when the whole urethra feels sore.

Compare: Sulphur, Thuja. (Blackwood)

Synopsis: Suppression of gonorrhoea. When the best selected remedy fails to relieve or permanently improve. Gout, rheumatism. For women-ovaritis, salpingitis, pelvis cellulitis, fibroids, cysts, scirrhus carcinoma or cancer with a history of sycosis. Children dwarfed, mentally dull and weak, heat and soreness - lymphatic glands all over body - state of collapse, wants to be fanned all the time - cold and bathed with cold perspiration - weakness of memory, cannot remember names, even forgets his own name, cannot speak without weeping, in a great hurry, ravenous hunger immediately after eating, craving for salt, sweets, ale, ice, acids, oranges, green fruits. Nocturnal enuresis, passes enormous quantity of ammoniacal high coloured urine in bed every night.

Sexual organs: Menses profuse, very dark, clotted - intense pruritus of labia and vagina agg: thinking of it - Asthma amel: by lying on stomach - lower limbs ache all night preventing sleep - intensely restless and fidgety legs and feet - burning of hands and feet, wants them uncovered and fanned - the burning feet of sulphur, and restless fidgety legs and feet of Zinc, are both found at the same time in Medorrhinum. Amel: at sea shore, lying on stomach, damp weather.

401. *Medusa*

(Jelly fish)

Female: The secretion of milk was established after lack of it in all previous confinements.

Skin: Numbness, burning pricking heat, vesicular eruption, especially on face, arms, shoulders and breasts. *(Boericke)*

Nettle rash: The effects of encountering jelly fish whilst bathing are well known - diseases of the stomach and leucorrhoea have been recorded - milk came into the breasts three years after the birth of her last child. *(JHC)*

This remedy is of service in oedema of the face, with numbness, burning, pricking heat, also in erythema.

Compare: Apis mel:, Chloral, Urtica urens. (Blackwood)

402. *Melilotus*

(Sweet clover)

Congestion and haemorrhages seem to be the special manifestations of this drug. Violent congestive and nervous headaches, infantile spasms; epilepsy from blow on head. Pain and debility point to it. Coldness but also increase of temperature, tenderness and pain. Muscular system depressed. Dreams and emissions.

Mind: Wants to run away and hide. Delusions, thinks every one is looking at her, fears to talk loud, wants to run away, etc.

Head: Sick headache, relieved by epistaxis or menstrual flow. Fullness all over head - neuralgia.

Nose: Dry, profuse epistaxis.

Female: Scanty, intermits, dysmenorrhoea.

Dose: Tr. for inhaling and lower potencies. *(Boericke)*

All the provers had fearful headaches and profuse haemorrhages except myself (Bowen) - In a school boy I cured with Meli. 30 very distressing recurrent headache accompanied by an intensely red face, amel: of haemorrhages by flow of urine. *(JHC)*

Constipation, the passage is difficult and painful, the anus feels constricted and throbs, there is no desire for stool till there is a large accumulation.

Compare: Bel., Ferr. phos.(Blackwood)

403. *Melitagrinum*

(The nosode of Eczema capitis)

Dr. Skinner has given a brief account of this nosode, introduced by him. He prepared it from the lymph and blood of a case of eczema capitis. Very severe case were cured with `melitagrinum' c.m. (Fc) given in single doses as considerable intervals. In one case there was an initial aggravation. *(JHC)*

404. *Menispermum*

(Moon seed)

A remedy for megrim, associated with restlessness and dreams. Pain in spine dryness, itching all over, dry mouth and throat.

Head: Pressure from within outward with stretching and yawning.

Dose: 3rd potency. *(Boericke)*

The most notable symptom was an intense headache combined with aching all down the back. Yawning and stretching were also a marked and frequent concomitant of headache and backache. Meni. is botanically related to Cocul. Vertigo and intoxication were not elicited. Dryness was a common feature in mouth, throat, skin. Itching was very intense, as with Coccul. *(JHC)*

405. *Mentha Piperita*

(Peppermint)

Stimulates the cold - perceiving nerves, so just after taking it, a current of air at the ordinary temperature seems cold. Marked action on respiratory organs and skin. Useful in gastrodynia, flatulent colic.

Respiration: Throat dry and sore as if pin crosswise in it - Dry cough worse from air into larynx, tobacco smoke, fog, talking, with irritation in supra - sternal fossa. Trachea painful to touch.

Dose: Tincture 1-20 drops to 30c. Locally in pruritus vaginae. *(Boericke)*

The most remarkable symptom of the proving was the cough and this has been fully confirmed. It was a dry cough excited by air entering larynx, by reading aloud, by exposure to cold, by shocks of any kind. `Demeures' says he cured with Menth. Pip. every case of influenza that came under his care in the winter of 1847-8. It is to dry cough, however caused, what `Arn' is to injuries and `Aco.' to inflammatory complaints. It relieved even the cough of consumptions. A single globule of 30th sufficed. `Demeures' gave it to singers a short time before singing and greatly helped them to hold the voice. *(JHC)*

This remedy is indicated in gastrodynia, flatulent colic, deranged digestion, broncho-tracheal catarrh and diseases of the skin.

Also in Hysteria when they are attended with nausea and vomiting.

It is of service when there is an irritation in the suprasternal fossa, when there is a dry, spasmodic cough which is worse in cold weather, and following the influenza, also vaginal pruritus, and herpes zoster. *(Blackwood)*

406. *Menyanthes*

(Buck bean)

A remedy for certain headaches, intermittent fever. Coldness of abdomen. Twitchings. Sensation of tension and compression. Fidgets and urinary difficulties in women. Diabetes.

Head: Better, hard pressure with hand.

Extremities: Icy coldness of hands and feet. As soon as patient lies down, legs jerk and twitch.

Dose: 3-30c *(Boericke)*

The Buck bean or Bog bean, as it is also called in Ireland and Lincoln shire, is a water plant and abounds in the ten districts, where it is in great local repute as a remedy for Ague. The main features of `Meny' are: -

1. Chill, 2. Sensations and pains of tension and compression and 3. spasmodic jerkings and visible twitchings, these are agg. during rest and may be associated with neuralgia. As soon as the patient lies down the legs jerk and twitch so that he cannot rest. Meny. has cured many cases of fidgets, jumps and urinary difficulties in women who are brunettes; leading indications for `meny' - with the headache there is often associated icy coldness of hands and fee. `Meny' - 30 *(JHC)*

This remedy is indicated in malarial disorders, when the coldness predominates. The hands and feet are icy cold, and there is coldness of the abdomen. There is a sensation of pressure on the vertex which is relieved by hard pressure with the hands.

Compare: Capsicum, Arsenicum alb. *(Blackwood)*

407. Mephitis

(Skunk)

A great medicine for whooping cough. In order to insure its full success, it should be given in the lower dilutions from 1x to 3x. Suffocative feelings, asthmatic paroxysms, spasmodic cough, cough so violent, seems as if each spell would terminate life, child must be raised up, gets blue in face, cannot exhale, Mucous rales through upper part of chest. Patient wants to bathe in ice-cold water.

Mouth: Coppery taste as after eating onions.

Respiratory: Sudden contraction of glottis, when drinking or talking, food goes down wrong way, false croup, cannot exhale, spasmodic and whooping cough. Few paroxysms in day time, but many at night with vomiting after eating. Asthma as if inhaling sulphur, cough from talking, hollow, deep, with rawness, hoarseness, and pain through chest. Violent spasmodic cough, worse at night.

Dose: 1st to 3rd potency - Has a very short action. *(Boericke)*

Mephitis was proved by Herring in the 30th. Among the symptoms he developed was choking while eating or drinking. Meph. will supersede all other remedies in whooping cough - Guernsey gives it as `Whooping or any other kind of cough, which is very violent, coming on spasmodically and seeming as though, each spell would terminate life. Decided agg: at night and after lying down - Meph. enables patients to endure extreme cold, makes them less chilly in cold water, washing in ice water is pleasant. Agg: night and day break. *(JHC)*

This remedy is indicated in whooping cough when the paroxysms are so violent that the child becomes blue and must be raised up in bed.

It is also of service in false croup and laryngeal spasms, when the child feels suffocated and cannot exhale.

Compare: Drosera, Corallium, Coccus cact. *(Blackwood)*

408. *Mercurialis Perennis*

(Dog's mercury)

Great exhaustion and drowsiness. Tumour at ensiform appendix, very sensitive. Affections of the muscular fibres of stomach, intestines, bladder.

Female: Amenorrhoea, scanty menses accompanied with orgasms. Pain and swelling of breasts. Dysmenorrhoea.

Dose: 3rd potency. *(Boericke)*

Dog's mercury is a common plant with poisonous properties on account of which it is avoided by cattle. Many of its symptoms resemble closely those of the more corrosive salts of mercury - prevalence of burning symptoms, irritation of eyes and nose, tenesmus after stool, etc. The dryness of the mouth and throat is more remarkabie than in any other remedy, even sugar refuses to melt in the mouth. Eating Agg: the dryness. A very remarkable action is that on the female generative organs and puts `Merls'; in the front rank of remedies for amenorrhoea, scanty and delayed menses and dysmenorrhoea, accompanied with orgasm, pains and swelling of breasts. *(JHC)*

This remedy is indicated in vertigo, which is worse while going downstairs. There is a sensation of heaviness in the head as if pressed down from a weight. The scalp seems light and difficult to move. It is useful in rheumatism. *(Blackwood)*

409. *Mercurius - Hydrargyrum*

(Quick Silver)

Every organ and tissue of the body is more or less affected by this powerful drug, it transforms healthy cells into decrepit inflamed and necrotic wrecks, decomposes the blood, producing a profound anaemia. This malignant medicinal force is converted into useful life saving, and life preserving service if employed homoeopathically guided by its clear-cut symptoms. The lymphatic system is especially affected with all the membranes and glands and internal organs, bones, etc. Lesions produced by mercury are very similar to those of syphilis. Very often indicated in the secondary stage of syphilis, where there is a febrile chloro-anaemia, rheumatoid pains behind sternum, around joints etc. ulceration of mouth and throat, falling of the hair, the eruptions and ulceration of mouth and throat etc. These are the special conditions and stages to which Mercur. is homoeopathic where the 2x will do surprising work. Again, hereditary syphilis manifestations are with in its range, bullae, abscesses, snuffles, marasmus, stomatitis, or destructive inflammations. Tremors everywhere, weakness with ebullitions and tremblings from least exertion. All mercury symptoms are worse at night, from warmth of bed, from damp, cold, rainy weather, worse during perspiration. Complaints increase with the sweat and rest, all associated with a great deal of weariness, prostration and trembling. A human `thermometer', sensitive to heat and cold. Parts are much swollen, with raw, sore feeling, the profuse, oily perspiration does not relieve. Breath, excretions and body smell foul. Tendency to formation of pus, which is thin, greenish, putrid, streaked with thin blood.

Head: Vertigo, when lying on back - Tension about scalp as if bandaged.

Eyes: Profuse burning acrid discharge. Floating black spots. After exposure to glare of fire, foundry men. Parenchymatous Keratitis.

Ears: Yellow discharge, otalgia worse warmth of bed, boils in external canal.

Nose: Sneezing in sun shine, nostrils raw ulcerated, coryza, acrid discharge, swelling of nasal bones and caries with greenish fetid ulceration.

Mouth: Sweetish metallic taste salivary secretions greatly increased, gums spongy, furrow in upper surface of tongue lengthwise, tongue heavy, thick moist coating, yellow, flabby, teeth indented, fetid odour from mouth, alveolar abscess, worse at night, great thirst with moist mouth.

Throat: Ulcers and inflammation appearing at every change in weather. Quinsy with difficult swallowing after pus has formed.

Stomach: Intense thirst for cold drinks, weak digestion with continuous hunger.

Abdomen: Flatulent distention with pain, liver enlarged, sore to touch, indurated, jaundice, bile secreted deficiently.

Stool: Bloody and slimy, worse at night with pain and tenesmus, never-get-done feeling.

Urine: Greenish discharge from urethra, burning in urethra on beginning to urinate.

Male: Vesicles and ulcers, prepuce irritated.

Female: Menses profuse, with abdominal pains, leucorrhoea excoriating, greenish and bloody, sensation of rawness in parts. Itching and burning worse after urinating, better washing with cold water.

Respiratory: Cannot lie on rt. side - cough with yellow muco-purulent expectoration worse night and warmth of bed.

Back: Tearing pain in coccyx.

Extremities: Oily perspiration, trembling extremities, especially hands, paralysis agitans - cold clammy sweat on legs at night - dropsical swelling of feet and legs.

Skin: Almost constantly moist. Persistent dryness of the skin, contra-indicates mercurius. General tendency to free perspiration but patient is not relieved by it - vesicular and pustular eruptions. Ulcers, irregular in shape, edges undefined. Itching worse from warmth of bed. Crustalactea, yellowish, brown crusts, considerable suppuration. Orchitis.

Fever: Generally gastric or bilious, with profuse nightly perspiration, debility slow and lingering. Heat and shuddering alternately. Profuse perspiration without relief, creeping chilliness.

Mod: Worse at night, wet damp weather, lying on right side, perspiring, warm room and warm bed.

Dose: 2nd-30c. *(Boericke)*

Though Merc. sol was the preparation Hahnemann proved, he recommended Merc. viv. as a superior preparation for homoeopathic prescribing in his preface to the proving. At night severe toothache. As the thermometer is sensitive to changes either to hot or cold, so is the Merc. patient.

1. Agg. heat and cold. (2) Agg. night. (3) Profuse sweat. (4) Mercurial odour. (5) Tremor - the best general remedy in paralysis agitans - Everything is done hastily - hurried and rapid talking - In the suppurative stage of small-pox, it is specific. Fetid ear discharge - Agg, lying on R. side - stomach disordered. Sweets disagree, aversion to meat, wine, brandy, beer, coffee, greasy food, butter - Merc. is rarely indicated when the tongue is dry. Slimy stools. Sliminess is general characteristic. Vibration in forehead. Head as if in a vice, as if growing larger. Voluptuous itching. Causation: fright, suppressed gonorrhoea, suppressed foot sweat. *(JHC)*

Mercurius vivus - This agent when applied to the skin is an antiparasitic, when absorbed there is a peculiar foetor in the mouth. The gums are swollen, the teeth are sore, there is an increase in the amount of saliva, and ptyalism, with a peculiar metallic taste.

When taken internally, large doses produce diarrhoea. The evacuation of bile is hastened in the duodenum. Tonic doses diminish the cardiac action, and produce anaemia and dissolution of the corpuscular elements of the blood. The breathing is labored and weak.

This remedy is indicated in those with light hair, whose skin and muscles are relaxed. They are weak and tremble from the least exertion.

The breath and body smells foul. There is a profuse perspiration attending nearly all the complaints, but it brings no relief. The pains are worse at night. There is intense thirst, while the tongue is moist, large and flabby, and shows paralysis agitans - should not be given before or after silicea - in low hastens suppuration. Mezereum is vegetable analogue - ailments from sugar - insect stings - vapours of Arsenic or copper - diseases occurring in winter. *(HC Allen)*

410. Mercuris Cor

(Corrosive sublimate)

Mercury is used in testing the temperature, and a Merc. constitution is just as changeable and sensitive to heat and cold. The patient is worst from the extremes of temperature, worse from both heat and cold. - Worse from the warmth of the bed - This applies to the pains, the fever, ulcers and eruptions and the patient himself.

Offensive patient. Odors very foetid, and it can be detected on entering the room. The perspiration is offensive, has a strong sweetish, penetrating odor.

Rheumatic inflammation of joints, aggravation while sweating. Rheumatism in old syphilitic, gonorrhoeal and gouty patients.

Tremor of the hands so that he cannot lift anything or eat or write. The trembling, weakness, sweat, foetor, suppuration and ulceration, the aggravation at night and from heat and cold, give the earlier impressions of the remedy.

A marked feature running all through is hastiness, a hurried, restless, anxious, impulsive disposition. Desire to kill persons contradicting her. Impulse to kill or commit suicide, sudden anger with impulse to do violence.

Think of Merc. if you are called to a child with sweating of the head, dilated pupils, rolling of the head, and aggravation at night, who has had scarlet fever or a suppressed ear discharge.

There is copious lachrymation with all eye symptoms, and the tears excoriate, causing a red line down the cheeks. Sometimes you will see a little fine growth on the iris, growing across the pupil and attached by a pedicle. It is really a syphilitic condyloma.

Ear troubles. Horribly stinking greenish discharge. Green thick acrid pus from the ears like the discharge from the nose and other parts. Stinking otorrhoea. With ruptured drum. Merc. is a frequently required remedy.

It has coryza with much sneezing with an opposite state, ameliorated lying, not at all during the night while lying in bed, only in the daytime while up and about.

Kali iod. is better for the same burning in the face, running coryza and aggravation from heat and warmth of the bed, and it will cure the coryza in a night when apparently Merc. is indicated.

Scorbutic gums in those who have been salivated. Toothache, looseness of the teeth, decay of the teeth. Copious salivation. The tongue is swollen as if spongy and presses in around the teeth. Merc. Ipec. and Acon are frequently indicated in epidemic dysentery, in hot weather, and Ipec. Dulc. and Merc. are indicated in cold weather. Stinging, itching and boring pains in the uterus and ovaries. Milk in the breast of the non-pregnant woman at the menstrual period. I once had a freak in a sixteen year old boy who had milk in his breasts. I cured him with Merc. With many complaints there is sore throat and rheumatism and stiffness of the neck; stiff neck with swollen glands and goitre.

Merc. especially affects the joints; inflammatory rheumatism with much swelling aggravated from the heat of the bed and from uncovering. Tremulous condition of the extremities, like paralysis agitans. Trembling of the hands with great weakness.

It acts wonderfully in catarrhal fever, grippe, etc. and when colds extend to the chest and there are copious discharges everywhere.

Scurfy eruptions, much itching of the skin, violent, in all parts of the body, as from fleas, especially when warm in bed at night. Rawness between the thighs and between the scrotum and thighs. Eruptions in such places. *(Kent)*

This salt leads all other remedies in tenesmus of the rectum, which is incessant and is not relieved by the stool. The tenesmus often involves the bladder as well. Bright's disease, Gonorrhoea, second stage with continuous tenesmus. Destroys the secreting portions of the kidneys. This process is slow but sure. Albuminurea in early pregnancy (Phos later and at full term).

Head: Frontal pain, congestion of head.

Eyes: Acrid lachrymation, Iritis, Iris muddy in color, thick and neither contracts nor dilates. lids oedematous, severe burning, soreness of the eyes.

Face: Lips black.

Mouth: Teeth loose, gums purple, swollen and spongy, salivation, pyorrhoea, ptyalism, tastes salty and bitter.

Throat: Red, swollen, painful, intensely inflamed, uvula swollen, swallowing painful. Burning pain with great swelling worse slight external pressure.

Stool: Dysentery, tenesmus, not relieved by stool, incessant, slimy, offensive and shreds of mucous membrane.

Urine: Suppressed, greenish discharge, albuminous, tenesmus, of bladder, stabbing pain extending up urethra into bladder. Perspiration after urinating.

Male: Penis and testes enormously swollen. Chancres assume phagedenic appearance, gonorrhoea, urethra orifice red, swollen, glans sore and hot. Discharge greenish thick.

Fever: Profuse perspiration. Surface cold.

Mod: Worse evening, night, acius. Better-while at rest.

Dose: 6th potency. *(Boericke)*

Merc. cor. is Merc. viv. with a much greater rapidity of action. The dysenteric straining is more excessive. For this reason Merc. cor is more generally prescribed in dysentery than Merc Viv. - Long uvulas sometimes give rise to irritating coughs. If to the uvula is applied on a brush a little of a low trituration of Merc. cor. it will in many cases immediately and permanently relieve the trouble. According to Teste Merc. cor. is suited to males and merc. sol. to females - Merc. cor will act in men on indication for Merc. sol. *(JHC)*

411. *Mercurius Cyanatus*

(Cyanide of Mercury)

Acute infections, pneumonia, nephritis. Its action is similar to that of the toxins of infectious diseases. Great and rapid prostrations, tendency toward haemorrhages from the different orifices, of dark fluid blood, cyanosis, rapid respiration and heart action, albuminuria and twitching and jerking of muscles, typhoid pneumonia. Livid states from great struggling, where suffocation is imminent and paralysis of lung threatening, great sweat. Affects most prominently the buccal cavity. This together with marked prostration gives it a place in the treatment of diphtheria, where it has achieved unquestioned great results. Malignant types, with prostration. Coldness and nausea. Syphilitic ulcers when perforation threatens.

Mouth: Ulcerations.

Throat: Necrotic destruction of soft parts of palate and fauces.

Rectum: Stools with tenesmus.

Skin: Moisture with icy coldness.

Dose: 6-30 potency. *(Boericke)*

The history of this remedy is a romantic one. When Dr. Alexander Villers was an infant he had diphtheria. Known remedies had failed to arrest the disease and his father Dr. Diminic Von Villers was in despair. Merc cy. has taken a sure place at the head of remedies for diphtheria. The local symptoms are very clearly defined and among the general symptoms profound prostration, coldness and cyanosis are leading indications. Villiers had better results with the 30th than with any lower attenuation. Diphtheritic membrane in throat, mouth and anus. Sore throat of public speakers - it hurts the patient to speak. (Nash) *(JHC)*

412. *Mercurius Dulcis*

(Calomel)

Has marked effect on catarrhal inflammation of ear and useful in Eustachian catarrh, deafness, diarrhoea, with soreness of anus. Prostatitis, remittent bilious attacks. Pallor, flabby bloatedness and turgid flaccidity. Inflammation with plastic exudate. Especially indicated in systems disposed to remittent, bilious fevers in peritonitis and meningitis with plastic exudate. Dropsies due to combined renal and cardiac diseases, especially with jaundice (Hale). Cirrhosis of liver, especially in the hypertrophic form (use 1x Jousset).

Stool: Scanty, bloody mucus, with bile and constant desire without tenesmus, dark green, watery with gripping. Anus sore and burning, dysentery, small stools, of mucus and blood, covered with bile.

Skin: Flabby and ill nourished, swollen glands, phagedenic ulcers, copper-coloured eruptions.

Relation: Kali-mur.

Dose: 3rd to 6th trituration. *(Boericke)*

The keynote of Merc Dulc. in this as in other complaints is pallor `Pallid as a corpse' and with this flabby bloatedness of appearance. Pale, scrofulous children who have swelling of cervical and other glands, skin flabby and ill nourished. Another leading feature of Merc. dulc. is inflammation with plastic exudation. I have seen calomel in old school practice rapidly resolve and cure a violent meningitis, with wild delirium in a girl of five. In this case, there was probably plastic exudation on the membranes. Plastic peritonitis, gluing up of Eustachian tube with catarrh. Eustachian tube closed, deafness of old age (Kali mur). *(JHC)*

This remedy is indicated in diarrhoea when the stools are scanty and bloody or are dark green and watery, and attended with griping. The anus is sore and burning. There is a constant desire for stool without tenesmus. It is also of use in dysentery when the stool is small in quantity and consists of mucus and blood, covered with bile.

It is of service in salivation with sore mouth and offensive breath. It should also be remembered that when the bowels must be evacuated, one-tenth of a grain every hour or more often for a few times is sufficient.
(Blackwood)

413.Merc Proto-Iodide

(Mercurius Iodatus Flavus)

Throat affections, with greatly swollen glands and characteristic coating of tongue. Worse right side. Chancre. Induration remains long time. Swollen inguinal glands, large and hard. Mammary tumors, with tendency to much warm perspiration and gastric disturbance.

Tongue: Coated thickly yellow at base.

Throat: Lacunar tonsillitis. When only the superficial part of the tonsil is involved cheesy exudate with offensive breath. Swelling begins on right side. Small ulcers on posterior pharynx and fauces. Worse on right tonsil. Much tenacious mucus. Sensation of a lump Constant inclination to swallow.

Dose: 2nd trituration. *(Boericke)*

The right to left direction was manifested in the throat. Agg: by warm drinks, cervical and parotid glands enormously swollen. The teeth feel too long. There is also irresistible desire to clench teeth. Lyco - follows well - (merc bin iod left to right)

414. Mercurius Iodatus Ruber

(Merc. bin - iodide)

Diphtheria and ulcerated sore throats especially on left side with much glandular swelling. Chronic suppurating buboes. Hard chancres. Old cases of syphilis on scrofulous patients. Early stages of cold, especially in children.

Throat: Fauces dark red, stiffness of muscles of throat and neck - worse on left tonsil - cough from elongated uvula with sore throat.

Dose: 3rd trituration. Merc. iodide is far more active as a bactericide than the other materials. Including the chloride.
(Boericke)

It acts more intensely on the lymphatic glands and cellular tissue than Merc. v. which it otherwise closely resembles. It has been extensively tested in throat affections. It acts more on the left side or primarily on the left. *(JHC)*

415. *Mercurius Sulph*

(Yellow sulphate of mercury)

Watery stools, burning in anus, sore tip of tongue, oedema of legs. Sneezing from direct rays of sun - diarrhoea early in the morning, stool bursts out in a hot stream of yellow matter. Intense evacuations, like rice water. Scanty clear scalding urine. Intense dyspnoea, must sit up. Respiration rapid short, burning in chest. Hydro-thorax (Ars). Cardiac pain and weakness. *(Boericke)*

Lippe is the chief clinical authority for this medicine. He considers it as important as "Ars" in dropsies of the chest. When Merc. sulph acts well, says Lippe, it produces a profuse watery diarrhoea with great relief to the patient. Oedema of legs agg. in afternoon 4-5 p.m. *(JHC)*

416. *Methylene Blue*

(One of the aniline Dyes)

A remedy for neuralgia, neurasthenia, malaria; typhoid, here it diminishes the tympanitis, delirium, and fever; pus infection. Tendency to tremor, chorea and epilepsy. Nephritis (acute parenchymatous), scarlatinal nephritis. Urine acquires a green color. Bladder irritation from its use antidoted by a little nutmeg. Surgical kidney with large amount of pus in urine. Gonorrhoeal rheumatism and cystitis. Backache, sciatica. Later states of apoplexy. (Gesevius)

Dose: 3x attenuation. 2 percent, solution locally, in chronic otitis with foul smelling discharge.

A. 1 percent aqueous solution for ulcers and abscesses of cornea. *(Boericke)*

It has been used in old school practice in doses of about 3 grains in capsules or pills in rheumatism of joints and muscles and in rheumatoid arthritis. Immunity from malaria seems to follow its continued use. It is apt to cause cystitis. An apparently hopeless case of typhoid was signally benefited by it. Tympanities disappearing as if by magic. Where ever there is pus infection it is indicated and it has made a record with him in gonorrhoea and cystitis. *(JHC)*

This agent changes the haemoglobin into methaemoglobin, causes irritation of the alimentary tract which results in nausea, vomiting, and diarrhoea upon the urinary tract it has produced retention of the urine, strangury, pyelitis, cystitis, spasmodic contraction of the bladder, albuminuria and hyaline casts. It has relieved neuralgia, and neurasthenia. It is considered an anti-malarial by many and has been used locally in cases of carcinoma.

It is of service in surgical kidney when there is a large quantity of pus in the urine.

It is indicated in cases of mania, periodic melancholia, paranoia and hystero epilepsy. One grain of the drug injected in the gluteal muscle and a sedative action that was manifest within theee to six hours and the effect remained from three to four days. This quieting action was neither attended nor followed by any unpleasant symptoms.

It is of servive in functional neuralgias and migraine of the angiospastic variety.

In nephritis of a haemorrhagic type in doses of from 2 to 3 grains, once, twice a day, it has been highly spoken of by Einhorn and others. The blood disappears from the urine, the albumin is greatly diminished and the patients condition is much improved. It has been employed in acute and chronic Bright's disease. There were present "bruit de galop", visual disorders, painful polyuria albuminuria and hyaline casts in the urine.

In several obstinate cases of rheumatic arthritis a two grain tablet was given twice a day after meals, resulting in great improvement, arresting the process, improving the nutrition and leading to an increase of the bodily weight.

It has been of service in pruritus vulvae, applied locally and given internally in grain doses.

It has been extensively employed in acute gonorrhoea, and in the treatment of interstitial nephritis. When it is administered in such cases it begins to show in the urine in about seven hours; in those with normal kidneys it shows in about on hour' and a third. In gonorrhoeal rheumatism it is of great service, as well as in cases of cystitis. *(Blackwood)*

417. Mezereum

(Spurge olive)

Skin symptoms, affections of bones, and neuralgias, most important, especially about teeth and face. Bruised weary feeling in joints with drawing and stiffness. Pains of various kinds with chilliness and sensitiveness to cold air. Bone pains, eruptions after vaccinations. Burning darting sensation in the muscles. Subsultus tendinum. Pains shoot upward and seem to draw patient up out of bed. Semilateral complaints. Patient is very sensitive to cold air.

Head: Covered with thick, leathery crusts, under which pus collects. Worse eating.

Ears: As if tympanum was exposed to the cold air and it blew into the ear.

Eyes: Ciliary neuralgia after operations, pains with cold feeling and stiffness of bone.

Stomach: Mouth waters, gastric ulcer.

Rectum: Green discharges.

Male: Enlargement of testicles.

Skin: Eczema, intolerable itching, chilliness with pruritus, worse in bed, ulcers itch and burn, surrounded by vesicles and shining, fiery red areola. Zona, with burning pain, eruptions ulcerate and form thick scabs under which purulent matter exudes (Chrysophanic acid).

Modalities: (Worse) Cold air, night, evening until midnight, warm food, touch, motion. (Better) open air.

Dose: 6-30. *(Boericke)*

Mezereum is the vegetable analogue of and is one of the most important antidotes to Mercurius - Merc and Mez antidote one another - they have the same sensitiveness to damp cold and warmth and the same nightly aggravations - eruption of thick whitish scabs, hard, almost, horny, covering the whole scalp. There were fissures through which exuded on pressure a thick yellowish pus often very offensive. "My stools are as hard as stone and as large as my arm, I feel as if they would split me open. They come in sections like mouthfuls and I become much exhausted and tremble with weakness.

Causation: anger, Mercury, Vaccination. *(JHC)*

It is of service in various lesions of the skin. These may be pustular, papular, vesicular or squamous. There is a tendency to form hard, dense crusts under which there is an acrid, irritating exudate. The crusts on the scalp are of a whitish colour and of a light yellow colour around the mouth. The discharge is very offensive, dries quickly and mats the hair in crusts. There is a sensation of burning, itching, stinging or tearing. Many of these cases are syphilitic or nervous in origin.

It is a most useful remedy in the neuralgia that attends and follows herpes zoster. It should be remembered in the pruritus of the aged when there is itching after getting warm in bed.

Compare: Phytolacca, Guaiacum, Causticum. *(Blackwood)*

418. Millefolium

(Yarrow)

An invaluable remedy for various types of haemorrhages, blood bright red. Incarcerated hernia, small pox, with great pain in pit of stomach. After operations for stone. Bad effects from fall from a height over-lifting. Continued high temperature. Haemoptysis.

Nose: Nose bleed (Erecht). Piercing pain from eyes to root of nose.

Stool: Haemorrhage from bowels, bleeding haemorrhoids, urine bloody.

Female: Menses early, profuse, protracted. Haemorrhage from uterus, bright red fluid. Painful varices during pregnancy.

Relation: Compare: Ficus venos (parker), Haemorrhage from bowels and lungs. Acalypha and Helix tosta (Snail) in haemoptysis, diseases of chest, consumption, also Secale, Ipecac., Erecht, Geran, Hamam.

Dose: Tr. to 3rd potency. *(Boericke)*

Yarrow was named Achillea by "Linnaeus" because the plant is mentioned in the Iliad as having been used by Achilles on the instruction of Chiron to heal the wounds of soldiers. It received its popular name "Nose bleed" because nose bleed comes on if the leaves are inserted into the nostrils. It was at length found that Ars. Iod 3x in solution was a complete antidote. Milli. is suited to all wounds which bleed profusely, sprains and over lifting agg. by coffee. *(JHC)*

This agent acts as a tonic and astringent. This remedy is of service in cases of active haemorrhage from any part of the body, such as the nose, lungs, bowels, or uterus, also in ailments that result from over lifting, over exertion, or a fall.

The haemorrhage is painless and not attended with fever. The blood is bright red and fluid in character, such as comes from a wound the result of a fall; haemoptysis after an injury in those suffering from incipient phthisis. It has also been of service in cases of haemoptysis following suppression of the menstrual or haemorrhoidal flow, when the blood is bright red and fluid in character. It has relieved cases of menorrhagia when the blood was bright red, fluid, and profuse. It has also relieved haematuria.

Compare: Hamamelis, Geranium, Acalypha. *(Blackwood)*

419. Mitchella

(Partridge Berry)

Bladder symptoms, accompany complaints especially uterine congestion.

Dose: Tincture *(Boericke)*

It belongs to same order as China, Coffea and Ipecac and shows its affinity with these in its power over haemorrhages. Indian women drink a decoction of it before confinement to make labor sage and easy. *(JHC)*

This remedy is indicated when the uterine cervix is swollen and presents upon inspection a dark red, engorged appearance; the uterus is enlarged and there is lack of tone of the uterine tissues. There may be a condition of amenorrhoea, delayed menstruation, dysmenorrhoea, menorrhagia with the dark, congested appearance of the parts.

It is of some service in the relief of the false labor pains of the last months of pregnancy. Its great use has been during the last few months of pregnancy to assist in securing a sage and easy delivery. In these cases it has been administered twice a day for three months before the expected event. The dose in these cases is from ten to fifteen minims.

It is also of service in the urinary difficulties of women who suffer from uterine derangements. There is catarrh of the bladder with dysuria and urging to urinate. The urine is highly coloured and contains a white sediment. There is a dull aching pain in the back referred to the renal region. The neck of the bladder and urethra are swollen and irritated.

In these cases there is often a depression of the spirits and a condition of forgetfulness.

Compare: Helonias, Aletris farinosa, Viburnum opulus. *(Blackwood)*

420. *Momordica*

(Balsam apple)

Griping, colicky pain in back and hypogastrium with painful and excessive menses. Accumulation of flatus in spenic flexure of colon. Dropsy.

Head: Contents of head feel lighter.

Abdomen: Rumbling, gripping colicky pains, starting from back, spreading over abdomen.

Dose: Tincture. Use also externally as a liniment and poultice for burns, chapped hands, etc. *(Boericke)*

Gripping and colic declared it relationship to Colocynth and Elater, as also severe pains in back and hypogastrium with painful and excessive menses. A peculiar sensation is: As if the whole contents of the head had greatly diminished in weight. *(JHC)*

This remedy is indicated when there is a large accumulation of flatus in the splenic flexure of the colon. *(Blackwood)*

421. *Morbillinum*

(The nosode of measles)

The well known symptoms, which characterise an attack of measles may all be taken as guides for its homeopathic use. Its chief use hitherto has been as a prophylactic against infection and to clear up after effects of an attack. My own use of it has been confined to the 30th and higher, but there is no bar upon lower potencies, and those who prefer them may begin with the 6th. As a prophylactic given to those who are or may be exposed to infection, I prescribe a dose of 30th thrice daily. For an attack of the disease, I find nothing better than Morbil. - 30, eight or ten globules in 6 oz of water, a dessert spoonful every two hours. The effect of this is heightened by giving alternately Bell. 30 in the same way. These two medicines will be sufficient to carry through any uncomplicated case, and in my experience do even better than Pulsatilla. As the measles poison has a great affinity for the mucous passes, the eyes, the ears and the respiratory mucous membranes, Morbil may be used in such cases like any other homoeopathic remedy, when the symptoms correspond.

Comple: Bell.

Compare: Pul., Hepar., Merc., Sul.

(JHC)

422. *Morphinum*

(An Alkaloid of Opium)

Morphine bears the same relation to Opium as Atrophine to Belladonna i.e. represents its nervous side. It is less stimulating, less convulsant and more decidedly hypnotic. Constipates less and affects contractility of the bladder more. It is less diaphoretic and more pruritic.

Mind: Profound depression, irritable, fault finding, hysterical, shock induced by terror, dream like state.

Head: Vertigo from the least movement of the head.

Eyes: Look unsteady, paresis of recti interni.

Ears: Left ear throbs painfully, better heat, seems to hear circulation all over body.

Face: Dusky red or pallid lividity of face, lips, tongue, mouth or throat.

Nose: Sneezing in paroxysms, itching and tingling on end of nose.

Mouth: Very dry, thirst, loss of appetite with aversion to meat.

Stomach: Nausea, incessant and deathly, faintness, constant retching, nausea and vomiting on rising up.

Abdomen: Tympanitis.

Urinary: Strangury, slow and difficult urination, uraemia.

Heart: Alternation of tachycardia and bradycardia, pulse small weak, dicrotic.

Respiratory: Faint and struggling for breath, diaphragmatic paralysis, hiccough, dyspnoea, paroxysmal on first falling asleep. Dry hard teasing, exhausting cough, worse at night, strangling cough with viscid mucus sputum.

Extremities: Numbness.

Skin: Livid. purple spots, Zoster, like herpes, itching, skin lost its elasticity, urticaria appearing at climaxis.

Nervous: Extremely susceptible to pain. Delirium, melancholic in character.

Neuralgia intense painful, multiple neuritis, bed feels too hard, aggravation after sleep. Neuralgia after Zoster/.

Sleep: Yawning, drowsy, prolonged deep sleep. Sleepless, restless sleep with frequent startings. Sleepy but cannot sleep.

Dose: 3-6 Trituration. *(Boericke)*

Cats and other felines, and fowls, are insensible to Morph. (JHC)

423. *Moschus*

(Musk)

A remedy for hysteria and nervous paroxysms, fainting fits and convulsions, catalepsy etc. The characteristic condition being aggravation by cold, there is great sensitiveness to air. Much nervous trembling and frequent fainting. Great flatulence. Diseases do not follow normal course. Coldness. Tension in muscles, skin and mind.

Mind: Uncontrollable laughter.

Stomach: Spasmodic, nervous hiccough.

Male: Violent desire, involuntary emissions, impotence associated with diabetes.

Urine: Profuse urination, diabetes.

Respiratory: Difficult respiration, chest oppressed, cough ceases, mucus cannot be expectorated, globus hystericus.

Heart: Hysterical palpitation.

Dose: 1-3 potency. *(Boericke)*

The well-known power of musk, the perfume, to produce fainting in some by the mere smell of it, gives the chief key note for its use in homoeopathy. Faints easily, faints dead away from the least excitement, scolds and rages till she falls unconscious, globus hystericus ending in unconsciousness, faints while eating, during menses, faints from heart disease, coldness is another keynote, epileptic fits where there is rigor or chilliness. Diabetes with impotence has been cured by mosch: Mosch is suited to spoiled, sensitive natures and hysterical women and men. Among the peculiar sensations are "as if falling from a height" As if nail pressed on occiput "the point piercing the brain". *(JHC)*

424. *Mucuna Urens*

(Horse Eye)

(Hot regions of Venezuela) N.O.

Leguminosae. The pulverised bean is macerated in five times its weight of alcohol.

Clinical - Haemorrhoidal discharges. Haemorrhoids.

In New, old and Forgotten remedies (P. 220) is a letter by Delgago Palacious, of Venezuela, pointing out that the name Dolichos, given to Cowhage or Cow-itch in homoeopathic literature (See Vol. I), is not in accordance with latest botanical terminology.

Cowhage is really in Mucuna, Mucuna and Dolichos being separate genera of the Leguminosae. They are so described in the Treasury of Botany. (Allen give Linnaeus as the authority for the name Dolichos pruriens.)

Palacios has used M. Urens, with which, he says, modern botanists consider Cowhage identical; but he does not name his plant M. pruriens, an alternative name of Cowhage, and as he says, further, that M. urens is a special plant which grows in the calid regions of Venezuela" and that the beans are very difficult to obtain. I think it best to give the plant a separate notice. This is more desirable as Palacios uses an entirely different preparation. In Dolichos (I retain the name for the sake of distinction) the entire Pod is used, the stinging hairs being the most important part of it. Palacious uses the puberised bean for making his tincture. His chief use for it is in haemorrhoids and complaints arising from the haemorrhoidal diathesis. The keynote symptom is burning. There may or may not be bleeding. Affections of liver, uterus, bladder, testicles, when accompanied by haemorrhoids, are likely to be cured by M. Urens. He gives one drop daily of the tincture, and sometimes makes an ointment of it as well. He places more reliance in it than in Hamamelis and Aesc.h. There is no pathogenesis. *(JHC)*

Mucuna Urens. Common name, Horse-eye. habitat, Venezuela. Preparations - Mother tincture of the pulverised bean; and dilutions.

Dosage: Dilutions from 3x up. This remedy is useful in haemorrhoids, in the hemorrhoidal diathesis, and haematurias. *(Blackwood)*

425. *Murex*

(Purple fish)

The symptoms of the female sexual organs are most prominent and have been clinically verified. Especially adapted to nervous, lively, affectionate women, patient, weak and run down.

Female: Conscious of a womb, pulsation in neck of womb. Desire, easily excited, feeling as if something was pressing on a sore spot in the pelvis, worse sitting. Pain from right side of womb to right or left breast. Nymphomania. Least contact of parts causes violent sexual excitement. Sore pain in uterus. Menses irregular, profuse, frequent, large clots, feeling of protrusion. Prolapse, enlargement of uterus, with pelvic tenesmus and sharp pains, extending towards breasts, aggravated lying down. Dysmenorrhoea and chronic endometritis with displacement. Must keep legs tightly crossed. Leucorrhoea green or bloody, alternates with mental symptoms and aching in sacrum. Benign tumors in breast. Pain in them during menstrual period.

Dose: 3-30 potency. *(Boericke)*

Petroz first proved the "purple fish" "Murex" which like the "Ink fish" `Sepia' produces the chief intensity of its action in the female generative sphere. They are chiefly distinguished in that Murex produces frantic sexual desire and tends to have excessive haemorrhage with large clots, Sepia having in general scanty flow, consciousness of the womb, bearing down and prolapse. The pains are frequently diagonal and shoot from ovary to opposite breast - as if something were pressing on a sore spot in the pelvis. The least contact with the parts causes violent sexual excitement - frequent necessity to rise at night to urinate. This nightly polyuria with the hungry craving of Murex and other symptoms has led to its successful use in diabetes. Climacteric sufferings. Amel: putting head back - must lie down from weakness but lying down agg. All symptoms. *(JHC)*

This remedy is indicated in lively and affectionate but exhausted women who are conscious of a womb. There is a sensation as though something was pressing on a sore spot in the pelvis. They must keep the legs tightly crossed to prevent a prolapsus.

The sexual desire is easily excited, there is nymphomania, the least touch of the genital organs causes violent sexual excitement. The menses are irregular, profuse, frequent and consist of large clots. There is a leucorrhoea which alternates with the mental symptoms, and aching in the sacrum.

Compare: Sepia, Platinum, Lilium tig. *(Blackwood)*

426. *Muriatic Acidum*
(Muriatic Acid)

The acid has an elective affinity for the blood, producing a septic condition similar to that found in low fevers with temperature and great prostration. patient becomes so weak, she slides done the bed. Decomposition of fluids. Involuntary stools while passing urine. Haemorrhages. Mouth and anus chiefly affected.

Mind: Loud moaning, suffers in silence.

Head: Worse lying on right side.

Nose: Haemorrhage.

Mouth: Sordes on teeth.

Stomach: Cannot bear sight or thought of meat. Ravenous appetite and constant desire to drink. Achlorhydria and fermentation of food.

Rectum: Tendency to involuntary evacuations, while urinating. Haemorrhoids most sensitive to all touch, even sheet of toilet paper is painful. Anal itching and prolapsus ani while urinating, haemorrhoids during pregnancy, bluish hot with violent stitches.

Heart: Feeble and small, intermits every third beat.

Dose: First to third potency.

(Boericke)

It is manufactured from salt (nat. mur) by the action of Sulphuric acid. Stupefying headache. Obscuration of sight and optical illusions. Whizzing noises in the ears and hardness of hearing, nose bleed and loss of smell, rough cracked lips and foul breath, scurvy of mouth, paralysis of tongue, loss of taste, distended, sensitive abdomen, pricking bruised pain in abdominal walls, serous, fetid diarrhoea, not very painful, involuntary stool, throat pains, paralysis of bladder, excited sexual desire, impotence, hoarseness, spasmodic cough, stitches about heart. Like Nit ac., Mur ac. is a powerful antidote to Merc. Piles like a bunch of grapes which look purple and burn when touched. Prolapse of rectum.

The skin is much affected and is sensitive to the sun's rays, eczema solare, freckles. Mur. ac. is a constituent of the gastric juice and must therefore be considered as allied to the sarcodes and proximate of the tissues eg: Cholesterin. Caustion: Sun.

(JHC)

It is of service in malignant affections of the mouth and throat, as are met with in certain cases of scarlatina, cancer, and diphtheria when the secondary septic condition is paramount. The mucous membrane is studded with ulcers, which are deep and perforating and have a black or dark base. The breath is foul and offensive.

It is indicated in achlorhydria and fermentation of the food when the tongue and mucous membranes are inclined to be pale; the papillae are greatly elongated and while red at the base are constantly tipped with white. The salivary secretion is scanty. Stool passes involuntarily while urinating. Haemorrhoids which are blue, swollen, and sensitive to touch; so sensitive that he cannot bear to have them touched ever so gently.

(Blackwood)

427. *Mygale Lasiodora*
(Black Cuban spider)

Weakness, palpitation, nervousness, fear, like other spider preparations. Chorea is the principal therapeutic field of this; sexual symptoms are important.

Face: Twitching of facial muscles, mouth and eyes open in rapid succession. Hot and flushed. Grating of teeth at night.

Extremities: Unsteady gait, constant motion of whole body, uncontrollable movements of arms and legs.

Dose: 3-30 potency. *(Boericke)*

The sphere of Myg. in chorea has been developed from the clinical side. In the cases cured with it, twitching and contractions of facial muscles have been very prominent, convulsive movements of head to right side, twitching of one side of body, mostly right. The limbs are quiet during sleep. Movements agg. morning, sitting (legs in constant motion) *(JHC)*

This remedy is indicated in chorea. The face is hot and flushed and there is twitching of the facial muscles, or one side of the body is convulsively twitched and uncontrollable. There is relief during sleep, but the symptoms return with greater severity in the morning.

Compare - Agaricin, Tarentula.
(Blackwood)

428. *Musa*
(Banana)

Jonner proved the tincture of Banana flowers produced costiveness and sensation of fullness about anus in a person of regular habits, and he cured with it a bad case of bleeding haemorrhoids. It also produced pain in the bladder and passage of mucus with urine. 'Crichton Campbell' commends bananas baked in their skin as an ideal food or even a cure for brain workers, nervous persons and anaemics. A syrup made with the juice of bananas extracted by heat is commended as a remedy in chronic bronchitis with insufficient expectoration and marked dyspnoea. *(JHC)*

429. *Myrica Cerifera*
(Bay bery)

Marked action on the liver with jaundice and mucous membranes. Persistent sleeplessness. Jaundice.

Mind: Despondent, Irritable, indifferent, gloony.

Head: Dull, heavy aching in temples and forehead on waking in the morning.

Mouth: Tenacious, thick, nauseous secretion. Tender, spongy and bleeding gums.

Stomach: Taste bitter and nauseous with offensive breath.

Abdomen: Dull pain in the region of liver. Complete jaundice with bronze yellow skin, loss of appetite.

Stool: Constant discharge of flatus when walking. Urging to stool with no other results than the expulsion of a great amount of flatus, loose, light-coloured stool, ash-coloured and destitute of bile.

Urinary: Dark, frothy, scanty, high-coloured, biliary.

Sleep: Insomnia.

Extremities: Pain under shoulder blades and back of neck in all muscles, in hollow of right foot.

Skin: Yellow and itching, jaundice.

Dose: Tincture to 3rd potency.
(Boericke)

According to Hale, though Myrica was known to older botanic practitioners, it was Samuel Thomson, of Lobelia fame who established its reputation. Thomson had a crude pathology of his own which served him to some extent. One of his ideas was that the digestive tract was liable to become fouled with a copious mucous lining. This he called canker and he stated of Myrica that it has the power of disengaging the thick, viscid secretions of the mucous membrane of the stomach. Myrica, says Hela, formed the chief ingredient in Thomson's powder. The provings confirm Thomson's observation, that Myrica produced abundant secretion of tenacious mucus in the throat, difficult to detach. This may be considered one of the Keynotes of the remedy. Profuse catarrhal discharges of old standing, of all kinds may require `Myrica', especially if offensive, tenacious and difficult to detach. Leucorrhoea, bronchorrhoea, intestinal catarrh, pharyngeal catarrh, stomatitis. Hale says as a local application in diphtheria it rivals Guaiacum. Perhaps allied to the catarrhal state of the intestinal tract is the liver disorder set up by the drug. These are the distinctive features: Aching pain in the liver, fullness, drowsiness, despondency, dull, heavy headache agg: in morning, dirty, dingy, yellowish white of eyes, lids abnormally red, weakness, ash-coloured stools, slow pulse, pains under scapulae (Agg: left), dirty yellow tongue, muscular soreness, aching in limbs, jaundice of all degrees. There is also the nasal obstruction, post-nasal catarrh which often accompanies disordered liver. It is in cases attended with jaundice that Myrica has had the greatest success, cases of black jaundice having been cured with it, and it meets the itching of jaundice as well. Urticaria is not unfrequently found associated with liver affections, and Douglass cured with it this case: Miss 0,18, complained of itching and stinging on face, neck, right forearm and leg. Sensation as if insects crawling on face, must brush them away. Skin yellowish. Tongue thickly coated yellow. Felt sick all over and rather irritable. Myrica 6x every two hours improved at once and cured in ten days. Burnett has used Myrica with excellent effect in cancerous and other grave diseases of the liver, especially when attended with jaundice. He has given material doses. It has generally been given in the lower attenuations. Myrica has also an action on the heart, and is thus closely related to Digitalis in several points. There are sharp pains about the heart with increased, audible pulsations but slow pulse. The heart pains are agg: on lying left side. Pains in left chest and under scapulae (especially left), and pain middle lobe of right lung. The symptoms are: Agg. by warmth of bed; after sleep; in morning; by motion. Amel: after breakfast; in open air.

430. Myristica Sebifera

(Brazilian Uncuba)

A remedy of great antiseptic powers. Inflammation of skin, cellular tissue and periosteum. Traumatic infections parotitis. Fistulas. Carbuncles. Specific action in panaritium. Pain in the finger nails with swelling of the phalanges. Hands are stiff, as if from squeezing something a long time. Coppery taste and burning in throat. Tongue white and cracked. Phlegmonous inflammations. Hastens suppuration and shortens its duration. Often does away with use of the knife. Inflammation of middle ear, suppurative stage. Fistula in ano. Acts more powerfully often than Hepar or Silica.

(Boericke)

Myr. seb. has evidently great power over suppurative process affecting joints. Hansen says Kippax regards it as the principal remedy in Elephantiasis Arabum. *(JHC)*

431. Naja Tripudians

(Virus of Cobra)

Naja produces a typical bulbar paralysis (L.J. Boyd), causes no haemorrhage but only oedema, hence the victims of this reptile frequently bear very little sign of external injury, a small scratch or puncture being the only indication, where the fangs have worked their havoc. The tissue lying beneath the wound is coloured dark purple, and a large quantity of viscid blood like fluid collects in the vicinity of the wound. An intense burning pain at the spot bitten is the first symptom. In man there follows an interval before fresh symptoms occur. The average is about an hour. Once developed the symptoms follow a rapid course. A feeling of intoxication is produced, followed by a loss of power over the limbs. The patient is bereft of speech, swallowing and the control over the movement of the lips. The saliva is ejected in large quantities, the respiration gradually becomes slower and slower and at length ceases. Conscious all the time. Is not a haemorrhagic or septic medicine like Lachesis and Crotalus. Its action settles around the heart, valvular troubles. Marked surging of blood upwards, marked dyspnoea, inability to lie on left side. Hypertrophy and valvular lesions. Organs seem to be drawn together. Very susceptible to cold with heart symptoms. Pain in forehead and temples. Diseases primarily depending upon degeneration of motor cells. Control of sphincters lost.

Head: Pain in left temple and in left orbital region extending to occiput with nausea and vomiting.

Respiratory: Irritating dry cough, dependent on cardiac lesions.

Heart: Dragging and anxiety in praecordia. Feeling of weight on heart. Angina pains extending to nape of neck, left shoulder and arm with anxiety and fear of death. With the heart symptoms, pain in forehead and temples. Pulse irregular in force. Threatened paralysis of heart, body cold, pulse slow, weak, irregular, tremulous. Acute and chronic endocarditis. Palpitation. Stitching pain in region of heart. Damaged heart after infectious diseases. Marked symptom of low tension.

Sleep: Profound like a log, with stertorous breathing, a typical reptilian state.

Modalities: Worse from use of stimulants. Better from walking or riding in open air.

Dose: 6-30 potency. *(Boericke)*

The hooded snake of Hindustan. The hot iron symptom and weight on the chest should be especially noted. After the first dose she felt awful heat in her system.

Majumdar has saved a number of apparently hopeless cases of cholera with Naja in the collapse stage, with pulselessness and difficulty of breathing - grasping at throat with the choking sensations.

Mahlon Preston cured himself with Naja 30 of asthma with difficult breathing.

Agg: lying down, amel: siting up. Causatio-grief. *(JHC)*

432. *Naphthaline*

(A chemical compound from coal tar)

Coryza, hay fever, phthisis - pulmonalis, also gonorrhoea have been influenced favourably by this drug. Pyelonephritis. Irritation of the periphery of the urinary apparatus. Whooping cough.

Eyes: It produces detachment of the retina, cataract, opacity of the cornea.

Respiratory: Sneezing, hay fever, spasmodic asthma, dyspnoea and sighing inspiration, emphysema in the aged with asthma, whooping cough.

Dose: 3rd trituration. *(Boericke)*

The hay fever sufferers who went into factories where Naphtha was much used were always cured. Leading indication for it are : Acute coryza with fluent excoriating discharge and much sneezing. Paroxysms of coughing following each other in rapid succession, so that the patient is unable to take his breath as in asthma and whooping cough. He has found it more often indicated than any other drug in whooping cough. The spasmodic action and the cyanosis of the drug are good indications here, though it is not necessary to wait till the child is blue before prescribing Naph. If any remedy is needed after Naph., Drosera follows admirably. In a case of phthisis of left lung, Naph removed these symptoms. Unable to sleep for cough, if he dozed off, it was sure to wake him. Exhausting night sweats and during the day, thin offensive diarrhoea. 'Hartmann' uses the 1x trit, having been disappointed with higher attenuations. Another action of Naph, is on the eyes, cases of opacity of the lens having been traced to its action by a cathartic, Naph is given in doses of gr. 1/4 to gr. 1/2 four times a day for 2 days. The dose should not be given after a meal and all fats and oils should be abstained from during the treatment, which may be repeated once or twice after leaving a week's interval. (The nose irritation in the poisoned cat is significant of the vermicide actin of Naph.) *(JHC)*

When given freely to dogs, cataracts have formed.

This remedy is indicated in whooping cough, when there are long-continued paroxysms of coughing. The patient is unable to breathe on account of the coughing. During the paroxysm the face becomes purple, the perspiration starts and there is expectoration of a quantity of thick, tenacious mucus.

Naphthalin is frequently preventive in its effects; while in its curative sphere it is second only to Allium cepa.

It is useful in spasmodic attacks of cough due to bronchitis, asthma and hay asthma, which are relieved while in the open air. There is fullness in the frontal region, soreness in the chest and stomach, so he has to loosen the clothing.

It should be remembered in pulmonary emphysema, dependent upon the playing of wind instruments. There is great dyspnoea with a sighing inspiration. The patient is better from violent motion.

It relieves gonorrhoea after the acute stage has passed; there is a violent desire to urinate, the meatus urinarius is reddened and tumefied and there is oedema of the prepuce. *(Blackwood)*

433. *Natrum Arsenicum*

(Arsenite of Sodium)

A remedy for nasal catarrh, with headache, pain at the root of the nose dry and painful eyes. Psoriasis (Ars., chrysoph.

Ac., thyroid). Bronchitis of children over seven years. Facilitates the termination of the cold and conserves strength and appetite.

Nose: Feels stopped, pain at root.

Throat: Purplish, swollen, oedematous, oppression of chest and about heart.

Dose: 3-30th potency. *(Boericke)*

The principal clinical use of Nat. ars has been in diphtheria (dark purple throat, great swelling, much prostration-not much pain, and in affections of the eyes and nose and root of nose. *(JHC)*

434. *Natrum Carb*

(Carbonate of sodium)

All the natrums stimulate cellular activity and increase oxidation and metabolism. Great debility, caused by summer heat, chronic effects of sunstroke exhaustion, anaemia, milky watery skin, very weak ankles are all peculiar natrum carbonicum conditions.

Head/mind: Sensitive to presence of certain individuals, headaches from slightest mental exertion, worse from sun or working under gas light.

Nose: Catarrh, bad smell of nasal secretion, posterior nasal catarrh. Hawking much mucus from throat, worse slightest drought.

Face: Freckles, yellow spots, pimples, swelling of upper lip. Pale with blue rings around eyes and swollen lids.

Stomach: Hungry at 5 a.m., very weak digestion. Averse to milk, old dyspeptics always belching, have sour stomach and rheumatism, dyspepsia relieved by soda biscuits.

Bowels: Sudden call to stool, escapes with haste and noise. Yellow substance like pulp of orange in discharge, diarrhoea from milk.

Extremities: Easy dislocation and spraining of ankles.

Skin: Inclination to perspire easily or dry, rough, cracked skin. Eruption on finger tips, knuckles and toes.

Mod: (Worse) sitting, from music, summer heat, mental exertion, thunderstorm, sun. (Better) by morning, by boring in ears and nose.

Dose: 6th potency. *(Boericke)*

Nat. C forms the alkaline basis in most soaps and most persons know by experience the effect of using soap with an excess of alkali leaves the skin dry and cracked - a true remedy for chapped hands and faces, rough, dry skins, eczema, herpes, warts, and scrofulous conditions of skin. Averse to society even that of their own family. The nearest analogue of Nat. c. in this and in the female sexual sphere is Sepia. The nervous system is strongly affected and symptoms of hysteria appear - he falls without any apparent cause. Ankle joints are weak and burn. Twitching in muscles and limbs - I have cured with Nat. c. jerking of hands on going to sleep. A peculiar symptom of nat. c. is discharge of mucus after an embrace in the woman and sterility as a result, the woman complained that she could not retain the semen, after the embrace. Agg. from sun, heat, gas light, amel. boring into ears and nose with fingers. *(JHC)*

This agent establishes a catarrhal condition of the alimentary tract.

It is useful in hypochlorhydria. There are sour eructations and a weak, gone feeling in the stomach. He is worse from eating starchy food. There are large quantities of gas formed. The slightest error of diet caused distress. *(Blackwood)*

435. Natrum Muriaticum

(Chloride of Sodium)

The prolonged taking of excessive salt causes profound nutritive changes to take place in the system, and there arise not only the symptoms of salt retention as evidenced by dropsies and oedemas, but also an alteration in the blood causing a condition of anaemia and leucocytosis. There seems also to be a retention in the tissues of effected materials giving rise to symptoms, loosely described as gouty or rheumatic gout. The provings are full of such symptoms. A great remedy for certain forms of intermittent fever, anaemia, chlorosis, many disturbances of the alimentary tract, and skin. Great debility, maximum weakness felt in the morning in bed. Coldness, emaciation most notable in neck. Great liability to take cold. Dry mucous membranes. Constrictive sensation throughout the body. Great weakness and weariness. Oversensitive to all sorts of influences.

Hyperthyroidism - Goitre - Addisons disease. Diabetes.

Mind: Consolation aggravates, gets into passion about trifles.

Head: Blinding headache, as if a thousand little hammers were knocking on the brain, after menstruation, sun rise to sunset, anaemic headache of school-girls, chronic headache, from sunrise to sunset, relieved by sleep.

Eyes: Feel bruised with headache in school children, muscles weak and stiff, stricture of lachrymal duct with suppuration. Escape of Muco-pus when pressing upon sac - Tears stream down face on coughing, asthenopia, insufficiency of internal recti muscles. Pain in eyes when looking down, cataract incipient.

Nose: Violent fluent coryza like raw white of egg, infalliable for stopping a cold commencing with sneezing, use 30th potency, loss of smell and taste.

Face: Oily, shiny as if greased, fever blisters.

Mouth: Numbness, tingling of tongue, vesicles like pearls on lips, deep crack in middle of lower lip, tongue mapped, immoderate thirst.

Stomach: Hungry yet loose flesh, sweats while eating, craving for salt, aversion to bread, to anything slimy, like oysters, fats.

Rectum: Constipation, stool dry crumbling. Painless and copious diarrhoea.

Urine: Has to wait a long time for it to pass if others were present.

Female: Menses irregular, usually profuse, vagina dry, leucorrhoea acrid, watery, bearing down pains, prolapsus uteri.

Respiratory: Cough, spurting of urine, shortness of breath especially on going upstairs, whooping cough with flow of tears.

Heart: Tachycardia, intermittent pulse, intermits on lying down.

Extremities: Pain in back, with desire for some firm support, palms hot and perspiring, hangnails, dryness and cracking about finger nails, numbness and tingling, coldness of legs.

Skin: Greasy, oily, especially on hairy parts, urticaria, itch and burn, crusty eruptions in bends of limbs, margins of scalp, warts on palms of hands, worse eating salt, at sea shore.

Fever: chill between 9 and 11 a.m., coldness of the body, hydraemia in chronic malarial states, with weakness, constipation, loss of appetite etc., sweats on every exertion.

Mod: (Worse) about 10 a.m., at sea shore, consolation, heat, (better) open air, cold bathing, going without regular meals.

Relation: Apis, Sepia, Ignatia.

Dose: 12 to 30 and higher.

Best results higher potencies - infrequent dosage. *(Boericke)*

If Nat. carb is the typical salt of the Natrum group (as Kali carb is of the Kalis), Nat. m. is the most important. Without restricting the amount of salt taken Nat. m. 30 will antidote most of the crude, and enable the patient to cut down the quantity taken afterwards. The relation to catarrh which Schussler brings out, is specific. Excessively fluent coryza with much sneezing, sore nose, especially the left wing, cold sores on lips and nose, loss of smell and taste are indications which I have verified repeatedly in acute colds and the tendency to them. With the coryza there is copious lachrymation. When ever there is a history of cauterisation and Arg. N. has been used Nat. m. will do great good. Lambert has recorded several cases of headache associated with errors of refraction and consequent eye strain cured with nat. m. 30. In aphthous and ulcerative condition of the mouth it is a leading remedy. The characteristic tongue of nat. m. is either a mapped tongue with red islands or a clean shining tongue with froth along each side. Nat. m. corresponds to children who are late in talking. One very characteristic effect is dryness of vagina, with painful coitus - aversion to coitus. Menses may be early and profuse, scanty and delayed. Backache generally accompanies this and the backache has this peculiarity that it is Amel. by pressure, by lying down with the back on something hard. The headaches come on in the morning on first waking up and last throughout the day - or else they come on at 10 or 11 a.m. Nat. m. is one of the first remedies for headaches of school girls. Nat. m. is a great heart remedy. Fluttering palpitation with faint feeling agg. lying down. In one case of huge hypertrophy with degeneration of most of the valves, the patient told me, nothing gave her so much relief as Nat. m. (which I had given for some incidental condition) - great hunger, with no appetite. Eats heartily but emaciates - grows thin especially about neck - it not only antidotes quinine but it causes intermittents on its own account. Chilliness predominates. Chill 10 to 11 a.m. with thirst. Agg. at seaside or cannot stay by the sea, nat. m. will probably be the remedy; but Amel. at sea side may also indicate it. Agg. after sleep, 10 to 11 am; during full moon.

Relations: Nat. m. is the chronic of Ignatia. *(JHC)*

Synopsis: Great emaciation, losing flesh while living well. Headache from sunrise to sunset - Amel. by perspiration. Children slow in learning to walk. Has to wait a long while for urine to pass, if others are present. For the bad effects of anger, acid food, bread, quinine, excessive use of salt or reserved displeasure. Craving for salt, great aversion to bread - Agg. from eating too much salt, at sea shore, from ocean voyage-complementary to Apis - N.M.

is chronic of Ign. - followed well by Sepia and Thuja. Cannot often be repeated in chronic cases - Amel: open air, cold bathing; going without regular meals.

436. *Natrum Nitricum*

(Nitrate of Sodium)

Nat. n. was 'Rademachers' Aconite. He used it in inflammations of all kinds, especially laryngo-tracheitis and croup, acute pneumonia, acute rheumatism and heart affections, purpura, haemorrhages, inflammations of the eye, exophthalmic Goitre. (Hansen). *(JHC)*

A Rademacherian remedy for inflammation - Influenza - nose bleed. Dose: 2x, also watery solution 1 dram of salt to 8 oz. water. Dram doses. *(Boericke)*

This remedy has been employed during the stage of congestion for much the same indications as those calling for Aconite. *(Blackwood)*

437. *Natrum Phos*

(Phosphate of Sodium)

Natrum phos. is the remedy for conditions arising from excess of lactic acid, often resulting from too much sugar. Ailments with excess of acidity. Sour eructations and taste. Sour vomiting. Yellow, creamy coating at the back of the roof of mouth and tongue. Inflammation of any part of the throat, with sensation of lump in throat. Flatulence with sour risings. Colic with symptoms of worms. Cracking of joints. Jaundice (1x). Oxaluria.

Mind: Fear.

Eyes: Discharge of golden yellow, creamy matter.

Ears: One ear red hot, frequently itchy, accompanied by gastric derangements and acidity.

Face: Paleness of bluish, florid appearance of face.

Mouth: Blisters on tip of tongue. Thin, moist coating on the tongue. Yellow creamy coating at the posterior part of the roof of the mouth.

Stomach: Sour eructations, sour vomiting, greenish diarrhoea.

Male: Weakness in back and trembling in limbs.

Extremities: Rheumatism of knee joint.

Back: Synovial crepitation, rheumatic arthritis.

Skin: Itching in various parts, especially of ankles, hives.

Relation: Natrum lactic (rheumatism and gout, gouty concretions, rheumatism with diabetes).

Dose: 3-12x, in Jaundice 1x. (Boericke)

Through the presence of Nat. p., lactic acid is decomposed into carbonic acid and water - nat. p. is the remedy for those diseases which are caused by an excess of lactic acid. It therefore answers to the diseases of infants who having been fed with excess of milk and sugar, and suffer from redundant acids. Uric acid is dissolved in the blood by two factors, the warmth of the blood and Nat. phos. If uric acid is deposited from its solution in the joints or near them, owing to a deficiency of Nat. p., or when it combines with the base of carbonate of soda into urate of soda, which is insoluble, then there arises podagra or acute arthritic rheumatism. Nat. p. also serves to saponify the fatty acids. It therefore cures those dyspeptic ailments which arise from eating fat food or which are aggravated thereby - he had much itching at the ankle joints with an eczematous eruption. Fear especially at night, that something would happen - nat. p. 6x cured promptly.

Causation: Sugar, milk, fat food, thunder storms.

Great itching of scrotum, prepuce and arms, Rheumatic pain in Rt. shoulder, feels nervous, shooting pains from neck over R. shoulder - Itching papules Rt. ear, about joints. Itching of scrotum, prepuce, and anus - chafing of skin - eczema with acidity, honey coloured secretion - crusta lactea. Golden yellow scabs. *(JHC)*

438. Natrum Salicylicum

(Salicylate of Sodium)

Has an extensive range of action affecting the head, ear, throat, kidneys and liver and on metabolism. Haemorrhages, especially epistaxis. Produces marked effects upon the internal ear, with vertigo, deafness, noises in ears and loss of bone conduction, hence its use in Menier's disease. One of the best remedies for the prostrating after-effects of influenza. Lassitude, drowsiness, listlessness, tremor. Incipient dementia. Increases the quantity of the bile. Follicular tonsillitis.

Head: All objects seem move to the right.

Ears: Tinnitus of a low tone, deafness, auditory vertigo.

Dose: 3rd potency.

Non-Homoeopathic uses: In acute articular rheumatism, lumbago, sciatica, etc. usual doses 10-20 grains every 3 hours. Must be used carefully, as it is often destructive of kidney tissue. Ordinary allopathic doses allay the pain of dysmenorrhoea and promote menstrual flow. *(Boericke)*

The most marked and persistent of the symptoms produced by Nat. Sal. is giddiness agg: on rising from lying, and intense tinnitus aurium with deafness. This combination of symptoms has led to the successful homoeopathic use of Nat. Sal. in Meniers disease and similar conditions. Nat. sal. has evidently an affinity for the joints, since it causes many of its poisoning symptoms, simultaneously with the removal of the joint pains of gout and rheumatism. *(JHC)*

While this agent possesses many of the properties of Salycylic acid, it is more readily soluble, it is irritating to the stomach to a limited extent. It is a diaphoretic and cholagogue and increases the fluidity of the bile and its secretion. Large doses (twenty grains) have produced suppression of the gastric fluids and an interference with digestion, alarming prostration, mental and physical; with a weak compressible slow pulse and a subnormal temperature, an erythema and urticaria developed which became petechial, with haemorrhagic extravasations, which subsequently formed slough and ulcers. This was attended with myalgic and arthritic pains.

It should be remembered in cases of progressive deafness due to a chronic catarrh. It is of service in Menier's disease, when there is vertigo, tinnitus aurium and deafness. It has been employed in relief of the prostration that follows influenza, when there are vertigo, noises in the head, with weakness and mental depression. *(Blackwood)*

439. *Natrum Sulph*

(Sulphate of Sodium)

A liver remedy, especially indicated for the so-called hydrogenoid constitutions, where the complaints are such as are due to living in damp houses, basements, cellars. They are worse in rainy weather, water in any form. Feels every change from dry to wet; cannot even eat plants growing near water, nor fish. Always feels best in warm, dry air. Clinically, it has been found tobe a valuable remedy for spinal meningitis. Head symptoms from injuries to head, mental troubles thereafter. Every spring return of skin affections. Tendency to warts. Fingers and toes affected. Chronic gout.

Mind: Periodical attacks of mania, suicidal tendency, must exercise restraint. Dreams of running water.

Mouth: Bitter taste.

Stomach: Brown, bitter coating on tongue, yellow complexion, acid dyspepsia with heart burn and flatulence.

Abdomen: Duodenal catarrh, hepatitis, icterus, vomiting of bile, liver sore to touch with sharp stitching pains, cannot bear tight clothing around waist, flatulence, diarrhoea, yellow watery stools, loose morning stools. Stools involuntary, when passing flatus. Great size of the faecal mass.

Urine: Excessive secretion, diabetes.

Female: Nose bleed during menses, leucorrhoea, yellowish green, following gonorrhoea in female.

Male: Condylomata, soft, fleshy excrescences.

Respiratory: Dyspnoea, during damp weather, must hold chest when coughing, humid asthma, rattling in chest at 4 and 5 a.m., asthma in children.

Back: Itching when undressing, violent pains in back of neck and at base of brain.

Extremities: Swelling of axillary glands, inflammation around roof of nails, burning soles, oedema of feet, compels frequent change in position. Pain in hip joints, worse left, stiffness of knees, cracking of joints, rheumatism worse in damp cold weather.

Skin: Itching while undressing, wart like red lumps all over body.

Relationship: Malaria officinalis — (Decomposed vegetable matter. Has evident power to cause the disappearance of the Plasmodium of Malaria - 6th potency and higher. Pulmo Vulpis - Wolfs lung - (persistent shortness of breath causing a paroxysm of Asthma on the slightest motion.)

Complementary: Ars., Thuja.

Dose: 1st to 12th trituration. *(Boericke)*

"Grauvogl" who found in it the typical remedy for his hydrogenoid constitution. Extreme sensitiveness to damp, wetting, bathing, watery foods and residence near fresh water, especially standing in water. Periodicity is also another feature of this state. This constitution, he considered, is providing the soil for gonorrhoeal infection. Nat. mur causes the splitting up of the cells necessary for their multiplication. Nat. sul withdraws water from the superannuated leucocytes and thus causes their destruction. The latter salt is therefore a remedy for leucaemia - Nat sul. is also intended to stimulate the functions of the nerves of the biliary apparatus of the pancreas and of the intestines. If the sensory nerves of the bladder are not stimulated by Nat. sul. the impulse to void urine does not come to man's consciousness, thence there follows involuntary micturition (wetting the bed). Nat. sul. is Schussler's specific for epidemic influenza

- Grauvogl and Schussler used Nat. sul in the lower triturations, but homeopaths need not confine themselves to any. When the correspondence is exact the highest attenuations will act better than the lower. When the likeness is more general the lower will give the best results. Irritability agg. morning. There is also cheerfulness after loose stools. A case of panaritum is reported. Amel: out of doors. Nat sul. 30 in water, a teaspoonful every two hours. Pain ceased rapidly. Attacks of Asthma frequently occur in the early morning hours Leonard has cured with Nat. sul 200x a very violent asthma - Sleep was disturbed by dreams of fighting - Pains flying from the chest beginning with a dry cough. *(JHC)*

This agent in small doses is a laxative, aparient and diuretic. It excites the secretions of the intestines and stimulates the activity of the intestinal glands, liver and pancreas.

He feels every change from dry to wet, and cannot eat even plants that grow near water. It is useful in morning diarrhoea, that is worse, when first rising and standing on the feet. The passage is sudden, urging, gushing, and is attended with much flatus. It is worse from damp weather or living in damp basements. It is one of the most useful remedies in epilepsy, and the mental effects from injuries of the cranium, when there is an osseous depression. *(Blackwood)*

440. *Niccolum*

(Metallic Nickel)

Periodic nervous sick headaches with asthenopia, weak digestion, constipation, catarrh. Suits debilitated, nervous, literary patients with frequent headaches, dyspepsia and constipation.

Head: Cracking in cervical vertebrae when moving the head. Pain on top as from a nail. Pressure on vertex, in morning, worse till noon. Objects appear too large. Migraine, first on left side, twitching of upper lip.

Nose: Violent sneezing.

Throat: Soreness to touch externally.

Gastric: Without desire for food, intense hiccough, sour, fetid secretions ooze from molar teeth, diarrhoea and tenesmus after milk.

Respiratory: Obliged to sit up and hold head. Must put arms on thighs, when coughing.

Skin: Itching all over, worse on neck, not relieved by scratching.

Dose: 3rd trituration. *(Boericke)*

Periodic headaches of a very severe character. Has cured cases when the pain is agg. 10 to 11 a.m, and may be so intense as to cause the patient to cry out. Appears first left side, may jump to right, disappears in evening - Herring says it is suited to "Literary men" and others who suffer from periodical nervous headaches. Peculiar sensations are - as if sweat would break out, must sit up and hold the head with both hands when coughing or has to put arms on thighs when coughing. *(JHC)*

441. *Nitric Acid*

Selects for its special seat of action, the outlets of the body, where the mucous membrane and skin meet; these pain as from splinters. Sticking pain. Marked improvement of all symptoms while riding in a carriage. Acts best on the dark complexioned and past middle life. Syphilis, after abuse of mercury. Pains appear and disappear quickly (Bell.). Hydrogenoid constitution, sycotic remedy.

Blisters and ulcers in mouth, tongue, genitals, bleed easily. Fissures with pain during stool as if rectum were torn. All discharges very offensive, especially urine, faeces and perspiration. Persons who have chronic diseases and take cold easily and disposed to diarrhoea. Excessive physical irritability. Cachexia due to syphilis, scrofula, intermittent fever with liver involvement and anaemia etc. Gravel, arthritis, capillary bleeding after currettage.

Mind: Irritable.

Head: Band around head.

Ears: Difficult hearing, better by riding in carriage or train, very sensitive to noise like the rattle of wagons over pavements.

Eyes: Sharp, sticking pains.

Nose: Nosebleed, corrosive discharge.

Mouth: Bleeding gums, tongue clean, red and wet with centre furrow. Teeth become loose, gums soft and spongy. Ulcers in soft palate, with sharp splinter-like pains, bloody saliva.

Throat: Sharp points as from splinters.

Stomach: Loves fat and salt.

Abdomen: Violent cutting pains after stools lasting for hours; Haemorrhoids bleed easily. Diarrhoea slimy and offensive.

Urine: Offensive, smells like horses' urine, cold on passing.

Male: Soreness and burning in glans and beneath prepuce, ulcers, burn and sting, exude offensive matter.

Female: External parts sore with ulcers. Leucorrhoea brown, flesh coloured, watery or stringy, offensive.

Respiratory: Short breath on going upstairs.

Extremities: Fetid foot sweat causing soreness of toes with sticking pain.

Sweating of palms, hands. Cold, blue nails. Offensive sweat in axillae at night.

Modalities: (Worse) evening and night, cold climate and also hot weather. (Better) while riding in carriage.

Dose: 6th potency.

As the Nitric acid patient begins to improve skin symptoms may appear for a time; favourable indication. *(Boericke)*

Hahnemann's three miasms, psora, syphilis, and sycosis, and Nit acid belongs almost equally to all three. In his directions about this remedy, Hahnemann makes the remark that it is rarely required by patients who suffer from constipation. "In my experience this is absolutely wrong. Constipation, as the symptoms of the Schema would indicate is a prominent indication for Nit. ac. and I have cured almost as many cases with this as with any other single remedy - slimy stools, from excess of mucus passed with much straining. A key note of Nit. ac. stools whether loose or constipated is "pain after stool." Among the haemorrhages of Nit. ac. is haematuria. Urine of strong odor, like horses' or extremely offensive. Fetid sweats on feet, hands, or in axilla, no less point to Nit. ac. - Nit. ac. has borborygmus as if a boiler was working in bowels. A characteristic accompaniment of Nit. ac. is profuse sweat breaks out on hands and feet. J.H. Fulton cured with one dose of Nit. ac. 200. R.M. 28 who had bleeding piles for eighteen months. He had frequent bloody and slimy stools, but always bright red blood after stools from a desert spoonful to half a teacupful - Brownish scattered spots in dark haired people. *(JHC)*

When this agent is applied to the skin in the diluted form it produces a yellow discoloration; when stronger preparations are applied it causes bulbous eruptions.

When administered internally the stronger preparation occasions vomiting, pain, and sloughing of the mucous membranes.

Small doses act as a stimulant to the intestinal glands, but should it be continued over a long period it will produce salivation, spongy and bleeding gums, foulness of the breath, loosening of the teeth, dyspepsia, colic, headache and debility. *(Blackwood)*

442. *Nitro-Muriatic acid*

(Aqua Regia)

Almost a specific in oxaluria. Removes the distressing skin symptoms, resembling psoriasis. Three to five drops TDS. So called bilious conditions, torpid liver, hepatitis and early cirrhosis of liver. More adapted to hepatic torpor and gastric catarrh common in hot and damp climate and aggravated by meat eating and alcohol, constricted anus, gravel.

Mouth: Ptyalism, constant drooling at night, salivation worse at night. Stool constipated, with ineffectual urging.

Urine: Cloudy, burning in urethra, oxaluria.

Dose: 5-10 drops well diluted. *(Boericke)*

Nit. mur. ac. has been proved in the lower dilutions and in the 30th, and some experiments have been made by Dr. Scott, who acidulated his bath with this acid - salivation and sore mouth and throat with dysphagia were produced in Scott and the provers - Scott noticed that the salivation was intermittent. Nat. mur. ac. has a clinical reputation in oxaluria and gravel. *(JHC)*

A yellow liquid, being the Aqua regia of the earlier chemists. It is a mixture of Nitric and Hydrochloric acids. This agent in toxic quantities acts as corrosive poison like its constituents. Small doses destroy the dental enamel and gold filling in the teeth and induce a gastric derangement. When employed over a prolonged period, diluted as a bath, it is absorbed and increases the renal and hepatic secretions, produces a feeling of burning in the mouth and fauces, and produces ptyalic redness and tumefaction of the gums, and ulcers of the bucccal mucous membrane and occasions diarrhoea. *(Blackwood)*

443. *Nuphar Luteum*

(Yellow Pond Lily)

Produces nervous weakness, with marked symptoms in the sexual sphere.

Male: Complete absence of sexual desire, parts relaxed, penis retracted.

Impotence with involuntary emissions during stool, when urinating. Spermatorrhoea. Pain in testicles and penis.

Relation: Agnus, Kali brom, Lycop., Selen, Yohimbinum

Dose: Tr. to 6th potency. *(Boericke)*

Nuphar Luteum, the yellow pond lily was proved by Pitet and many of his symptoms have been clinically confirmed. Most marked was yellow diarrhoea coming on in the early hours of the morning - with the diarrhoea is great exhaustion. Nuph. has cured many cases of diarrhoea, so characterised - excessive depression of the male generative system and Nuphar has done good work in analogous conditions.

Agg: 4 to 6 a.m. *(JHC)*

This remedy is indicated in impotence. There is complete absence of all sexual desire, with involuntary emission during stool and when urinating. The organs are relaxed, the penis is retracted, and there is pain in the testicles.

It is of service in morning diarrhoea. The stool is liquid, of a light yellow color. The call is urgent. There are three or four stools and no more till the next morning.

Compare: Gamboge, Sulphur, Agnus castus, Selenium. *(Blackwood)*

444. Nux Moschata

(Nut meg)

Marked tendency to fainting fits with heart failure. Cold extremities, extreme dryness of mucous membranes and skin. Strange feeling, with irresistible drowsiness. Indicanuria - General inclination to become unconscious during acute attacks. Lypothymia (Ignatia), staggers on trying to walk.

Mind: Changeable, laughing and crying.

Head: Bursting headache, better hard pressure.

Mouth: Very dry. Tongue adheres to roof of mouth, but no desire for water. Saliva like cotton.

Stomach: Excessively bloated, flatulent dyspepsia.

Abdomen: Paralytic weakness of intestines. Enormously distended, stool is soft and yet unable to expel it. Faintness during or after stool.

Female: Variability of menstruation, irregularity of time and quantity.

Sleep: Complaints cause sleepiness, coma.

Fever: Want of perspiration.

Relation: Ornithogalum (flatulence, swollen feeling across lower chest whenever she turns in bed, feels as if a bag of water turned. Also, gastric ulcer and cancer).

Dose: 1-6th potency. *(Boericke)*

Nux Mosch. is one of the many examples of powerfully poisonous and medicinal substances used as a common article of food. The Nut meg has a popular repute for putting off the menstrual period or else for bringing it on; as a remedy for diarrhoea and also for boils. Nux. m. is one of the most profoundly active of psychical remedies in the materia medica, producing states of exaltation resembling hysteria and the mesmeric state with exalted sense and consciousness of double personality. One hypersensitive patient to whom I gave a single dose of Nux m 30, said it seemed to put a coat of cotton wool over her. Chilliness may be considered the second keynote, and third dryness. Tongue so dry it adheres to the roof of the mouth. The saliva seems thick like cotton. I cured with Nux m. 30 a very bad case of indigestion with acne in a youth who had this symptom - Eyes dry; too dry to close the lids. The use of Nut meg as a condiment has doubtless its origin in the fact that Nux. m. is specifically related to weak digestion. *(JHC)*

This agent produces a disturbance of a nervous character of the digestive tract, uterus, and ovaries.

This remedy is indicated in nervous, hysterical people, and pregnant women whose complaints are attended with sleepiness in some cases, and a tendency to faint in others.

It is useful in flatulent dyspepsia. The abdomen is enormously distended after every meal. There is a nervous irritation of the intestinal tract; all the symptoms are worse after every unpleasant emotion. The mouth and throat are dry and stiff.

It is of service in diarrhoea when the stools are soft and like chopped eggs. There is loss of appetite, great sleepiness, and a tendency to faint. It should be remembered during the menstrual period, when the menses are too early and too profuse. The flow is thick and black; there is vaginal flatulence. The throat is especially dry after sleeping and there is pain in the back.

It should be remembered during pregnancy; when the stomach is distended there is difficulty in breathing, and the patient is hysterical.

It is beneficial in nervous , dry, hysterical coughs, with sudden hoarseness, nervous aphonia, oppression of the chest, and frequent fainting spells.

Compare: Asafoetida, Ignatia, Nux vomica. *(Blackwood)*

445. *Nux Vomica*

(Poison Nut)

Is the greatest of polychrests, because the bulk of its symptoms correspond in similarity with those of the commonest and most frequent of diseases. It is frequently the first remedy, indicated after much dosing, establishing a sort of equilibrium of forces and counter-acting chronic effects.

Nux is pre-eminently the remedy for many of the conditions, incident to modern life. The typical Nux patient is rather thin, square, quick, active, nervous and irritable. He does a good deal of mental work, has mental strains and leads a sedentary life, found in prolonged office work, over study, close application to business with its cares and anxieties. This indoor life and mental strain, seeks stimulants, coffee, wine, possibly in excess, or again, he hopes to quiet his excitement, by indulging in the sedative effects of tobacco, if not really a victim, to the sedactive drugs, like opium etc. These things are associated with other indulgences, at table, he takes preferably rich and stimulating food, wine and women play their part to make him forget the close application of the day. Late hours area consequence, a thick head, dyspepsia, and irritable temper are the next day's inheritance. Now he takes some cathartic, liver pills, or mineral water, and soon gets into the habit of taking these things, which still further complicate matters. Since these frailties are more yielded to by men than women. Nux is pre-eminently a male remedy. These conditions produce an irritable, nervous system, hypersensitive and over-impressionable, which Nux will do much to soothe and calm. Especially adapted to digestive disturbances, portal congestion and hypochondriacal states depending thereon. Convulsions, with consciousness, worse, touch, moving. Zealous, fiery, temperament. Nux patients are easily chilled, avoid open air etc. Nux always seem to be out of tune. Inharmonious spasmodic action.

Mind: Irritable - cannot bear noises, odors, light, etc., sullen, fault finding.

Head: Vertigo with momentary loss of consciousness, worse morning, mental exertion, tobacco, alcohol, coffee, open air, Head in the sunshine.

Nose: Stuffy colds, snuffles, stuffed up at night and out doors.

Mouth: Small aphthous ulcers with bloody saliva. Gum, swollen, white and bleeding.

Throat: Rough, scraped feeling, tickling, sensation of roughness - stitches into ear.

Stomach: Nausea in the morning after eating, weight and pain in the stomach, worse eating, some time after, flatulence and pyrosis, nausea and vomiting. Region of stomach very sensitive to pressure. Epigastrium bloated with pressure as of a stone. Several hours after eating - difficult belching of gas.

Abdomen: Bruised soreness of abdominal walls - Weakness of abdominal ring region - Umbilical hernia of infants.

Stool: Constipation with frequent ineffectual urging, feeling as if part remained un-expelled, frequent ineffectual desire, or passing but small quantities at each attempt. Absence of all desire for defaecation is a contra-indication. Itching, blind, haemorrhoids. Diarrhoea after a debauch, worse morning, frequent small evacuations, scanty stool with much urging. Dysentery, stools relieve pains for a time. Constant uneasiness in rectum.

Female: Menses too early, last too long, always irregular, blood black, prolapsus uteri, dysmenorrhoea. Metrorrhagia. Sensation as if bowels wanted to move.

Respiratory: Scraping in throat. Asthma with fullness in stomach, morning or after eating. Shallow respiration. Oppressed breathing. Tight, dry, hacking cough. Cough brings on bursting headache.

Back: Backache in lumbar region worse 3-4 a.m., must sit up in bed in order to turn.

Extremities: Arms and hands go to sleep. Legs numb - feel paralysed, cramps in calves and soles-cracking in knee joints during motion - sensation of sudden loss of power of arms and legs in the morning.

Sleep: Cannot sleep after 3 a.m. until towards morning, awakes feeling wretched-better after a short sleep.

Skin: Body burning hot specially face, yet cannot move or uncover without feeling chilly. Urticaria with gastric derangement. Acne.

Fever: Chilly, must be covered in every stage of fever. Perspiration sour. Chilliness on being uncovered, yet he does not allow being covered.

Mod: Worse - Morning, mental exertion, after eating, touch, spices, stimulants, narcotics, dry weather, cold. (Better) from a nap, if allowed to finish it, in evening while at rest, in damp wet weather, strong pressure. Nux seeds contain copper (notice the cramp causing proclivities of both.)

Comple: Sulphur, Sepia. Inimical - Zinc.

Nux is said to act best given in the evening. *(Boericke)*

Dose: 1 to 30th potency and higher.

If nitric acid be added to the seeds, a deep orange - yellow colour is produced. The wood of the tree is very bitter. It is used in India in cases of intermittent fever and snake bites. A decoction of the leaves is used externally in rheumatism. Spasms with tetanic rigidity of nearly all the muscles of the body, with interruption of a few minutes during which the muscles were relaxed. The pulse became soft and the patient recovered consciousness and speech, the spasm was renewed by the slightest touch, though at times it would immediately cease when the patient was tightly grasped or the elbow was straightened up. During the spasm, relief was afforded by forcible extension of the body - the general effect of the spasms was to cause opisthotonus and throwing back of the head, though in some, the body was spasmodically drawn sideways. Spasms is the key note of Nux and the second is exaggerated sensitiveness. The irritability and excessive sensitiveness of Nux depicted in the tetanic seizures and drawn facial expression applied to mind as well as body. Nux is especially suited to (1) Very particular, zealous persons inclined to get angry and excited or of a spiteful, malicious disposition. (2) Ardent persons or disposed to anger, spite or deception, always irritable or impatient, (3) Nervous melancholic people troubled with indigestion, venous constitution with tendency to haemorrhoids. (4) Thin, irritable, cholereic persons with dark hair, who make great mental exertion or lead a sedentary life (5)vigorous persons of dry habit, tense fibre, ardent and irascible temperament and tenacious disposition. (6) Bilious temperament. (7) Persons addicted to wine, coffee, or pepper or condiments who live a sedentary life with much mental exertion. (8) Debauches, thin, irritable, venous. (9) Drugged subjects. Spasms after eating unripe fruit and other digestive irregularities, and sometimes they take the form of incipient hernia. Hernia, inguinal, and umbilical has been cured with Nux and I have seen a case of strangulated hernia resolved by Nux, whilst preparations for operation were in progress. Constipation - Frequent ineffectual desire for stool, after the usual evacuations. The diarrhoea of Nux is sudden and drives the patient out of bed. In the dysentery the straining ceases as soon as the motion passes. Nux has proved curative in epilepsy when the fit occurred during pregnancy, hiccough, morning sickness. Lochia, scanty, offensive, nipples sore, white spot in centre. The slightest provocation suffices to excite the sexual passion. Spasms is the chief note of Nux in the respiratory sphere, where it produces a variety of asthmatic states, a dry persistent fatiguing cough. Excitement with trembling. Nux is a drowsy medicine and also produces sleeplessness. Wakes at 3 a.m. and lies awake for hours, falls asleep when it is time to rise. It is curative in cases where sleep in unattainable except from a stimulant. Amel: after undisturbed sleep. Agg: when sleep disturbed. The third key note of Nux is chilliness. It is a great remedy in intermittent fevers - cannot get warm in bed at night - coldness of whole body with blue hands - Repugnance to cold or cold air. Nux has hunger with aversion to food, loss of appetite and sudden satiety. The red face of Nux is a characteristic feature. Sour breath, I have noticed to be a very leading indication of Nux. The pressure in stomach two or three hours after eating distinguishes Nux from Nux m. and Kali bi. which have it immediately after. Nux has many eye symptoms. "Sircar" cured cases of night-blindness with Nux 6. He connected the disorder with the liver. His plan was to give Nux 30 four times daily for 4 days and see the patient again and take a new picture. The best time to give Nux is in the evening at bed time that is well away from the time of its chief aggravation. When all medicines disagree Nux will often cure the morbid sensitiveness and other troubles with it. Agg: from music. There is very great amel: for a short time after a stool - Nux and Puls have many symptoms in common, but are opposite in temperament and conditions. In clearly Nux cases, Sep. follows better than Puls - Carbo veg. often follows Nux well in ill effects of debauchery. Causation - Anger. Coffee, Alcohol, Debauchery, Masturbation, Sexual excess, injury. *(JHC)*

Adapted to irritable, careful, zealous, persons with dark hair and bilious or Sanguine temperament. Quarrelsome, spiteful, malicious, nervous and melancholic. Debauchers' ardent character, hypochondriac, literary studious persons. Over sensitive to noise, odors, light or music, every harmless word offends. Bad effects of coffee, tobacco, alcoholic stimulants, spiced or seasoned food, over-eating, mental over exertion, sedentary habits, loss of sleep. Convulsions with consciousness, Agg: anger, emotion, touch, moving - cannot keep from falling asleep in the evening, while sitting or reading hours before bed time and awakes at 3 or 4 a.m., falls into a dreamy sleep at day break from which he is hard to arouse and then feels tired and weak (rev. of Puls). Snuffles of infants - coryza, dry at night, fluent by day, Agg: in warm room, Amel: in cold air. Stomach-pressure an hour or two after eating - tightness, must loosen clothing, cannot use the mind for 2 or 3 house after a meal. Constipation with frequent unsuccessful desire, passing small quantities of faeces - sensation as if not finished, frequent desire for stool, anxious, ineffectual, amel: for a time after stool, in morning after rising, after mental exertion. Menses - too early, profuse, last too long, irregular, labor pains, cause urging to stool or to urinate, strangulated hernia, especially umbilical, backache, must sit up or turn over in bed, lumbago, from sexual weakness, from masturbation, repugnance to cold or to cold air, chilly on least movement, from being uncovered, must be covered in every stage of fever - fever, great heat, whole body burning hot, face red and hot, yet patient cannot move or uncover without being chilly. Nux should be given on retiring or what is better, several hours before going to bed, it acts best during repose of mind and body. Agg: morning, waking at 4 a.m. mental exertion, after eating or over eating, touch, noise, anger, spices, narcotics, dry weather, in cold air, amel: in evening, while at rest, lying down and in damp wet weather. *(HCA)*

Physiological action: In small does this agent is a stomachic tonic, increasing the vascularity of the gastric mucous membrane, and increasing the gastric juice, as well as the biliary and pancreatic secretions. It stimulates the peristalsis of the intestines and renders them irregular. The motor nerve cells of the spinal cord, cardiac ganglia, respiratory and vasomotor centers in the medulla are stimulated. The reflex excitability is increased. The respirations are quickened and deepened, the action of the heart is increased and the blood pressure raised. The senses are all rendered more acute. The desire to urinate is increased. It excites uterine contractions, promotes menstruation, and excites the sexual organs. *Blackwood)*

(1) Cord: (Gray Port'n) Tetanic Convulsions; Death from asphyxia. (2) Motor Nerves: exhaustion; paralysis (3) Sensory Nerves: hyperaesthesia (4) Eyes - Pupils contracted, Hyperaesthesia, vision increased (5) Ears: Hearing Augmented. (6) Nose: Sense of smell increased (7) Circulation: Vaso motor spasm; increased arterial blood pressure. (8) Heart: Paresis of Inhibitory nerves. (9) Stomach: Increased Appetite; acid vomiting; gastralgia; (10) Intestinal canal: constipation; haemorrhoids (11) Bladder: paralysis of Muscular Coat; incontinence (12) Sexual organs - male: increased sexual desire; impotence (13) Sexual organs Female: Menses too soon, last too long (14) Lungs: Dry cough; flatulent asthma (15) Blood: Oxidation arrested.

The arrest of the respiratory movements suspends oxidation of the blood, and the skin becomes cyanosed; strong erections of the penis occur, and frequently involuntary evacuations of semen, urine and faeces take place.

Strychnia affects the peripheral and organs of special sense locally. Small arteries can be seen to contract under the influence of Strychnia, and conclude that the rise of the pressure is due to vasomotor spasm. Modern experimentation has confirmed this observation, showing that strychnia contracts the arterioles and greatly increases the blood - pressure and does this by direct stimulation of the vasomotor center at the base of the brain.

In the abdomen we have much flatulence, with all varieties of colicky pains. Nux vomica assists in rather small evacuations mixed with mucus, attended by tenesmus and straining. Often the stool is soft, mixed with mucus and streaked with blood, or there is clear blood along with the faeces. The power of producing and curing haemorrhoids is one of the most prominent features in the action of Nux vomica.

The menses occur too soon, and continue much longer than they should; accompanied by nausea, chills, faintness, and spasmodic pains in the abdomen.

In the nose, it produces obstructive catarrh, Nux vomica is useful in Dyspeptic asthma.

It has been employed in treatment of atrophy of the optic nerve and various forms of amblyopia.

Let no man forget the use of Strychnia, 3rd trituration, in dyspepsia where there is an atonic state of the digestive organs, with its manifold symptoms of a nervous nature; it greatly excels Nux vomica for chronic dyspepsia.

The slightest irritation, especially if a woman is touched, produces lascivious thoughts, and frequently emissions, followed by nervous exhaustion. (Use the 30 up to the 1000th for spermatorrhoea).

Strychnia is indicated in all cases of paralysis from exhaustion of the spinal cord, spinal anaemia; reflex paraplegia, hemiplegia, or white softening (Hale).

(Willium, H. Burt)

446. *Ocimum Can*

(Brazilian Alfavaca)

Is to be remembered in diseases of the kidneys, bladder and urethra. Uric acid diathesis. Red sand in the urine is its chief characteristic and frequently verified. Swelling of glands, inguinal and mammary. Renal colic, especially right side. Symptoms of renal calculus are pronounced.

Urine: Brick dust red or yellow sediment, odor of musk, pain in ureters.

Female: Vulva swollen, darting pain in labia. Nipples painful to least contact. Breasts feel full and tense, itching; prolapsus vagina.

Dose: 6-30 potency. *(Boericke)*

Renal colic, with violent vomiting every fifteen minutes. One wrings one's hand and moans and cries all the time. Red urine with brickdust sediment after the attack. The urine may be Saffron colour or thick purulent, with an intolerable smell of musk. Majundar adds that Ocimum. can is the sacred Tulsi of India and that the Kaviraj is use it in the diseases of the liver and bilious remittent fevers. All the members of the Ocimum genus are aromatic. The sweet or common basil; Basilicum is one of the best known. The vaginal prolapse, excessive sensitiveness of the breasts and pain on nursing are important symptoms. *(JHC)*

There is an impression gaining ground amongst us that the American Ocimum Can is nothing but Ocimum Gratissimum (Ram Tulsi). The therapeutic properties that have been attributed to Ocimum Sanctum (Shiva Tulsi) are present in this variety also.

This herb can be found in abundance all over Indian and no less than half a dozen varieties are found. The black and the white varieties possess identical qualities.

With lime juice, the leaves are rubbed over ring worm.

Ayurveda found it very efficacious in cough, cold, catarrh, nose affections, Ozaena, scorpion-bites, remittent and intermittent fevers and constipation.

Homoeo provings - 'Ocimum can' is a species of this shrub, which grows abundantly in Brazil. Dr. Mure has proven and introduced this remedy into homoeopathy. Dr. Mure tells us that it is largely used in Brazil as a specific for diseases of the kidneys, bladder and urethra. He has given a short list of nineteen symptoms which are partially clinical and partially pathogenetic.

It is an excellent remedy in nasal catarrh associated with frequent sneezing, secretions being white or yellow.

Forgetfulness is a special key note symptom of this drug.

Ocimum Sanctum plays its parts very well and in this respect, it can be closely compared with Baptitia (Slumber or drowsiness while answering questions).

In asthma of children it is also an excellent remedy. It yields good results even when Aralia Racemosa, Lobelia and Blatta orientalis fail to do any good.

In toothache it is a grand remedy. The pains are terrible, worse at night, cold. Offensive smell comes out of mouth and offensive salivation is present.

Ocimum is an excellent remedy in influenza and in fevers, acute pains in the body. In this respect it resembles Eupatorium Perfoliatum. *(Dr. S.C. Ghose)*

447. Oenanthe Crocata

(Water Dropwart)

Epileptiform convulsions, worse during menstruation and pregnancy. Puerperal eclampsia, uraemic convulsions. Burning in throat and stomach, nausea and vomiting. Red spots in face. Convulsive facial twitching. Skin affections, especially lepra and Ichthyosis.

Head: Sudden and complete unconsciousness, furious delirium, eyes fixed, pupils dilated, convulsive twitching of facial muscles.

Respiratory: Frothy expectoration, heavy, spasmodic stertorous breathing.

Extremities: Convulsions, Opisthotonus, pain along crural and sciatic nerves.

Dose: 1st to 6th potency. *(Boericke)*

In homoeopathic practice, it has been given with much success in case of epilepsy. The cases of epilepsy in which it is particularly indicated are those in which there is during the fit, vomiting, tympanitis or semi-priapism. Epilepsy arising from disorders of the sexual sphere. Hysterio-epilepsy-Oen.c. ϕ - 5 drops in six ounces of water. A teaspoonful every 3 hours and later less often. *(JHC)*

448. *Oleander*

(Rose Laurel)

Has a marked action on the skin, heart and nervous system, producing and curing paralytic conditions with cramp-like contractions of upper extremities. Hemiplegia, difficult articulation.

Head: Eruption on scalp. Humid fetid spots behind ears, corrosive itching on forehead and edge of hair.

Eyes: Sensation as if eyes were drawn back into the head.

Stomach: Canine hunger with hurried eating.

Abdomen: Undigested faeces, stool passes when emitting flatus.

Chest: palpitation.

Extremities: Weakness of lower limbs.

Skin: Very sensitive skin, violent itching eruption, bleeding, oozing, want of perspiration. Pruritus especially of scalp.

Mod: Worse - Undressing, rest, friction of clothes.

Dose: 3rd to 30th potency. *(Boericke)*

In the Cape de Verde Islands, the petals of Oleander blossoms are used with dried orange peel in all kinds of fevers to promote perspiration and drive out the rash.

Hahnemann says of Olean - It will found to be, if not a complete remedy, yet an indispensable intermediate remedy in some kinds of mental derangements eg. absence of mind, and in certain kinds of painless paralysis, in eruptions on the head and in some external head affections. Desquamation of the epidermis of the scalp, violent gnawing itching on the scalp as from lice, after scratching, a smarting as if scratched raw. Cooper's experience in one very bad case, in a school boy, that a single dose of the ϕ may give the best possible result on such cases. Olean. ϕ-2 drops in a powder at bed time. *(JHC)*

This remedy is indicated in eczema. There is a violent itching, bleeding, oozing eruption. The skin is very sensitive, the slightest friction causing soreness and chapping. While this condition may appear at any point, it is often at the margin of the hair.

It is also useful in paralytic conditions, hemiplegia, paraplegia, painless paralysis with swelling, burning, and stiffness of the fingers.

Compare: Conium mac., Rhus tox., lathyrus. *(Blackwood)*

449. *Oleum Animale*

(Dippel's Animal oil)

Acts on the nervous system, especially on pneumo-gastric region. Useful in migraine and neuralgia of spermatic cord. Burning pains and stitches. "Pulled upward and from behind forward pains".

Face: Twitching of lips, toothache better pressing teeth together.

Stomach: As if water were in.

Urine: Polyuria.

Male: Pain along spermatic cord to testicles. Testicles feel seized and pulled forcibly upward. Pressure in the perineum.

Female: Early and scant menstruation.

Respiratory: Stitches in breast from behind forward.

Dose: 3 to 30 and higher. *(Boericke)*

As is usually the case with combustive products Ol. an. has burning pains and burning sensations in almost all parts and like the carbons and K. carb. It has also stitches and sometimes combination of the two-stitches as with red hot needles. Gave great relief in a case of Scirrhus of right breast in which pains darting forward out of the nipple were complained of - Both testicles are drawn up and very painful - Desire for soft boiled eggs or for bread only with aversion to meat.

Causation: Suppressed foot sweat. *(JHC)*

450. *Oleum Jecoris Aselli*

(Cod-Liver oil)

Internally a nutrient and a hepatic and pancreatic remedy (Burnett). Emaciation, lassitude, scrofulous diseases, rheumatic affections, atrophy of infants, emaciation, with hot hands and head, restless and feverish at night. Pains in liver region. Tuberculosis in the beginning.

Chest: Dry, hacking, tickling cough, especially at night, whooping cough in miserable, scrofulous children. Here give drop doses. Increasing daily one drop up to twelve then descend in the same way. Soreness through chest - yellowness, children who cannot take milk.

Extremities: Aching in elbows and knees, in sacrum, chronic rheumatism with rigid muscles and tendons, burning in palms.

Fever: Constantly chilly towards evening. Hectic fever, night sweats.

Dose: First to third trituration, locally in ring worm and nightly rubbing for dwarfish, emaciated babies. *(Boericke)*

Oil obtained from the livers of 'Gadus Morrhua' and some other allied fishes. The number of people who cannot make cod liver oil is very great, which means that Ol. J.A. is a pathogenetic as well as curative agent. It is a liver remedy. Very decided pains in the liver and liver region with great soreness were noted in "Neidhard's" provings - a remedy for phthisis and scrofulous affections - dry hacking cough - night cough-cough with tough expectoration - yellow or white-soreness of chest especially on coughing - sharp stitches here and there - through chest, burning through to back - burning in spots. Fever agg: towards evening with burning in palms. The yellowness of O.J.A. appears not only in the expectoration, but in the coating of the tongue. Yellow mucus from sore throat and a yellow leucorrhoea. Burnett has shown that ringworm generally has its constitutional bases in a consumptive habit and Bacil. has again proved the remedy. In recent ringworm the application of the plain oil at bed time is at once the most innocent and most effectual of local measures that I know. Before the application the part should be washed well with soft soap. Another use of the remedy taught me by the same authority is as general application in the case of emaciated, dwarfish, chilly babies and children. A nightly rubbing with the oil soon revolutionises their condition. Defective nutrition, anaemia, weakness and emaciation, deficiency of animal heat. Children who cannot take milk. One curious symptom was abnormal growth of hair on the face of a woman. *(JHC)*

451. *Oleum Santali*

(Oil of Sandal wood)

The action in the urinary and sexual spheres is most utilizable, especially in gonorrhoea. It is also a stimulating, disinfectant expectorant. Two or three drops on sugar will frequently relieve the hacking cough, when but little sputum is expectorated.

Male: Painful erections, swelling of the prepuce. Thick yellowish, mucopurulent discharge, deep pain in perineum.

Urine: Frequent burning, smarting, swelling and redness of meatus, stream small and slow. Acute aching in kidney region. Sensation of a ball pressing against the urethra, worse standing.

Gleet with profuse, thick discharge. Chronic cystitis.

Dose: 2 to 10 m in capsules. *(Boericke)*

This remedy is indicated in gonorrhoea. The discharge is thick and yellow. There is a swelling of the prepuce. The erections are painful, the urine is passed slowly and causes burning and smarting of the urethra.

It is of service in these cases when the prostate gland is implicated and there is a pain deep in the perineum.

It should be remembered in bronchitis when the cough is dry and hacking.

Compare: Cannabis sativa, Buchu, Copaiva. *(Blackwood)*

452. *Onosmodium*

(False Gromwell)

Want of power of concentration and cordination. Vertigo, numbness and muscular prostration. Marked association of head and eye symptoms with muscular tiredness and weariness. A remedy for migraine. Headaches from eye strain and sexual weakness. It produces diminution of sexual desire in both sexes, hence its homoeopathicity. Depressed or lost sexual life in women. Neuralgic pain. General prostration. Acts as if born tired.

Eyes: Ocular muscles tense, pain in eye balls.

Male: Constant sexual excitement, physical impotence, loss of desire, speedy emissions, deficient erections.

Female: Sexual desire completely destroyed.

Dose: 30 c. *(Boericke)*

The most remarkable feature of 'Greens' striking proving is the want of power or coordination produced by the drug. This appears in inability to concentrate thought, to focus eyes, to co-ordinate muscles, to judge the height of impedimenta on stepping - "Jones" quotes Hahnemann's canon that only the primary symptoms of a drug afford the indications for its therapeutical application (a canon which Jones endorses as far as the infinitesimal dose is concerned)- Yingling many times verified 'complete loss of sexual desire' as a leading indication - Yingling had an interesting experience in the case of a woman to whom he gave 'Onos' for dryness of nose and throat. Not only did it cure this but it also restored the breasts which were diminutive and almost absent, to their normal size.

Yingling's desires were obtained mostly from the C.M. attenuation. He had no results from the ϕ and not marked from the 30c.

Causation: Eye strain, Sexual excess. *(JHC)*

453. *Oophorinum*

(Ovarian Extract)

Suffering following excision of the ovaries. Climacteric disturbances generally. Ovarian cysts. Cutaneous disorders and acne rosacea. Prurigo.

Dose: Low triturations. *(Boericke)*

Ovarian Extract. A sarcode. Trituration of expressed juice of ovary of sheep or Cow Ooph. has been used with much success in cases of suffering following excision of the ovaries, and for the climacteric sufferings of women. Acne rosacea and other skin disorders of the climacteric. A woman, 20, after double oophorectomy had lichen - like eczema. This was greatly relieved by Ooph, along with the accompanying nervous symptoms and adiposity. He obtained good results also in some non-climacteric cases (1) Acne and Seborrhoea in chlorotic women. (2) A case of prurigo which had lasted from childhood in a woman of 20. In this case the itching was amel: for a short time after the period. This amel: during menses may prove a keynote and relate the remedy to Zinc. *(JHC)*

454. *Opium*

(Dried latex of the poppy)

Hahnemann says that it is much more difficult to estimate the action of Opium than of almost any other drug. The effects of the opium as shows in the insensibility of the nervous system, the depression, drowsiness, stupor, painlessness, and torpor, the general sluggishness and lack of vital reaction, constitute the main indications for the drug when used homoeopa-thically. All complaints are characterised by sopor. they are painless and are accompanied by, heavy stupid sleep, stertorous breathing, sweaty skin. Dark mahogany brown face. Serous apoplexy. Venous passive congestion. Want of sensitiveness to the action of medicines. Reappearance and aggravation from becoming heated. Opium lessens voluntary movements, contracts pupils, depresses higher intellectual powers, lessens self control and power of concentration, judgement, stimulates the imagination, checks all secretions except that of the skin. Want of susceptibility to remedies even though indicated. Diseases that originate from fright.

Mind: Complete loss of consciousness, apoplectic state.

Head: Lightness of head in old people.

Eyes: Contracted.

Face: Swollen, dark, suffused, hot, hanging down of lower jaw.

Mouth: Paralysed.

Stool: Obstinate constipation, no desire to go to stool. Round, hard, black balls. Faeces protrude and recede, spasmodic retention of faeces in small intestines.

Urine: Slow to start, feeble stream, retarded or involuntary.

Respiratory: Breathing stops on going to sleep, deep snoring, rattling, stertorous breathing.

Sleep: Falls into a heavy stupid sleep. Very sleepy, but cannot go to sleep. Distant noises, cocks, crowing etc. keep him awake.

Back and extremities: Twitching of limbs.

Skin: Hot perspiration over whole body except lower limbs.

Mod: Worse - heat, during and after sleep - Better - cold things, constant walking.

Dose: 3-30 to 200 potency. *(Boericke)*

Death takes places by asphyxia, the heart continuing to beat after breathing has ceased. Op-30 has helped me in case of sleeplessness as often as coffea. The grand characteristic of Opium is the drowsiness, inertia, torpor, absence of sensation, absence of reaction. Intestinal obstruction. Opium has won many triumphs. Also in uterine inertia, during labour opium is often needed. Opium is one of the chief remedies for foetal movements, when they become excessive. Sweat as a concomitant is a characteristic of Opium. Complaints appearing with perspiration - the skin is hot and damp. "Snow" Contends that it has a certain degree of power over the cancer process. Constipation of inertia (little, hard, dry, black balls). *(JHC)*

The concrete milky exudation obtained by incising the unripe capsules of the poppy. Its principal alkaloids are morphine and Codeine; an artificial alkaloid derived from these is Apomorphine.

This agent is a narcotic, hypnotic, analgesic, antispasmodic and diaphoretic. It arrests all the secretions except the milk and sweat, increasing the latter. The mucous membranes are drier than normal. There is loss of appetite and the digestion is retarded. The heart's action and the arterial tension are increased, and the cerebral function is active. There is an exhilaration that borders on intoxication, which is followed by a calm. The sleep that follows is disturbed by dreams. This is followed by headaches, exhaustion, constipation and digestive disturbance.

When a toxic dose is taken, the pulse is slow, there is slow and stertorous breathing which becomes feeble and irregular. The face is cyanosed, the reflexes are lost and coma gradually deepens. The pupils that at first are contracted, dilate as death approaches. Post-mortem shows a wet brain, the lungs congested and the venous trunks engorged. This remedy is indicated when there is a lack of vital reaction and the well chosen remedy does not have the desired effect. Diseases that originate in fright. He is very sleepy, but cannot sleep. The face is purplish and swollen. There is great stupor, patient complains of nothing and wants nothing. It is useful in cerebral haemorrhage when the pulse is slow, the breathing stertorous, and there is tetanic rigidity.

It is also useful in constipation of children, and corpulent women when the stools are composed of round, hard, black balls, the stool protrudes and recedes. The abdomen is distended and tympanitic. At times the stools are involuntary, especially after a fright. They are black and offensive.

It is of service in retention of the urine, when the bladder is full and distended, following confinement, and in fevers or acute illnesses. Also in spasms of children caused by the approach of strangers; from nursing after fright or anger of the mother. Their eyes are half open. There is screaming before and during the spasm.

It should be remembered whenever there is a heavy, stupid sleep, with stertorous breathing, the face is red, the eyes are half closed and bloodshot, the skin is covered with hot sweat; also in insomnia when he is sleepy but cannot sleep, sleepiness with acuteness of hearing, a clock striking at a distance is heard distinctly.

It is of benefit in twitching of the muscles with trembling of he head, arms and hands and ptosis when the lids hang down as if paralyzed.

Compare: Belladonna, Gelsemium, Nux moschata. *(Blackwood)*

455. *Origanum*

(Sweet Marjoram)

Acts on nervous system generally and is effective in masturbation and excessively aroused sexual impulses. Affections of the breasts. Desire for exercise. Impelling her to run.

Female: Erotomania, powerful lascivious impulses, leucorrhoea, hysteria, lascivious, ideas and dreams.

Dose: 3rd potency. *(Boericke)*

All kinds of sexual excitement, in females, especially have been remedied by "Orig". The sexual symptoms were developed chiefly in female provers, and were these: sadness followed by joyfulness and thoughts of marriage, increased desire for coitus. Swelling and itching of nipples and pains in breasts. Impulse to run. *(JHC)*

This remedy is indicated in erotomania and obscure nervous disorders of women that are dependent upon irritation of the sexual organs.

Compare: Platinum, Valeriana, Cantharis. *(Blackwood)*

456. *Ornithogalum Umbellatum*

(Star of Bethlehem)

To be considered in chronic gastric and other abdominal indurations, possibly cancer of intestinal tract, especially of stomach and caecum. Center of action is the Pylorus, causing painful contraction and duodenal distention.

Depression of spirits. Complete prostration, feeling sickness, keeps patient awake at night.

Stomach: Tongue coated, agonizing feeling in chest and stomach, starting from pylorus with flatus that rolls in balls from one side to other, loss of appetite, phlegmy retchings and loss of flesh. Gastric ulceration even with haemorrhage. Pains increased when food passes pyloric outlet. Vomiting of coffee ground looking matter. Distention of stomach. Frequent belching of offensive flatus. Painful sinking across epigastrium.

Dose: Single dose of mother tincture and await action. *(Boericke)*

A plant of which, there are many varieties, nearly allied to Garlic (Allium Sativum). Tincture of fresh plant.

'Cooper' particularly insists on his method being followed. A dose of a single drop being allowed to act till all trace of its action has disappeared. *(JHC)*

This remedy has been employed in the relief of inoperable cancer of the stomach and ulcer of the stomach. The pylorus was the seat of the lesions. But one dose of the tincture was employed. *(Blackwood)*

457. *Osmium*

(The element)

Irritation and catarrh of respiratory organs. Eczema. Albuminuria. Pain in trachea. Increases and gives odor to local perspiration. Causes adhesion of the nail fold.

Eyes: Glaucoma, green colours surround candle light. Increase in intraoccular tension, dim sight, photophobia.

Respiratory: Noisy, dry, hard cough in violent short bursts. Pain in larynx.

Skin: Eczema with pruritus, irritated skin, itching pimples, bromidrosis, sweat in axilla, smelling of garlic.

Dose: 6th potency. *(Boericke)*

Osmium is a metal of the Platinum group in association with which it is always found. G.S. Norton suggests that "Osm" may be a remedy in many cases of Glaucoma. *(JHC)*

458. *Ovigallinae Pellicula*

(Membrane of egg shell)

Sudden pains. Bearing down sensation. Intolerance of bands on wrists, arms, waist etc. Backache and pain in left hip. Debility. Pain in heart and left ovary.

Relation: Ova tosta, (Roasted egg shells). Leucorrhoea and backache. A feeling as if the spine were broken and wired or tied together with a string. Pain of cancer. Warts. *(Boericke)*

Under Calc. Ov. Test. - I have given an account of the action of egg shells in leucorrhoea, and "Swans" adds that, it has an ancient reputation for immoderate flux of the courses (like our Calc. carb) and for nocturnal enuresis. The egg shells were anciently used powdered fresh or roasted and as such were and are much used in the treatment of Oxyuris Vermicularis. `Swan' prepared the membrane. As an ovarian product it might be expected that all parts of the egg should have an action on ovaries. It is recognised that as an article of diet in some forms, eggs have a stimulating effect on the sexual functions. The provings of Ovi. G.P. bear out this relation. *(JHC)*

This remedy is indicated when there is a dull heavy aching pain in the region of the heart, which at times extends to the left ovary. *(Blackwood)*

459. *Oxallicum Acidum*

(Sorrel Acid)

Although certain oxalates are constant constituents of vegetable food and of the human body, the acid itself is a violent poison when taken internally producing gastro-enteritis, motor paralysis, collapse, stupor and death. Influences the spinal cord, and produces motor, paralysis. Pains very violent in spots, (Kali bich), worse motion and thinking of them. Periodical remissions. Spasmodic symptoms of throat and chest. Rheumatism of left side, neur-asthenia. Tuberculosis.

Eyes: Hyperaesthesia of retina.

Male: Terrible neuralgic pains in spermatic cord.

Respiratory: Hoarseness, left lung painful, aphonia, dyspnoea, short, jerking inspiration.

Heart: Angina pectoris, sharp lancinating pain in left lung, coming on suddenly, depriving of breath.

Extremities: Lancinating pains, back-ache.

Modalities: Worse left side. Aroused about 3 a.m. with gastric and abdominal pain. All conditions made worse by thinking about self. Lime water antidotes the poisoning of Oxal acid.

Dose: 6-30th potency. *(Boericke)*

If Opium is the painless remedy, Oxal. ac. may be considered its antithesis. It causes pains excruciating beyond descrip-tion and it has this grand key note distinction, that its pain are all agg: when the patient thinks of them.

And not only that, thinking of pains and conditions will bring them on when they are not actually present . If the patient thinks about urinating he must go instantly and relieve the bladder.

Pains in small spots (especially linear spots). Pains agg: when thinking of them. Sharp pains through the lower lobe of the left lung. It matters not what the name of the disease may be-pleurisy, pneumonia, phthisis - when the pain is present Oxal. ac. will do its work. Among the peculiar sensations are - Jerking pains, like short stitches, confined to small spots, lasting only a few seconds. *(JHC)*

This agent is an irritant poison to the nervous system and blood, producing gastro-enteritis. There is intense burning of the parts over which it passes with pain that is excruciating beyond description, with destruction of the mucous membrane. There is a bloody vomit and stool. The pulse becomes feeble, there is motor paralysis, so that he is unable to assume the upright posture; there is collapse, stupor and death.

In the milder type of poisoning there is excruciating pain in the lower back and loss of power in the lower limbs. Thinking of the pains makes them worse.

This remedy is indicated in those cases in which there is excruciating pain that is beyond description. The pains are worse when the patient thinks of them. They are excruciating in spots, are worse from motion and have periods of remission.

It should be thought of in oxaluria, when there is pain in the region of the kidney, with frequent and copious urination. The urine is a clear straw color. There is burning in the urethra and pains in the glans of the penis when urinating. The urine contains calcium oxalates, and albumin; when the patient thinks of urination he must go at once to urinate.

It is to be remembered in spermatic neuralgia when there are terrible neuralgic pains along the spermatic cord. These are made worse from motion and the urine contains oxalates.

It should be studied in seminal vesiculitis when there is exhaustion, increased frequency in micturition which is attended with pain and burning, the testicles are usually very sensitive, there is great sexual excitement, while the urine contains oxalates.

It has been of service in Multiple cerebral sclerosis when there are lancinating pains which are like electric currents in various parts, now in the forehead, again in the occiput, with tremor of the limbs, they may be jerking pains confined to small spots and lasting only a moment. The patient complains of muscular prostration, dyspnoea and a general weakness and numbness.

It has been found beneficial in myelitis when there is a general weakness about the hips and loins that extends down the legs which are apt to be cold and bluish. There are pains that come and go in small circumscribed spots and are aggravated from thinking of them.

Under picric acid there is a sensation of heaviness while under oxalic acid it is a sense of numbness.

It has relieved gastralgia. The attack appears after eating, there is pyrosis and sensation of coldness between the epigastrium and umbilicus.

Compare: Picric acid, Argentum met., Arsenicum album. *(Blackwood)*

460. Oxydendron-Andromeda Arborea

(Sorrel Tree)

A remedy for dropsy, ascites and anasarca. Urine suppressed. Deranged portal circulation. Prostatic enlargement. Vesical calculi. Irritation of neck of bladder. Great difficulty in breathing.

Dose: Tincture. *(Boericke)*

Ascites and Anasarca, which dated from an attack of measles - After the failure of Apocy. and several carefully chosen medicines. The legs having burst in several places, Douglass was about to tap the abdomen, but before doing so put Oxydend. ϕ in a tumbler of water and gave 3 teaspoonfuls every 3 hours. In forty eight hours the breathing was better and urine increased. *(JHC)*

461. Oxytropis

(Loco-weed)

Marked action on nervous system. Trembling, sensation of emptiness, walks backwards. Congestion of spine and paralysis. Pain come and go quickly. Sphincters relaxed. Staggering gait. Reflexes lost.

Mind: Mental depression.

Rectum: Lumps of jelly.

Urine: Profuse flow.

Extremities: Staggering gait.

Relation: Loco plant is rich in Baryta.

Dose: 3rd potency and higher. *(Boericke)*

The animal affected loses flesh, has a feeble staggering, uncertain gait, a rough coat and general appearance which is said to be characteristic. It loses all sense of distance or direction and is liable to fits of rearing, plunging and wild excitement. Pregnant animals drop their offspring prematurely. Dr. Mary Gage Day made experiments with a decoction of roots, leaves and stems gathered in September. She is convinced by experiments made with materials gathered in different months, that the greatest amount of poison is present in autumn and winter after the seeds have ripened. *(JHC)*

This agent produces congestion of the spinal cord and paralysis. The sphincters are relaxed and the stools escape from the rectum. The gait is staggering, there is lack of co-ordination, the reflexes are lost, and the pains come and go quickly.

Compare: Lathyrus. *(Blackwood)*

462. Paeonia

(Peony)

The rectal and anal symptoms are most important. Chronic ulcers on lower parts of body, leg, foot, toe, also breast, rectum.

Rectum: Biting, itching in anus, orifice swollen, burning in anus after stool, then internal chilliness, fistula and diarrhoea with anal burning, painful ulcer, oozing offensive moisture on perineum. Haemorrhoidal fissures covered with crusts. Atrocious pains with and after each stool. Sudden pasty diarrhoea, with faintness in abdomen.

Relation: *Hamam., Sil., Aesc., Ratanh,* great constriction of anus, stools forced with great effort.

Dose: 3rd potency. *(Boericke)*

The symptoms are well characterised, but it is principally the anal and skin symptoms which have been verified in practice. One of the symptoms of the proving is this. A small ulcer on perineum near anus, that constantly oozes very offensive moisture, painful for eight days. Anal symptoms. Biting, itching, swelling, burning, clearly point to Paeon. as a remedy in anal affection, such as abscess, fissure, fistula and piles. The leading indications are intolerable pain during and after stool, and oozing moisture. Experience has proved that varicose veins as well as anal varices are amenable to Paeon. *(JHC)*

463. Palladium

(The Metal)

An ovarian remedy. Produces the symptoms — Complex of chronic oophoritis. Useful where the parenchyma of the gland is not totally destroyed. Acts also on mind and skin. Motor weakness, averse to exercise.

Mind: Love of approbation, easily offended, keeps up brightly when in company.

Head: Pain across top of head from ear to ear.

Abdomen: Shooting pain from navel to pelvis. Sensation as if intestines were bitten off. Intestine feel strangulated. Soreness of abdomen. Swelling in right groin. Flatulence.

Female: Uterine prolapse and retroversion. Subacute pelvic peritonitis with right sided pain and backache, menorrhagia, cutting pain in uterus, relieved after stool. Pain and swelling in region of right ovary. Shooting or burning pain in pelvis and bearing down, relieved by rubbing. Soreness and shooting pain from navel to breast. Glairy leucorrhoea, menstrual discharge while nursing. Stitches in right breast near nipple. It is indicated in that gynaecological condition where the disease had its inception in the right ovary, the uterine prolapse and retroversion, the subacute pelvic peritonitis and concomitant symptom being secondary.

Extremities: Pruritus. Tired feeling in small of back. Fleeting neuralgic pains in extremities. Heavy and tired in limbs. Darting pains from toes to hips. Rheumatic pain in rt. shoulder, in right hip. Sciatica.

Relation: Comple: Platina.

Dose: 6-30 potency. *(Boericke)*

The chief charactᵊristic of Palladium is affections of the Rt. Ovary attended with pains which are amel: by pressure. Palladium in the mental sphere is 'Love of approbation' which lays its victim an easy prey to slights, real or imaginary, and easily gives place to a state of wounded pride and fancied neglect, irritability which often finds vent in violent expression. There is much uterine bearing down and even prolapse-undressing causing itching all over body. Amel: Rest, after sleep. Agg.: Motion, after social excitement, concerts, etc.

***Comple:** Plat.*

Compare: Rt. ovary - Apis, Graph, Pod., Plat; Left ovary-Arg. met., Lach.; Agg: pressure; Lil tig, Act. r, Sul; tired backache; Helon - Hysteria, Introverted state of mind - Tarentula. *(JHC)*

A metallic element. A white metal when compact, or a gray powder of spong, according to method of reduction.

This remedy is indicated in those who are inclined to weep. They love approbation, but are easily offended and employ abusive language. It is of service in headache when the pain extends across the top of the head from one ear to the other. This is apt to appear the day after an evening entertainment. It is useful in neuralgia of the right ovary. There is a sensation of bearing down in the pelvis. The pain is worse while standing and moving, and is better from lying down.

Compare: Helonias, Lilium tig.

(Blackwood)

464. *Paraffine*

(Purified Paraffin)

Valuable in uterine affection. Particularly serviceable in constipation. Knife-like pains. Pains extend from one part to another, and alternate. Pain in stomach alternates with pain in throat and spine.

Rectum: Frequent desire for stool. Obstinate constipation in children. (Alumina, Nyctanthes). Chronic constipation, with haemorrhoids and continual urging to stool, without result.

Dose: Lower triturations and thirtieth potency. (Boericke)

Paraffine as a generic term includes all those substances which have no affinity for sulphuric acid, and cannot be destroyed by it, Petroleum itself coming within this designation. Specifically Paraffin is a tasteless, inodorous, fatty matter, which resists the action of acids and alkalis, obtained by the dry distillation of wood, peat, bituminous coal, petroleum, etc. In the distillation of petroleum, naphthalin is the first substance that comes off; Paraffin is the next. The symptoms of the proving which was made on persons of both sexes, are very striking. The pains are: Knife like stabs; twitching, wrenching pains; stinging and twisting; electric pains. The pains extend from one part to another and alternate. With these pains there was leucorrhoea, pruritus vulvae, and other disturbances of the female generative organs. The homoeopaths of Rome have found it serviceable in uterine and other troubles, particularly constipation. Cooper has seen swollen joints lessen considerably from its use as a liniment. *(JHC)*

465. *Pareira Brava*

(Virgin Vine)

The urinary symptoms are most important. Useful in renal colic, prostatic affections and catarrh of bladder. Sensation as if bladder were distended. With pain. Pain going down thigh.

Urinary: Black, bloody, thick mucous urine. Constant urging, great straining. Pain down thighs during efforts to urinate. Can emit urine only when he goes on his knees, pressing head firmly against the floor. Feeling of the bladder being distended and neuralgic pain in the anterior crural region, dribbling after micturition. Violent pain in glans penis. Itching along urethra, urethritis, with prostatic trouble. Inflammation of urethra, becomes almost cartilaginous.

Dose: Tr to 3rd potency. *(Boericke)*

C.M. Fox of Denver, brought out some characteristic symptoms which have been clinically confirmed. Among these are violent pains with strangury, must go on all fours and press head against floor to pass water at all - violent pain in glans penis - Pareira b. 1x gave rapid relief. *(JHC)*

This remedy is indicated when there is a constant urging to urinate. There are violent pains in the glans penis, that extend down the thighs during the effort to urinate. The urethra and prostate glands are inflamed. The urine is dark and bloody and is passed only with great efforts upon the hands and knees. The bladder feels as if it were distended. The urine passes in dribbles.

Compare: Chimaphila, uva ursi, Hydrangea, Berberis vulgaris. (Blackwood)

466. *Paris Quadrifolia*

(One berry)

Head symptoms marked and verified. Sensation of expansion and consequent tension. Coldness of right side of body, left hot. Catarrhal complaints, stuffed feeling at root of nose. Disorder of sense of touch.

Mind: Garrulous.

Head: Aches, as from pulling a string from eyes to occiput.

Eyes: Sensation of string through eyeballs.

Mouth: Tongue dry when awaking, coated white without thirst.

Respiratory: Hoarseness.

Extremities: Weight and weariness in nape of neck. Fingers often feel numb.

Dose: 3rd potency. *(Boericke)*

The eyes feel as if much too large for their sockets; as if they were projecting and were being drawn tightly backward by a sting to the middle of the brain. A case of loquacious insanity cured with Paris-3 was recorded by B. Nath Banerjee - her looks became wandering and her eyes appeared as if protruding from their sockets. *(JHC)*

467. *Parotidinum*

(The nosode of Mumps)

Parotidinum has been used as a prophylactic against infection by Mumps. In this instance it is generally given in the 6th or 30th, 2-3 times a day to those exposed to infection. In the disease itself or alternated with other indicated remedies. The well known complications which some times occur with mumps, cerebral inflammation and orchitis, suggest its possible use in these conditions. *(JHC)*

Relation - Compare - Merc.

468. *Parthenium-Escoba amargo*

(Bitter Broom)

A Cuban remedy for fevers, especially malarial. Increased flow of milk. Amenorrhoea and general debility. Cheyne-Stokes breathing. After quinine.

Head: Teeth feel on edge. *(Boericke)*

It is a Cuban remedy of great repute in the treatment of fevers. She noticed a marked increase of milk in the breasts. It antidotes quinine. *(JHC)*

This remedy and its alkaloid is employed in the relief of malarial fever in the tropics (Cuba and Panama). It has not only controlled the early attack, but has reduced the enlarged liver and spleen, which are painful to the touch. It has controlled the periodical neuralgia that attends many of these cases after quinine has failed. It has been employed in the tincture and 6x, also the alkaloid in 1/6 to 1/5 of a grain, administered every hour or two.

(Blackwood)

469. Pentorum

(Virginia Stone Crop)

A remedy for coryza, with rawness and wet feeling in nose. Throat feels raw. Chronic post-nasal catarrh, chronic pharyngitis, mucous membrane purple and relaxed. Posterior nares feel moist and raw, nose and ears feel full. Aphonia, hoarseness, relaxed vocal cords. Hyper-secretions of mucous membranes. Itching of anus and burning in rectum. Trouble in pharyngeal vault and eustachian tube,

Nose: Constant wet feeling in nose, which no amount of blowing will relieve. Discharge thick pus like, streaked with blood. Post nasal catarrh of puberty.

Dose: Not very active, and better adapted to chronic affections, its use should be persisted for some time - Lower potencies. *(Boericke)*

This remedy is indicated during the incipience of coryza. There is rawness of the nose and throat, with a sensation of fluid in the nose. Later the discharge becomes thick and purulent. (Blackwood)

470. Pertussin

(Coqueluchin)

Taken from the glairy and stringy mucus containing the virus of whooping cough. Introduced by John H. Clarke for the treatment of whooping cough and other spasmodic coughs.

Dose: 30th potency. *(Boericke)*

In all cases of whooping cough suspected or defined, I give the remedy in the 30th attenuation every four hours as a matter of routine and as a rule it quickly assumed control of the case and does all that is necessary. In my experience it agrees well with all other whooping-cough remedies and when their specific indications appear, I give them also in alternation or else alone.

(JHC)

471. Passiflora Incarnata

(Passion-flower)

An efficient anti-spasmodic. Whooping cough. Morphine habit. Delirium tremens. Convulsions in children. Neuralgia. Has a quieting effect on the nervous system. Insomnia, produces normal sleep, no disturbance of cerebral functions, neuroses of children, worm fever, teething, spasms, tetanus, hysteria, puerperal convulsions, painful diarrhoea, acute mania, atonic condition generally present. Asthma 10-30 gtt every 10 mts. for a few doses. Locally in erysipelas.

Sleep: Restless, wakeful, resulting from exhaustion. Especially in the feeble infants and the aged. Insomnia of infants and the aged and the mentally worried and over worked with tendency to convulsions. Nocturnal cough.

Dose: Large doses of M.T. are required. 30-60 drops repeated several times.

(Boericke)

Farrington considers Passif. suited especially to tetanus of hot countries and refers to two cures with the ϕ and 1x. It has also been used in convulsions of children and other complaints of dentition and even in epilepsy. Passif. has been also used for ordinary sleeplessness, for restlessness of fevers, for tedious labours when the patient becomes nervous and excitable. *(JHC)*

This agent is narcotic and antispasmodic. In large doses it causes spasm and convulsions in animals.

This remedy is indicated in insomnia, which is dependent upon worry, exhaustion, overwork, and nervous erethism from any cause; this wakefulness may be observed in infants or the aged. It should not be relied upon when the insomnia is dependent upon pain. It is useful in muscular twitching and nervous excitement of children, when convulsions are threatened. It will often prevent convulsions while the cause is still operative, and during its removal. It should be remembered in tetanus, with opisthotonus, trismus, and the convulsions in children. It is of service in the nervous effects of alcoholism, morphinism and following the acute symptoms of spinal meningitis, when he cannot sleep or rest in bed, and yet is too weak to sit up.

Compare: Piscidia, Hyoscyamus.
(Blackwood)

472. Petroleum

(Crude Rock Oil)

Strumous diathesis, especially the dark type who suffer from catarrhal conditions of the mucous membranes, gastric acidity and cutaneous eruptions.

Very marked skin symptoms, acting on sweat and oil glands. Ailments are worse during the winter season. Ailments from riding in cars, carriages, ships, lingering gastric and lung troubles, chronic diarrhoea, long lasting complaints follow mental states - fright, vexation etc. Chlorosis in young girls with or without ulceration of the stomach.

Mind: Feels that death is near and must hurry to settle affairs. Irritable, easily offended, vexed at everything. Low spirited with dimness of sight.

Head: Sensitive, as if a cold breeze blowing on it. Vertigo on rising - moist eruption on scalp, worse back and ears. Use 30th.

Eyes: Loss of eye lashes, dim sight, far sighted, cannot read fine print without glasses, blenorrhoea of lachrymal sac, marginal blepharitis. Skin around eyes dry and scurfy.

Ears: Noise unbearable, eczema intertrigo etc. in and behind ears with intense itching.

Nose: Nostrils ulcerated, cracked, burn.

Stomach: Strong aversion to fat food, meat, worse eating cabbage. Hunger immediately after stool. Nausea with accumulation of water in mouth. Gastralgia when stomach is empty, relieved by constant eating.

Abdomen: Diarrhoea only in the day time, itching of anus agg: after cabbage.

Extremities: Tips of fingers, rough, cracked, fissured every winter. Skin dry, constricted, very sensitive, rough and cracked, leathery. Intertrigo, psoriasis of hands.

Skin: Thick greenish crusts burning and itching, redness, raw, cracks, bleed easily. Eczema. rhagades worse in winter.

Mod: Worse, dampness, passive motion, in winter.

Complementary. Sepia.

Dose: 3-30. *(Boericke)*

The affections met with in petroleum extractors and refiners are (1) Diseases of the skin and subcutaneous tissue, depressed nutrition, anaemia, dyspepsia, nerve troubles, irritability, insomnia, respiratory affections. In my experience no remedy corresponds to more cases of chlorosis in young girls with or without ulceration of stomach. Irritability of skin and irritability of mind are both found in petrol. Illusions as if there is another person or another baby in bed. Falling out of the hair. Agg: by motion in a carriage or on the sea. The localities of petrol are very like those of Graph; Scalp, behind ears, scrotum, genitals. Agg: in winter - Nash has given Pet - 200 for several cases of eczema, chapped hands, chilblains, and one case of chronic diarrhoea as soon as he discovered that the patient had eczema of the hand in winter. *(JHC)*

It is to be thought of in the nausea and vomiting that attends pregnancy, as well as the salivation. At times a sensation of weakness and relaxation in the region of the stomach in complained of; there is a tendency to diarrhoea, and a sensation of chilliness in the abdomen. It has been employed in sea-sickness, and as a prophylactic against it. It should be given hourly for a day or two before going abroad.

It should be remembered in foetid sweats of the axilla, and of the feet, when the latter are tender and there is a general unhealthy condition of the skin.

Compare - Graphites, sulphur, Phosphorus. *(Blackwood)*

473. *Petroselinum*

(Parsley)

The urinary symptoms give the key notes for this remedy-piles with much itching. Burning, tingling, from perineum throughout whole urethra, sudden urging to urinate. Frequent, voluptuous tickling in fossa navicularis (end of urethra). Gonorrhoea, sudden irresistible desire to urinate, intense biting itching deep in urethra, milky discharge.

Relation: Canth, Sars, Cannab, Merc. (Compare)

Dose: 1st to 3rd potency. *(Boericke)*

Petrosel is referred to by Hahnemann as a gonorrhoeal remedy when frequent desire urinate exists. Leading indication is: sudden urging to urinate, and drawing, tingling and crawling, or itching in navicular fossa. During micturition, burning and tingling from perineum, through whole urethra. Milky or yellow discharge - Parsley eaten after meals with or without salad oil is reputed to act as a solvent on Uric acid if there is a tendency to its formation in the urine. An old Edinburgh surgeon used to give it in all nephritic and vessel diseases that were chronic. (JHC)

Petrosel. contains an oily principle called Apiol. This is an active principle of Petroselinum and has been employed in cases of amenorrhoea, menstrual derangements and neuralgic dysmenorrhoea. It is given in five drop doses before the expected menstrual period.

Compare - Cantharis. *(Blackwood)*

474. *Phaseolus*

(Dwarf-bean)

Heart symptoms quite pronounced. Diabetes.

Head: Aches chiefly in forehead or orbits from fullness of brain; worse any movement or mental exertion.

Eyes: Pupils dilated, insensible to light. Eyeballs painful to touch.

Chest: Breathing slow and sighing; pulse rapid. Palpitation. Sick feeling about heart, with weak pulse. Right ribs sore. Dropsical effusion into pleura or pericardium.

Urine: Diabetic urine.

Heart: Fearful palpitation and feeling that death is approaching.

Relationship: *Compare: Crataeg; lach.*

Dose: Sixth and higher. A decoction of the shells as a drink for diabetes, but look out for severe headache.

(Boericke)

Ramm. considers Phas. a most important remedy in Gout and in Diabetes - The inside of the pod rubbed on warts is said to cure them - Did Phas. antidote Morph?

(JHC)

This remedy is indicated in weak heart. There is a feeling of impending dissolution. The heart action is irregular, there is palpitation and general dropsy. The pulse is scarcely perceptible, while the respirations are slow and irregular.

Compare - Digitalis, Crataegus.

(Blackwood)

475. *Phellandrium*

(Water drop-wort)

The respiratory symptoms are most important and have been frequently verified clinically. A very good remedy for the offensive expectoration and cough in phthisis, bronchitis and emphysema, tuberculosis, affecting generally, the middle lobes. Everything tastes sweet. Haemoptysis, hectic and colliquative diarrhoea.

Head: Weight on vertex, aching and burning in temples and above eyes.

Female: Pain in milk ducts.

Chest: Sticking pain through right breast near sternum, extending to back near shoulders. Dyspnoea and continuous cough, early in morning. Cough with profuse and fetid expectoration compels him to sit up. Hoarseness.

Fever: Hectic, profuse and debilitating perspiration, intermittent, with pain in arms. Desire for acids.

Dose: Tincture to 6c. In phthisis not below the sixth. *(Boericke)*

Phelland, which like Oenanthe Croc, grows in moist places and even in the water itself has not shown the poisonous properties of the latter. Clinical experience in nursing women has further brought out its characteristics. The keynote is intolerable pain in lactiferous tubes between the acts of nursing. It has also pain in nipples on each application of child. Either breast may be affected, but the right breast and nipple were more affected than the left. The breast and chest symptoms have led to the use of phelland in phthisis and other chest affections and it is right side affections that Phelland. has done its best work in. The cough is continuous and suffocating, the sputa purulent and horribly offensive. There are also offensive eructations, smelling of bed bugs - Desire for acid is a leading symptom - Goullon jr. calls attention to the value of Phelland. as a cough remedy. He regards it as a universal cough remedy, but particularly useful in phthisical coughs. *(JHC)*

Phellandrium Aquaticum - This remedy is indicated in persons of a feeble, irritable, lymphatic constitution, with weak and defective reaction, who suffer from a chronic bronchial catarrh, with more or less profuse expectoration. The cough returns and increases during the cold season of the year, and only abates upon the return of warm weather. It is continuous for an hour or more early in the morning, and is accompanied by dyspnoea and prostration. The cough at night is not relieved by sitting up. The secondary changes, such as emphysema and dilatation of the right heart, have often taken place. There are coarse rales; the respirations are short; cough continues at all times, day and night; there being great thirst, with loss of appetite and sleeplessness. It should be studied during the last stage of pulmonary tuberculosis, when the expectoration is very offensive.

It is also of service in neuralgic headaches, the pain involving the nerves going to the eyes. The pains are worse on attempting to use the eyes. Bright lights cannot be borne. It should be remembered in mastodynia, when the pain is in the milk ducts and is worse between periods of nursing. *(Blackwood)*

476. *Phlorizin*

A bitter crystalline principle found in the bark and more abundantly in the bark of the root of the apple, pear, cherry and plum trees.

This agent causes sugar to disappear in the urine and has been employed in the relief of diabetes mellitus.

Preparation - Trituration and dilutions.

Dose: 3x. *(Blackwood)*

Phlorizin exists in fine, silky, four sided, colourless needless, soluble in water. It has a bitter and slightly astringent taste, and has been used in the old school practice as a remedy for intermittent fever and whilst being administered for this it has produced glycosuria. This observation has led to its successful use by homoeopaths in cases of diabetes. Successes with the 3x and 6 have been report. Er. V. Mering produced glycosuria in dogs with Phlor. but if Syzygium was given simultaneously with Phlor, no glycosuria appeared. *(JHC)*

477. *Phosphoricum acid*

The common acid debility is very marked in this remedy producing a nervous exhaustion. Mental debility first, later physical. A congenial soil for the action of Phos acid is found in young people who grow rapidly and who are overtaxed, mentally or physically. Whenever the system has been exposed to the ravages of acute disease, excesses, grief, loss of vital fluids, we obtain conditions calling for it. Pyrosis, flatulence, diarrhoea, diabetes, rhachitis and periosteal inflammation. Neurosis in stump after amputation. Haemorrhages in typhoid. Useful in relieving pain of cancer.

Mind: Apathetic, indifferent.

Head: Confused, worse shaking or noise, crushing headache, pressure on top. Hair: Grey early in life, falls out. Vertigo toward evening, when standing or walking.

Eyes: Blue rings around eyes. Pain as if eyeballs were forcibly pressed together and into head.

Nose: Itching.

Stomach: Symptoms following sour food and drink, thirst for cold milk.

Abdomen: Aching in umbilical region.

Stool: Diarrhoea, white, painless.

Urine: Milky, diabetes, frequent urination at night.

Male: Sexual power deficient. Eczema of scrotum, oedema of prepuce and swollen glans penis, sycotic excrescences.

Respiratory: Weak feeling in chest from talking, pressure behind the sternum.

Extremities: Great debility, pains as if bones were scraped.

Skin: Falling out of the hair (N.M. Selen).

Sleep: Somnolence.

Fever: Profuse sweat.

Mod: (Better) - from keeping warm (Worse) - everything impeding circulation causes aggravation of symptoms.

Dose: 1st pot. *(Boericke)*

As if her feet were rising to the ceiling. Exalted sensitiveness to light, sound and odours. Odours take away his breath. Persistent painless, watery diarrhoea, often containing undigested particles of food and which does not debilitate. Patient is rested by a short sleep. Involuntary biting of tongue in sleep. Hair turns grey. Growing fast and tall. Patient will think a little while about to answer a question. *(JHC)*

By loss of vital fluids, sexual excesses. Eyes sunken, blue margins, listless, indifferent to the affairs of life, prostrated and stupefied with grief; headache of school girls from eye strain or overuse of eyes; of students who are growing too fast. Diarrhoea, painless, not debilitating white or yellow. Urine profuse at night clear watery. Emission profuse debilitating - watery. Despair of cure. Irresistible tendency to masturbate *(H.C Allen)*

478. Phosphorus

Phosphorus irritates, inflames and degenerates mucous membranes, irritates and inflames serous membranes, inflames spinal cord and nerves, causing paralysis, destroys bone, especially the lower jaw and tibia, disorganises the blood, causing fatty degeneration of blood vessels and every tissue and organ of the body and this gives rise to haemorrhages and haematogenous jaundice.

Produces a picture of destructive metabolism, causes yellow atrophy of the liver and subacute hepatitis. Tall, slender persons, narrow chested, with thin, transparent skin, weakened by loss of animal fluids, with great nervous debility, emaciation, amative tendencies, seem to be under the special influence of Phosphorus. Great susceptibility to external impressions, to light, sound, odors, touch, electrical changes, thunder storms. Suddenness of symptoms, sudden prostration, faints, sweats, shooting pains, etc. Polycythaemia, blood extravasations, fatty degenerations, cirrhosis, caries, are pathological states often calling for phosphorus. Muscular pseudo-hypertrophy, neuritis, inflammation of the respiratory tract. Paralytic symptoms. Ill effects of Iodine and excessive use of salt, worse lying on left side. Tertiary syphilis, skin lesions, and nervous debility. Scurvy, pseudo-hypertrophic paralysis. Ataxia and adynamia. Osteomyelitis. Bone fragility.

Head: Vertigo, after rising, heat comes from spine, coldness of occiput, itching of scalp, dandruff, falling out of hair in large bunches.

Eyes: Cataract, patient sees better by shading eyes with hand. Green halo about the candle light. Letters appear red. Atrophy of optic nerve. Pearly white conjunctiva and long curved lashes partial loss of vision from abuse of tobacco, diplopia, amaurosis from sexual excess, glaucoma.

Ears: hearing difficult.

Nose: Epistaxis instead of menses, chronic catarrh, with small haemorrhages, handkerchief is always bloody, polypi, bleeding easily (Calc., Sang.).

Face: Blue rings under eyes, swelling and necrosis of lower jaw.

Mouth: Bleeding gums, tongue dry smooth red. Persistent bleeding after tooth extraction. Thirst for very cold water.

Stomach: Hunger soon after eating, throws up ingesta by the mouthfuls, water is thrown up as soon as it gets warm in the stomach, post-operative vomiting. Cardiac opening seems contracted to narrow, the food scarcely swallowed, comes up again. Bad effects of eating too much salt.

Abdomen: A very weak, empty, gone sensation.

Stool: Very fetid stools and flatus. Stool long, narrow, hard, like dogs. Difficult to expel. Great weakness after stool.

Male: Irresistible desire.

Respiratory: Larynx very painful, clergyman's sore throat, violent tickling in larynx while speaking. Aphonia, worse evenings, with rawness. Cannot talk on account of pain in larynx. Cough from tickling in throat, worse cold air. Hard, dry, tight racking cough, tightness across chest, great weight on chest, respiration quickened, oppressed, much heat in chest, worse lying on left side, tuberculosis in tall rapidly growing young people. Repeated haemoptysis.

Heart: Dilated especially right.

Back: Heat between the shoulder blades.

Extremities: Can scarcely hold thing with his hands. Arms and hands become numb, joints suddenly give away.

Sleep: Short naps and frequent wakings.

Fever: Adynamic with lack of thirst.

Skin: Wounds bleed very much, even if small, purpura haemorrhagica, scurvy.

Compare: Tuberculinum follows Phosphor well, and complements its action. Phos. antidotes the nausea and vomiting of chloroform and Ether.

Dose: 3-30th potency. Should not be given too low or in too continuous doses especially in tuberculosis cases. It may act as Euthanasia here. *(Boericke)*

Constitution of Phos.

1. Tall slender persons of sanguine temperament, fair skin, blonde or red hair, quick lively perceptions and sensitive nature.
2. Young people who grow too rapidly and are inclined to stoop, chlorotic, anaemic.
3. Persons of waxy translucent skin, half anaemic, half jaundiced.
4. Tall, slender, narrow chested, phthisical patients, delicate eye lashes, soft hair.
5. Tall slim dark haired persons, especially women disposed to stoop.

6. Nervous week persons who like to be magnetised.
7. Haemorrhagic patients, slight wounds bleeds profusely. Phos has burning thirst for cold water, cold water relieves, but as soon as it becomes warm in the stomach it is vomited. Phos remedies the effects of excessive salt eating. Suffocative pains in upper part of chest with constriction of larynx and engorgement of lungs, mucous rales, panting and laboured breathing, even emphysema. After the cough an asthmatic attack. Phos affects all parts of the eye. Retina, choroid, vitreous and crystalline lenses, cornea and conjunctiva. Phos has cured more cases of headache always coming on when thunder storms are about than any other remedy in my experience. It has also cured blindness from lightning stroke - the venous more than the arterial system. Asthma after cough. *(JHC)*

Anaemic old people with morning diarrhoea - over sensitiveness to light, noise, odors, touch - haemorrhagic diathesis, small wounds bleed profusely. Great weakness and prostration - with nervous debility and trembling of whole body. Diarrhoea as soon as anything enters the rectum. Perspiration has the odor of sulphur. Phos removes the bad effects of Iodine and excessive use of table salt. Hahnemann says it is most beneficial when the patient suffers from chronic loose stool or diarrhoea. *(HC Allen)*

The alkalinity of the blood is increased and the amount of urea excreted is diminished. There are caries of the nasal bones, with stoppage of the nose, haemorrhage and nasal polypi. There is a halo around the light, a red appearance of objects, flashes of light. It is also of service in retinal apoplexy. In diarrhoea, when the passage is painless and involuntarily pours away as if from a hydrant. When constipation is present the stools are long and slender, like a dog's and are voided with much straining. It relieves nephritis when there is a profuse discharge of bloody urine which contains many granular casts.

It is of service in laryngitis, when there is hoarseness and aphonia, with great sensitiveness of the larynx. The voice is hoarse and there is a distressing cough upon attempting to talk. The cough is dry, and is caused by an irritation and tickling. It is worse in the evening, and on coming from a warm room into the cold air.

The cough is dry and hacking, with burning and tickling of the air passages. There are frequent haemorrhages from the lungs. *(Blackwood)*

Synopsis: Tall slender persons, loss of animal fluids, nervous debility, susceptibility to light, sound, odors, touch, electrical changes, ill effects of iodine and excessive use of salt, agg: lying on left side, cataract, amaurosis from sexual excesses, glaucoma, haemorrhage, bleeding gums, stool long narrow, hard like a dog's, aphonia, cough from tickling in throat, worse cold air, racking cough, can scarcely hold anything with his hands, burning thirst for cold water, cold water relieves, but as soon as it becomes warm in the stomach it is vomited, emphysema. Phos. affects all parts of eyes, blindness from lightning stroke. perspiration has the odor of sulphur. Most beneficial when patient suffers from chronic loose stool or diarrhoea.

479. Physalia

(Physalia pelagica - Portuguese man-of-war)

The sensation as if stung by a nettle, succeeded in a few minutes by violent aching affecting the finger joints and spreading up arm, involving elbow joint. The pain was agg: by application of water, by motion, when joints became affected.

Compare: Medusa, Urtica. ur. (JHC)

480. Physalis-Solanum Vesicarium

(Winter cherry)

Marked urinary symptoms, confirming its ancient uses in gravel etc. Lithiasis, marked diuretic action. Languor and muscular weakness. Urine acrid, foul, retained abundant, polyuria, sudden inability to hold it in women. Nocturnal incontinence. Enuresis. Dose: Tincture to 3rd attenuation. The juice of the berries is used in dropsical conditions and irritable bladder. *(Boericke)*

This remedy has been employed in Paralysis of the facial nerve. *(Blackwood)*

481. Physostigma

(Calabar bean)

This remedy and its active principle, Eserine, form a valuable addition to Materia medica. Stimulates heart, raises blood pressure and increases peristalsis. Causes contraction of the pupil and of the ciliary muscles. Induces a condition of short sightedness. Spinal irritation, loss of motility, prostration, with very sensitive vertebrae. Fibrillary tremors, rigidity of muscles, paralysis. Depresses the motor and reflex activity of the cord and causes loss of sensibility to pain, muscular weakness, followed by complete paralysis, although muscular contractibility is not impaired. Paralysis and tremors, chorea, meningeal irritation with rigidity of muscles. Tetanus and trismus. Poliomyelitis anterior. Eserine is used locally to produce contraction of pupil.

Head: Cannot bear to raise eyelids.

Eyes: Contraction of pupils, twitching of ocular muscles. Glaucoma, spasm of ciliary muscle with irritability after using eyes, increasing Myopia.

Mouth: Tongue feels sore on tip.

Heart: Fluttering of heart felt in throat.

Extremities: Pain in right popliteal space.

Relationship: Eserine - the alkaloid of physostigma - slows action of heart and increases arterial tension. Used locally to contract the pupil - Eserine contracts the pupils - dilated by Atropin, but not those dilated by Gelsemium. Internally 6x.

Dose: 3rd potency. *(Boericke)*

Its seeds are very poisonous and are used by the Calabari as an ordeal; suspected persons being compelled to eat them until they either vomit or die. In the latter case they are considered guilty, in the former innocent. It is for its action on the eye especially for its power of contracting the pupil and thereby antagonising atropine, that Phys. and its alkaloid Eserine are best known in old school-practice. In glaucoma it has been used with signal success to diminish intraocular tension and especially when glaucoma has been the result of injury - Paralysis and tremors predominate over the cramps, twitchings, stiffness and tension of physo, but these are also characteristic and tetanus has been cured by Physo. The inability to get the will into the muscles is a striking feature of many paralysis. One of the provers (a water drinker) developed a perfect disgust for cold water and cold drinks, other provers felt uncomfortable after bathing and had great reluctance to their bath. *(JHC)*

Vision dim, from blur or film, objects mixed - pain after using eyes, floating black spots, flashes of light, twitching of lids and muscles of the eyes. Idiopathic or traumatic tetanus, brought on or agg: by slightest breath of air from a person passing. *(HCA)*

This remedy is indicated in spinal and nervous irritation. There is great prostration of the muscular system and tenderness of the spine. It has also been employed in general paralysis of the insane and progressive muscular atrophy; also in tetanus of traumatic or idiopathic origin, when the slightest draught of air renews the spasm.

It is claimed to relieve acquired myopia, the result of ciliary spasm; also night blindness, with twitching of the ocular muscles and contraction of the pupils. *(Blackwood)*

482. *Pytolacca*
(Poke Root)

Aching, soreness, restlessness, prostration are general symptoms guiding to Phytolacca. Pre-eminently a glandular remedy. Glandular swellings with heat and inflammation. Has a powerful effect on fibrous and osseous tissues, fasciae and muscle sheaths. Acts on scar tissue. Syphilitic bone pains, chronic rheumatisms, Sore throat, quinsy and diphtheria. Tetanus and opisthotonus. Decrease of weight. Retarded dentition.

Eyes: Smarting. Abundant lachrymation, hot.

Nose: Flow of mucus from one nostril and from posterior nares.

Mouth: Bites the teeth together. Tongue has red tip.

Throat: Dark, red or bluish red, throat feels rough, narrow, hot, tonsils swollen, especially right, shooting pain into ears on swallowing. Cannot swallow anything hot - throat feels very hot, pain at root of tongue extending to ear, quinsy, tonsils and fauces swollen. Mumps, follicular pharyngitis.

Urine: Scanty, suppressed, with pain in kidney region.

Female: Mastitis, mammae hard, very sensitive. Tumors of the breasts with enlarged axillary glands. Cancer of breast. Breast is hard, painful and purple hue. Mammary abscess. When child nurses, pain goes from nipple all over body. Cracks and small ulcers about nipples, Galactorrhoea.

Male: Painful induration of testicles. Shooting along perineum to penis.

Extremities: Pains fly like electric shocks. Aching of heels amel: by elevating feet, pain like shocks.

Skin: Disposition to boils, venereal buboes, warts and moles.

Mod: Worse, sensitive to electric changes, damp cold weather. *Better:* Warmth, dry weather.

Relation: Tincture of Phytolacca berry (sore throat and in the treatment of obesity)

Dose: Tincture. to 3rd potency. Externally for mastitis. *(Boericke)*

Phyt. dec. is a branching herbaceous plant with a thick perennial root, some times larger than a man's leg in diameter. The young shoots, though extremely acrid, are rendered harmless by boiling and are eaten like asparagus in the United States. The berries have a popular repute as a remedy for cancer and rheumatism - wild pigeons and other birds which eat the berries acquire a highly red colour and lose their fat. This last observation has led to the use of a Tincture of Phyt. berries as an anti-fat and many successful results have been reported. This observation may be taken as the key to one of the great spheres of the action of this remedy. The absorption of tissues, especially new growths. There are few remedies which gave a wider range in the cure of tumors and indurations, particularly of the female breast. But its chief repute is in caked udders. In breast, induration and abscesses of nursing women and even in cancers, its action has been well confirmed. The intense action of the drug on the throat has led to its being used as a routine remedy in diphtheria. The nervous irritability of phyt has led to its successful use in disorders of dentition, a key note symptom being: Irresistible inclination to bite the teeth or gums together "NASH" has removed many breast tumors by giving a single dose of Phyt. C.M. during the wane of moon. Hunger soon after eating (This is like the deadly sinking so often met with in the cancerous diathesis) - I have found a gargle of a few drops of the ϕ to a tumbler of water useful in many throat cases. Sensation of apple core in throat. Brings loss of fat. Opposite to Sabal Serrulata. *(JHC)*

Patients of a rheumatic diathesis. Emaciation, chlorosis, loss of fat. Occupies a position between *Bryonia* and *Rhus,* cures when these fail, though apparently well indicated. Irresistible desire to bite the teeth or gums together, during dentition. Sore throat of dark colour, uvula large, dropsical, almost translucent (*Kali bi. Rhus*) - Mammae full of hard painful nodosities. Breast shows an early tendency to cake, is full stony hard and painful nodosities, especially when suppuration is inevitable. Mammary abscess, fistulas, gaping angry ulcers, pus sanious, ichorous foetid, unhealthy - Nipples sensitive, sore, fissured, agg: when it rains, exposure to damp cold weather.

Compare: Kali Iod is its analogue. *(HCA)*

This remedy is indicated in subacute and chronic rheumatism, located in the periosteum and fibrous tissue of the neck and back, or he feels sore all over from head to foot. The muscles are sore and stiff. Rheumatic pains in the lower extremities, with nightly bone pains, the patient is worse at night and during damp weather, and while he is restless and desires to move, motion aggravates. It is useful in tonsillitis and diphtheria. The throat is covered with a dark coloured membrane, and feels as though a ball of fire had lodged there. The breath is offensive. The glands of the parts are enlarged. The fever is high, and there are aching pains in the back and legs, and he feels as though he were pounded all over. There is great prostration and a pain shoots from the throat into the ears on swallowing. It is also useful in pharyngitis, when the parts are of a dark red colour. The uvula is large and almost translucent.

It is of service in inflammation of the breasts, when the glands are hard and painful. The pains shoot all over the body when the child nurses. It is also of service in the hard, painful nodosities that appear independent of lactation, when it should be applied locally and taken internally. It should be remembered during dentition, when the child bites the teeth together. It is employed in syphilis during secondary stages. *(Blackwood)*

483. *Picricum Acidum*

(Tri-nitrophenol)

Causes degeneration of the spinal cord with paralysis. Brain fag and sexual excitement. Acts upon the generative organs, probably through the lumbar centers of the spinal cord, prostration, weakness and pain of back, pins and needle sensation in extremities. Neurasthenia (Oxal acid). Muscular debility. Heavy tired feeling. Myelitis with spasms and prostration. Writers' palsy. Progressive, pernicious anaemia, uraemia with complete anuria. A one percent solution applied on lint is the best application for burns until granulation begins to form. Sallow complexion.

Mind: lack of will power, disinclined to work, sits still and listless.

Head: Pain amel: bandaging tightly, occipital pains, boils within ears, after prolonged mental strain with anxiety and dread of failure of examination, brain fag.

Urinary: Scanty, complete anuria, dribbling micturition, uraemia.

Male: Priapism, satyriasis, hard erections with pain in testicles and up cord. Prostatic hypertrophy.

Extremities: Spine-great weakness, tired, heavy feeling all over body, especially limbs, worse exertion, feet cold, cannot get warm.

Mod: (Worse) least exertion, especially mental, after sleep, wet weather, hot weather. *Better:* cold air, cold water, tight pressure.

Dose: 6th potency. *(Boericke)*

It is formed by the action of Nit. ac. and carbolic acid, salicin, silk and many other substances. Pulse slow, small, very feeble. Great weakness, compelling to lie down, no anxiety, vivid colouration of sclerotics and integuments, urine coloured blood red. a stenographer and typist after using her right hand finger continuously for 6 years noticed weakness of her thumb and index finger and inability to hold pen or pencil. Next there was difficulty in striking correctly the keys of the type writer and some wrist drop. Massage, electricity had failed to give any relief. Pic. ac. 3x - 6 times daily cured the case. Priapism, penis distended almost to bursting. Terrible erections disturbing sleep - Great sexual desire with emissions. Amorous fancies. Pic. acid solution is a remedy for burns. Among other affections it has cured diabetes, intense thirst and copious urination especially at night. (Urine 1040 - 7½ percent of sugar and some albumin. Pic ac. 6x - 6 times daily). Brain fag. Inability to study. Gastric symptoms:-- sour eructations, *Agg:* morning.

Compare: Nux, brain fag, occipital headache, sexual neurasthenia, writers cramp, *Gels, Plat.*

Causation: Study, fatigue, mental exertion. *(JHC)*

Nervous prostration, neurasthenia, brain fag of literary or business people.

Headache of students, teachers and over worked businessmen, occipital cervical region, satyriasis, burning along spine and great weakness of spine, tired heavy feeling all over body, especially of limbs, Agg: exertion. *(HCA)*

This remedy is indicated in restoring the wasted and worn out systems of those who are suffering from the effects of close application to study or business and become anaemic and neurasthenic and asthenic. It is indicated in progressive pernicious anaemia, people who complain of a heavy tired feeling over the body. Brain fag of students and businessmen. Indicated in myelitis, when there are tonic and clonic spasms with exhaustion and prostration. It should be thought of in acute, ascending paralysis. It is of service in satyriasis and priapism, which are violent and last a long time with profuse seminal emission. The penis is so distended that it feels as though it would burst. There are amorous fancies and erections that disturb the sleep. This is often associated with spinal or cerebral affections. It has been employed locally in eczema in the proportion of one part of the acid to eighty-six of water. Found useful in neurasthenics with glycosuria, in which the mental condition is one of indifference and loss of will power.

Compare: Oxalic acid, Gel., Phos. acid.
(Blackwood)

484.Pilocarpus Microphyllus

(Jaborandi)

Pilocarpus is a powerful glandular stimulant and the most efficient diaphoretic. Its most important effects are disphoresis, salivation and myosis. Hot flushes, nausea, salivation and profuse perspiration. The face, ears and neck become, in a few minutes after a dose of Jaborandi, deeply flushed and drops of perspiration break out all over the body, whilst at the same time, the mouth waters and saliva pours out, in an almost continuous stream. Other secretions - lachrymal, nasal, bronchial and intestinal also but in less degree. The sweat and saliva produced by a single dose is often enormous in quantity, not infrequently half a pint.

Is homoeopathic to abnormal sweats and has achieved great success in night sweats of consumptives. Acts upon the thyroid and its sudorific action may possibly be due to it. Exophthalmic goitre with increased heart's action and pulsation of arteries, tremors and nervousness, heat and sweating, bronchial irritation. A valuable remedy in limiting the duration of Mumps.

Eyes: Strain - pupils contracted, near sighted, white spots before eyes, smarting pain in eyes, lids twitch.

Mouth: Saliva viscid, like white of eggs, free salivation with profuse sweating.

Skin: Excessive perspiration from all parts of body.

Dose: 3rd potency. *(Boericke)*

South American Indian use as an antidote to the bite of serpents of the Trigenocephalus group - Hale commends its use in women or young girls who have always a dry skin, scanty menses and tendency of blood to the head - eye weakness - especially hypometropia - Cooper has seen a violent leucorrhoea caused by jaborandi, also the discharge of a quantity of thread worms. Stimulant of the mammary secretions. Suffer from extreme nervousness and by a fixed idea that she should murder all her family with a hatchet. Jaborandi has been used as a remedy for baldness and it forms the principal ingredient in some of the popular hair restorers. In a number of patients, who have been taking it, white hair and blonde hair have been observed to turn black. *(JHC)*

This remedy is indicated in dropsical effusions of the lung and in cardiac dropsy, where it produces free and rapid diaphoresis, renal ascites, hydrothorax and pleuritic effusions.

It should be remembered in sialorrhoea (Ptyalism) and the salivation of pregnancy, especially when the secretion is characterized by profuseness.

It has been employed extensively, with marked success in puerperal and uraemic eclampsia.

It has been extensively used in the lower potencies during the afternoon and evening to control the night sweats of slow convalescence and that of pulmonary phthisis.

It is claimed to have a favourable influence in cases of alopecia and if continued over a prolonged period to restore the original colour of gray hair. It has been found curative in the hot flushes that attend the climacteric period, when these are attended with nausea, salivation and profuse perspiration.

It acts as a prompt and efficient galactagogue but should be given with care to asthenic patients owing to its mydriatic properties. It has been extensively employed by ophthalmologists, much after the manner of eserine. Its beneficial effects have been observed in iridiocyclitis, in plastic, traumatic and rheumatic iritis, in simple glaucoma, optic neuritis, retinal haemorrhages, detachment of the retina.

It has been employed during parturition, especially when the skin is dry, the pains hard, the muscular system tense and the os uteri rigid.

It is employed in South America as an antidote to the bite of the serpents of the Trigonocephalus group.

Physiological action

This agent produces a free sweating and salivation. The sweat produced has been estimated at from nine to fifteen ounces. The chlorides are increased in the sweat, while the urine is increased about five times its normal amount. It has been estimated that in the hour following the employment of the drug, one quart of saline is secreted, while the secretion of the whole glandular system is stimulated. The secretion of milk is promoted. *(Blackwood)*

485. Pilocarpinum

Pilocarpin is one of the most characteristic of several alkaloids which have been isolated from Jaborandi (Pilocarpus) to produce and cure profuse sweating and by oculists to produce contraction of the pupils, which it does whether it is injected subcutaneously or applied directly to the eye. Good effect in labyrinthine deafness, tinnitus and auditory nerve vertigo, in which the hearing was amel: in a noise as of a train etc. The hair as well as the skin is affected by pilo, which is an ingredient in many hair restorers. Schmidt of Cologne treated two bald men with injection of Pilomur to produce absorption of inflammatory residue within the eye. As a secondary effect - growth of young downy hair black. Pilomur 3x is Burnett's chief remedy for mumps - He regards it (and Jaborandi) as an organ remedy of the sweat gland, parotid and pancreas. *(JHC)*

Pilocarpin-mur-Meniere's disease, rapidly progressive phthisis, with free haemorrhages, profuse sweating, 2x trit. Atropine is the antagonist to Pilocarpin, in dose of one, one hundredth grain for one-sixth of Pilocarpin. *(Boericke)*

486. *Pinus Sylvestris*

(Scotch Pine)

Has been found of real use in the treatment of weak ankles and tardiness in walking, in scrofulous and rachitic children. Emaciation of lower extremities. Pinus sylvestris combines rheumatic, bronchial, and urticarious symptoms, the chest seems thin and to give way.

Extremities - Stiffness, gouty pain in all joints, especially finger joints. Cramps in calves.

Skin: Nettle rash, itching all over especially about joints and on abdomen. Nose itches.

Dose: Tincture to 3rd potency.

(Boericke)

Pine baths may also be made by adding Oleum pini sylvestris to an ordinary bath in the proportion of one minim to the gallon. These baths have a reputation in the treatment of rheumatism, gout, paralysis, scrofula and skin disease. Itching of the nose and discharge of round worms was noted. Emaciation of lower extremities and weak ankles in children, is indication for it. The ϕ may be used externally, whilst the attenuations are given internally. *(JHC)*

This remedy is indicated in scrofulous and rachitic children, whose ankles are weak and who are late in learning to walk. The lower extremities are emaciated.

It should be remembered when there is a sensation of violent boring, burning pains in the region of the kidneys that extend along the ureters. The urine is increased in quantity, has a strong odor, and there are severe, burning pains upon urinating. There are gouty and arthritic pains in the extremities, and a sensation as though the parts would give out.

There is itching of the whole body, but especially about the joints and abdomen.

Compare: Terebinthina, Benzoic acid.

(Blackwood)

487. *Piper Methysticum*

(Kava-Kava)

The intoxication produced by Kava is of a silent and drowsy character, with incoherent dreams, loss of muscular power.

Urinary and skin symptoms have been verified. Marked modality. Arthritis deformans, colic with flatulence.

Mind: Amelioration of pains for a time by diverting attention.

Urine: Chordee.

Skin: White spots, leprosy.

Relationship: Chaulmoongra Taraktogenos - the oil and its derivatives are to a certain extent effective in the treatment of leprosy, especially in early cases. Bixa orellana, a South American plant related to Chaulmoongra recommended for leprosy, eczema and elephantiasis.

Dose: Tincture to lower potencies. *(Boericke)*

The natives use it as a stimulant, either showing the root or drinking a beverage made of it before undertaking any important business or a religious rites. Excessive indulgence in it produces a skin disease, like leprosy called at Tahiti Arevareva - The drug causes a feeling of buoyancy as if every nerve was strung up to the highest pitch - feels he can work without fatigue, quickly followed by a feeling of tired brain. Skinner gave fractional doses of drops

Tincture in water to a highly excitable young girl who had severe toothache and earache and had worn out her family by the incessant day and night attendance she required. Oh! my tooth or ear. *(JHC)*

This remedy is indicated in subacute gonorrhoea, and gleet; also cystitis and catarrh of the bladder. In these cases twenty drops should be given in a glass of water four times a day. It is of service in nocturnal enuresis of the aged, the feeble, and in children, dependent upon muscular weakness.

It is useful in nephritis with dropsy. The urine is loaded with albumin and contains many casts; the heart is feeble and irregular. It has been recommended in leprosy. The skin is covered with scales, which when drop off, leave white spots that may ulcerate.

Compare - Cannabis sativa, Copaiba.
(Blackwood)

488. Piperazinum

Piperaz. is a synthetic product which was intended to replace Spermin C2 H5 N and was named Dispermine. It was found, however, to be different, both in chemical and physiological properties. It occurs in well-defined, colourless, acicular crystals (Helbing), or in lustrous tables (J. Gordon); is deliquescent and mostly soluble in water. It readily unites with Uric acid, forming a very soluble compound (urate of piperazine). When taken by the mouth it is not entirely oxidised, as part is discoverable unchanged in the urine. John Gordon experimented with Piperaz and found that a 1% solution in normal urine at body temperature dissolved to a large extent a fragment of uric acid calculus, and converted undissolved portions to a granular and pulpy condition. The amount of urea is increased in the urine of those taking it; and Helbing (Modern Materia Medica) says it has been used with success in mental diseases, and in a case of lead paralysis with very remarkable results. J.H. Hamilton, of Hawisk (Lancet, Dec. 30. 1893), reports success in treating renal colic with Piperaz; and Walter, of Odessa (Quoted H.W. XXV. 10), cleared up the symptoms disappearing within three weeks. (After a teaspoonful dose of an effervescing preparation of Piperaz, a patient complained that he was seized with a bad attack of acute gout, that was quite unexpected. (Cooper)

Compare: Phloriz, Hydrang., Urt. u.
(JHC)

This agent is non-toxic and non irritating to the mucous membranes with which it comes in contact. It has but little or no effect upon the digestive, circulatory or respiratory system and within two hours is detected in the urine in a state of combination with uric acid. Full doses induce nausea, loss of muscular power and irregular respiration in the lower animals.

In man in full doses (grs. xxxvii) it has produced severe headache, tremor, convulsions, and clonic spasms. Under its influence there is an enormous increase in the amount of urea and a likely decrease in the amount of uric acid eliminated. It is said to have twelve times the power of carbonate of lithia in its solvent effect upon uric acid.

This remedy is indicated in cases where there is a persistent excess of uric acid and urates in the urine. There is a constant backache, the skin is dry, the urine scanty and contains a brick. dust sediment. It should be remembered in cases of chronic rheumatic arthritis, gout and acute rheumatism when there is an excessive formation of uric acid.

It is also found to be of service in cases of constant sickening pain in the back.

Compare: Lithia, Berberis vulgaris.
(Blackwood)

489. *Piper Nigrum*
(Black pepper)

Sensation of burning and pressure everywhere. Heavy headache as if temples were pressed in. *(Boericke)*

The peppers are tropical climbing shrubs. Piper nig. yields the pepper of commerce. The fruit when ripe is red. It is gathered before it is fully ripe and spread on mats in the sun, when it loses its red colour and becomes black and shrivelled. This is black pepper. White pepper is the same fruit freed from its outer skin by maceration in water and subsequent rubbing. The symptoms of the proving are Houat's. The only additional symptom is one recorded by Berridge as having occurred in a lady on two occasions from taking a large quantity of pepper. Feeling as if temples and malar bones were pressed in. Agg: on left side. This confirms one of Houat's symptoms. The full, heavy headache of Houat's provings I can confirm by personal experience: I get the headache whenever I take food highly peppered and I know others who do the same. Sensations of foreign round body rising to stomach. The symptoms are Agg: by change of temperature; in damp weather; in evening; by motion. *(JHC)*

This remedy is employed in malarial regions as a stimulant to overcome the depression that attends the malarial paroxysm. It is indicated in nausea and vomiting when the latter is attended with extreme exertion as though every thing would be brought up. There is continuous thirst. It is of service in blenorrhoea (Gonorrhoea) when the discharge is greenish and offensive. There is inflammation of penis with priapism and at burning pains in the organ. It should be remembered when there is soreness of chest and at each coughing spell, it appears that the part will be torn.
(Blackwood)

490. *Pituitary Gland*

Pituitary gland exercises a superior control over the growth and development of the sexual organs, stimulates muscular activity and overcomes a uterine inertia. Its influence over unstripped muscular fibre is marked. Cerebral haemorrhage. Will check haemorrhage and add absorption of clot. Uterine inertia in second stage of labor where os is fully dilated. High blood pressure (30 potency), chronic nephritis, prostatitis. Ten drops after meals (Dr. Geofuller). Vertigo, difficult mental concentration, confusion and fullness, deep in frontal region. Use 30th potency. (Boericke)

Posterior lobe (Metabolism of sugar)

If there is a hyper-secretion, glycosuria may result. If there is a hyposecretion an undue tolerance of sugar results, may cause diabetes insipidus. An extract from this lobe is an active diuretic as a result of its action on the heart and its power of raising the blood pressure.

Anterior lobe

This is enlarged during pregnancy. If it is not enlarged, there are marked disturbances of metabolism as such deposits of fat, puffing of the hands and feet or a derangement of the calcium metabolism, as is observed in the loss of the teeth and hair, brittle nails in the mother and a defective bone formation in the foetus. Such disturbances of this gland are often associated with those of the thyroid and parathyroid. A hypersecretion of anterior lobe during childhood results in a condition of Gigantism. If this condition persists, till the person is 20 or over, the epiphyses of the bone become united and the acromegalic type takes place.

If there is a hyposecretion of anterior lobe, in young children the bones do not grow and the child remains dwarfed. If this condition is present at the adolescent, there is a lack of hair on the pubes, in the axilla and on the genitals and the child remains underdeveloped. If hyposecretion develops later in life, there is testicular atrophy and male assumes the feminine type.

Under its influence the uterine contractions are brisk and frequent. It should never be used until the cervix is completely dilated and it is known that there is no obstruction to the passage of the child.

In incontinence of the urine both in adults and children, it has been of service, also in nocturnal enuresis, both when administered by the mouth and injected.

These preparations are derived from the pituitary of cattle. *(Blackwood)*

491. *Pix Liquida*

(Pine tar)

Tar and its constituents act on various mucous membranes. Its skin symptoms are most important. A great cough medicine. Bronchial irritation after influenza (Kreosot, Kali bich.). Scaly eruptions. Much itching, constant vomiting of blackish fluid, with pain in stomach. Alopecia (Fluor. ac.).

Chest: Pain at a spot about the third left costal cartilage where it joins the rib. muco-purulent sputum.

Skin: Cracked, itches intolerably, bleeds on scratching, eruptions on back of hands.

Dose: 1st to 6th potency. *(Boericke)*

In old school practice, Tar is known as 'stimulant expectorant' in chronic bronchitis and phthisis, a stimulant to the skin in psoriasis and scaly eczema. Pain at the third left costal where it joins the rib. This is really a pain on the left bronchus and when associated with offensive mucopurulent expectoration, the indication of Pix are complete. Pix often cures the enuresis somni of children. In chest pains, Iliac. has pain at 3rd right costal cartilage. *(JHC)*

This remedy is indicated in skin diseases, when the eruption is scaly and is attended with intolerable itching. The eruption is most pronounced upon the back of the hands. It is useful in chronic bronchitis with rales through the lungs and a muco-purulent sputum of an offensive odor and taste. There is a painful spot where the third left costal cartilage joins the sternum. *(Blackwood)*

492. *Plantago Major*

(Plantain)

Has considerable clinical reputation in the treatment of earache and enuresis. Sharp pain in eyes, reflex from decayed teeth or inflammation of middle ear. Eye ball very tender to touch. Pain plays between teeth and ears. Pyorrhoea alveolaris.

Depression and insomnia of chronic Nicotinism. Causes an aversion to tobacco.

Ears: Pain goes from one ear to the other through the head.

Mouth: Toothache, worse cold air and contact - better while eating.

Urine: Nocturnal enuresis.

Dose: Tincture and lower potencies. Local use in toothache, in hollow teeth, otorrhoea, pruritus. *(Boericke)*

Plantago maj. not to be confounded with musa, sometimes called Plantain which belongs to a different class, viz the endogens. In A.D. 1558 the Herbal of Dodens recommended the juice of leaves or roots for toothache and bleeding of gums. John Parkinson in his Theatre of plants says the root taken fresh out of the ground, washed and genty scraped with a knife, then put into the ear, cures the toothache like a charm. In switzerland the leaf fibres are frayed out and put into the ear for the same purpose, and if they relieve the pain they turn black and have to be removed, if there is no relief they remain green. A case is related of a man who allowed himself to be bitten by rattle snakes and cured himself by drinking the juice of the plant and applying bruised leaves to the bites changing them frequently. The neuralgic pains of teeth, ears and face were especially pronounced. The very copious discharge of urine along with the thirst suggests diabetes and the laxity of sphincter has led to the cure of a number of case of enuresis. In common with others, I have used it with success in numberless cases of toothache and earache. Plantago 'ϕ' applied locally to gums, temple, and check, removed the pain in a few minutes. Toothache with earache. Toothache with salivation are leading indications - Plant. has a relation to tobacco - it produces disgust for it in chewers. In enuresis, Bell has irregular action of sphincter, Plant. and Caust. cause relaxation. *(JHC)*

493. Platanus Occidentalis

(Sycamore. Buttonwood)

Tarsal tumors (eye lid) - apply the tincture. Both acute and neglected cases where destruction of tissue occurred and cicatrical contraction caused marked deformity of lid, restored to practically normal conditions. Acts best in children. Must be used for some time. Ichthyosis.

(Boericke)

The tree commonly grown in and about London as P. Occidentalis - Burnett has recorded a case of Ichthyosis in an aged lady in which Platanus caused considerable improvement in the condition of the skin - Girl 5 1/2, blind from double cataract due to the shock of a fall in the first instance, the lenses having gradually silted up - In this case Platanus ϕ was given (five drops) night and morning for a number of months with very evident improvement in the nutrition of the child's lenses. (Burnett) named the remedy Plat. occ. but his tincture was made from the London tree which is Plat. Acer. It sheds its bark annually, which was the signature of its skin action. (JHC)

494. Platina

(The metal)

Is pre-eminently a woman's remedy. Strong tendency to paralysis, anaesthesia, localized numbness and coldness are shown. Hysterical spasms. Pains increase and decrease gradually (Stannum). Tremulousness.

Mind: Irresistible impulse to kill. Self exaltation. Contempt for others, Arrogant, proud, weary of everything, everything seems changed. Mental troubles associated with suppressed menses. Physical symptoms disappear as mental symptoms develop.

Head: Tense, pressing pain confined to a small spot, cramplike, squeezing pain, constriction about forehead and right temples. Numbness with headache.

Eyes: Objects look smaller than they are, twitching of lids (Eyes feel cold, cramplike pain in orbits).

Face: Prosopalgia, pain at root of nose as if squeezed in a vise. Coldness, creeping and numbness.

Stomach: Fermentation, much flatulence, constriction, ravenous hunger, nausea with anxiety and weakness.

Abdomen: painters colic, pain in umbilical region extending through to back. Pressing and bearing down in abdomen, extending into pelvis.

Stool: Retarded, faeces scanty, evacuated with difficulty, adheres to rectum, like soft clay, sticky stool, constipation, stool as if burnt.

Female: Parts hypersensitive, tingling internally and externally, ovaries sensitive and burn. Menses too early, too profuse, dark clotted, with spasms and painful bearing down, chilliness and sensitiveness of parts. Vaginismus. Nymphomania, excessive sexual development, vaginismus, pruritus vulvae, ovaritis with sterility, abnormal sexual appetite and melancholia.

Extremities: Tightness of thighs as if too tightly wrapped. Numb and weary sensation. Feels paralysed.

Sleeps: With legs apart.

Mod: Worse, sitting and standing, evening.

Better: Walking.

Dose: 6X to 30c. *(Boericke)*

(The patient, generally a woman) looks down on everything and everybody. This is a Keynote of Plat. Another is occurrence of cramps, cramping pains and spasms. As physical symptoms disappear mental symptoms appear and vice versa. Laughs at serious things - Inspiration to kill her child, to kill her husband, whom she loved passionately. Sensitiveness of the external genitals is often so great as to make coition impossible Digital examining of such a patient causes great pain impulse to pederasty and sodomy. Tendency to uncover completely in sleep is a leading note of it. Excessive itching in uterus, pruritus vulvae - Constipation scarcely less marked than that of Pb. Stool may be hard as if burnt. Constipation comes on whilst travelling. As if she did not belong to her own family. Plat is suited to women with dark hair, thin sanguine, bilious, with too frequent and too profuse menses. Hysterical and haemorrhoidal patients. Headache commences on waking Agg: in warm room Amel: In open air. Sees ghost and demons.

The mind is deranged and has distorted superiority over those associated with her. The menses are premature and profuse with spasmodic and neuralgic conditions. Also in Nymphomania, vaginismus, pruritus vulva. It is of service in constipation. There is an inertia of the bowels and frequent unsuccessful attempts to stool, which are like putty and adhere to the anus. It is also of service in the constipation of emigrants and travellers. *(JHC)*

495. *Plumbum Met*

(Lead)

The great drug for general sclerotic conditions. Lead paralysis is chiefly of extensors, forearm or upper limb, from center to periphery with partial anaesthesia or excessive hyperaesthesia, preceded by pain. Localised neuralgic pains, neuritis. The blood, alimentary and nervous systems are the special seats of action of plumbum. Hematosis is interfered with rapid reduction in number of red corpuscles, hence pallor, icterus, anemia. Constrictive sensation in internal organs.

Delirium, coma and convulsions. Hypertension and arteriosclerosis. Progressive muscular atrophy. Infantile paralysis. Locomotor ataxia. Excessive and rapid emaciation. Bulbar paralysis. Important in peripheral affections. The points of attack for plumbum are the neurons and the anterior horns. Symptoms of the Multiple Sclerosis, posterior spinal sclerosis. Contractions and burning pain. All the symptoms of the acute nephritis with amaurosis and cerebral symptoms. Gout (Chronic).

Mind: Mental depression, fear of being assassinated.

Head: Tinnitus.

Eyes: Glaucoma.

Face: Pale and cachectic, yellow, corpse-like, cheek sunken, skin of face greasy, shiny.

Mouth: Distinct blue lines along margins of gums.

Stomach: Gastralgia.

Abdomen: Excessive colic, radiating to all parts of body. Abdominal wall feels drawn by a string to spine, intussusception, strangulated hernia. Abdomen retracted.

Rectum: Constipation, stools hard, lumpy, black, with urging and spasm of anus. Anus drawn up with constriction.

Urinary: Albuminous, chronic interstitial nephritis.

Male: Loss of sexual power.

Female: Vaginismus, induration of mammary glands.

Skin: Yellow, dark brown liver spots. Jaundice.

Extremities: Paralysis of single muscles, pain in muscles of thighs, come in paroxysms, wrist drop.

Mod: Worse at night, motion. Better-rubbing hard, pressure, physical exertion.

Dose: 3-30 potency. *(Boericke)*

Plumbum, the saturn of Alchemists. Among painters and lead manufacturers, the best known symptoms are the colic and drop wrist. With albuminuria, there is an excess of uric acid in the blood of persons under the influence of lead and actual gouty deposits and gouty attacks have been observed. A state of anemia is set up and dry inactive scaly skin and inveterate constipation - the hands became paralysed, which led to the testing of the drinking water and the discovery of lead. According to taste, Plumb is particularly adapted to adults, males, rather than females. Sense of retraction, as if abdominal wall were drawn back by a string to the spine - constant urgent call to stool, only small hard black balls passed. The excessive emaciation of Plumb and action on the spine make it a remedy of the first importance in progressive muscular atrophy. *(JHC)*

Intussusception, with colic and faecal vomiting, strangulated hernia, femoral, inguinal or umbilical. Podophyllum in retraction of navel. Pod. is the vegetable analogue. *(HCA)*

Slowing of the heart's action and enteralgia. The calibre of the smaller blood vessels is contracted. Albuminuria, cirrhosis and contraction of the kidneys with diminished excretion of uric acid. Gout has been observed in acute cases. They often complain of everything tasting sweet. At times there is faecal vomiting. It has benefitted many cases of progressive muscular atrophy, locomotor ataxia and infantile paralysis. Also in rapid and excessive emaciation following the paralysis.

Compare - Alumina, Opium, Mercurius. *(Blackwood)*

496. Podophyllum

(May Apple)

Is especially adapted to persons of bilious temperament. It affects chiefly the duodenum. Small intestines, liver and rectum. The Podophyllum disease is a gastro-enteritis with colicky pain and bilious vomiting. Stool is watery with jelly- like mucûs, painless, profuse. Gushing and offensive. Many troubles during pregnancy, pendulous abdomen after confinement, prolapsus uteri, painless cholera morbus. Torpidity of the liver, portal engorgement with a tendency to haemorrhoids, hypogastric pain, fullness of superficial veins, jaundice.

Head: Headache, dull pressure, worse morning, with heated face and bitter taste, alternating with diarrhoea, rolling of head from side to side.

Mouth: Intense desire to press the gums together. Difficult dentition, tongue broad, large, moist, burning sensation of tongue.

Abdomen: Sensation of weakness or sinking, can lie comfortably only on stomach, better rubbing part.

Rectum: Cholera infantum and morbus, diarrhoea of long standing, early in morning, during teething with hot glowing cheeks, while being bathed or washed, in hot weather, after acid fruits. Morning painless diarrhoea when not due to venous stasis or intestinal ulceration, fetid profuse, prolapse of rectum.

Female: Right ovary, with shifting noises along ascending colon. Prolapsed uteri.

Fever: Chill at 7 a.m., great loquacity during fever, profuse, sweat.

Mod: Worse in early morning, in hot weather, during dentition.

Dose: 200-1000. Seems to do good work in cholera infantum. when indicated. *(Boericke)*

Pod. grows throughout the United States in damp shady places in woods, has leaves which are five to nine — lobed, large with nodding flowers, yellowish fruits, egg shaped, not unlike a small lemon, hence the plant is sometimes called wild lemon. The botanic and eclectic practitioners adopted the remedy and used it as a vegetable mercury. The early morning agg:, the profuse stool, faint gone sensation. I have many times cured with Podo prolapsus ani in children. Sensation at stool as if the genital organs would fall out. In the pregnant and puerperal state, Pod. is frequently indicated, in the vomiting of pregnancy, swelling of labia, severe after-pains with strong bearing down sensation, haemorrhoids and prolapsus recti-after confinement. A peculiar symptom of pregnancy indicating Podo. is - can lie comfortably only on stomach (Early months). Great desire to press gums or teeth together. Podo. is one of the important antidotes to Merc. Fevers of many kinds are met by Podo. - remittent, chiefly bilious remittent, intermittent. Delirium is not rare and is apt to be loquacious. Moaning and whining during sleep - alternating conditions are noted. Diarrhoea alternating with constipation. Headache in winter. Diarrhoea in summer. Inflammation of scrotum or the eyes. The concomittance of diarrhoea with other affections points to Pod. Loquacity during chill and heat is key note in fevers. Chills violent, followed by intense fever with great loquacity, when the fever passed the patient fell asleep, and on waking remembered nothing of his loquacious delirium. Podo is suited to bilious temperaments, especially after mercurialisation - notable symptoms are thirst for large quantities of cold water. Intense desire to press the gums together. Viscid mucus in mouth coating teeth. Diarrhoea whilst being bathed or washed, of dirty water soaking through napkin, with gagging. Patient is constantly shaking and rubbing region of liver with his hands - Great loquacity during chill and heat - Pod is predominantly right sided. Right throat - Hypochondrium-ovary. Guernsey mentions that it is often called for in complaints of pregnant and parturient women, with sensation as if intestines were falling down.

Agg: Morning especially early morning 2-4 a.m. Some symptoms Agg: night, open air, while washing. Antidote to merc. Diarrhoea. Cham. < evening. Podo. - *agg:* Morning, in one gush. Veratrum has much pain. Pod may have absence of pain. *(JHC)*

This agent, known as the vegetable calomen, when applied to ulcers and raw surfaces, produces its purgative effects. It is a gastrointestinal irritant, often excites nausea, produces salivation, increases the intestinal secretion and the flow of bile. There is pronounced intestinal peristalsis, with gripping pains, and in a few hours a complete evacuation of the bowels. The stools are copious, watery and contain much bile.

Gastro-enteritis - Rectum prolapsed - Colon as if it were ulcerated. Stools contain bile Morning diarrhoea. There may be a normal stool later in the day. Congestion of the liver and cirrhosis. Diarrhoeas that attend dentition. Grinding of the teeth, whining and moaning during sleep - Tongue is coated white - Certain cases of Jaundice. When there is constipation the stools are hard, dry and coloured.

Compare: Aloe, Chelidonium, Mercurius, Sulphur. *(Blackwood)*

497. Polygonum Punctatum

(Smart weed)

Metrorrhagia, also amenorrhoea in young girls. Varicosis, haemorrhoids and rectal pockets. Burning in stomach followed by feeling of coldness in the pit of the stomach.

Abdomen: Flatulent colic.

Rectum: Interior of anus studded with itching eminence. Haemorrhoids. Liquid faeces.

Female: Aching pains in hip and loins, sensation as if hips were being drawn together. Sensation of weight and tension within pelvis. Shooting pains through breasts - amenorrhoea.

Skin: Superficial ulcers and sores on lower extremities, especially in females at climacteric.

Dose: Tincture. *(Boericke)*

Smart weed, says "Hale," is a popular remedy (domestic) throughout, U.S.A.. Applied externally it has the effect of mustard plaster and the leaves saturated with hot water are applied to relieve cramps and colic and as an emoliment in inflammation and sprains. Clinical experience has shown a definite action in the female generative sphere, amenorrhoea, aversion to coitus and congestion of the ovaries having been cured by it-left side more so than right. As if whole intestinal contents were fluid. *(JHC)*

This remedy is indicated in the amenorrhoea of young girls, when there are aching pains in the hips and loins and a sensation of weight and tension within the loins. It is also of service in rectal diseases.

Compare: Caulophyllum, Pulsatilla, Seneca. *(Blackwood)*

498. Populus Candicans

(Balm of Gilead)

Seems to have remarkable power over acute colds, especially when accompanied by a deep hoarse voice or even aphonia. General insensibility of surface (worse back and abdomen); rubbing and pounding borne without pain and is grateful on account of warmth produced. Finger ends thickened, horny, insensible to pinching and pricking. Instantaneous voice producer (Coca).

Respiratory: Acute hoarseness, throat and nostrils burn, sits bent forward with dry cough. Pharynx and larynx feel dry and the voice weak and toneless. Rawness and soreness of chest and throat. Cough of children caused by naso-pharyngeal catarrh, mucus drops from posterior nares.

Dose: Tincture 1-5 drops. *(Boericke)*

The resinous gum exuding from buds and stalks, deliciously aromatic in perfume, is widely used to heal wound, open sores and eruptions and often suppresses the latter to the harm of the patient. As an application Nichols say it is like Arnica, dangerous though most people are not susceptible to its poisonous effect. He has never seen blisters of the size of those of Pop. C. produced by any other drug, blisters hand down like bags of water the size of Walnuts. Able to speak in hoarse whispers. Among the peculiar symptoms observed by Nichols is surface anaesthesia with or without numbness. The finger-ends are actually thickened, horny, insensible to pinching and pricking. *(JHC)*

This remedy is indicated in acute colds when there is a deep, hoarse voice, or aphonia; also in anaesthasia of the surface of the body, with thickening of the finger ends, which are horny and insensible. *(Blackwood)*

499. Populus Tremuloides

(American Aspen)

The gastric and urinary symptoms point to its usefulness in dyspepsia and catarrh of the bladder, especially in old people. Good remedy in vesicle troubles after operations and in pregnancy, cystitis, fullness of head and sensation of heat of the surfaces of the body. Night sweats. Ague.

Stomach: Indigestion, with flatulence and acidity.

Dose: Tr. 1-30 drops. *(Boericke)*

Pine used Pop. t. in affections of the bladder, urethra and prostate. Hale conforms its action in vesical tenesmus and inflammation of the neck of the bladder. In the cases cured by Hale he says there was little pain during urination, but as soon as the last drops were voided or a little before, a severe cramp-like pain just behind pubes, lasting 10-15 minutes. *(JHC)*

This remedy is indicated in urethritis when micturition is painful and scalding during pregnancy. It is also useful in catarrh of the bladder when the urine contains much mucus and pus. There is severe tenesmus, and vesical irritation following laparotomy or ovariotomy.

Compare: Cornus flor., Nux vomica, Chimaphila umbellatus. *(Blackwood)*

500. Pothos Foetidus

(Skunk cabbage ictodes)

For asthmatic complaints, worse from inhaling any dus. Hysteria. Erratic spasmodic pains. 'Will-o'-the-wisp' like character of its subjective symptoms and its physometric property are special features. Inflation and tension in the abdomen. Millar's asthma.

Head: Absent minded, irritable. Headache in single spots, with violent pulsation of temporal arteries. Outward drawing from glabella. Better in open air (Puls), red swelling across the bridge of the nose.

Abdomen: Inflation and tension in abdomen.

Respiratory: Spasmodic croup, troublesome respiration, with sudden feeling of anguish and sweat. Sneezing with pain in throat, pain in chest with difficult breathing. Tongue feels numb. Asthma relieved by stool.

Dose: Tincture and lower potencies. (Tincture 1-60 drops-Blackwood) *(Boericke)*

The roots in cases of asthma, the leaves as an application to ulcers. The seeds are also considered to be anti-spasmodic and useful in coughs - Arum family - Burning sensations from fauces down throat, enlarged glands of throat, swelling of nose and sneezing, spasmodic cough and skin affections are common to 'Ictod' and the Arums. Amel: Open air. Asthma agg: Dust. *(JHC)*

This remedy is indicated in asthma and respiratory troubles that are precipitated by the inhalation of dust. The distress is relieved by stool. It is of service in hysteria, characterized by distention of the abdomen. *(Blackwood)*

501. Primula Obconica

(Primrose)

The poison of the Primrose occurs in its glandular hairs, which break easily and discharge an irritating fluid which is absorbed into the skin.

But the skin symptoms of poisoning appear in sensitive patients, even without coming in direct contact with the plant, mere nearness being sufficient, just like poison ivy. Intermittent symptoms, worse right side, pain in liver and spleen. Deep infiltration and tension of tissues, blisters, paralysed sensation. Weakness. Pharyngeal soreness, alternates with diminished facial irritation.

Face: Moist eczema. Papular eruption on chin, burns at night, urticaria-like eruption, eyelids swollen.

Extremities: Eczema on arms, wrists, forearms, hands, papular and excoriated.

Rheumatic pain around shoulder. Palms dry and hot. Cracking over joints and fingers. Eruption between fingers. Purple blotches on back of hands, palmar surface stiff. Blisters on fingers.

Skin: Great itching, worse at night, red and swollen like erysipelas, tumefied, small papules on a raised base. Skin symptoms accompanied by febrile symptoms.

Dose: 6x (Blackwood). *(Boericke)*

Primula obconica is an ornamented variety of primrose. Gardeners, amateur and professional, have discovered after much suffering that it has with some persons a most powerful action on the skin, its action taking place, chiefly by contact but partly by effluvia. *(JHC)*

This agent produces eruptions on the skin, moist eczema, erythema vesicles and small bullae.

It has been employed in eczema, chapped hands, itching affections of the skin. There is also pain in the liver and spleen. *(Blackwood)*

502. Propylamin

(Trimethylaminum)

(Distilled Herring-brine)

In acute rheumatism, dissipated fever and pain in a day or two. Rheumatic prosopalgia and rheumatic metastasis, especially heart lesions.

Extremities: Pain in wrists and ankles, worse, slightest motion (Bry). Great restlessness and thirst, rheumatism, needle held in fingers gets too heavy. Tingling and numbness of fingers. Pain in wrist and ankle, unable to stand.

Relationship: Chenopodium Vulvaria - The plant has an odor of decaying fish and contains a large amount of propylamine - weakness in lumbar and lower dorsal region.

Dose: 10-15 drops, in about six ounce of water, teaspoonful doses every two hours. *(Boericke)*

Trimethyl, which is prepared from Herring-brine among other sources, has a very unpleasant and penetrating fish like odour. At one time it was regarded as panacca in cases of acute rheumatism. Experiments on patients and others show that it diminishes the amount of Urea excreted. Hansen gives these as characteristics: great pains in wrist-joints, also great restlessness, pains in ankle joints from standing. Agg: slightest movement. Rheumatism when the needle held in the fingers gets so heavy she cannot sew. Copious diarrhoea with pains in ankle joints but not in wrists, thirst for large quantities of cold water, like Bry. *(JHC)*

503. Prunus Spinosa

(Black thorn)

Special action on the urinary organs and head. Very valuable in certain neuralgias, anasarca and especially oedema pedum. Ankle and foot feel sprained. Ciliary neuralgia.

Head: Shooting from right frontal bone through brain to occiput - Pain in right eyeball as if it would burst. Opacity of vitreous humor. Eyes feel as if bursting.

Urine: Hurriedly impelled to urinate, the urine seems to pass as far as glands and then returns and causes pain in urethra. Neuralgic dysuria. Must press a long time before urine appears.

Dose: 3-6. *(Boericke)*

The pains are felt in skull, eye, root of nose and ears, the teeth feel raised out of their sockets. These pains occuring in and around the eyes have led to its successful use in Glaucoma, ciliary neuralgia, choroide-retinitis, Irido-choroiditis, Irido-cyclitis. Felt as if air inhaled did not reach pit of stomach. Strangury of the most painful description was produced and the symptom is quite characteristic. Hurriedly impelled to pass urine, which however seems to pass forward into glands penis and then return and cause most violent pain in urethra-spasmodic tenesmus of bladder and rectum at close of urination with pains in glans. *(JHC)*

504. Psorinum

(Scabies vesicle)

The therapeutic field of this remedy is found in so-called psoric manifestations. Psorinum is a cold medicine, wants the head kept warm, wants warm clothing even in summer. Extreme sensitiveness to cold. Debility independent of any organic disease, especially the weakness remaining after acute disease. Lack of reaction. Phagocytes defective, when well chosen remedies fail to act. Scrofulous patients. Secretions have a filthy smell, profuse sweating, cardiac weakness, skin symptoms very prominent. Often gives immunity for cold catching; easy perspiration when walking. Syphilis, inherited and tertiary, offensive discharges.

Mind: Melancholy.

Eyes: Chronic ophthalmia, that constantly recurs.

Ears: Oozing scabs around ears, offensive discharge from eczema around ears, intolerable itching, moist fetid pus from ears.

Face: Humid eruption on face.

Throat: Eradicates tendency to quinsy.

Stomach: Very hungry always, must have something to eat in the middle of the night.

Stool: Mucous, bloody, excessively fetid dark fluid, constipation of infants.

Female: Leucorrhoea, fetid, lumpy with much backache and debility.

Respiratory: Asthma, with dyspnoea, worse sitting up, better lying down and keeping arms spread wide apart, dry hard cough, with great weakness in chest. Feeling of ulceration under sternum.

Extremities: Eruption around finger nails, fetid foot sweats.

Skin: Intolerable itching. Herpetic eruptions, especially on scalp and bends of joints with itching, worse from warmth of bed, enlarged glands, sebaceous glands secrete excessively, oily skin, indolent ulcers, slow to heal. Eczema behind ears, crusty eruptions all over, urticaria after every exertion, pustules near finger nails.

Fever: Profuse offensive perspiration, night sweats.

Sleep: Sleepless from intolerable itching, easily startled.

Mod: Worse - coffee, in hot sun shine, from cold, dread of least cold air or draft. Better - heat, warm clothing, even in summer.

Relation: *Complementary-Sulphur.*

Pediculus: Head louse. (Psoric manifestations in children, eruptions on dorsum of hands, feet, neck, prurigo, pellagra, unusual aptitude for study and work.) In lack of reaction.

Compare: Calcarea, and Natrum Ars., Gaertner.

Dose: 200 and higher potencies, should not be repeated too often. Psorinum requires some thing like 9 days before it manifests its action and even a single dose may elicit symptoms lasting for weeks. *(Boericke)*

Constitutional itch-psorinum has been proved entirely in the potencies and I know of no more trustworthy proving in the materia medica - I have frequently seen 'Psor' develop some of its own symptoms in patients whom it has benefitted in other ways. One great mark of distinction between 'Sul and Psor' is that the Psor patient is exceedingly chilly, likes to have a fur cap on in summer, whilst the Sul. patient is predominatingly hot - Psor specially suited to - scrofulous, nervous, restless persons who are easily startled. Psoric constitutions, lack of reaction after severe diseases. Patient emits a disagreeable odour. Pale sickly delicate children-peevish, unhealthy looking children - Those subject to diseases of the glands and skin and who have had eruptions suppressed - Lack of vital reaction - night sweats - Foulness may be considered the second keynote of 'Pso' - Otorrhoea is horribly offensive. Diarrhoea putrid, smelling like carrion. Always very hungry during headaches. Sick babies will not sleep day or night - worry, fret, cry or good and play all day, restless troublesome screaming all night. Great sensitiveness to cold air, change, storm, to sun, restless for days before a thunderstorm - Feels unusually well day before attack. Dry lustreless hair Acne agg: during menses, from fats, sugar, coffee, meat. Psor has cured more cases of hay fever in my practice than any other single remedy. Many cases have a psoric basis and when the basic taint is corrected the irritating agent has no effect - Psor cannot bear to have the limbs touch each at other at night, or weight of arms on chest. Amel: when eating, Agg: immediately after (rush of blood to head) - Antidoted by coffee.

Comple: *Sulphur, Bac. is the acute of Psor. Inimical-Lachesis.*

Compare: Sick babies fret day and night (Jalap) - good all day, screams all night (Lyco. opposite) (JHC)

Teething in children. Constipation obstinate with backache from inactivity of rectum. When sulphur fails to relieve - Asthma, dyspnoea Agg: in open air, in sitting up (Laur) Amel: lying down and keeping arms stretched apart (Rev of Ars.) - Sulphur follows Psorinum well in mammary cancer. *(HCA)*

505. Ptelea

(Wafer Ash)

Is a remarkable remedy in stomach and liver affections. The aching and heaviness in the region of the liver is greatly aggravated by lying on the left side. Atonic states of stomach. Asthma.

Head: Pain from forehead to root of nose, pressing outward-pain, frontal headache.

Mouth: Excess of saliva, with dry bitter taste-tongue coated white or yellow, feels rough, swollen papillae red and prominent-coating may be brownish yellow.

Stomach: Weight and fullness. Griping in epigastric region. Stomach and liver symptoms associated with pain in limbs.

Respiratory: Asthma.

Modalities: Worse lying on left side, early morning.

Better: Eating, sour things.

Dose: First to 30th potency. *(Boericke)*

Ptelea is the Greek name for the Elm - Hop tree, Wafer ash. In Cannada the young green shoots of Pte. tri. are used as an anthelmintic in the form of an infusion. One of the provers of Pte confirmed its anthelmintic powers by a very copious expulsion of Ascarides. Says Hale, in hepatic difficulties and in those erysipelatous and urticarious eruptions, that are so often concomitant with affection of the liver, bilious headache, dyspepsia, gastralgia, congestion of the liver, chronic hepatitis and chronic erysipelas. Others have used it in chronic rheumatism, dysentery and constipation. Hale says the oily constituent of Pte. resembles turpentine; and one of the most marked symptoms of the proving is: "Pressure as from a stone in pit of stomach." J. Preston cured a case of jaundice, following gall stones with great emaciation. Amel: after eating acid things. Agg: lying down, lying left side. Amel: R. side. Stool small hard balls. Predominating bitter taste, Nux - sour. Pte. feels effect of food at once. Nux two hours after. Dreams of fighting - Nat. Sulph. *(JHC)*

This agent acts upon the liver, stomach and lungs. The tongue is coated yellow, or brownish yellow. There is relief from lying upon the right side, and aggravation from lying upon the left side.

Compare: Mercurius, Chelidonium majus, Nux vomica. *(Blackwood)*

506. *Pulex Irritans*

(The common flea)

This remedy is employed when there is frequent desire to urinate. The urine is foul. It is also of service in delayed menstruation with burning in vagina and an increased flow of saliva, during the menses. Between the periods there is a profuse leucorrhoea and backache.

Dose: Dilutions 6 and higher. *(Blackwood)*

Marked urinary and female symptoms. Frontal headache, with enlarged feeling of eyes. Face wrinkled and old looking.

Mouth: Metallic taste. Sensation of a thread in throat. Thirsty especially during headache.

Stomach: Breath and taste foul, intense nausea, with vomiting, purging, and faintness. Stool very offensive. Abdomen bloated.

Urine: Scanty with frequent urging with pressure on bladder and burning in urethra. Must attend to the call without delay.

Female: Increased flow of saliva during menses. Intense burning in vagina. Leucorrhoea, profuse, staining a greenish yellow; stains of menses and leucorrhoea very hard to wash out. Backache.

Fever: Feels a glow all over like being over steam; chilly while sitting beside the fire.

Skin: Prickly itching. Sore spots all over. Skin emits foul odor.

Dose: The higher potencies. *(Boericke)*

507. *Pulmo Vulpis*

(Fox's lung) Trituration

Recent discoveries in the use of tissues and organs as remedies have thrown light on many curiosities of ancient medicine. As the Fox is probably the longest winded of all animals the doctrine of signatures pointed to his lungs as a likely remedy for short breath. Humid asthma. Chronic catarrh and symptom of oedema of the lungs. Strong sonorous bubbling, now rattling, now whistling sounds over whole chest. Accelerated short breath amounting to suffocation - frequently with cough and inability to expectorate (some times in light cases, there is no catarrh present and only persistent shortness of breath, becoming a paroxysm of asthma on the least bodily exertion). The patient could live only sitting up, bent forward. Constant lividity of face, lips and extremities and dropsy of legs. Heart's pulsation irregular and death seemed imminent. Pulmo vulpis 1x gr. was given and repeated in an hour - After a third powder, the patient was able to lie down and fall into a refreshing sleep - in eight days, she engaged in her domestic duties. *(JHC)*

508. *Pulsatilla*

(Wind flower)

The weather Cock among remedies. The disposition and mental state are the chief guiding symptoms to the selection of Puls. It is pre-eminently a female remedy, especially for mild, gentle, yielding disposition, sad, crying, readily weeps when talking, changeable, contradictory. The patient seeks the open air, always feels better there, even though he is chilly. Mucous membranes are all affected. Discharge thick, bland and yellowish green. Often indicated after abuse of iron tonics and after badly managed measles.

Symptoms everchanging, thirstless, peevish and chilly. When first serious impairment of health is referred to age of puberty. Great sensitiveness, wants the head high. Feels uncomfortable with only one pillow. Lies with hand above head.

Mind: Weeps easily, fears, in evening to be alone, dark, ghosts, likes sympathy, children like fuss and caresses, morbid dread of the opposite sex, religious melancholy, highly emotional, mentally an April day.

Head: Neuralgic pains, commencing in right temporal region, with scalding lachrymation of affected side. Headache from over work.

Ears: Otorrhoea, thick bland discharge, otalgia, worse at night, diminishes acuteness of hearing.

Eyes: Thick, profuse, yellow, bland discharges, itching and burning in eyes. Profuse lachrymation, lids inflamed, agglutinated, styes, worse in warm room.

Nose: Coryza, stoppage of right nostril, large green fetid scales in nose, stoppage in evening, yellow mucus, abundant in morning.

Face: Right sided neuralgia, swelling of lower lip, which is cracked in middle.

Mouth: Greasy taste - dry mouth without thirst, wants it washed frequently - Frequently licks the dry lips. Crack in middle of lower lip. Yellow or white tongue, covered with a tenacious mucus. Toothache relieved by holding cold water in mouth - offensive odor from mouth - food, especially bread tastes bitter. Much sweet saliva. Alterations of taste, bitter, bilious, greasy, salty, foul, loss of taste, desire for tonics.

Stomach: Averse to fat food, warm food and drink. Eructations, taste of food remains a long time, after ices, fruits, pastry, bitter taste, diminished taste of all food - flatulence. Dislikes butter - thirstlessness with nearly all complaints. Pain in stomach an hour after eating.

Stool: Rumbling, watery, worse night, no two stools alike, dysentery, mucus and blood with chilliness. Two or three normal stools daily.

Urine: Increased desire, worse when lying down.

Female: Suppressed menses from wet feet, nervous debility or chlorosis, tardy menses, too late, scanty, thick, dark, clotted, changeable, intermittent, leucorrhoea, acrid, burning, creamy, pain in back, tired feeling.

Male: Orchitis, pain from abdomen to testicles, thick yellow discharge from urethra, late stage of gonorrhoea, acute prostatitis, worse lying on back.

Respiratory: Dry cough in evening and at night, must sit up in bed to get relief and loose cough in the morning. Pressure upon the chest and soreness - Pain as from ulcer in middle of chest, expectoration bland, thick, bitter, greenish.

Sleep: Wide awake in the evening, sleeps with hands over head.

Extremities: Chilliness, pain in limbs, shifting rapidly, tensive pain letting up with a snap, numbness around elbow. Hip joint painful-knees swollen with tearing drawing pains. Boring pain in heels toward evening; suffering worse from letting the affected limb hang down; veins in forearms and hands swollen.

Skin: Urticaria after rich food, with diarrhoea from delayed menses worse undressing, measles, acne at puberty, varicose veins.

Fever: Chilliness, even in warm room, without thirst, chilly with pains in spots, chill about 4 p.m., external heat is intolerable, veins are distended.

Modalities: (Worse) from heat, rich fat food, after heating, towards evening, warm room, when allowing feet to hand down. (Better) open air, motion cold applications, cold food and drinks, though not thirsty.

Relationship: Penthorum often indicated after pulsatilla in colds. Jonasia Ashoka, Saraca Indica (Amenorrhoea, menorrhagia) acts powerfully on female organs. Abdominal pain.

Comple: Coffea, Chamom.,nux.

Dose: 3rd to 30. *(Boericke)*

Perhaps its tearful propensities gave rise to the legend that it sprang from the tears of venus. Of the numerous provings left us by Hahnemann, says Taste, that of Pul. seems to be the one to which he has contributed himself more than any other. One is obliged to lie with the head much higher than the rest of the body. It is useful in acute as well as in chronic diseases, as its action, even in small doses lasts from 10-20 days. It is particularly suitable for females, when their menses come on some days after the proper time, and especially when the patient must be long in bed at night before he can get to sleep- when the patient is worse in the evening. Sandy hair, blue eyes, pale face, easily moved to laughter or tears, affectionate, mild, timid, gentle, yielding disposition, women and children-women inclined to be fleshy-changeability is one of its most important keynotes. When one set of symptoms comes on another vanishes. The Puls patient is chilly, but at the same time there is extreme aversion to heat. Amel: in open air, cold air, or cold room, eating or drinking cold things, cold applications. metastases of mumps to testes or mammae. As a prophylactic against measles, Puls has a reputation almost equal to that of Bell. Suppressed gonorrhoea, orchitis, and cystitis, prostatitis, sarcocele, varicocele, hydrocele, all come within the sphere of Puls-in the female Puls ranges over the whole sexual period, from puberty to climacteric including disorders of menstruation, pregnancy, the puerperium and lactation. Secretions (of eye, ear, nose, vagina) are generally thick, bland and yellowish green. Great dryness of mouth without thirst. In chlorotic girls who have been damaged by iron, Puls has excellent effect-Tearfulness (Puls cries when telling her symptoms, Sep. weeps when questioned about her symptoms, Sep irritability and anger, indifference to household affairs. Nat mur *Agg:* by consolation- Ignatia hides her grief - Cycl. has spasmodic sneezing - Desire for lemonade Cyc., Sabi., Bell. - Ant. C tongue as if white washed, vomiting predominates - Puls stool greenish and slimy, non-appearance of milk Urt. u., Ric. com., Agn. c - Uterine affections Caul., Helon, Senec., Alet. f., Cycl., Hydr., lil — Measles - Morbil, K. Bi - Backache Agg: sitting Zn., Cobalt., Sep., Can. i., Earache-borax- Puls and Nux-m. dry mouth without thirst. Coccul - as if sharp stones rubbed together with every movement. Menstrual pain begins with the flow (Opp) Lach., pain subsides as flow begins. Puls is a close analogue of Cycl. in many respects, but cycl has profuse menses, the flow being agg: sitting and amel: walking. Puls agg: during day - Kreos. agg: lying down and cycl Agg: in open air - Puls and nux are in most respects antidotal, though they follow each other well - Silicea is the chronic of puls.

Causation: Chill, wetting feet, eating pork, fats, pastry, ice cream, mixed diet, thunder storm, tea. *(JHC)*

Ailments from abuse of chamomile, quinine, tea drinking, iron, mercury, sulphur tonics etc. *(HCA)*

Diuretic, diaphoretic and emenagogue, indecisive and slow, easily moved to tears or laughter, easily frightened, mild, gentle and timid, seldom thirsty, relief from motion, open air, agg. after eating, during rest, evening, in a close warm room, discharges are bland and yellow or greenish, sluggish circulation, constantly changing their position, headache, bursting and throbbing often from over eating, bad taste in the mouth, rich fat foods or ice cream, diarrhoea worse at night. In orchitis, testicles and spermatic cord are greatly swollen. Scanty menstruation, dysmenorrhoea, amenorrhoea, regulate the position of the child in utero, albuminous leucorrhoea. Bronchitis, copious expectoration, mucopurulent character during the day, tight at night, phlebitis, varicose, rheumatism, pains shift rapidly from one part to another, catarrhal inflammation of the eyes.

Compare: Antimonium crudum, Caulophyllum, chamomilla, Cyclamen, Hamamelis, Rhus Toxicodendron.

(Blackwood)

509. Pyrogenum

(Artificial Sepsin)

This remedy was introduced by English Homoeopathists, prepared from lean beef allowed to stand in the sun for two weeks and then potentised. The provings and most of the clinical experience have been obtained from this preparation. But subsequently, Dr. Swan potentised some septic pus which preparation has also been proved and clinically applied. There does not seem to be any marked difference in their effects.

Pyrogen is the great remedy for septic states, with intense restlessness. In septic fevers especially puerperal, Pyrogen has demonstrated its great value as homoeopathic dynamic antiseptic (H.C. Allen). Hectic, typhoid, typhus, ptomaine, chronic malaria, after effects of miscarriage, all these conditions at times may present symptoms, calling for this unique medicine. All discharges are horribly offensive, menstrual, lochial, diarrhoea, vomit, sweat, breath etc. Great pain and violent burning in abscesses, chronic complaints that date back to septic conditions. Threatening heart failure in zymotic and septic fevers. Influenza, typhoid symptoms.

Mind: Full of anxiety and insane motions, loquacious, thinks he is very wealthy. Restless, feels as if crowded with arms and legs. Cannot tell whether dreaming while awake or asleep.

Mouth: Tongue red and dry, clean, cracked, smooth, as though varnished.

Heart: Palpitation, can always hear her heart beat. Pulse abnormally rapid out of proportion to the temperature.

Fever: Septic fevers, temperature rises rapidly, sweating does not cause a fall in temperature.

Complementary: Bry.

Dose: 6-30 and higher potencies. Should not be repeated too frequently. *(Boericke)*

John Drysdale was the first in 1880 to suggest the use of this substance as a medicament. From a non-fatal dose, the animal shivers and begins to move about restlessly. The temp. rises from 2 deg. to 3 deg. C, the max. being reached in 3 hours. Thirst and vomiting come on followed by thin mucous and finally bloody diarrhoea and tenesmus. Yingling erroneously describes Pyro. as prepared from pus from septic abscess. This is septicaemin - Burnett's were cases of fully developed typhoid, all cut short at the height by Pyro-6 given every 2 hours. I have had ample opportunity of observing the power of Pyro. over typhoid fever and hectic states. "Sherbino" cured a case of puerperal fever with Pyro., being led to its selection by the very high pulse rate. Relapse of typhoid, pulse 150, temp. 102 deg. F., both were normal in 24 hours. As the fever left the pulse kept, mounting up - The most summary indication of Pyro. would be to term it the Aconite of the typhoid quality of Pyrexia and wherever there is poisoning by bacterial products - As pyro is a product of carrion, the carrion like odor of bodily emaciations, secretions and excretions is a keynote for its use. Under its action a sweating at the seat which the man had for many years, disappeared and the skin of his hands, which were subject to dry eczema, assumed a much cleaner aspect. *(JHC)*

Chill begins in the back, between scapulae, severe, general, of bones and extremities marking onset of septic fever, temperature 103 to 106, heat sudden, skin dry and burning, pulse rapid, small, wiry, 140 to 170, cold clammy sweat follows. *(HCA)*

A product of the decomposition of chopped lean beef in water; it is allowed to stand in the sun for two or three weeks.

Typhoid and Septic conditions. Septicaemia, ptomaine and severe gas poisoning, diarrhoea, frequently involuntary. Septic conditions following abortions and confinements, pulse is rapid. *(Blackwood)*

510. Quassia - Picraena Excelsa

(Quassia-Wood)

Acts on gastric organs as a tonic (Gentian, Hydr). Seems to posses, marked action on the eyes, producing amblyopia and cataract pain in right intercostal muscles above the liver. Pressure and stitches in liver and sympathetically in spleen.

Stomach: Acid dyspepsia with gas and acidity, heart burn and gastralgia.

Urinary: Excessive desire, impossible to retain urine, copious micturition day and night. As soon as the child wakes up the bed is drenched.

Dose: 1-3 potency or spoonful doses of Aqua Quassia. *(Boericke)*

The name Quassia was given by Linnaeus to Quassia excelsa of Surinam from the name of a Negro, Quassi or Coissi, who employed its bark as a remedy for fever. In the old school the infusion is used as a bitter tonic in dyspepsia and as a cluster for clearing the rectum of thread worms. *(JHC)*

Quassia Amara - the ϕ 1-30 drops -The wood is bitter and yields properties best into a cold distilled water. It has long been employed in the form of an infusion as a bitter tonic and as a clyster for clearing the rectum of pin worms - It is indicated in atonic dyspepsia, when there is an excessive fermentation and acidity with gastralgia and regurgitation of food. *(Blackwood)*

511. *Quercus Glandium Spiritus*

(Spirit distilled from Tr. of Acorn Kernels)

Used by Rademacher for chronic spleen affections, spleen dropsy. Antidotes effects of Alcohol, Vertigo, deafness with noises in head. Takes away craving in alcoholics, give dose as below for several months. Dropsy and liver affections. Useful in gout, old malarial cases with flatulence. Relationship: Angelica 5 drops Tr. TDS produces disgust of liquor, also for atony of different organs, dyspepsia, nervous headaches etc. Chronic bronchitis to increase expectoration.

Dose: Quercus. 10 drops to a teaspoonful of the distilled spirit 3-4 times a day. A passing diarrhoea often appears for a time when using it. Curative effect. Quercus acts well in trituration of the Acorn 3x in splenic cases. Flatulence, old malaria and alcoholic history. *(Boericke)*

Rademacher gave the Tr. of Acorns to an old brandy drunkard, who had long suffered from the spleen which was at times very painful and there was ascites and dropsy of the legs. Rademacher noticed that not only was the flow of urine increased, there was also especially, in old spleen engorgements, an eliminative diarrhoea, with amelioration of the symptoms generally. *(JHC)*

512. *Quillaya Saponaria*

(Chile Soap bark)

Produces and cures symptoms of acute catarrh, sneezing and sore throat. Most effective in the beginning of coryza, frequently checking its further development. Colds with sore throat, heat and dryness of throat. Cough with difficult expectoration. Squamous skin.

Dose: Tincture to 1st Potency.

(Boericke and Blackwood)

513. *Radium Brom*

An important addition to the materia medica, especially since the provings by Diffenbach have precisioned its use. Radium Brom of 1,00,000 radio activity was employed. Found effective in the treatment of Rheumatism and gout, in skin affections generally, acne rosacea, naevi, moles, ulcers and cancers. Lowered blood pressure, severe aching pain all over; with restlessness, better moving about. Chronic rheumatic arthritis. Lateness in appearance of symptoms. Ulcers due to radium burns, take a long time to heal. Marked increase in the polymorpho-nuclear neutrophils. Great weakness.

Mouth: Metallic taste.

Stomach: Aversion to sweets, ice creams.

Abdomen: Stool-alternating constipation and loose movements, pruritus ani and piles.

Female: Pruritus vulvae, right breast sore, relieved by hard rubbing.

Respiratory: Dry spasmodic cough, throat dry, sore, chest constricted.

Back: Aching in back of neck, pain and lameness in cervical vertebrae and sacral backache, pain appears to be in bone, continued motion relieves, backache between shoulders and lumbar sacral region, better after walking.

Extremities: Legs, arms and neck feel hard and brittle as though they would break on moving. Arthritis, aching pains worse at night. Dermatitis of the fingers.

Skin: Itching all over body burning of skin as if a fire.

Sleep: Restless, sleepiness, dreams of fire.

Mod: Better open air, continued motion, hot bath, lying down, pressure.

Relation: *Compare:* Anacardium (the ulceration produced by it is like Radium)

Dose: 30-12 trituration. *(Boericke)*

In 1904, I began to make a few provings with the 30th and in 1908, I published them in Radium as an internal remedy —Pure radium is a white metal which oxidises in water, burns paper, turns black on exposure to air and has the property of adhering firmly to iron. This last quality is not without significance and shows a close affinity with ferrum. A girl employed in the X-ray department of the hospital with which she is connected developed dermatitis of the R. hand and fingers - 2 doses of Radium B. 30 were given - the following day the patient came out in a rash, which the matron mistook for measles, eyes watering, fingers very sore, and she felt very ill. By the following day the rash had disappeared and she felt well. Among the most successful local uses of Radium may be mentioned cases of lupus, epithelioma, carcinoma of cervix uteri and urethral caruncle - cases of cure of skin cases with Radium in potencies are numerous. A retired excise officer had an intractable eruption on the genitals, inner surfaces of thighs and legs, which had prevented him from getting any refreshing sleep for 3 years. One tablet of Rad. B. 30 each morning was prescribed for a month. Defaecation at noon, stool soft, dark, or offensive, slate colour, clay colour, pains in extremities wakes at 4 a.m., pains in all joints, knees, ankles, feet, could not walk, had to lie down. Rad brom. was given and cured entirely. Intolerance of tobacco was produced. Agg: from warmth of bed, amel in open air, agg: by smoking. Rad brom is antidoted by Rhus and Nux mos.

Causation - Effects of X-ray burns. *(JHC)*

It is an important remedy in the relief of Arthritis, both acute and chronic, when focal lesions can be discovered as a cause. The

pain is severe in the various joints. Any or all the joints may be involved. The parts may have a sensation as though they were hard and brittle and would break if moved. Myalgia, muscular rheumatism, lumbago. Increasing the red blood cells and reducing the white blood count. In common with the uranium nitrate, this remedy has relieved glycosuria and has modified diabetes mellitus - The urine is extremely acid and there are severe pains in various parts of the body.
(Blackwood)

514. *Ranunculus Bulbosus*

(Butter cup)

Acts especially upon the muscular tissue and skin and its most characteristic effects are upon the chest walls, like pleurodynia. Bad effects of Alcohol, delirium tremens. Spasmodic hiccough. Hydrothorax. Shocks throughout the whole body. Sensitive to air and touch. Chronic sciatica.

Eyes: Day blindness, mist before eyes. Herpes on cornea. Intense pain.

Chest: Soreness as if bruised in sternum, intercostal rheumatism. Chilliness in chest when walking in open air. Tenderness of abdomen to pressure.

Muscular pain along lower margin of the shoulder blade.

Skin: Burning and intense itching, worse contact. Herpetic eruptions, shingles, bluish vesicles, itching in palms, blister like eruption in palms. Corns sensitive. Horny skin. Finger-tips and palms chapped. Vesicular and pustular eruptions.

Mod: (Worse) open air, atmospheric changes, cold air brings on all sorts of ailments.

Relationship - Sulphur, Staph.

Dose: Mother Tincture in 10-30 drop doses in delirium tremens; 3-30 generally. Chronic Sciatica-apply tincture to heel of affected leg. (M. Jousset) *(Boericke)*

One of our most effective remedies for the bad effects of alcoholic beverages - spasmodic hiccough, delirium tremens, day blindness, mist before eyes, pressure and smarting in eyeballs.

Muscular pains about margins of shoulder blades in women of sedentary employment, often burning in small spots - from needle work, typewriting, piano playing.

Pains, stitches, sharp, shooting, neuralgic, myalgic or rheumatic in walls of chest, coming in paroxysms, excited or brought on by atmospheric changes, inflammatory, depending upon spinal irritation.

Pleurisy or pneumonia from sudden exposure to cold, while over-heated or vice versa.

Corns sensitive to touch, smart, burn, intercostal rheumatism, chest sore, bruised. Agg: from touch, motion, or turning of body, in wet stormy weather.

Shingles, preceded or followed by intercostal neuralgia. Vesicles may have a bluish appearance.

Incompatible: Sulph and Staphis. Agg: Contact, motion, atmospheric changes, especially wet stormy weather.

515. *Ranunculus Scleratus*

(Marsh buttercup)

Is more irritating than others of this botanical family, as seen in the skin symptoms. Borning, gnawing pain very marked. Pemphigus. Periodical complain. Fainting with pain in stomach.

Mouth: Tongue mapped, burning and rawness of tongue.

Abdomen: Pain over region of liver, with sensation as if diarrhoea would set in.

Chest: Sore burning behind xiphoid cartilage.

Skin: Vesicular eruption, with tendency to form large blisters. Acrid exudation which makes surrounding parts sore.

Extremities: Boring pain, in right tow.

Dose: 1-3 potency. *(Boericke)*

The best known characteristic of R. Sc. (which is a well proved drug) is the mapped or peeled tongue and when this is associated with smarting, burning and rawness R. Sc will be the remedy. Continual gnawing in left palm. The right toe is the seat of many acute pains giving the remedy a high place in acute attacks of gout and also painful corns. As if face covered with cob webs. *(JHC)*

516. Raphanus

(Black garden Radish)

Produces pain and stitches in liver and spleen. Increases bile and salivary secretion. Symptoms will not appear if salt is used with Radish. Great accumulation and incarceration of flatulence. Globus symptoms. Seborrhoea with greasy skin. Pemphigus, Hysteria, chilliness in back and arms. Sexual insomnia. Nymphomania. Post operative gas pains.

Abdomen: Tympanitic, hard, no flatus emitted upward or downward. Griping about navel, stool liquid, frothy, profuse, brown, with colic and pad-like swelling of intestines.

Female: Nervous irritation of genitals. Menses very profuse and long lasting. Nymphomania, with aversion to her own sex and to children and sexual insomnia.

Dose: 3-30 potency. *(Boericke)*

Burning sensation in epigastrium, followed by hot eructations, lasting a whole day and ending in a headache - The leaves of Rap. are said to antidote its root and the Arum root is to antidote the effects of Radish leaves (Cooper) - Rap. is one of the most flatulent of remedies, wind accumulates so that it almost stops the breathing. Aversion to her own sex and to children, especially girls. Among the peculiar symptoms of Rap. are oedema of lower eye lids. In flatulence - Carbo v. - accumulation and retention of flatulence - Lyco (Raph) flatus does not pass away, bowels move but no flatus passes. Masturbation in females. Sexual insomnia (K. Bro). *(JHC)*

517. Ratanhia

(Krameria-Mapato)

The rectal symptoms are most important and have received much clinical confirmation. It has cured pterygium. Violent hiccough. Cracked nipples. Pin worms.

Head: Bursting in head after stool.

Stomach: Pain like knives cutting the stomach.

Rectum: Aches, as if full of broken glass. Anus aches and burns for hours after stool. Feels constricted. Dry heat at anus with sudden knife-like stitches. Stools must be forced with great effort. Protrusions of haemorrhoids, fissure of anus, with great constriction, burning like fire, as do the haemorrhoids, temporarily relieved by cold water, fetid thin diarrhoea, stools burn, burning pains before and after stools, oozing at anus, pinworms, itching of anus.

Relation: Paeon, Croton (Rectal neuralgia), Sanguin nit. (Disease of rectum), Mucuna prurens - Dolichos - piles with burning haemorrhoidal diathesis.

Dose: 3-6 potency. Locally the cerate has proved invaluable in many rectal complaints. *(Boericke)*

Possessed of great power in passive, bloody or mucus discharges - it acts as a tonic in weakness of digestive organs and muscular debility - Used as an astringent and tonic, this root sometimes arrests passive haemorrhages (epistaxis, haemoptysis, metrorrhagia). It has successfully been used against scurvy, mucous discharges, such as chronic catarrh of the bronchia, vagina, large intestines, etc. - straining, stool so hard she cried out, with great protrusion of haemorrhoids, followed for a long time by burning in anus. Another peculiarity in connection with the stool is bursting headache. The eye symptoms are striking, burning, smarting twitching of lids, obscured vision. This symptom has led to the cure of cases of pterygium. Rat. both causes and prevents abortion, metrorrhagia and leucorrhoea. It also meets fissure of the breasts in nursing women as well as fissure of the anus. As if splinters of glass in rectum and anus. Cushing who made a proving of Rat. says, it caused great itching in the rectum and he has cured with it since nearly every case of pin worms in his practice. Cushing considers that next to Sang. Not Rat. meets more rectal cases than any other remedy.

Relation: Fissure of anus - Nit. ac. - Anal symptoms Sul., Ir. v., Canth., Paeon., Graph., (Graph is the nearest but has not the constriction of Rat) - Splinters of the glass in rectum, Thuja, Aesc. Hip. *(JHC)*

Terrible toothache during early month of pregnancy, tooth feels elongated. *(HCA)*

518. Rhamus Californica

(California coffee Tree)

One of the most positive remedies for rheumatism and muscular pains. Pleurodynia, lumbago, gastralgia, vesical tenesmus, dysmenorrhoea of myalgic origin, pain in neck, head and face. Inflammatory rheumatism, joints swollen, painful, tendency to metastasis, profuse sweat, rheumatic heart. (Provings of students - 2x potency).

Head: Dizzy, bursting feeling with every step, twitching eyelids.

Ears: Dullness of hearing.

Bowels: Constipation with some flatus. Tenesmus and dry stool, flatulent diarrhoea.

Heart: Variation of pulse-slow pulse.

Extremities: Unable to control muscular action - legs sore - walked like a drunken man.

Modality: Symptoms worse in evening.

Dose: Tincture in 15 drop doses every four hours. *(Boericke)*

This remedy is indicated in myalgia and muscular rheumatism. This may be in the form of pleurodynia or lumbago when there is great soreness and distress of the part.

519. *Rheum*

(Rhubarb)

Of frequent use in children with sour diarrhoea, difficult dentition, whole child smells sour.

Head: Sweat on hairy scalp, constant and profuse. Cool sweat on face, especially about mouth and nose.

Mouth: Difficult teething, restless and irritable. Breath smells sour.

Abdomen: Colicky pain about navel.

Rectum: Stools smell sour, pasty, with shivering and tenesmus and burning anus. Sour diarrhoea during dentition. Colicky, even ineffectual urging to evacuate, altered faecal stools.

Mod: Worse uncovering, after eating, moving about.

Dose: 3-6 potency. *(Boericke)*

In its homoeopathic form, it has no terrors, but it remains a great remedy of sucklings and children especially during dentition, to whom as well. as to pregnant and nursing women, it is particularly suited. In small doses, it improves digestion and appetite, and renders the renal secretions more healthy. In disorders of children, such as flatulence and irritation of the alimentary canal, it renders the serum of the blood yellow, the urine is almost of a blood-red colour. The grand key note of Rhe is sourness. The stools are sour, the taste is sour, the body has a sour smell. No amount of washing will wash the sourness out of a characteristic Rheum baby. Such a condition may occur in sucklings or at the period of dentition. The Rheum child is as acid in temper as he is in body, peevish, impatient, screams for things, dislikes even his favourite play things. Screaming of children with urging and sour stools is characteristic - Shivering with stool should draw attention to Rheum - Sweat on hairy scalp, constant and very profuse, whether asleep or awake, in motion or quiet, hair always sopping wet, may or may not be sour. *Agg:* uncovering from cold. Uncovering arm or leg *agg:* Colic; *amel:* Wrapping up; from warmth - Rheum has twitching of muscles of face and fingers during sleep - also puts arms over head - Screaming children with diarrhoea - difficult dentition - Kreos., Chamo., sour body smell - Hep, Mag. c - Mag-c is deeper acting than Rhe - children cry and toss all night - Pso. *(JHC)*

It is an important remedy in chronic diarrhoea and dysentery, when there are loose evacuations of a sour smell as if fermented. *(Blackwood)*

520. *Rhododendron*

(Snow Rose)

Rheumatic and gouty symptoms well marked, Rheumatism in the hot season. The modality (worse before a storm) is a true guiding symptom.

Mind: Dread of a storm, particularly afraid of thunder, forgetful.

Head: Ciliary neuralgia.

Male: Testicles, worse left, swollen, painful, drawn up, orchitis, glands feel crushed. Induration and swelling of testes after gonorrhoea, Hydrocele (Sil.).

Extremities: Joints swollen, Gouty inflammation of great toe-joint. Rheumatic tearing in all limbs, especially right side, worse at rest and in stormy weather.

Stiffness of neck. Pain in shoulders, arms, wrists, worse when at rest. Pain in bones in spots, reappears by change of weather, cannot sleep unless legs are crossed.

Mod: Worse before a storm - all symptoms re-appear in rough weather, night, towards morning. *Better* - after the storm breaks, warmth and eating.

Dose: 1 to 6 potency. *(Boericke)*

Growing among the storms of the siberian mountains, shows that it produces sensitiveness to storms and weather changes - has a strong effect on the kidneys, producing increased urine - the scrotum shrinks, testes are retracted, or else they swell especially at night and are the seat of a bruised pain as if they had been crushed violently - it has cured cysts in the vagina and has caused the rupture of an ovarian cyst. *(JHC)*

Cannot get sleep or remain asleep unless legs are crossed - Amel: from wrapping the head warmly, dry heat and exercise. *(HCA)*

It is of service in Orchitis and epididymitis due to gonorrhoea and rheumatism when there is a sensation as though the testicles were being crushed. *(Blackwood)*

521. *Rhus Aromatica*

(Fragrant Sumach)

Renal and urinary affections, especially diabetes. Enuresis due to vesical atony, senile incontinence. Haematuria and cystitis come within the range of this remedy.

Urine: Pale, albuminous, incontinence. Severe pain at beginning or before urination, causing great agony in children. Constant dribbling, diabetes, large quantities of urine of low specific gravity.

Dose: Tincture in rather material doses. *(Boericke)*

A woman, 37, had diabetes mellitus with increased urine, weakness, pain in back, thirst, appetite, now ravenous, now deficient, skin sallow, temp. 101.5°F. Rh.a. half teaspoonful doses every four hours - Qty of urine diminished next day and this diminution progressed. The doses of Rh. a. were given at increasing intervals, and in three months it was discontinued, proper diet having been observed in the meantime. Cod liver oil and hypo-phosphites were given after the Rh. a. was discontinued. *(JHC)*

This remedy is indicated in urinary incontinence both in children and the aged, in dribbling of the urine and nocturnal enuresis. It has been employed in interstitial nephritis and diabetes insipidus, when the quantity of urine is increased and the specific gravity is low. *(Blackwood)*

522. *Rhus Glabra*

(Smooth sumach)

Epistaxis and occipital headache. Fetid flatus. Ulceration of mouth. Dreams of flying through the air. (Sticta). Profuse perspiration arising from debility. (China). It is claimed that this remedy will so disinfect the bowels that the flatus and stools will be free from odor. It acts well in putrescent conditions with tendency to ulceration.

Mouth - Scurvy; nursing sore mouth (Veronica). Aphthous stomatitis.

Relationship: Said to be antidotal to the action of Mercury, and has been employed in the treatment of secondary syphilis after mercurialization.

Dose: Tincture. Usually locally to soft, spongy gums, aphthae, pharyngitis, etc. Internally, first potency. *(Boericke)*

Rhus glabra, R. Tryphina, and R. Coriaria have acid fruit and astringent bark which is used in tanning. Rh. g. is a deciduous shrub with stem 2 to 12 feet high and has terminal flowers, and fruit clothed with acid crimson hairs, like the other non-poisonous Rhoes. The tincture of the bark was proved by Dr. A.V. marshall on himself with very substantial doses. The symptoms of the Schema are his and they bear out the traditional uses of the remedy. One of these is, profuse perspiration arising from debility and Marshal had profuse sweat during sleep and such a degree of debility that he was obliged to leave off the proving. Hale mentions that an infusion of the root has a popular repute in diarrhoea and dysentery, especially when the discharges are fetid, and that the berries are used for chronic cough, wheezing cough and laryngeal asthma. A tincture made of the whole pannicle (Sumach-bobs) cured a patient of his, who had every spring an attack of laryngeal cough with dyspnoea and almost complete loss of voice. Farmers observed an aggravation in a case of psoriasis: the patient felt irritable and despondent, and the skin became irritable. In the proving there were dull, heavy headaches amel: by exercise. (Hale says it has cured occipital headaches). There was agg: of stomach symptoms by either food or drink. Agg: by touch (Abdomen; ulcers in mouth). Agg: after sleep, amel: by movement. *(JHC)*

523. *Rhus Toxicodendron*

(Poison Ivy)

The effects on the skin, rheumatic pains, mucous membrane affections, and a typhoid type of fever, make this remedy frequently indicated. Rhus effects fibrous tissues markedly, joints, tendons, sheaths, aponeurosis, etc. Producing pains and stiffness. Post operative complications. Tearing asunder pains. Motion always limbers up the Rhus patient and hence he feels better for a time from a change of position. Ailments from strains, over lifting, getting wet, while perspiring. Septic conditions. Cellulitis and infections, carbuncles in early stages. Rheumatism in the cold season. Septicaemia.

Mind: Extreme restlessness, with continued change of position - delirium with fear of being poisoned. Sensorium becomes cloudy - great apprehension at night, cannot remain in bed.

Head: Vertigo on rising - Headache in occiput - Pain in forehead and proceed thence backward - Humid eruptions on scalp, itching greatly.

Eyes: Swollen, red, oedematous, orbital cellulitis, pustular inflammations.

Nose: Sneezing coryza from getting wet.

Face: Jaws crack when chewing, swollen face, parotitis, facial neuralgia with chilliness, cursta lactea.

Mouth: Tongue, red and cracked, coated except red triangular space at the tip, dry and red at edges. Corners of mouth ulcerated - fever blisters around mouth and chin, pain in maxillary joint.

Throat: Swollen glands, sticking pain on swallowing, parotitis, left side.

Stomach: Want of appetite for any kind of food with unquenchable thirst, bitter tastes - desire for milk - Great thirst with dry mouth and throat. Drowsy after eating.

Abdomen: Excessive distention after eating, rumbling of flatus on first rising but disappears with continued motion.

Rectum: Diarrhoea of blood, slime and reddish mucus, dysentery, with tearing pains down thighs, stools of cadaverous odor. Frothy painless stool. Will often abort at beginning suppurative process near the rectum. Dysentery.

Male: Swelling of glans penis and prepuce - dark-red, erysipelatous, scrotum thick, swollen, oedematous, itching intense.

Female: Swelling, with intense itching of vulva - Menses early, profuse and prolonged, acrid, lochia thin, protracted, offensive, diminished, with shooting upwards in vagina.

Respiratory: Dry teasing cough from midnight until morning, during a chill or when putting hands out of bed. Haemoptysis from over exertion, blood bright red. Influenza, with aching in all bones. Hoarseness from over straining voice. Bronchial coughs in old people worse on waking and with expectoration of small plugs of mucus.

Heart: Hypertrophy from over-exertion, pulse quick, weak, irregular, intermittent with numbness of left arm. Trembling and palpitation when sitting still.

Back: Pain and stiffness in small of back, better motion, or lying on something hard, worse while sitting, stiffness of the nape of the neck.

Extremities: Hot painful swelling of joints. Pains tearing in tendons, ligaments and fasciae. Rheumatic pains spread over a large surface at nape of neck, loins and extremities, better motion. Limbs stiff, paralysed. The cold fresh air is not tolerated, it makes the skin painful. Pain along ulnar nerve. Tearing down thighs. Sciatica, worse cold damp weather at night. Numbness and formication, after over-work and exposure, paralysis, trembling after exertion. Tenderness about knee joints. Loss of power in forearm and fingers, crawling sensation in the tips of fingers. Tingling in feet.

Fever: Adynamic, restless, trembling. Typhoid, tongue dry and brown, sordes, bowels loose, great restlessness. Intermittent, chill with dry cough and restlessness, during heat urticaria, hydroa, chilly as if cold water were poured over him followed by heat and inclination to stretch the limbs.

Skin: Red, swollen, itching intense, vesicles, herpes, urticaria, pemphigus erysipelas, vesicular suppurative forms, glands swollen, cellulitis, burning eczematous eruptions with tendency to scab formation.

Sleep: Dreams of great exertion. Heavy sleep as from stupor, sleepless before midnight

Modalities: Worse during sleep, cold, wet, rainy weather and after rain at night, during rest, drenching, when lying on back or right side.

Better: Warm dry weather, motion, walking, change of position, rubbing, warm applications, from stretching out limbs.

Relationship: Bry, Calc fluoride, Phytol. (Rheumatism), in urticaria follow with Bovista.

Inimical: Apis. *(Boericke)*

It was brought to the notice of Dufresnoy of Valenciennes by the cure of a young man having herpetic eruption of 6 years duration, through his being accidentally poisoned with the plant. He used it successfully in eruptive diseases, paralysis, rheumatism and amaurosis. The milky juice, which turns black on exposure, is used as a marking ink and as an ingredient of varnishes for finishing boots. It is more poisonous during the night. An acrimonious vapour, combined with carburetted hydrogen exhales from a growing plant of the poison oak during the night. It can be collected in a jar and is capable of inflaming and blistering the skin of ·rsons of excitable constitution who plunge their arms into it. Rheumatoid pains develop about the joints and a painful stiffness asserts itself in the lumbar region, while the legs and arms become numb-tongue with triangular red tip, swelling of parotids, agg: by rest, amel: exercise. Eczema on perineum and scrotum with sweat in cleft of nates - relieved in a week with Rhus rad. 12 twice daily. The severest symptoms and sufferings are excited when the body or the limb is at rest and kept as much as possible without movement. Rhus and Bry. have almost identical rheumatic pain with opposite conditions. Rheumatism of the hip joints and wrist seem to be most effectually controlled by its action, the greatest rigidity and pain is experienced on first moving the joints after rest and on waking up in the morning - the more he moves the better he is where as Bry has - the more he moves the worse he is - Rhus has not only agg: during rest but agg: after resting also - However Rhus and Bry complement each other - it is not unusual for the conditions of a case to change under one of these remedies and then the other will be required.

The characteristic tongue of Rhus is dry or dark coated with triangular red tip. In intermittent fever a characteristic is cough during the chill. Fatal effects of over lifting in ordinate exertions of the muscles and contusions. There is an analogy to this in the dreams - dreams of great exertion, rowing, swimming, working hard at his daily occupation. Rhus has cured many forms of paralysis. Paraplegia from getting wet-ptosis - paralysis of single limbs. Numbness of parts paralysed. Facial neuralgia, lumbago and sciatica of left side. Heels as if stepping on pins, as if nails under skin of heels, as if walking on needles. Scalp sensitive, agg: turning hair back. *(JHC)*

Synopsis - Rhus.

Adapted to persons of Rheumatic diathesis, bad effects of getting wet, especially after being over heated. Ailments from spraining or straining, a single part, muscle or tendon, over-lifting, particularly from stretching high up to reach things, lying on damp ground, too much summer, bathing in lake or river, right side more than the left - worse after midnight. Pain on first moving after rest or on getting up in the morning. Amel: by walking or continued motion. Great restlessness. Must change position often to obtain relief from pain - Amel: by motion or lying on something hard. Great sensitiveness to open air. Putting the hand out from under the bed-cover brings on cough - muscular rheumatism, sciatica, left side. Dreams of great exertion-corners of mouth ulcerated, fever blisters, tongue dry, sore, red, cracked, triangular red tip, takes imprint of teeth. Great thirst, with dry tongue, mouth and throat. External genitals inflamed. When acute diseases assume a typhoid form. Diarrhoea with beginning typhoid-paralysis with numbness, paresis of limbs - ptosis-skin-vesicular, burning, itching, stinging. *(HCA)*

524. *Rhus Venenata*

(Poison-Elder)

The skin symptoms of this species of Rhus are most severe. Itching relieved by hot water. Vesicles, erysipelas, skin dark red, Erythema nodosum, with nightly itching and pains in long bones. *(Boericke)*

According to Hale - it is more poisonous than Rh. t. - A most severe itching and burning (more burning) set in the scrotum and penis. The glans was very painful. Slight friction amel: for a moment the itching but not the burning. I have frequently used Rh. V. with good effect in skin disease. I have found Rhus an excellent remedy for arsenical over-dosing. *(JHC)*

525. *Ricinus Communis - Bofareira*

(Castor oil)

Has marked action on gastro-intestinal tract. Increases the quantity of milk in nursing women. Vomiting and purging. Languor and weakness.

Stomach: Profuse vomiting.

Abdomen: Diarrhoea and purging. Rice water stools with cramps and chilliness.

Stool: Loose, incessant, painless, with painful cramps in muscles of extremities.

Anus inflamed, stool green slimy and bloody, fever, emaciation, somnolence.

Dose: 3rd potency - 5 drops every four hours for increasing flow of milk-also locally a poultice of the leaves. *(Boericke)*

The leaves have an especially powerful action on the breasts and female generative organs. In acute and chronic dysentery and in those cases, in which there is an impaction of faeces. Hale has seen the oil promptly curative. Ric. has great power over lactation. The leaves of the plant were applied to the breast to increase the flow of milk, if it were delayed and even to produce it in women, who had never borne children or who had not suckled for years. In increasing the flow of milk in nursing women the breasts were fomented with a decoction of the leaves of the plant, the boiled leaves being afterwards thinly spread on the breasts. For producing milk in others more vigorous measures were resorted to. The women had to sit over a boiling decoction of the leaves, care being taken to prevent the escape of steam. When the decoction was sufficiently cool, the parts were bathed with it and also the breasts, to which the leaves were applied as in the other case. Women with well developed breasts are more easily influenced. When the breasts are small and shrivelled, this treatment acts more on the uterine system, bringing on the menses, long before their time or causing immediate flow if the time is near. Tyler Smith in his application, produced swelling of the breasts, throbbing and other pains in them, swelling of axillary glands, with pains running down the arms. Pains in the back, like after-pains were caused in every case. Leucorrhoea was increased. Soon discharges from the breasts became milky and menses came on too soon. The radiating pains; bar sensation, constricting and cramping pains are the most peculiar. *(JHC)*

This remedy is employed as a galactogogue when the flow of the milk is scanty or suppressed. It is also of service in diarrhoea when the stools are loose, incessant and painless. The anus is inflamed and stools are green, slimy and are frequently attended with cramps in the muscles and extremities.

Compare: Urtica Urens, Agnus Castus, resorcin. *(Blackwood)*

526. *Robinia*

(Yellow locust)

The remedy for hyperchlorhydria. In cases where albuminoid digestion is too rapid and starch digestion is perverted. The gastric symptoms with the most pronounced acidity are well authenticated, and are the guiding symptoms. The acidity of Robinia is accompanied by frontal headache. Intensely acrid eructations. Acrid and greenish vomiting, colic and flatulence, nightly burning pains in stomach and constipation with urgent desire - Acidity of children. Stool and perspiration sour. Incarcerated flatus.

Head: Gastric headache.

Stomach: Sour eructations, vomiting of an intensely sour fluid - Sour stools - child smells sour.

Female: Nymphomania, acrid fetid leucorrhoea. Discharge of blood between menstrual periods. Herpes on vagina and vulva.

Dose: 3rd potency - must be continued a long time. *(Boericke)*

The chief keynote of Rob. is acidity especially if the time of aggravation is night. Sour stomach, vomiting of intensely sour fluid which set the teeth on edge. Eructation of a very sour fluid. Sour stools of infants, with sour smell of body and vomiting of sour milk. Heart burn and acidity, coming on when lying down at night and preventing sleep. The combination of gastric and head symptoms has placed Robinia among the chief remedies in migraine and sick headaches. A.L. Fisher has relieved with Robinia when everything else failed, the intensely acid vomiting in four cases of gastric cancer. Agg: from fat, gravies, flatulent food, cabbages, turnips, new bread, ice cream, raw fruit etc. cause gastric headache. *(JHC)*

This agent acts upon the stomach producing a hyperacidity of the gastric juice, large doses acting as an emetic and purgative.

This remedy is indicated in hyperchlorhydria when there is an excessive acidity of the stomach with constant eructation and vomiting of a sour fluid that sets the teeth upon edge. There is pain and distress in the gastric region which is worse while the stomach is empty, but is relieved by taking food. Accompanying these gastric symptoms the patient is low spirited and irritable, and there is a dull headache which is made worse from motion.

Compare: Acidum sulph. *(Blackwood)*

527. *Rosa Damascena*

(Damask Rose)

Useful in the beginning of hay-fever, with involvement of Eustachian tube.

Ear: Eustachiam catarrh.

Relation: Phleum pratense - Timothy grass (Hay fever with Asthma, watery coryza, itching of nose and eyes, frequent sneezing, dyspnoea).

Dose: Lower Potencies 6-30. *(Boericke)*

Farrington mentions that R. Dam. was introduced by Jeans as a remedy at the beginning of Rose-cold, when the eustachian tube is involved, with some degree of deafness and Tinnitus. *(JHC)*

This remedy is indicated during the early stages of Hay - fever. The eustachian tubes are closed, there is hardness of hearing and tinnitus aurium. *(Blackwood)*

528. *Rumex Crispus*

(Yellow Dock)

Is characterised by pains, numerous and varied, neither fixed nor constant any where. Cough caused by an incessant tickling in the throat pit, which runs down to the bifurcation of the bronchial tubes. Touching the throat pit brings on the cough. Worse from the least cold air, so that all cough ceases by covering up all the body and head with the bed clothes. Rumex diminishes the secretions of mucous membranes and at the same time exalts sensibility of mucous membranes of the larynx and trachea. Its action upon the skin is marked producing an intense itching. Lymphatics enlarged and secretions perverted.

Stomach: Cannot eat meat, it causes eructations, pruritus, flatulence, pain in left breast after meals.

Respiratory: Nose dry, tickling in throat pit, causes cough, copious mucous discharge. Dry teasing cough, preventing sleep, aggravated by pressure, talking, and especially by inspiring cool air and at night. Thin watery frothy expectoration by the mouthful, later, stringy and tough.

Stool: Brown, watery diarrhoea, early in morning, with cough driving him out of bed.

Skin: Intense itching of the skin, especially of lower extremities, worse exposure to cold air when undressing. Urticaria, contagious, prurigo.

Modalities: Worse in evening, from inhaling cold air, left chest, uncovering.

Relation: Rumex contains "Chrysophanic acid" to which the skin symptoms correspond.

Dose: 3-6 potency. *(Boericke)*

Rumex crispus according to Joslin, quoted by Hale, was used by allopaths internally and externally for the cure of itch. Among the constituents and salts of Rx. c. are sulphur and Calc. Ph. and sul, Calc, and Phos are strongly represented in its action. Rx. c. is a close ally of Rheum and has analogous purgative and other properties - sensitiveness to cold air. Cough and skin symptoms are agg: by uncovering or exposure to air - by covering up all the body and head, with bed clothes; there is no cough. This symptoms has led to many cures of the skin cases - while undressing and for some time after considerable itching of surface of lower limbs. Where exposure to air is again the exciting cause—the characteristic diarrhoea of Rx. c occurs in the early morning, driving the patient out of bed. It comes on after catarrh, and is often associated with the characteristic cough of the remedy. The Rx. c. cough causes expulsion of urine and it may even cause expulsion of the foetus in pregnant women. (Rx. c. 30 and 200 promptly relieved) - cough is excited by pressure on throat pit. Paroxysms exhaust him - the flatulence and rumbling of Rx. C are well marked and I have found it the best general remedy for the painless but annoying borborygmi frequently complained of by women. Sensation as if a feather swaying to and fro in bronchi. *(JHC)*

Dry, incessant, fatiguing cough, worse from changing air or room - from slightest inhalation of cold air, covers head with bed clothes to make air warmer. Urine involuntary with the cough, early morning diarrhoea, driving out of bed in morning, 5-10 a.m. - skin itching agg: cold, undressing, amel: warmth - amel: Cough, mouth covered to exclude cold air. *(HC Allen)*

This remedy is indicated in those of a tubercular diathesis who are extremely sensitive to the open air. *(Blackwood)*

529. Ruta Graveolens

(Rue-Bitterwort)

Acts upon the periosteum and cartilages, eyes and uterus. Complaints from straining flexor tendons especially. Tendency to the formation of deposits in the periosteum, tendons, and about joints, especially rist. Overstrain of ocular muscles. All parts of the body are painful, as if sprained. Lameness after sprains. Jaundice. Feeling of intense lassitude, weakness and despair - injured bruised bones.

Eyes: Eyes red, hot and painful from sewing or reading fine print (N.M., Arg. nit), disturbance of accomodation.

Rectum: Difficult faeces, constipation, alternating with stool. Carcinoma affecting lower bowel-prolapsus ani.

Extremities: Spine and limbs feel bruised. Small of back and loins pain. Legs give out on rising from a chair, hips and thighs so weak. Contraction of fingers. Pain and stiffness, in wrists and hands. Ganglia (Benz. ac.). Sciatica, worse, lying down at night; pain from back down hips and thighs. Tendons sore. Thighs pain when stretching the limbs.

Mod: Worse lying down, from cold, wet weather.

Dose: 1-6 potency - locally the Tincture for ganglia and as a lotion for the eyes. *(Boericke)*

It certainly acts strongly on deposits of scirrhous material in both the breasts and in the vagina and sometimes lessens the size of these. Ruta is one of the chief remedies for injured bones and especially bruised bones - Impaired sight due to straining the eyes was an old use of the remedy - Caused prolapse of rectum in the provers - Prolapse agg: stooping - Prolapse preceding a very difficult stool - A sensation of nausea located in the rectum. Rheumatic paralysis of wrists and ankles. Ruta is specially suited to robust sanguinous persons, haemorrhages from nose, gum, rectum, peculiar symptom is cramp in the tongue with embarrassed speech. A prolonged use of Ruta 3x has cured ganglion in front of left wrist — slow pulse, contracted pupil, salivation and swollen tongue are features of its action.

Comp: Calc. phos in joint affection and symphytum in bone injuries.

Causation: Bone, injuries of, bruises, fractures, sprains, carrying heavy weights, over-exertion of eyes. *(JHC)*

This agent produces pain in the limbs and eyes that simulate rheumatism. It is an emmanagogue and an abortifacient.

Mechanical injuries of the bones and periosteum - a fall or blow- bruised lame sensation especially of the wri~ts and ankles - asthenopia and amblyopia, over use of the eyes - fine sewing or reading - hot like a ball of fire - faulty refraction.

Compare - Phytolacca, Rhus toxicodendron, Arnica montana. *(Blackwood)*

530. *Sabadilla*

(Cevadilla seed.
Asagraea officinalis)

Action on mucous membrane of the nose and the lachrymal glands, producing coryza and symptoms like hay-fever, which have been utilised homoeopathically. Chilliness, sensitive to cold. Ascarides, with reflex symptoms (nymphomania). Convulsive symptoms. Children's diarrhoea with constant cutting pains.

Head: Oversensitiveness to odors. Thinking produces. Headache and sleeplessness - Eyelids red, burning, lachrymation.

Nose: Spasmodic sneezing, with running nose - coryza.

Throat: Sore begins on left side - warm food and drink relieve - sensation of lump in throat with constant necessity to swallow.

Stomach: No thirst, canine appetite for sweets and farinaceous food, desire for hot things - sweetish taste.

Fever: Chill predominates.

Extremities: Cracking of skin under and beneath toes, inflammation under toe nails.

Skin: Thickened nails.

Dose: 3-30 potency. *(Boericke)*

At first it was almost exclusively used for destroying lice and also worms in putrid ulcers and in the intestines - the periotidicity of Saba. may be as clock-like as that of Cedron and renders it a leading remedy in intermittent fevers and neuralgias - Saba. is a chilly remedy, the symptoms, especially the coryza being generally agg: in the open air. The catarrhal symptoms are very severe, and correspond to many cases of hay asthma. I have often relieved cases with Saba. though it does not cure the diathesis. Sore throats characterised by a sensation of a lump or foreign body in the throat and a constant necessity to swallow, I have frequently cured with Sab. - Kent says, old chronic sore throats agg: from cold air - tonsillitis going from left to right, the desire for hot drink distinguishes Saba. from Lach - Violent itching of hairy scalp compelling her to scratch till blood comes out. Itching of anus and rectum as from ascarides - itching of anus alternating with itching of alae nasi and meatus auditorius - vertigo early in the morning after rising - After a dose of Saba. in high potency, I astonished myself by falling back on the bed with giddiness on rising the following morning. *(JHC)*

Suited to persons of light hair, fair complexion with a weak, relaxed muscular system-worms' affections of children - nervous diseases, twitching, convulsive tremblings, catalepsy, from worms - illusions, that he is sick - parts shrunken, that she is pregnant, when merely distended from flatus, that she has some horrible throat disease - that will be fatal - sneezing in spasmodic paroxysms, followed by lachrymation, copious watery coryza, face hot and eyelids red and burning - sensation of a skin hanging loosely in throat, must swallow over it - dryness of fauces and throat - parchment - like dryness of skin. *(HCA)*

This remedy is indicated in hay fever and influenza, when there is violent, spasmodic sneezing and lachrymation upon going into the open air. There is a burning watery discharge from the eyes and nose, the throat and tonsils are swollen.

It is of service in delirium. She believes she is pregnant or that there is some incurable disease.

It is to be remembered in headache that results from too much thinking or close application.

It is useful for worms; ascarides and lumbricaria; when nervous affections, such as twitching, convulsions, and trembling result from these conditions. *(Blackwood)*

531. *Sabal Serrulata*

(Saw Palmetto)

Sabal is homoeopathic to irritability to the genito-urinary organs. General and sexual debility-promotes nutrition and tissue building. Head, stomach and ovarian symptoms marked. Of unquestioned value in prostatic enlargement - epididymitis and urinary difficulties. Acts on membrano-prostatic portion of urethra - Iritis with prostatic trouble - valuable for undeveloped mammary glands. Fear of going to sleep. Languor, apathy and indifference.

Urinary: Constant desire to pass water at night. Enuresis-chronic gonorrhoea - difficult urination - cystitis with prostatic hypertrophy.

Male: prostatic troubles - enlargement, discharge of prostatic fluid, wasting of testes and loss of sexual power coitus painful at the time of emission - sexual neurotics - organs feel cold.

Female: Breasts shrivel - suppressed or perverted sexual inclination.

Dose: Mother Tincture 10-30 drops - 3rd potency often better - The Tincture must be prepared from the fresh berries to be effective. *(Boericke)*

While on a hunting trip through the wilds of Florida Hale observed the great fattening properties of the berries on animals. During summer food is scanty and the wild animals become very thin, but as soon as the Palmetto fruit ripens they improve rapidly, and in a few weeks have put on so much fat that they become an easy prey to the Hunter. Fears to fall asleep lest something should happen, starts up with this fear as he is dozing. Sbl. is an organ remedy of great power, selecting the uterus and prostatic gland, ovaries and testes and bladder - It is indeed an anti lean and well deserves the name of "The Homoeopathic catheter" - 5 drops Tincture TDS, in about a month the menses came (nine months without a period) and the breasts began to increase in size - an impotent man was cured in thirty days. A Man, 76, enlarged prostate had to use catheter for 3 years, cured in 4 months. Antidoted by Sil. (Sabal. grows on sandy shore) - Sbl. is most fruitful nearest the sea - Compare Sil., Mariana. *(JHC)*

This agent is a tonic which improves the digestion, and as a result there is an increase of strength, weight and flesh. It has a most favourable influence upon the mucous membrane of the respiratory tract and reproductive organs.

Prostatitis - difficult urination-weakening of the sexual powers - epididymitis-testicles may be wasted - restoring the size and secreting powers of the mammary glands - uterine and ovarian-atrophy attended with dysmenorrhoea - re-establishing menstruation - impotence - in those who have practiced masturbation - sexual perversion. *(Blackwood)*

532. *Sabina*

(Savine)

Has a special action on the uterus, also upon serous and fibrous membranes, hence its use in gout. Pain from sacrum to the pubis. Haemorrhages, where blood is fluid and clots together. Tendency to miscarriage, especially at 3rd month, violent pulsations, wants windows open.

Mind: Music in intolerable - produces nervousness.

Stomach: Heart burn, desire for lemonade.

Abdomen: Colic mostly in hypo-gastric region.

Rectum: Pain from back to pubis. Haemorrhoids, with bright red blood, bleed copiously.

Female: Menses profuse, bright- uterine pains extend into thighs. Threatened miscarriage. Sexual desire increased. Leucorrhoea after menses, corrosive, offensive. Discharge of blood between periods with sexual excitement. Retained placenta, internal after-pains. Menorrhagia in women, who aborted readily. Inflammation of ovaries and uterus, after abortion. Promotes expulsion of moles from uterus. Pain from sacrum to pubis and from below upwards - shooting up the vagina. Haemorrhage, partly clotted, worse from least motion.

Back: Pain between sacrum and pubes from one bone to another. Paralytic pain in joints. Shooting in heels and metatarsal bones.

Skin: Warts, black pores in skin.

Male: Gonorrhoea, with pus-like discharge. Sycotic excrescences - burning sore pain in glans. Prepuce painful with difficulty in retracting it - increased desire. Sanguisuga: The leech (haemorrhage, especially bleeding from anus) use 6x.

Rosmarinus: (Menses too early, violent pain followed by uterine haemorrhage, head heavy, drowsy, chilly with icy coldness of lower extremities, without thirst, followed by heat. Memory deficient).

Antidote: Pulsatilla for Sabina.

Dose: Locally for warts Tincture internally 3-30 Potency. *(Blackwood)*

Hahnemann and his son were among the provers. The action of sabina on the generative organs of both sexes is pronounced. It produces figwarts with itching and burning of the external genitals, phimosis of the male, swelling of the dorsum of the penis, gonorrhoea, in the female-uterine haemorrhages and in the case of pregnant women abortion. The haemorrhage is partly pale red and partly clotted. Agg: From the least motion but *amel:* by walking - The flow is in paroxysm and is accompanied by labour-like pains. A grand characteristic of Sab. is a pain from Sacrum to pubis and this will be a guiding symptom in a large number of uterine cases requiring Sabina - like Thuja it removes wart-like growths from the muco-cutaneous surfaces - suited to chronic ailments of women, arthritic pains, tendency to miscarriage, gouty diathesis, discharge of blood between periods with sexual excitement. Sabina is one of the remedies which affect the heels, rheumaic inflammation of the heels. Pains are paroxysmal and labour like - Haemorrhage comes in gushes - Comple: to Thuja. *(JHC)*

It induces hyperaemia of the uterus and ovaries; and contractions of the pregnant uterus that may result in abortion. It is eliminated by the lungs, skin and kidneys.

Haemorrhages when the blood is partially fluid, and partially clotted; habitual abortion at the third month; arthritic affections and gout - Haemorrhages may appear from any orifice but are most frequently uterine. The menses appear too early, are profuse, and protracted, they are partially fluid and partially clots. Begins menstruating early in life; attended with colic and pain that extends from the sacrum to the pubes, or from below upwards, shooting up into the vagina. Discharge of blood between the periods.

Threatened abortion about the third month - habit of aborting. Arthritic affections and gout in women who suffer from uterine and ovarian derangements. Rectum haemorrhoids bleed profusely. The patient is aggravated by music which makes her nervous, she is also made worse from the least motion, from heat and warm air and is better in the cool frosty air.

Compare - Trillium, Ipecacuanha
(Blackwood)

533. *Saccharum officinale*
(Cane Sugar)

According to the great Dr. Hering, a large proportion of chronic disease cf women and children are developed by using too much sugar. Sugar is an antiseptic, combats infection and putrefaction - has a solvent action in fibrin and stimulates secretion by the intense osmotic changes induced, thus rinsing out the wound with serum from within outward, favoring healing leg ulcers.

Sugar must be considered a sustainer and developer of the musculature of the heart and hence useful in failure of compensation and a variety of cardiovascular troubles. Acts as a nutrient and tonic, in wasting disorders, anaemia, neurasthenia etc. increasing weight and power.

Opacity of cornea. Dim sight. Acidity and anal itching. Cold expectoration. Myocardial degeneration. Fat, bloated, large limbed children, who are cross, peevish, whining, capricious, want dainty things, titbits and refuse substantial food. Oedema of feet. Headache every seven days.

Relation: Saccharum lactis - Sugar of milk - Lactose (diuresis amlyopia, cold pains, as if produced by fine icy cold needles with tingling as if frost bitten great physical exhaustion. Sugar of milk in large doses to develop the bacillus acidophilus to correct putrefactive intestinal conditions and also constipation).

Dose: 30th potency and higher - Locally in gangrene. One ounce of lump sugar morning and evening is a valuable adjunct in the treatment of obstinate case of heart failure due to deficient heart muscle without valvular lesion. Epilepsy, blood with reduced sugar content irritates the nervous system with tending to convulsions. Sugar: As an oxytocic has its most suitable application toward the end of labor when there is no mechanical obstruction, and delay is due to uterine inertia. 25 grams dissolved in water, several times, every half hour.

Compare: Saccharin: (Hinders both the salivary and peptic ferment actions with consequent dyspepsia. Prof. Lewin believes its action to be on the secretory cells themselves and it has caused pain (right hypogastrium), loss of appetite, diarrhoea and wasting. *(Boericke)*

Sac. l. Scientific and clinical studies have shown it to be possessed of very great diuretic powers when given in full doses - Sac. l. causes sensations of both coldness and heat. Sensation of extreme cold passing in a fine line from centre of pubes to a point 2-3 inches above - Swan regards cold pains as a key note.

Acidity of the stomach and itching at the anus are common effects of taking too much sugar - Miss.L. was continually eating candies of which she was very fond till her digestive organs were affected - A few doses of Sac. a. 30 m changed her taste so that she ate no more and could not even bear the sight of them - Farrington traces a great similarity between Sac off. and Calc - Sac. off. is indicated, he says, in children who are large limbed, fat and bloated with a tendency to dropsy. It has produced opacity of the cornea and ought to cure it. *(JHC)*

This remedy is employed when the child is fat, bloated and is cross, whinning, and wants nick-nacks but no solid food. There are opacities of the cornea. *(Blackwood)*

534. *Salicylicum Acidum*

(Salicylic acid)

The symptoms point to its use in rheumatism, dyspepsia, and Meniere's disease. Prostration after influenza, also Tinnitus aurium and deafness. Haematuria.

Eyes: Retinal haemorrhage.

Ears: Roaring and ringing in ears, deafness with vertigo.

Stomach: Canker sores, flatulence, hot, sour, belching - fermentative dyspepsia, tongue purplish.

Extremities: Knees swollen and painful, acute articular rheumatism, worse touch and motion, profuse sweat, pain shifts, sciatica, burning pain worse night, copious foot sweat and ill effects where suppressed.

Skin: Itching vesicles and pustules, better by scratching - sweat without sleep - urticaria. Herpes zoster. Necrosis and softening of bones.

Relation: Spiraea and Gaultheria contain salicyl acid.

Dose: 3rd decimal trituration. In acute articular rheumatism 5 gr. every 3 hours (old school dose).

Salicyclic acid is found in nature in the leaves and barks of willows, in oil of winter green (Gaultheria) which is one chief source of its supply - Meniere's disease (auditory nerve vertigo) - an excellent remedy for affections following suppression of foot - sweat fermentative dyspepsia and diarrhoea with putrid smelling stools.

Causation: Suppression (foot sweat) *(JHC)*

Salicyclic acid, or Ortho-oxybenzoic acid, is found in the flowers of spiraea ulmaria, also in the leaves of wintergreen (Gaultheria procumbens).

This agent is an antipyretic and antiseptic. When taken internally, in small doses, it stimulates the stomach, heart and respiration; in larger doses it deranges the stomach, causing nausea and vomiting, depressing the heart action, the respiration and producing a profuse sweat. If fever is present the temperature is reduced.

There is vertigo, tinnitus aurium similar to that produced by quinine, dilated pupils, a sensation of distension in the frontal cerebrum and delirium. There is deafness and impaired vision, strabismus or ptosis may occur and temporary amaurosis has been noticed. There is restlessness, difficult breathing, feeble pulse, and loss of control of the natural evacuations.

The functions of the central nervous system are depressed. The circulation is so weakened that bed sores may result. It destroys the oxygen carrying power of the red blood corpuscles. It stimulates the action of the kidneys and increases the urine. This stimulation may pass to the stage of irritation, producing congestion, haematuria with partial suppression of the urine, with a degree of albuminuria. The urine of patients taking this acid or its compounds may show a reaction with tests similar to that of sugar and is often misleading. Under its prolonged use an excess tissue salt is found to be present in the urine and the skeletal bones are softened.

This remedy has been extrensively employed in acute articular rheumatism with serious effusions. The condition is aggravated by motion and touch, The pains shifting, burning in character and worse at night. Five grains every three hours. Relapses are more liable to accur after this agent than after almost any other remedy.

Cardiac depression and in some cases delirium has been attributed to its excessive use.

It should be remembered in rheumatic pharyngitis, lumbago and tonsillitis. The parts are sensitive and painful upon motion.

It is useful in fermentation, dyspepsia and putrid fermentation, when there is an excessive acidity of stomach with a tendency to vomit. The tongue is purplish or lead colored, the breath is foetid, and there are canker sores in the mouth that are painful and have a sensation of burning.

It should be studied in the gastrointestinal derangement of children when the stools are acid and green like frog's spawn.

It has been employed in management of ulceration and cancerous condition of the stomach and lungs, when there was a persistent foul breath and offensive expectoration.

It has been of service in Meniere's disease when there is vertigo, roaring in the ears and deafness.

It has been employed extensively locally in powder form or as an ointment, in old indolent ulcers, pruritus and in tubercular and epitheliomatous conditions of the skin.

In small doses it has been found of service in necrosis and softening of the bones; as well as in the ill effects of suppressions of the foot sweat.

Compare - Salicylate of Soda.

(Blackwood)

535. *Salix Nigra*

(Black Willow)

Has a positive action on the generative organs of both sexes. Hysteria and nervousness. Libidinous thoughts and lascivious dreams. Controls genital irritability - Moderates sexual passion. Satyriasis and erotomania. In acute gonorrhoea with much erotic trouble - Chordee. After masturbation. Spermatorrhoea.

Relation: Yohimbin; Canth.

Dose: Material doses of Tincture 30 drops. *(Boericke)*

(1) Man 35, lost control of his sexual appetite, and the more he indulged the worse the craving became and indulgence made him a physical wreck. Sal. N. Q. in teaspoonful doses thrice daily, cured in 5 weeks.

(2) Youth 23, had masturbated since he was a boy Sal N.XX. gtt. QID was given for a fortnight, the quantity being gradually diminished until in a few weeks, the young man was quite cured.

(3) A negro, 53, had sexual desire but without ability, yet during the night he would have emissions without erections. Sal. N.Q. gtt. xiv. QID cured in three weeks. *(JHC)*

Pronounced sexual excitement, satyriasis, erotomania and spermatorrhoea-erotic conditions during acute gonorrhoea. In cases of chordee with great irritation a dose on retiring and possibly one towards morning is of great service as well as in cases of cystitis, prostatitis and nocturnal emissions. In the female there is nymphomania dependent upon a local irritation, ovarian irritation, congestion and neuralgia when it is accompanied by hysteria and erotomania - It is useful in hysteria with marked excitability, nervousness and globus hystericus. *(Blackwood)*

536. *Salvia Officinalis*

(Sage)

Controls excessive sweating, when circulation is enfeebled; often used in phthisis with night sweats and suffocating tickling cough - Galactorrhoea - exerts a tonic influence on the skin.

Respiratory: Tickling cough especially in consumption.

Skin: Soft, relaxed, with enfeebled circulation and cold extremities. Colliquative perspiration.

Dose: Tincture in 20 drop doses in a little water. The effects manifest themselves quickly 2 hours after taking a dose and they persist for 2-6 days. *(Boericke)*

The tickling cough of consumptives and the night sweats were entirely relieved by doses of 20-40 drops in a table spoon of water. *(JHC)*

This remedy is employed in the tickling, suffocating, cough and night sweats of pulmonary tuberculosis. It is useful in galactorrhoea. *(Blackwood)*

537. *Sambucus Nigra*

(Elder)

Acts especially on the respiratory organs. Dry coryza of infants. Snuffles, oedematous swelling. Profuse sweat accompanies many affections.

Mind: Constant fretfulness - fright followed by suffocative attacks.

Abdomen: Colic frequent, watery, slimy stools.

Urine: Profuse urine.

Respiratory: Paroxysmal, suffocative cough, coming on about midnight with crying and dyspnoea, spasmodic croup. Dry coryza-sniffles of infants, nose dry and obstructed - When nursing child must let go of nipple, nose blocked up, cannot breathe - child awakes suddenly, nearly suffocating, sits up, turns blue, cannot expire.

Fever: Dry heat while sleeping, dreads uncovering, profuse sweat over entire body during waking hours. Dry deep cough precedes the fever paroxysm.

Skin: Dry heat of skin during sleep. Bloated and swollen, general dropsy, profuse sweat on waking.

Mod: *Worse* sleep, during rest, after eating fruit. *Better* - Sitting up in bed, motion.

Dose: Tincture to 6th potency. *(Boericke)*

Spasms of Larynx, chest and nasal passages. Proved by Hahnemann. One of the chief notes of the remedy is oedema, dropsical swellings in various parts of the body, especially legs, in step and feet. This oedema, when it affects the nose may give rise to obstruction as in the snuffles of infants with dry coryza, preventing breathing and nursing. When its occurs lower down in the tract it causes dyspnoea, the child awakens suddenly nearly suffocated, face livid, blue, sits up in bed, turns blue, gasps for breath, which it finally gets, attack passes off but is again repeated, child inspires but cannot expire, sleeps into the attack. The breathing is rattling. Croup, whooping cough, asthma, may all manifest this group of symptoms. 'Nash' once relieved with the 200th a very bad case of asthma, having attacks of suffocation of the above kind. The patient was an old lady. The relief was accompanied by a profuse flow of urine which carried off a large amount of dropsical effusion in her legs and abdomen. This tendency of attacks to recur is another note of the remedy. Another grand characteristic is: profuse sweat during waking hours, dry heat when asleep-other fever peculiarities are deep dry cough, precedes the fever paroxysm-fever without thirst. Dreads uncovering. Agg: about midnight, after midnight 2-3 a.m. (roused with sense of stoppage of air tubes)

Conium - Sweats as soon as he closes his eyes to sleep (Opp. of sambucus).

Thuja: Sweats on uncovered parts.

Puls: One sided sweats. *(JHC)*

This remedy is indicated in catarrhal affections of the air passages with suffocative attacks. There is much mucus in the bronchi, while expectoration is difficult. It is of service in spasmodic cough, with paroxysms that come on about midnight, with dyspnoea; also snuffles of infants. The nose is dry and obstructed. There are profuse and debilitating sweats. A strong infusion is employed to remove dropsical effusion.

Compare - Mephitis, Ipecacuanha.
(Blackwood)

538 Sanguinaria Can.
(Blood Root)

It is a right sided remedy preeminently, and affects chiefly the mucous membranes, especially of the respiratory tract. It has marked vaso-motor disturbances as seen in the circumscribed redness of the cheeks, flashes of heat, determination of blood to head and chest, distention of temporal veins, burning sensations like from hot water. Influenzal coughs. Phthisis. Sudden stopping of catarrh of respiratory tract followed by diarrhoea. Burning in various parts is characteristic.

Head: Worse right side, sun headache, periodical sick headache, pain begins in occiput, spreads upwards, and settles over eyes, especially right. Veins and temples are distended. Pain better lying down and sleep. Headaches return at climacteric, every seventh day. Pain in small spot over upper left parietal bone. Burning in eyes. Pain in the back of head like a flash of lightning.

Face: Redness and burning of cheeks. Hectic flush.

Nose: Hay-fever, ozaena, nasal polypi, coryza followed by diarrhoea, chronic rhinitis, membrane dry and congested.

Throat: Swollen, worse, right side, dry and constricted, ulceration of mouth and fauces with dry burning sensation-tongue white, feels scalded, tonsillitis.

Stomach: Aversion to butter-craving for piquant things. Unquenchable thirst. Nausea with salivation.

Abdomen: Diarrhoea as coryza improves. Pain over region of liver. Cancer of rectum.

Female: Leucorrhoea fetid corrosive - Menses offensive profuse, soreness of breasts. Uterine polypi. Before menses itching of axillae. Climacteric disorders.

Respiratory: Oedema through abdomen and diarrhoea is a strong indication for Sang - Circumscribed hectic flush on the cheeks - Violent dry cough, wheezing, whistling, metallic sputa almost impossible to raise-like Cheli, Sang, is a right sided medicine. Like Cheli, it has a reputation for curing cancer, polypi and new growths. I have seen breast tumors diminish under its action. The headaches of Sang are of great intensity and have some striking characteristics. (1) periodic - every seventh day. (2) begin in the morning, increase to noon and then diminish. (3) are bursting or as if the eyes would be pressed out. (4) begin at occiput, spread upwards and forwards and settle over right eye. (5) like a flash of lightning in occiput. (6) Amel: by sleep (7) return at climacteric. Neuralgia of the face Amel: by kneeling down and pressing head firmly against the floor. Headache agg: by day, sunrise to sunset. *(JHC)*

It is also of service in whooping cough that returns whenever the patient takes cold, it should be remembered in nasal catarrh, and fluent coryza, when the slight odour aggravates and causes the patient to faint. There is burning and rawness of the nose, also nasal polypi which bleed easily. Beneficial at climacteric period - flushes of heat - burning of the hands and feet.

(Blackwood)

539. Sanguinaria Nit

(Nitrate of Sanguinarine)

Is of use in polypus of the nose. Acute and chronic catarrh. Acute pharyngitis (Wyethia), smarting and burning in throat and chest especially under sternum. Influenza, lachrymation, pains in eyes and head, sore scalp, sense of obstruction. Chronic follicular pharyngitis.

Nose: Feels obstructed, profuse, watery mucus with burning pain dry and burning nostrils, watery mucus, with pressure over root of nose. Nostrils plugged with thick yellow bloody mucus, sneezing.

Throat: Dry, constricted, burning.

Respiratory: Hawking of thick yellow, sweetish mucus. Pressure behind center of sternum, tickling cough, chronic, nasal, laryngeal and bronchial catarrh. Voice altered, deep, hoarse.

Dose: 3rd trituration. *(Boericke)*

The catarrhal symptoms of Sang. appear in great intensity-nose, eyes, throat, and bronchi being affected. Lachrymation, pains in eyes and head, sore scalp, obstructed nose and burning pains, throughout all regions were experienced.

A sense of obstruction is very characteristic, sensation of obstruction and fullness in the head, accumulation of mucus obstructing nose, awakes frequently with dry mouth, the nose being obstructed. Accumulation of mucus behind centre of sternum, sense of suffocation, feeling as if air passages lined with thick, stiff mucus or pus. Heat and tension behind sternum is characteristic, and so is expectoration of quantities of sweet-tasting mucus - Adenoids and polypi have been cured with it.

There is great craving for air, bathing with warm water amel: heat in forehead.

(JHC)

Cause: - Driving in cold wind, winter weather, exposure.

This remedy is indicated in nasal polypus, and in chronic nasal catarrh. The nostrils are dry and burning, or are filled with a thick, yellow, bloody mucus.

It is useful in bronchitis, with hoarseness and a dry, hacking cough. The expectoration consists of a thick yellow, sweet mucus. There is a sensation of pressure behind the center of the sternum.

It should be remembered in megrim. The pain is severe on the left side of the head and through the left temple.

(Blackwood)

540. Sanguisuga

(The Leech)

Burnett was the first to use Sanguisuga as a homoeopathic medicine. Dangerous haemorrhages have not unfrequently followed the application of leeches and it has been ascertained that the leech does not merely bite, it poisons the bitten part in such a way as to render the blood too watery. Having a case of persistent bleeding from the rectum, the blood being watery and all the usual haemorrhagic remedies having failed to arrest it, Burnett thought that Sanguisuga might prove the similimum. He had a tincture made and attenuated, gave the 5th attenuation and made a brilliant cure. I have had frequent opportunity of confirming the value of Sags. in cases of the kind.

541. Sanicula

(Aqua)

(The water of Sanicula springs of Ottawa)

Has been found a useful remedy in enuresis, sea sickness, constipation etc. Rickets.

Head: Dread of downward motion *(Borax)*. Profuse sweat on occiput. Profuse scaly dandruff.

Mouth: Tongue large, flabby, burning, must protrude it to keep cool - Ringworm on tongue.

Stomach: Is vomited as soon as it reaches the stomach.

Rectum: Pain in whole perineum - no desire until a large accumulation. Crumbles at verge of anus - excoriation of skin about anus perineum and genitals.

Female: Bearing down as if contents of pelvis would escape - desire to support parts. Leucorrhoea with odor of fish brine or old cheese - Vagina feels large.

Extremities: Burning of soles of feet - Offensive foot sweat - cold, clammy sweat of extremities.

Skin: Dirty greasy, brownish, wrinkled, eczema, fissured hands and fingers.

Mod: Worse moving arms backward.

Dose: 30th potency. *(Boericke)*

We have in Sanic. one of the best proved remedies of the Materia Medica, a polychrest and antipsoric of the wide range. Cachexia. Dirty, greasy, and brownish appearance of body. Scrofulous ophthalmia and scrofulous cruptions, cold, clammy hands and feet, foul smelling foot sweat, profuse sweat of back of head and neck, hair dry and lustreless, thick dandruff of scalp and eyebrows, slow digestion, constipation or else diarrhoea, stools turning green, pot bellied, rickety children.

The foot sweat occurs between the toes, making them sore, as well as on the soles, which are as if one had stepped in cold water. On the other hand there may be burning of soles, must uncover or put them in a cool place and child kicks off clothing, even in coldest weather. The odours of sanic. are characteristic. The stool has an odour of rotten cheese and no amount of washing will get rid of it. The flatus has the same odour. Vaginal discharges and condylomata of penis have an odour of fish brine. This has led to a number of cures. Eating causes desire for stool, must leave the table. Sanic. is a remedy in constipation and in diarrhoea. There is no desire for stool till a long accumulation has occurred. Stools square as if carved with a knife. There is excoriation of skin about anus, perineum and genitals.

Compare: Dread of downward motion - Borox.

Head sweat - *Calc., Silicea.*

Soreness behind ears, viscid discharge - *Graph., Psor.*

Ringworm on tongue: *Nat. m., Ranc. sc., Tarax.*

Drinks little, often vomits when it reaches stomach - *Ars.*

Symptoms change constantly - *Lac. c., Puls.*

Sphincter not under control - *Aloe.*

Stool recedes - *Sil., Thuja.*

Must be removed mechanically - *Sel.*

Crumbling at anus - *Mag-mur.*

Odour of stool follows despite bathing - *Sul.*

Excoriation about anus - *Sul., Lyco., Chamo.*

Places hand on vulva for support - *Lil Tig., Murex.*

Offensive foot sweat - *Sil., Psor.,Graph.*

Burning soles - *Lach., Medo., Sang., Calc.*

Kicks off clothing in coldest weather - *Hep., Sul.*

Skin of neck wrinkled, hangs in fold - *Abrot, Iod., Nat- m., Sars.*

Vomits "schmierkase", falls asleep after vomiting - *Aethusa.*

Fish brine odour - *Calc.* (Rectum), *Graph* (Scab of ulcer), *Med.* (Moisture from anus)

Tell. (Ear discharge).

Stool when eating - *Fer., Tromboid.*

Cough from laughing or talking - *Pho., Arg. n.*

Sweet expectoration - *Sant., Stan.*

Agg: lifting arms - *Bar-c., Con.,Cup., Fer., Led.*

Symptoms increase to noon and decrease after - *Sang., Spig.*

Dreams of Robbers - *Nat. mur.*

Cries before urinating - *Lyco.*

Fears darkness - *Grindel, Stram.*

Fears touch - *Cina, Ant.t., Arn.*

Sea sickness and train sickness - *Ars., Cocc., Tab.*

Headache from nape to eyes - *Sil., Sang.*

Wraps up head - *Mag. m., Sil., Psor.*

Mental restlessness when reading - *Dros.*

Depression with feeling of impending misfortune - *Calc.*

Irritability - *Cham., Con.*

Child rubs nose and eyes on waking - *Scil.*

Hair lustreless - *Alm., K. Ca.*

Clinkers - *K. bi.* *(JHC)*

542. *Santoninum*

(Santonin)

Is the active principle of Santonica, the unexpanded flower head of Artemisia Maritima - Cina - The eye symptoms and those of the urinary tract are most prominent. It is of unquestioned value in the treatment of worm diseases, such as gastro - intestinal irritation, itching of nose, restless sleep, twitching of muscles. Ascaris lubricoides and thread worms but not tape worms. Night cough of children - Chronic cystitis - Laryngeal crisis and lightning pains of tabes.

Head: Chromatic hallucinations - itching of nose.

Eyes: Sudden dimness of sight - color blindness, Xanthopsia - strabismus due to worms - Dark rings about eyes.

Mouth: Fetid breath, depraved appetite, thirsty, tongue deep red, grinding of - teeth-nausea better after eating - choking feeling.

Urinary: Incontinence and dysuria, enuresis.

Dose: 2nd to 3rd trituration - do not give to a child with fever or constipation. *(Boericke)*

Santonin is the favourite anthelmintic of the old school and it is chiefly against lumbrici that it has been given. Visions of figures have been produced and coloured vision is a frequent phenomenon, even when the lower trituration have been used. Yellow is the predominant colour, but green and violet vision are also marked. Hale mentions enuresis, strangury, chronic cystitis as having been cured by it. *(JHC)*

A neutral principle prepared from Santonica. The unexpanded flower heads) of Artemisia maritima. This agent acts as an anthelmintic to the round worm and to a less degree on the thread worm. It has no action on the tape worm.

Intestinal or gastro-intestinal irritation. This group of symptoms is usually complained of when worms are present, but the symptoms may appear and this remedy will relieve them when worms are not to be found. Dark rings about the eyes, itching of the nose-bores the fingers into the nostrils - sleep is restless - cries out in a fright, grinds the teeth and groans during sleep-wetting the bed-urine is whitish and cloudy-dry hacking cough with tickling in the larynx and trachea-reflex irritation-enuresis and dysuria. Albuminuria of pregnancy, the face and head are hot and there is great restlessness and twitching of the muscles - post puerperal, post scarlatinal and post diphtheritic nephritis - choroiditis and atrophy of the optic nerve and amblyopia - Compare: Cina, Teucrium marum. *(Blackwood)*

543. *Saponaria*

(Soap root)

Of great use in the treatment of acute colds, coryza, sore throat etc., will often break up a cold.

Mind: Depressed with sleepiness.

Head: Stitching pain, supra-orbital, coryza.

Eyes: Glaucoma. *(Boericke)*

One prover, who took the 30th, for many years a sufferer from articular rheumatism had none of his usual pains during the proving and a great enlargement of the left knee was entirely removed.

Among the peculiar symptoms of Sap. are involuntary emission of urine when walking, roughness of mucous membrane of mouth, with raised papillae on palate and strawberry tongue. *(JHC)*

544. *Sarcolatic acid*

Is apparently formed in muscle tissue during the stage of muscle exhaustion. Differs from ordinary lactic acid in its relation to polarised light. It represents a much broader and more profoundly acting drug and its pathogenesis is quite dissimilar from the normal acid. Proved by Wm. B. Griggs M.D. who found it of great value in the most violent form of epidemic influenza, especially with violent retching and greatest prostration, when Arsenic had failed. Spinal neurasthenia, muscular weakness, dyspnoea with myocardial weakness.

Stomach: Nausea, uncontrollable vomiting even of water followed by extreme weakness.

Dose: 6-30 potency. The 15x most marked action (Griggs). *(Boericke)*

545. *Sarracenia Purpurea*

(Pitcher plant)

A remedy for variola. Visual disorders. Congestion to head, with irregular heart action. Chlorosis, contains a very active proteolytic enzyme. Sick headache, throbbing in various parts, especially in neck, shoulders and head, which feels full to bursting.

Skin: Variola aborts the disease, arrests pustulation.

Dose: 3-6 potency. *(Boericke)*

The spotted appearance of the plant probably suggesting a resemblance to the disease. Hale has collected much confirmatory evidence of its power to antidote the smallpox poison. In an epidemic occurred in the environs of Wavre, Sarr., was given to two thousand persons living in the very middle of the disease and coming in constant intercourse with it, but all who took Sarr. escaped during the same epidemic, 200 cases were treated with Sarr. without a death. Bilden, who used the 1x tincture in an epidemic with success concluded that Sarr. is to smallpox what Gels. is to bilious fever. *(JHC)*

This remedy is indicated in Variola; it aborts the disease and prevents pustulation. The head is congested. The limbs are weak and there are pains in the knees and hips.

Compare: Tartar emetic, Variolinum.
(Blackwood)

546. *Sarsaparilla*

(Smilax)

Renal colic, marasmus and periosteal pains due to venereal disease. Eruptions following hot weather and vaccination, boils, and eczema, urinary symptoms well marked.

Head: Pains cause depression. Pains from occiput to eyes. Periosteal pain due to venereal disease - influenza - eruptions of face and upper lip - moist eruption on face and upper lip-moist eruption on scalp.

Mouth: aphthae, salivation, metallic taste, no thirst.

Abdomen: Rumbling and fermentation, colic and backache at same time much flatus.

Urinary: Urine scanty, slimy, flaky, sandy, blood, gravel. Renal colic, severe pain at conclusion of urination. Urine dribbles while sitting. Bladder distended and tender - child screams before and while passing urine - sand on diaper - renal colic and dysuria in infants - pain from right kidney downward - tenesmus of bladder - urine passes in thin, feeble stream. Pain at meatus.

Male: Intolerable stench on genitals. Herpetic eruption on genitals. Itching on scrotum and perineum, syphilis.

Female: Nipples small, withered, retracted. Before menstruation, itching and humid eruption on forehead. Menses late and scanty. Moist eruption in right groin before menses.

Skin: Emaciated, shrivelled, lies in folds. Dry, flabby. Herpetic eruptions, ulcers dry itching, comes on in spring, become crusty, rhagades. Cracked hands and feet - skin hard indurated - summer cutaneous affections.

Extremities: Trembling of hands and feet-onychia, ulceration around ends of fingers, cutting sensation under nails deep rhagades on fingers and toes - ulceration around ends of fingers.

Modalities: *Worse* dampness, at night, after urinating, when yawning, in spring, before menses.

Cucurbuta Citrelbus - Water melon: Infusion of the seed acts promptly in painful urination with constriction and backache, relieves pain and stimulates flow.

Dose: 1-6 potency. *(Boericke)*

It is given in scrofula and secondary syphilis and the concomitants of these diseases, such as ulcers, cutaneous eruptions, nodes, indurated glands, caries, necroses, articular swellings and rheumatism often improve under a protracted course of it. Some think it a kind of restorative after an exhausting course of Mercury. This well summarises the ancient reputation of Sars. as a blood purifier - The chief localities of the action of Sars. are - The urinary organs, genitals, rectum, skin and bones, right lower extremity - right lower side - inner semilateral head. There is great pain at end of micturition, just as the urine ceases to flow, when sitting only it dribbles. Passage of gravel which looked like grey sand, many cases of renal colic and dysuria in infants with passage of sand. Spermatorrhoea with swollen cords. Moist eruption in right groin before menses. There are moist eruptions also on scrotum and thigh of the male and offensive odours about genitals in both sexes. In all cases if the other symptoms are associated with the peculiar urinary symptoms of Sars - this will be a strong corroborative indication - The skin is severely affected by Sars - One of its popular uses is for clearing the complexion. Sars produces herpetic eruptions in all parts, and tettery eruptions, moist and dry rhagades - itch like eruptions prone to appear in spring - itching eruption on forehead during menses - it causes great emaciation causing the skin to be shrivelled and lie in folds. Farrington gave these indications—Sycotic eruption, little spots scarcely raised above the skin often scaling a little but looking like the roseola of syphilis and itching intolerably, agg: in spring. Moist eruption on scalp, the pus from which causes inflammation of any part it touches. Sycotic headache beginning at back of head, coming forward and setting at root of nose with swelling of nose. Moist eruption about genitals or between scrotum and thighs. Scirrhus of the breast has been cured with it. The nipples are soft, unexcitable, they are retracted and cannot be made to come out. *(JHC)*

Renal colic and vesicle calculi - excruciating pain at the close of urination. Marasmus, the neck is greatly emaciated Periosteal pain - Compare: Berberis vulgaris, Lycopodium, Petroselinum. *(Blackwood)*

547. *Scarlatinum*

(Nosode of Scarlet fever)

Scarlatina has been used, like other nosodes, for the prevention and cure of the disease from which it takes origin; but its well known affinity for the skin, throat and kidney suggests its applicability for affections of these organs.

Relation : Bell. is the nearest analogue and should be its antidote and various Mercuries come next.

548. *Scilla Maritima*

(Squill. Sea onion)

Physiological dose: The agent in large doses acts as an emetic and purgative and may cause severe and fatal gastro-enteritis. It acts upon the kidneys, causing a diminished flow of urine which may contain blood, the urine may be suppressed. It contains two heart poisons, one scillipierin and the other scillitoxin, the latter slowing the heart and raising the arterial tension. In smaller doses, it acts upon the mucous membrane of the respiratory tract and may establish an inflammatory state. It is eliminated by the bowels, kidneys and bronchial mucous membrane.

Therapeutics: This remedy is of service in cases of bronchial catarrh with a scanty tenacious sputum. The cough is dry harsh and irritating, although there appears to be much mucus in the chest. When he coughs, there is involuntary escape of urine. There are sharp stitching pains in the side with dyspnoea. The cough is precipitated by taking a deep breath or a cold drink and is often followed by sneezing. It is of service in sub-acute and chronic pleurisy when the sticking pains are present. *(Blackwood)*

Scilla maritima grows on the shores of the Mediterranean sea and has had a place in medicine from the most ancient times - Its cardiac action is exactly the same as that of Digitalis - And old rule runs put Squilla in every cough mixture - Butnett quotes - I have found it quickly and surely helpful in painful spleen diseases - affections painful and beyond any doubt in and of the spleen. The gushing of tears, with the cough is another scil. Indication. The cough causes sneezing, flow of tears, spurting of urine and even involuntary stools. The kidneys are powerfully acted on by Scil. and many of the traditional uses of the drug have been with the idea of eliminating dropsical effussions by producing a great flow of urine. Boger adds the heart to the organs primarily affected by Scil. - profuse urine - Stitching pain in the left chest - frequent hot scanty urine. Teeth show black marks, consistantly rubs eyes and sneezes - Lippe notes Black teeth as a symptom of Scil. Boger adds that the nails become brittle and split and that the veterinarians use Scil. for cracked hoof in horses. *(JHC)*

549. *Scirrhinum*

(Nosode of Scirrhous cancer)

Burnett is my authority for this nosode. He proved it on himself, and produced a tremendous sinking at the navel, which he regarded as a keynote for its use. Scirrh. has aided the cure of many cases of breast tumour in Burnett's hands. With it he cured a man of hard glands which appeared on the left side of the neck after other glands had been removed by the patient's brother, a surgeon. Haemorrhages and varicosis of legs and feet with purple points, have also been cured by Burnett with Scirrh. A patient to whom Burnett had given scirrh. mentioned to him that it had caused the passage of an enormous number of thread worms. On this hint Burnett gave it with great success in many cases of this troublesome complaint and I have verified this experience. In inveterate cases where Cina and Teucr. have given little relief Scirrh has wrought a great change for the better. The time of agg: of Scirrh is from 5-6 p.m. and irregularly on through the night. *(JHC)*

550. *Scrophularia Nosodea*

(Knotted Figwort)

A powerful medicine whenever enlarged glands are present - Hodkins disease. A valuable skin remedy. Has a specific affinity for the breast - very useful in the dissipation of breast tumours. Eczema of the ear. Pruritus vaginae. Lupoid ulceration, scrofulous swellings. Painful haemorrhoids. Tubercular testis. Ephithelioma. Nodosities in the breast (Scirrh.) Pain in all flexor muscles. Abdomen: Pain in liver on pressure - Colic below navel. Pain in sigmoid flexure and rectum - painful bleeding, protruding piles. Sleep: great drowsiness.

Dose: Tr. and 1st potency - apply locally to cancerous glands. also semper. Viv. *(Boericke)*

The plants of the genus Scrophularia have generally an unpleasant smell - Gerarde mentions: Hard Kernels and painful and swollen piles as indicating it - Nodosities in the breast is another indication of Coopers. *(JHC)*

This remedy is of service in diseases of the skin, eczema, crusta lactea, eruption of a vesicular character, pruritus vaginae, herpetic ulceration, and scrofulous swelling, when there is a tendency to ulceration following the slightest contusion and indications of perverted nutrition.

Dosage: 1-60 drops Tincture.

(Blackwood)

551. *Scutellaria Lateriflora*

(Skull cap)

(Mad dog skull cap)

This is a nervous sedative, where nervous fear pre-dominates-cardiac irritability - chorea - nervous weakness after influenza.

Mental: Fear of some calamity - inability to fix attention - confusion.

Head: Dull frontal headache-eyes feels pressed outwards-flushed face, restless sleep and frightful dreams. Must move about - night terrors-migraine worse over right eye-aching in eyeballs - explosive headache of school teachers with frequent urination - headache in front and base of brain-nervous sick headaches - worse noise, odor, light; better: night rest. (5 drops of Tincture)

Stomach: Nausea, sour eructations, hiccough-pain and distress, abdomen gas, fullness and distention, colicky pain and uneasiness, light coloured diarrhoea.

Male: Seminal emission and impotence with fear of never being better.

Sleep: Night-terrors, sleeplessness, sudden wakefulness, frightful dreams.

Extremities: Twitching of muscles, must be moving, chorea, tremors, sharp stinging pains in upper extremities, nightly restlessness, weakness and aching.

Dose: Tincture and lower potencies.
(Boericke)

Scutel, says Hale who introduced it into homoeopathy, is in the domestic practice of North America what valerian in that of Europe - Its calming effects on the nervous system have been known ever since the settlement of New England - Nervo-bilious headache with nervous symptoms uppermost and nothing the matter with her - Royal. He found the patient screaming - every few minutes she had to urinate, and passed only a few drops - stools frequent, loose, watery. Pulse irregular - Scut-ϕ was given - 10 drops - every 1/2 hour, patient was better after the second dose, slept after the fourth - Hale quotes - Depression of nervous and vital powers after long sickness, over-exercise, over-study, long continued and exhausting labours. It controls nervous agitation. Scudder mentions chorea, delirium tremens and hydrophobia (as its popular name suggests). Hale has used it with success in sleepless ness, night terrors, hysteria, nervous agitation from pain or exciting emotions, cerebral irritations of children from dentition or intestinal irritation. It has been found useful in the weak heart resulting from cigarette smoking - gave 60 drops of the Tincture every 2 hours in a case of rapid hiccough which chloroform, morphia and pilocarpine had failed to relieve permanently. After the eighth dose, the patient slept and the spasms gradually diminished and stopped for good by the fourth day. The hemicrania is amel: moving about in open air - All symptoms are amel: sleep - (Cypr. according to Hale acts more on brain, Scut. on spinal cord) - Over worked women - mag. c.
(JHC)

This remedy is indicated when there is a nervous fear that predominates every thing. The patient fears some calamity.

It is useful in migraine and dull frontal headaches. The face is flushed. The patient must move about - the pain is worse over the right eye.

It should be remembered in chorea, irregular muscular twitching and paralysis agitans, also in insomnia and night terrors of children and nervous palpitations of the heart.

Compare: cypripedium. *(Boericke)*

552. *Secale Cornutum*

(Claviceps Purpurea - Ergot)

Produces contraction of the unstriped muscle fibres, hence a constringent feeling throughout the whole body. This produces an anaemic condition, coldness, numbness, petechiae, mortification, gangrene. A useful remedy for old people with shrivelled skin - thin scrawny old women. All the Secale conditions are better from cold. The whole body is prevaded by a sense of great heat. Haemorrhages, continued oozing, thin, fetid, watery black blood. Debility, anxiety, emaciation, though appetite and thirst may be excessive. Facial and abdominal muscles twitch - Secale decreases the flow of pancreatic juice by raising the blood pressure (Hinsdale).

Head: Passive congestive pain (rises from back of head) - falling of hair, dry and gray-nose bleed, dark, oozing.

Eyes: Incipient cataract. Eyes sunken and surrounded by a blue margin.

Face: Pale, pinched, sunken. Cramps commence in face and spread over whole body - spasmodic distortion.

Mouth: Tongue dry, cracked, blood like ink exudes. Tingling of the tip of the tongue, which is stiff - Tongue swollen, paralysed.

Stomach: Unnatural ravenous appetite, craves acid, thirst unquenchable, nausea, vomiting of blood and coffee grounds fluid, burning in stomach and abdomen.

Stool: Cholera like stools with coldness and cramps, olive green, thin putrid, bloody, with icy coldness and intolerance of being covered, with great exhaustion, involuntary stools, no sensation of passing faeces, anus wide open.

Urine: Paralysis of bladder, retention, discharge of black blood from bladder, enuresis in old people.

Female: Brownish offensive leucorrhoea, menses irregular, copious, dark, continuous oozing of watery blood until next period, threatened abortion about the third month, during labor no expulsive action, though everything is relaxed after pains, suppression of milk, breasts do not fill properly, dark offensive lochia.

Sleep: Insomnia of drug and liquor habitues.

Extremities: Fingers, spread apart or bent backwards, numb, violent cramps. Icy coldness of extremities. Violent pain in finger tips, tingling in toes.

Skin: Dry gangrene, varicose ulcers, burning sensation, better by cold, wants parts uncovered, though cold to touch, slight wounds continue to bleed. Skin feels cold to touch, yet covering is not tolerated, great aversion to heat, formication under skin.

Fever: Coldness, cold dry skin, cold clammy sweat, excessive thirst - sense of internal heat.

Modalities: *Worse* heat, warm, covering, *better* cold, uncovering.

Relation: Ergotin. Increased blood pressure 2x trit.

Dose: 1 to 30 potency. *(Boericke)*

Rye and grasses are apt to be affected with the Ergot disease in damp seasons, and when grown on damp, ill drained lands. If breeding cows are turned on pastures, where infected grasses grow they are very liable to drop their calves. Ergot has been known as a hastener of parturition from remote times. Its other actions have been for the most part learned from the terrible epidemics of Ergotism which have occasionally devastated districts in which Rye infected with Ergot has been ground into flour and eaten by the population. Death takes place in convulsions or else from gangrene and consequent exhaustion or from exhausting haemorrhages or discharges as diarrhoea. The nervous symptoms of Secale are convulsive-rigid-alternates with relaxation. Hands which are either clenched or have the fingers spread widely apart (A keynote symptom). The muscles of the face and abdomen twitch-incontinence or retention of urine. Spasmodic retching. The stomach is violently contracted. Fingers turn bluish black, dry gangrene of the parts. Sec. shrivels up the skin, makes it dry and harsh. Women of very lax muscular fibre, everything seems loose and open, no actions, vessels flabby, passive haemorrhages, copious flow of thin, black, watery blood lessens the coagulating power of the blood, and produces a haemorrhagic diathesis. Persistent offensive bleeding, small wounds bleed persistently—grand characteristic agg. by external heat - In cholera, patient is cold, almost pulseless - spasmodic twitchings of muscles in various parts - Surface harsh - shrivelled, dry, as though no moisture were left in the body-though cold to the touch, cannot bear to be covered, in spite of this coldness Sec. has burning among its characteristic sensations, burning in all parts of the body as if sparks were falling on the patient - Another characteristic is numbness, tingling as if ants crawling all over Amel: by rubbing. Diarrhoea is peculiar, involuntary, with wide open anus -catarrh has been caused in many instances - exopthalmic goitre, heart being acted on by 'sec'-violent palpitation induced-great affinity for the uterus - it may be used on its homoeopathic indications with perfect safety-in threatened abortion, especially at 3rd month, prolonged bearing down, forcing pains, labourpains are irregular, too weak, feeble or ceasing, everything seems loose and open but there is no expulsive action, fainting — after pains too long, too excessive, hour glass contraction of the uterus, non-appearance of milk-menses irregular, copious, dark, fluid, labour-like pains, continuous watery discharge of blood during the whole time between the periods. One drop of 6th the flooding ceased immediately and permanently - as if intoxicated while undressing, as if fingers asleep-as if sparks of fire falling on different parts - as if mice creeping under skin - Desires lemonade. Averse to fat and meat.

Relation: Post partum haemorrhage, Cinnamon increases labour pains, controls profuse or dangerous flooding, is always sage, while Ergot is always dangerous - cold skin, cannot bear to be covered Camph - Erigeron flow in fits and starts with dysuria. *(JHC)*

A fungus growing on the seed bud of rye and several other cereals. Causes a fall of the blood pressure due to the direct action of the agent upon the heart muscles. This is followed by a rise of the blood pressure as a result of its action upon the vasomotor centers, and the unstriped muscular fibres in the arterioles. Tinnitus aurium - cramps of the abdominal muscles - dry gangrene which destroys more or less of the extremities and may involve the nose and other portions of the body. Thin, scrawny, cachectic women, bearing down in the uterus, passive haemorrhages - always cold, and desire to uncover - worse from warmth - putrescence and gangrene. Congestive headache - putrid, foetid diarrhoea - cramps - skin is shrivelled - cold, clammy perspiration - urine is suppressed - paralysis of the sphincter ani. Service in labour and prolonged haemorrhage, flow is dark, patient is wrinkled, scrawny, cold and often unconscious. Beneficial in gangrene - skin is shrivelled, dry, and brittle - relief from cold applications.

Compare - Arsenicum album, cinnamon, Colchicine. *(Blackwood)*

553. *Selenium*

(The Element Selenium)

Selenium is a constant constituent of bones and teeth. Marked effects on the genito-urinary organs and often indicated in elderly men, especially for prostatitis and sexual atony. Great debility-worse heat. Easy exhaustion, mental and physical in old age. Debility after exhausting diseases.

Mind: Lascivious thoughts, with impotency, extreme sadness.

Head: Hair falls out, pain over left eye, worse walking in sun, strong odors and tea, headache from tea drinking.

Throat: Hoarseness, cough in morning with expectoration of bloody mucus, hoarseness of singers.

Abdomen: Chronic liver affections, enlarged with fine rash over liver region. Stool constipated, hard and accumulated in rectum.

Male: Dribbling of semen during sleep, dribbling of prostatic fluid, loss of sexual power, increased desire, decreases ability, on attempting coition penis relaxes, hydrocele.

Skin: Dry scaly eruption in palms with itching-itching about the ankles - Hair falls out from brows, beard and genitals, comedones with an oily surface of the skin, alopecia, acne.

Sleep: Prevented by pulsation in all vessels.

Modalities: Worse after sleep.

Compare: Agnus, Calad., Sulphur, Tellu., Phos. ac.

Dose: 6-30 potency. *(Boericke)*

Selenium was discovered in 1818 by Berzelius and was named by him after the Moon - when precipitated it appears as a red powder, which melts when heated and on cooling forms a brittle mass, nearly black but transmitting red light when in thin plates - when heated in air, it takes fire, burns with a blue flame, giving a gaseous oxide of selenium, which has a most penetrating and characteristic odour of putrid horse raddish - The hotter his body the weaker he is, strength rises as the sun sinks - cannot bear any nervous drain hence agg: after coitus or seminal emissions - impotence-headache agg: by strong odours as of musk, roses etc., above the left eye. There is constipation from atony with impacted faeces and dribbling of semen after stool and also after micturition-hoarseness of singers, appearing as soon as they begin to sing or after long use of the voice-Sel causes itching in folds of skin as between fingers and about joints especially the ankle-joint-hair falls off scalp and all parts of body - I have frequently relieved 'Psoriasis palmaris' with Sel., which shows that it has a relation to syphilis. Irresistible desire to lie down and sleep, strength leaves him suddenly, especially in hot weather - Aversion to salted food, agg: from tea, sugar, salt, lemonade, wine agg: towards noon. Amel: as sun declines. Impotence, (Sul.). Sul. has more coldness and shrivelling of the organs - Sel. more total relaxation, so that semen escapes involuntarily and dribbles. *(JHC)*

This remedy is indicated in prostratitis and the sexual atony of middle aged and old men when there is dribbling of the semen and prostatic fluid. There are lascivious fancies and loss of sexual power. Compare: Phosphorus, Agnus castus, Caladium. *(Blackwood)*

554. *Sempervivum Tectorum*

(House leek)

Is recommended for herpes, zoster, and cancerous tumors. Scirrhous induration of tongue. Mammary carcinoma, ringworm, Haemorrhoids.

Mouth: Tongue has ulcers, bleed easily, stabbing pains.

Skin: Warts and corns.

Relation: Cotyledon, Ficus Carcica (Fig.). The milky juice of the freshly broken stalk, applied to warts, causes their disappearance.

Dose: Tr. and 2x. *(Boericke)*

In many countries Semp. has a popular reputation for indurations and sores on the tongue. *(JHC)*

It is applied locally to the bites of insects and stings of bees and poisonous wounds. *(Blackwood)*

555. *Senecio Aureus*

(Golden Ragwort)

Its action on the female organism has been clinically verified. Urinary organs also affected in a marked degree. Backaches of congested kidneys. Early cirrhosis of liver.

Head: Wave like dizziness, sharp pains over left eye and through left temple.

Abdomen: Straining at stool, thin dark bloody with tenesmus.

Urinary: Scanty, high coloured, bloody, with much mucus and tenesmus. Great heat and constant urging. Nephritis, irritable bladder of children with headache, Renal colic.

Male: Lascivious dreams - prostate enlarged.

Female: Menses retarded, suppressed, functional amenorrhoea of young girls with backaches. Before menses inflammatory conditions of throat, chest and bladder. After menstruation commences, these improve. Anaemic dysmenorrhoea with urinary disturbances. Premature and too profuse menses.

Respiratory: Cough loose, dry teasing cough, stitching chest pains.

Dose: Tr. to 3rd potency. *(Boericke)*

A very definite relation has been traced between the nose and the female sexual organs, and Senec. is indicated when epistaxis or nasal catarrh takes the place of menses when suppressed from any cause. The menses may be profuse and early or they maybe retarded or absent. Senec. may be required in a great variety of conditions traceable to non-appearing menses. "Lyman Watkins" quoted, females taking senec, generally improve in health and strength, accumulate flesh, become light hearted and cheerful. This may be due to some tonic influence. *(JHC)*

Especially of females - Atonic states of the reproductive organs - uterus is enlarged, cervical leucorrhoea replaces the menses, catarrhal headache, enlarged prostate.

Compare: Mitchella, Cimicifuga. *(Blackwood)*

556. *Senega*

(Snakewort)

Catarrhal symptoms, especially of the respiratory tract and distinct eye symptoms of a paralytic type, are most characteristic.

Circumscribed spots in chest left after inflammations.

Head: Dullness, with pressure and weakness of eyes. Pain in temples. Bursting pain in forehead.

Eyes: Hyperphoria, better by bending head backwards. Acts on the rectus superior, Blepharitis, lids dry and crusty, dryness with sensation as if too large for orbits, opacities of vitreous humor. Promotes absorption of fragments of lens, after operation.

Nose: Dry coryza, much watery mucus and sneezing, nostrils feel peppery.

Throat: Catarrhal inflammation of throat and fauces, with scraping hoarseness, burning and rawness. Sensation as if membrane had been abraded.

Respiratory: Hoarseness, hurts to talk, bursting pain in back on coughing, catarrh of larynx, loss of voice, hacking cough, throat feels too narrow, cough often ends in a sneeze, rattling in chest, chest oppressed on ascending, bronchial catarrh, with sore chest wall, much mucus, sensation of oppression and weight of chest, difficult raising of profuse mucus in the aged. Asthenic bronchitis of old people with chronic interstitial nephritis or chronic emphysema. Old asthmatics with congestive attacks, exudations in pleura, hydrothorax. Pressure on chest as though lungs were forced back to spine. Voice unsteady, vocal cords partially paralysed.

Mod: Worse walking in open air, during rest, better from sweat, bending head backwards.

Dose: Tincture to 30 potency. *(Boericke)*

Other old school practitioners used it as an expectorant in chronic respiratory catarrh, acute phthisis, rheumatic fever, dropsies, incipient cataract, croup. It is at present regarded as a stimulant, diaphoretic and expectorant especially in chronic bronchitis. It is in affections of the chest, eyes and bladder that homoeopaths have found it of most service. Taste considers it specially suited to females of slender and tall make, thin, but having retained a good deal of sprightliness and moral power - other observers, including myself have found Seneg more suited to plethoric, phlegmatic persons, persons tending to obesity, fat persons of lax fibre, fat chubby children and old persons. Guernsey outlines its action thus where there is a great burning in the chest, either before or after coughing, profuse secretion of mucus-general affections of the wind pipe, left side of chest particularly - right eye, lower eyelids. Nash has cured many cases of cough with great accumulation of mucus which seems to fill the chest with much rattling, wheezing and difficult breathing. I have used Seneg only in the 30th and have found it answer to its indications exceedingly well - Leading indications (1) Great accumulations of clear albuminous mucus which is difficult to expel (2) Great soreness of walls of chest. (3) Pressure on chest as though lungs were forced back to spine, whooping cough in fat chubby children, clear mucus like white of egg, difficult to raise, cough agg: towards evening, the soreness of the chest walls makes Seneg appropriate to cases of pleurodynia - There is hoarseness, and the throat is so dry and sensitive, it hurts the patient to talk - cough often ends in sneezing. A case - there was hoarseness hawking of thick, tenacious mucus, profuse, a quart in twenty four hours from larynx especially in morning with burning sensation. Seneg acts on eyes, even more powerfully than on the nose, producing pains, inflammation both of the exterior and interior of the eye and lids and much disorder of vision - Amel bending head backwards - violent rush of blood to head when stooping, especially to eye balls, where a painful pressure is experienced. Peculiar sensation - Eyes as if they were pressed out Amel: Sweat. *(JHC)*

This agent is a stimulating expectorant, diuretic and diaphoretic. This remedy is indicated in chronic bronchitis when secondary changes have resulted, and emphysema and bronchiectasis are present. There is great rattling of mucus in the bronchial tubes, which is accompanied by a loose, rattling cough, though there is but little expectoration, and that is tough. There is a sensation of burning in the chest, which is painful and sore.

It is of service in muscular asthenopia, and opacities of vitreous humor; objects look shaded, there is double vision. It is credited with promoting the absorption of fragments of the lens after operation of cataract.

Compare: Spongia tosta, Phosphorus.
(Blackwood)

557. Senna
(Cassia Acutifolia)

Is of much use in infantile colics when the child seems to be full of wind. Oxaluria, with excess of urea; increased specific gravity. Where the system is broken down, bowels constipated, muscular weakness, and waste of nitrogenous materials, senna acts as a tonic. Ebulitions of blood at night. Acetonaemia, prostration, fainting, constipation with colic and flatulence. Liver enlarged and tender.

Stool: Fluid yellowish, with pinching pains before. Greenish mucus; never get done sensation, (Merc). Burning in rectum, with strangury of bladder. Constipation, with colic and flatulence. Liver enlarged and tender, stools hard and dark, with loss of appetite, coated tongue, bad taste and weakness.

Urine: Specific gravity and density increased; hyperazoturia, oxaluria, phosphaturia, and acetonuria.

Relationship:*Compare: Kali carb; Jalapa.*

Antidote: Nux, Cham.

Dose: Third to sixth potency.
(Boericke)

Used as a laxative in ordinary practice. Senna has proved an excellent remedy in the colic of infants with incarcerated flatulence and sleeplessness. Infantile colic when the patient seems full of wind. The symptoms are mostly derived from over dosings. A peculiar symptom is repeated sneezing which causes heat especially of hands, exhaustion and panting breathing. Exhaustion is typical of Senna. Farrington says, it is one of the best remedies in the materia medica for simple exhaustion with excess of nitrogenous waste. The exhaustion is exemplified in the sinking immediately after meals. The pods cause a nasty unclean smell from the body of a woman taking them for constipation. *(JHC)*

This agent is an active cathartic, produces a copious yellow stool. It is a mild hepatic stimulant and excites the menstrual flow.
(Blackwood)

558. Sepia
(Inky Juice of Cuttle fish)

Acts specially on portal system with venous congestion. Stasis and thereby Ptosis of viscera and weariness and misery.

Weakness, yellow complexion, bearing down sensation, especially in women, upon whose organism, it has most pronounced effect. Pains extends down to back, chills easily. Tendency to abortion. Hot flashes at menopause with weakness and perspiration. Upward tendency of its symptoms. Easy fainting. Ball sensation in inner parts. Sepia acts best on brunettes. All pains are from below up. One of the most important uterine remedies. Tubercular patients with chronic hepatic troubles and uterine reflexes. Feels cold even in warm room, pulsating headache in cerebellum.

Mind: Indifferent to those loved best. Averse to occupation, to family, irritable, easily offended, dreads to be alone, very sad, weeps when telling symptoms, miserly, anxious towards evening, indolent.

Head: Coldness of vertex, headache in terrible shocks at menstrual nisus, with scanty flow. Hair falls out; open fontanelles, pimples on forehead, near hair.

Nose: Thick greenish discharge, thick plugs and crusts, yellow saddle across nose, chronic nasal catarrh, especially post nasal.

Eyes: Tarsal tumors, ptosis, ciliary irritation.

Ears: Herpes behind ears on nape of neck.

Face: Yellow blotches, pale or sallow, yellow about mouth, saddle like brownish distribution on nose and cheeks.

Mouth: Tastes salty, tongue foul but clears during menses, swelling and cracking of lower lip.

Stomach: Feeling of goneness, not relieved by eating, nausea at smell or sight of food, tobacco dyspepsia, longing for vinegar, acids and pickles, worse after milk, especially when boiled, acid dyspepsia, loathes fat.

Abdomen: Flatulent, liver sore and painful, relieved by lying on right. Many brown spots on abdomen, feeling of relaxation and bearing down in abdomen.

Rectum: Bleeding at stool and fullness of rectum, constipation, large hard stools, feeling of a ball in rectum, cannot strain with great tenesmus and pains shooting upward, dark brown, round balls glued together with mucus, soft stools, difficult, prolapsus ani. Almost constant oozing from anus, infantile diarrhoea, worse from boiled milk and rapid exhaustion. Pains shoot up in rectum and vagina.

Urinary: Red adhesive, sand in urine, involuntary urination during first sleep, chronic cystitis, slow micturation, with bearing down sensation above pubis.

Female: Pelvic organs relaxed, bearing down sensation as if everything would escape from vulva (Bel, Kreos, Lac. c., Lil. t., Nat. c., Pod.) Must cross limbs to prevent protrusion or press against vulva, leucorrhoea yellow, greenish with much itching. Menses too late and scanty, irregular, early and profuse, sharp clutching pains. Violent stitches upward in the vagina from uterus to umbilicus. Prolapse of uterus and vagina. Morning sickness, vagina painful especially on coition.

Respiratory: Dry fatiguing cough, cough in morning with profuse expectoration, tasting salty.

Back: Weakness in small of back- Pains extend into back, coldness between shoulders.

Extremities: Restlessness in all limbs, twitching and jerkings night and day. Pain in heel, coldness of legs and feet.

Fever: Frequent flushes of heat, sweat from least motion, general lack of warmth of body, feet cold and wet, shivering with thirst, worse towards evening.

Skin: Herpes circinatus in isolated spots. Itching, not relieved by scratching, worse in bends of elbows and knees, chloasma, herpetic eruption on lips, about mouth and nose. Ringworm like eruption every spring. Urticaria in going in open air, better in warm room, hyperidrosis and bromidrosis, sweat on feet, lentigo in young women, ichthyosis with offensive odor of skin.

Modalities: *Worse,* forenoons and evenings, washing, laundry work, dampness, left side, after sweat, cold air, before thunder storm, *better* by exercise, pressure, warmth of bed, hot applications, drawing limbs up, cold bathing, after sleep.

Dose: 12, 30, 200 potency. Should not be used too low or be repeated too frequently. On the other hand Dr. Joussets unique experience is that, it should be continued for some time in strong doses. 1x twice a day. *(Boericke)*

Sepia is predominantly, but by no means exclusively, a woman's remedy. It affects the generative organs of both sexes and a large number of the symptoms occurring in the other organs have some relation thereto. Taste describes the type, between pubescence and the critical period of life, of delicate constitutions, with white pure skins, or skin having a rosy tinge, blonde or red hair, nervous are disposed to sexual excitement or have been exhausted by sexual excesses. Hering gives these types. (1) Persons of dark hair, rigid fibre, but mild and easy disposition. (2) Women during pregnancy, in child birth and, while nursing (3) Children who take cold readily when the weather changes (4) Scrofulous persons (5) Men who have been addicted to drinking and sexual excesses (6) Pot bellied mothers, yellow saddle across nose, irritable, faint from least exertion. Farrington says - puffed flabby persons, with yellow or dirty yellow brown blotched skin, inclined to sweat, especially about genitals, axillae and back. Sepia disturbs the circulation causing flushes and other irregularities - Hands hot and feet cold - or vice versa-sensation of a ball in rectum. The menses are generally scanty, as with Murex they are the reverse. Uterus either prolapse or retroversion, morning sickness - thought of food sickens her, prone to abortion should take Sepia and Zinc. The relaxed sphincters of Sep. favour enuresis. The bed is wet almost as soon as the child goes to sleep; always during the first sleep- in some cases the discharge of urine may be difficult and the patient may have to wait a long time. Skin is delicate, the least injury tends to ulceration. Itching which often changes to burning when scratched - chloasma - Herpetic eruption on lips and about mouth. Ringworm like Herpes circinatus - the nettle rash of Sep appears on going to open air - Amel: in warm room - the itching of Sepia may be desperate especially when it effects the genitals and anus - Sepia is a chilly remedy from lack of vital heat. Chills so easily. Peculiarities - Anxiety, with fear, flushes of heat over face and head, about real or imaginary evils, towards evening, great sadness and weeping, dread of being alone, of men, of meeting friends, with uterine troubles, indifferent even to one's family; one's occupation; to one's nearest and dearest. Greedy, miserly - indolent - The sepia patient weeps, when asked about her symptoms. Faints easily. A very peculiar symptom- Involuntary jerking of head backward and forward especially forenoons when sitting - This may occur in hysteria sitting with legs crossed - Sep. is the washer woman's remedy - Chloasma, Lyco., Nux, Cruar - Ringworm - Bac, Calc, Tell -Sep, weeps when asked about her symptoms, Puls weeps when telling her symptoms - Heat of vertex - Calc., Graph., Sul. (Bell Agg: lying down Sep. Amel:) (Bel. Amel: standing up Sep. Agg:) (Prolapse - Ust.,Sec., Vib. Op., Inula) *(JHC)*

General venous congestion, portal system, genito urinary system - gastro intestinal canal - skin earthy-yellow and cachectic-eczema and herpes develop-sluggishness, thinks slowly and forgets - dark rings about the eyes - yellow saddle across the upper parts of the cheek and nose- dark hair rigid fibre but mild and easy disposition - Tall Slender women with narrow pelvis - pains better continued exercise - return while resting - chills so easily - indifferent even to one's occupation, to those whom she loves best, dreads to be alone - spiteful, greedy, miserly - Yellowness of the face. Yellow spots on the chest-tell-tale face of uterine ailments - washer woman's remedy - Agg: laundry work - sweat about the genitals, arm pits and back. Ankles feel tired - To relieve backache keeps book or some object in the chair to lean against - catarrhal conditions - thick yellow green; eyes, nose, leucorrhoea-hands hot, feet cold-feet hot, hands cold-imaginary evils it is an exertion to think-headache-scanty flow-hysterical women - relief external pressure - continued hard motion. Falling of hair - chronic headache - at the climacteric dyspepsia associated with uterine disease-all gone feeling in epigastrium-Amel: eating, longs for acids and pickles-tongue coated but clear at menstrual period-constipation during pregnancy - stools hard knotty balls, insufficient. Prolapsus, uterus, vagina, sensation of bearing down-menses irregular-leucorrhoea-fetid odor-like pus - itching vagina, amenorrhoea - urine deposits - reddish clay coloured sediment - sexual organs weak and relaxed. *(Blackwood)*

559. *Serum Anguillar Ichthyotoxin*

(Eel Serum)

The serum of the Eel has a toxic action on the blood, rapidly destroying its globules. The presence of albumin and renal elements in the urine, the haemoglobinuria, the prolonged anuria (24-26 hrs) together with the results of the autopsy, plainly demonstrate its elective action on the kidneys. Secondarily, the liver and heart are affected and the alteration observed are those usually present in infectious diseases.

From all these facts it is easy to infer, a priori, the therapeutical indications of the serum of Eel. Whenever the kidney becomes acutely infected, either from cold or infection or intoxication and the attack is characterised by oliguria, anuria and albuminuria we will find the Eel's serum eminently efficacious to re-establish diuresis and in rapidly arresting albuminuria. When during the course of heart disease, the kidney previously working well should suddenly become affected and its function inhibited and when besides we observe cardiac irregularities and a marked state of asystolia, we may yet expect good results from this serum. But to determine here the choice of this remedy is not an easy matter. While digitalis presents in its indication the well known symptomatic triology - arterial hypertension, oliguria and oedema, the serum of Eel's seems better adapted to cases of hypertension and oliguria without oedema. We should bear in mind that the elective action of the Eel's serum is not on the kidney and I believe we can well assert that if digitalis is a cardiac, the Eel's remedy is a renal remedy. So far, at least, the clinical observations published seem to confirm this distinction. The serum of the Eel has given very small results in attacks of asystolia, but it has been very efficacious in cardiac uremia. There, where digitalis is powerless, the serum of the Eel has put an end to the renal obstruction and produced an abundant diuresis. But its really specific indication seems to be for acute nephritis a frigori.

Subacute nephritis. Heart diseases, in cases of failure of compensation and impending asystole. The experiments of Dr. Jousset have amply demonstrated the rapid haematuria, albuminuria and oliguria caused by it. In the presence of acute nephritis with threatening uremia we should always think of this serum. In functional heart diseases. Mitral insufficiency, asystolia with or without oedema, dyspnoea and difficult urinary secretion.

Relationship: Great anology exists between eel serum and the venom of the vipera.

Compare: also Pelias, Lachesis.

Dose: Attenuations are made with glycerine or distilled water, the lower 1x to 3 in heart disease, the higher in sudden renal attacks. *(Boericke)*

560. Silicea

(Terra) - Silica - Pure flint.

Imperfect assimilation and consequent defective nutrition. It goes further and produces neurasthenic states in consequence and increased susceptibility to nervous stimuli and exagerated reflexes. Diseases of bones, caries and necrosis. Silicea can stimulate the organism to reabsorb fibrotic conditions and scar tissue. In phthisis - must be used with care, for it may cause the absorption of scar tissue, liberate the disease, walled in, to new activities (J. Weir). Organic changes, it is deep and slow in action. Periodical states, abscesses, quinsy, headaches, spasms, epilepsy, feeling of coldness before an attack. Keloid growth, scrofulous, rachitic children with large head, open fontenelles and sutures, distended abdomen, slow in walking, ill effects of vaccination, suppurative processes. It is related to all fistulous burrowings. Ripens abscesses, since it promotes suppuration. Silica patient is cold, chilly, hugs the fire, wants plenty of warm clothing, hates drafts, hands and feet cold, worse in winter, lack of vital heat. Prostration of mind and body. Great sensitiveness to taking cold. Intolerance of alcoholic stimulants. Ailments attended with pus formation. Epilepsy, want of grit, moral or physical.

Mind: Faint hearted, anxious, nervous and excitable, sensitive, thinks only of pins, fears them.

Head: Aches from fasting, vertigo when looking up, better wrapping up warmly, when lying on left side - profuse sweat of head, offensive and extends to neck. Pain begins at occiput, and spreads over head and settles over eyes.

Eyes: Angles of eyes affected, swelling of lachrymal duct. Aversion to light especially day light. Styes - Abscess in cornea - Cataract in office workers. Use 30th potency for months.

Ears: Fetid discharge, caries of mastoid, pistol like raport, roaring in ears.

Nose: Dry, hard crusts form, bleeding when loosened, sneezing in morning. Obstructed and loss of smell - Perforation of septum.

Face: Skin cracked on margin of lips.

Mouth: Sensation of a hair on tongue, boils on gums - abscess at root of teeth pyorrhoea - sensitive to cold water.

Throat: Periodical quinsy - pricking as of a pin in tonsil - parotid glands swollen, stinging pain on swallowing - hard, cold swelling of cervical glands.

Stomach: Disgust for meat and warm food.

Abdomen: Colic, cutting pain, with constipation, yellow hands and blue nails.

Rectum: Feels paralysed, fistula in ano, fissures and haemorrhoids, painful and spasm of sphincter, stools come down with difficulty, when partly expelled recede again, rectum stings, closes upon stool - constipation always before and during menses.

Urinary: Prostatic fluid discharged, when straining at stool - noctural enuresis in children with worms.

Male: Eruption on inner surface of thighs, gonorrhoea, with thick fetid discharge, elephantiasis of scrotum, hydrocele.

Female: Acrid leucorrhoea, itching of vulva and vagina, discharge of blood between menstrual periods - menses with icy coldness over whole body nipples very sore, ulcerated easily, drawn in, fistulous ulcers of breast -Abscess of labia, discharge of blood from vagina every time child is nursed, vaginal cysts, hard lumps in breast.

Respiratory: Colds fail to yield, sputum persistently muco-purulent and profuse. Cough and sore throat, with expectoration of little granules like shot, which when broken, smell very offensive - violent cough when lying down, with thick yellow, lumpy expectorations.

Back: Pain in coccyx - diseases of bones of spine.

Sleep: Night walking, gets up while asleep - Frequent starts in sleep - Anxious dreams.

Extremities: Sciatica, pains through hips, legs and feet. Tremulous hands when using them. Affection of finger nails, especially if white spots on nails, in growing toe nails - icy cold and sweaty feet. The parts lain on go to sleep - offensive sweat on feet, hands and axillae - sensation in tips of fingers as if suppurating - panaritium. Soreness in feet from instep through to the sole - suppurates.

Skin: Felons, abscesses, boils, old fistulous ulcers, cracks at end of fingers - painless swelling of glands. Rose coloured blotches - scars suddenly become painful - promotes expulsion of foreign bodies from tissues. Every little injury suppurates. Long lasting suppuration and fistulous tracts. Dry finger tips. Eruptions itch only in day time and evening - crippled nails. Indurated tumours, abscesses of joints. After impure vaccination - nodes and coppery spots - Keloid growths.

Fever: Chilliness, very sensitive to cold air, creeping, shivering over the whole body, cold extremities, even in a warm room, sweat at night, worse towards morning, suffering parts feel cold.

Modalities: *Worse* - New moon, in morning, from washing, during menses, uncovering, lying down, damp, lying on left side. Better - warmth, wrapping up head, summer, in wet or humid weather.

Relation: *Comple: Thuja, Sanic., Puls, Fluor. ac - Mercurius and Silicea* do not follow each other well.

Compare: Black Gun powder. 3x.

Dose: 6-30 potency.

The 200 and higher of unquestioned activity. In malignant affection the lowest potencies needed at times. *(Boericke)*

Silica forms one of the most important remedies of the chronic diseases. The spicules (Prickles) of many sea sponges are made up of Silica - Equesetum generally contains as much as 18% of silica to the fresh plant - Want of grit, moral or physical is a leading indication for Sil. - according to Taste, Sil. is the chronic of Puls - Rush of blood to the head especially to the right temple and vertex, headache every day, photophobia, lachrymation, loss of taste, aversion to fat food with rancid or oily taste in mouth. Taste points out that Puls, flourishes best on sandy soils - as Bell does on Calcarea soil -Schusslers, tissue remedy point of view is as follows: Silicic acid is a constituent of the cells of the connective tissue, the epidermis, the hair and the nails through a supply of molecules of Sil, these cells are thereby enabled to throw off inimical substances (the pus) - Sil will also cure chronic arthritic rheumatic affections as if forms a soluble combination (Sodium silicate) with the soda, of the urate of Soda, this combination is then absorbed and removed through the lymphatics. For the same reason, it may also be used in renal gravel. Sil can also restore the perspiration of the feet when this has been suppressed and is thus an indirect remedy in diseases arising in consequence of such suppression (Amblyopia, cataract, paralysis) - Schussler adds that he generally gives the 12x trituration - Sil. is a great evacuant - sensation of splinter in the finger; of a pin in the throat - foreign bodies embedded in the tissues - tonsils which refuse to heal after the pus has been evacuated - abscesses which leave sinuses and fistulae - Sil. affects the nails, cripples them and produces inflammation around and under them - sensation as if the finger tips were suppurating - every little injury ulcerates - Hands and feet are sweaty, generally offensive - The feet may give off an intolerable odour without any sweat the head sweats and may be offensive. Corresponds to many cases of rickets - children with large heads, which must be kept warm, distended abdomen, weak ankles, slow in learning to walk - This constitutes type (1). Silica is also suited to (2) nervous irritable persons with dry skin, profuse saliva, diarrhoea, night sweats (3) weakly persons, fine skin, pale face, light complexion, lax muscles, (4) Constitutions which suffer from deficient nutrition due to lack of assimilating power; over-sensitive physically and mentally (5) Scrofulous children who have worm diseases during dentition (6) Stone cutters ailments' (Chest affections and total loss of strength). Recurrent keloid - stitching aching pain in the spot where an ulcer had been formerly on the leg - over worked brain - epileptic convulsions - Agg: at full and newmoon - the neck is stiff causing headache. The part of the body lain on goes to sleep - the headaches of Sil present one of the grand characteristics of the remedy - Chronic kind - may owe their origin to some severe disease of youth. They ascend from the nape of the neck to the vertex, as if coming from the spine and locate in one eye, especially the right, agg: from draught of air, uncovering head, amel: pressure and wrapping head up warmly, amel: profuse urination - sensative to noise - sensitive, weeping mood, yielding, faint hearted - children become obstinate, headstrong, cry when kindly spoken to - thinks only of pins, fears them yet look every where for pins. Sil-30 - discharge of blood from the vagina, every time the child takes breast. Cancer - nipple is drawn in like a funnel - always before and during menses there is constipation - as if rectum was paralysed - when partly expelled recedes again - vertigo as if drunk - Eyes as if too dry and full of sand - as if a splinter in upper lid - as if a panaritum would form in index finger - as if tips of fingers were suppurating writing causes tonic spasm of hand. Amel: Summer; Agg: approach of winter, averse to warm food, amel: from magnetism and electricity - in compitable Merc. *(JHC)*

Nervous, irritable, psoric sanguine temperament - dry skin - lax muscles - deficient nutrition - oversensitive - children with large heads, open fontanelles and sutures - sweating head, distended abdomen - suppressed foot sweat-bad effects of vaccination —want of vital heat -chilly-suppuration of glands - obstinate-cry when spoken to kindly - vertigo looking up. sick headache - ascending from nape of neck, to vertex, locating in eyes- right, amel: head wrapping, pressure, profuse urination. Constipation Agg: menses - inactivity of symptoms - nipple is drawn in like a funnel - night walking - crippled nails of fingers, toe nails - panaritium - blood boils - ulcers of all kinds - fistulae ani-great pain after stool - Promotes expulsion of foreign bodies - fish bones - needles etc. Complementary: Thuja, Sanicula. *(HCA)*

561. Silphium

(Rosin weed)

Is used in various forms of Asthma and chronic bronchitis, catarrh of bladder. Catarrhal influenza. Dysentery, attack preceded by constipated stools covered with white mucus.

Respiratory: Cough with expectoration, profuse, stringy, frothy, light coloured. Excited by sense of mucus rattling in chest and worse by drafts of air. Constriction of lungs, catarrh with copious, stringy, mucous discharges, desire to hawk and scrape throat. Irritation of posterior nares, involving mucous membranes of nasal passages with constriction of supra - orbital region.

Relation: *Aral, Copaiv, Tereb, Cubeb, Samb - Arum dracontium* (Loose cough at night on lying down), Justicea adhatoda (bronchial catarrh, hoarseness, oversensitive).

Dose: 3rd potency - lower triturations preferred by some. *(Boericke)*

The leaves of this plant, when they first come up, present their faces uniformly north and south, later on when the leaves become heavy, the winds carry them in different directions and the polarity is not observed. The stem of the plant exudes an abundance of resin as some of its name indicates (Rosin wood). Hale mentions that it has been used in all forms of asthma and in chronic bronchitis with large quantities of stringy, frothy, light coloured mucus and in catarrh of the bladder. *(JHC)*

562. Silphium Laciniatum

(Compass plant)

This remedy is employed in the various forms of asthma when it is associated with chronic bronchitis and large quantities of stringy, frothy expectoration. There is a sensation of constriction of the lungs, and a desire to scrape and clear the throat.

Compare: Copaiva, Cubeba. (Blackwood)

563. *Simaruba*
(Mountain Damson)

My first practical experience with Simb. as a homoeopathic remedy was in the case of a much travelling patient, who suffered from a chronic tendency to looseness of the bowels. He had stools like yellow ochre for which Gamboge has been very helpful - prescribed Simruba with excellent effect. Since then I have used it in similar cases.

564. *Sinapis Nigra*
(Black Mustard)

Is of use in hay fever, coryza and pharyngitis - dry nares and pharynx, with thick, lumpy secretion - Small pox.

Head: Sweat on upper lip and forehead, tongue feels blistered.

Nose: Mucus, acrid discharge - stoppage of left nostril all day or in afternoon and evening. Dry hot with lachrymation, sneezing, hacking cough, better lying down, nostrils alternately stopped.

Cough: Is relieved by lying down.

Throat: Feels scalded. Asthmatic breathing.

Stomach: Offensive breath smelling like onions - colic pains come on while bent forward, better sitting up straight.

Urinary: Frequent copious flow day and night.

Back: Rheumatic pain in intercostal and lumbar muscles - sleeplessness from pain in back and hips.

Relation: Sinapis alba - white mustard (throat symptoms marked especially pressure and burning with obstruction in oesophagus; sensation of a lump in oesophagus behind the manubrium sterni and with much eructation, similar symptoms in rectum).

Mustard oil: By inhalation (acts on the sensory nerve endings of the trigeminal, relieves pain in middle ear disease and in painful conditions of nose, nasal cavities and tonsils)

Dose: 3rd potency. *(Boericke)*

The yellow colour of mustard suggests Sulphur, a large amount of which is contained in the seeds. Like many other crucifers Sin. n. has antiscorbutic properties and it has cured cases of ague, mucosis, fever, catarrh of bladder, of stomach and of air passages. It is in the treatment of hay fever, that it has been most used. Acute coryza with thin watery excoriating discharge, lachrymation, sneezing, hacking cough, amel: lying down. Acute pharyngitis, throat feels scalded, hot, inflamed. Cooper suggests the use of Sin. as an aperient - He considers that the chief agent in constipated states, in flatus. Sweat on upper lip and forehead, is a symptom worth noting, also these, mucus hawked or coughed from posterior nares felt cold.

Causation: Damp weather, summer season. *(JHC)*

This remedy is indicated in acute coryza when there is a thin, watery, excoriating discharge, with lachrymation, sneezing, and a hacking cough.

It is useful when the mucous membranes of the nose are dry and hot, the discharge is scanty and acrid. The left nostril especially is stopped.

It is of service in acute pharyngitis, when the parts feel as though they were scalded hot and inflamed.

Compare - Colocynthis, Capsicum, Sinapis alba. *(Blackwood)*

565. *Skookum - Chuck*

(Salts from water from medical lake near Spokane, Washington)

Has strong affinity for skin and mucous membranes. An antipsoric medicine - otitis media, profuse ichorous, cadaverously smelling discharge, lithaemia, catarrh, urticaria, skin affections, eczema, dry skin, hay fever, profuse coryza and constant sneezing.

Dose: 3rd trituration. *(Boericke)*

Generally has himself cured with 'skoo' many cases of catarrh and he considers it as a remedy in hay fever. The cure of many cases of inveterate skin disease is on record, the external use of 'Skoo' soap or ointment has been employed as well as the internal administration. *(JHC)*

566. *Solanum Lycopersicum*

(Lycopersicum - Esculentum) - Tomato.

Marked symptoms of rheumatism and influenza, severe aching pains all over body, pains left after influenza - Head always shows signs of acute congestion. Hay fever with marked aggravation from breathing the least dust. Frequent urination and profuse watery diarrhoea.

Nose: Profuse watery coryza, drops down throat. Itching in anterior chamber, worse breathing any dust, better indoors.

Heart: Decided decrease in pulse rate with anxiety and apprehension.

Respiratory: Hoarseness, constant desire to clear throat - Chest oppressed, dry, hacking cough coming on at night and keeping one awake.

Urine: Constant dribbling in open air must rise at night to urinate.

Extremities: Sharp pain in right deltoid and pectoralis muscles.

Mod: *Worse* - right side, open air, continued motion. *Better* - warm room, tobacco.

Dose: 3-30 potency. *(Boericke)*

There is a popular impression that eating tomatoes is a cause of cancer. The impression is not strong enough to prevent the universal use of them and I have been unable to discover any basis for the idea - Cooper-comends the use of them in cases of obesity - some women cannot eat tomatoes without getting backache, leucorrhoea, or metrorrhagia - she was obliged to rise in the night to urinate. The rheumatic and congestive symptoms were mostly produced by the 3x, the nervous symptoms mostly by the 30x. The right deltoid was markedly affected and should make Lycopers a useful alternative to Cepa which has amel: Out of doors. The headache in one instance was completely Amel: by tobacco smoke. Polyuria was a feature of both provings and with the great thirst should give Lycopers a place in diabetes. *(JHC)*

567. *Solanum Nigrum*

(Black Night shade)

Used with success in ergotism, with tetanic spasms and stiffness of whole body, with mania. Marked action on head and eyes. Meningitis. Chronic intestinal toxaemia. Brain irritation during dentition. Restlessness of a violent and convulsive nature. Formication with contraction of extremities.

Head: Furious delirium, congestive headache.

Nose: Profuse, watery discharge from right nostril, left stopped up.

Dose: 2-30 potency. *(Boericke)*

Sol. n. is a common weed found in waste places. It has white flowers and black berries - The leaves applied externally cause pain and abate inflammation. Too large a quantity occasions violent sickness and headache, giddiness, drowsiness and other dangerous symptoms. The Arabians apply the leaves to burns and ulcers, skin diseases, scrofulous and cancerous affections, they are diaphoretic, diuretic and purgative. Hale says, some country practitioners used it with much success under the impression that it was an indigenous Belladona having been mislead by the name night shade - Hale verified its use in meningitis and headache, in scarlatina, when the eruption is blotchy - Hale justly points out the close affinity of Sol. n. with Bell - Delirium, headache, flushed face, sparkling eyes, pains coming and going suddenly, fiery rashes, burning skin and sweat. A curious feature of the skin effects of the black night shade is that they have a tendency to blackness. The swelling is very painful, it enlarges, becomes shiny hard and deep red and in several places quite black. The tip of the nose, the hands from the finger tip to the knuckles and the toes of the tarsal joints become quite black as if regularly dyed. The delirium is characterised by the cephalic cry, efforts to escape and by stammering speech - spasms, convulsions, tetanic rigidity of the whole body have been induced. In the midst of these convulsions the children frequently stretch out their little hands, then carry them eagerly to their mouths and go through the motions of mastication and swallowing. *(JHC)*

Relation: *Compare* - Solanum Carolinese (Horse-nettle) convulsions and epilepsy, 20-40 drop doses, is of great value in grandmal of idiopathic type, where the disease has begun beyond age of childhood, hystero-epilepsy, also in whooping cough. *(Boericke)*

Tincture of fresh ripe berries - Solan Car. is a domestic remedy in the southern states for convulsions - and it has been tested by several old school authorities, in cases of epilepsy with some success. Doses of 30-60 drops were given, three times a day, the only unpleasant effects being a mild diarrhoea in some cases. *(JHC)*

It has been used in epilepsy that was brought on or agg: at the menstrual period, used in chorea, non-traumatic tetanus, puerperal eclampsia and hysterical convulsions. *(Blackwood)*

Solan Mammosum - Apple of Sodom - Pain in left hip joint. *(Boericke)*

Hering is the authority for Sol. mam. The chief symptoms were: irritability and inability to think, sleepiness without being able to sleep, a kind of stupor agg: at time of flood tide, at the full moon, amel: with ebb tide, hawking of blood streaked mucus, sensitivity to tobacco. *(JHC)*

Solan Oleraceum: Swelling of mammary gland, with profuse secretion of milk. *(Boericke)*

This remedy has been employed in congestions of mammary glands, with a profuse secretion of milk. *(Blackwood)*

Solan Tuberosum: Potato berries - Cramps in calves and contraction of fingers, spitting through closed teeth. *(Boericke)*

Solan Vesicarium: Recommended in facial paralysis. *(Boericke)*

Solaninum Aceticum: Threatening paralysis of the lungs in the course of bronchitis in the aged and children, must cough a long time before able to raise expectoration. *(Boericke)*

Had frequent threatening of respiratory paralysis with accumulation of mucus which he was unable to expel. Solan-acet more than any other remedy rescued him from danger and prolonged his life. It exists in potatoes, and under certain conditions of germination, potatoes may contain a poisonous amount. Slowed and oppressed respiration was a marked feature. Respiration was slowed in inverse proportion to the increase in the pulse rate.

Relation: Compare in respiratory paralysis—Dulc., Bel. *(JHC)*

This remedy has some reputation in albuminuria, but its field of usefulness is in threatened paralysis of the lung in the aged and in children. Old people have to cough for a long time to raise the sputum (Senega) *(Blackwood)*

Solan Tuberos Agrotans: Diseased potato.

Prolapse of the rectum, patulous anus, offensive breath and odor of body, tumors of rectum look like decayed potatoes, dreams of pool of blood. *(Boericke)*

Effects of eating diseased potatoes, some of them fatal, have been observed. The symptoms of the proving were pretty severe and one of the most important - prolapse of rectum - has been confirmed by the poisoning cases. Prolapsus ani, which was probably caused by the violent and ineffectual efforts to discharge the contents of the rectum. The foul odour of the diseased potato is reproduced in the breath and body odour of the patients.

Relation - Compare: prolapsus ani — Podo, Ruta. *(JHC)*

•

568. Solidago Virgo

(Golden rod)

Inhalation of the pollen has caused haemorrhage from the lungs in phthisis. Repeated colds of tuberculosis (2x), feeling of weakness, chilliness alternating with heat, naso-pharyngeal catarrh, burning in throat, pains in limbs and thoracic oppression. Pain in region of kidneys, with dysuria. Kidneys sensitive to pressure. Brights disease. Hay fever when solidago is the exciting cause - Here give 30th potency or higher.

Nose: Nares irritated, with abundant mucus secretion, paroxysms of sneezing.

Respiratory: Bronchitis, cough with much purulent expectoration, blood streaked, oppressed breathing, continuous dyspnoea. Asthma with nightly dysuria.

Female: Fibroid tumors.

Urine: Scanty, reddish brown, thick sediment, dysuria, gravel, difficult and scanty, albumen, blood and slime in urine. Pain in kidneys extends forward to abdomen and bladder - clear and offensive urine. Some times makes the use of the catheter unnecessary.

Dose: Tincture to 3rd potency-oil of solidago 1 oz to 8 oz alcohol - 15 drop doses to promote expectoration in bronchitis and bronchial asthma in old people. *(Boericke)*

This herb says Rademacher is a very old and good kidney medicine. It is a specific for kidneys and brings the patients back to the normal condition - The grand key note of this remedy lies in the condition and the action of the kidneys and the quality of their secretions. Diseases arising from or complicated with the defective action of the kidneys are very likely to be benefitted by solid. Pain and tenderness in kidney region, pain extending from kidneys, to abdomen, bladder and down limbs, urine dark, red brown, scanty, thick, voided with difficulty, albuminous, mucus and phosphatic urine. I have seen very sharp attack of conjunctivitis produced in a patient who was taking solid for prostatic troubles.

Compare. In prostatic and urinary affections, Sabal, Santal, Hydrang, Trictum, Kidney ache. Santal, gonorrhoea and its effects, sciatica, Medor. *(JHC)*

569. *Spartium Scoparium Cystisus Scoparius*

(Broom)

Sparte in sulphate increases the strength of the heart, slows it and reduces the blood pressure. It continues the good effects of Veratrum and Digitalis without any of the undesirable effects of either (Hinsdale).

The effect of sparte in sulphate (the alkaloid of broom) is to cause a lowering of the systolic and diastolic pressures of the provers. Sphygmograms also show a condition of lowered blood pressure. It depresses the heart by poisonous action exerted on the myocardium and this, with the stimulating action of the drug upon the vagus, accounts for the lowered blood pressure and reduced pulse rate. It weakens the cardiac contraction. The drug has therefore, diuretic properties and is useful in dropsy.

Albuminuria, cheyne stokes respiration, irregular heart following grip and various infections, hypotension (in potency). Used palliatively in physiological dosage to combat arterial hypertension, arteriosclerosis. Very useful hypodermically 1/10 to 1/4 grain in sustaining heart after stopping habit of Morphia.

Spartium is indicated when primarily the muscles of the heart and especially the nervous apparatus is affected. Acts rapidly and lasts 3 to 4 days. Does not disturb digestion. Nephritis.

Heart: Tobacco heart. Angina pectoris. Irregular action, disturbed rhythm due to gas etc, feeble in nervous hysterical patients. Myocardial degeneration, failing compensation, hypotension (in potency). Spartium in 2 gr. doses for water - logged cases, cannot lie down. Here it produces much comfort. Has specific action upon the kidneys, enabling them to eliminate and relieve the distress upon the heart.

Stomach: Great accumulation of gas in gastrointestinal canal, with mental depression.

Urinary: Burning along urinary tract or in pudendum. Profuse flow of urine.

Dose: For non-homoeopathic use (Palliative as above) one or two grains TID by mouth, exerts a definite action upon the kidneys that will enable them to relieve the distress upon the heart. It is a safe drug and prompt in its action. Hypodermically, not less than 1/4 of grain. Dose as high as 2 grains by mouth three times a day are safe. (Hinsdale).

Homoeopathically - 1st to 3rd trituration. *(Boericke)*

This is a volatile alkaloid contained in spartium scoparium (Broom). It comes as a heavy yellowish, syrupy liquid. Mother tincture .the solution of the alkaloid in alcohol; and dilutions. Dosage: of the pure alkaloid. Gr. 1/10 to 1/4.

Physiological action - This agent produces an increase in the blood pressure, augments the ventricular contractions of the heart, and quickens the pulse rate. The action of the kidneys is stimulated. Large doses produce muscular tremor, lack of co-ordination, emesis, catharsis and paralysis of the respiratory and motor centers. (This statement is contradictory to Boericke)

This remedy is indicated in functional derangement and organic diseases of the heart that are attended with marked irregularity of its action, also in feeble hearts that are met with in nervous, hysterical individuals. In some cases there are indications of myocardial degenerations, especially of the fatty type, when it should be employed cautiously if compensation is failing.

It is of service in assisting to establish a compensation where there are valvular lesions. When there is pronounced cardiac weakness with anasarca and a disturbance of the rhythm.

When this disturbance of the rhythm is dependent upon dyspepsia and accumulations of gas in the intestinal canal, and there is great mental depression its action is favourable; as it is in the albuminuria that attends nephritis, and organic heart lesions. In the feeble heart's action that attends the various pulmonary lesions, its action is favourable.

Compare - Digitalis, Strophanthus.
(Blackwood)

570. Sphingurus
(Tree Porcupine)

The old world porcupines have the name Histricinae, those of the new world Sphingurinae. Mure proved the 3x trituration of the prickles. The most noteworthy symptoms were - falling out of the hair, of whiskers especially, pain in the jaw and joint and right zygoma. Itching of the pubes after taking tea. Embarassed speech. Nausea at sight of food. The symptoms are Agg: lying down, after tea, Amel: walking in open air, after dinner. *(JHC)*

571. Spigelia
(Pink Root)

Spigelia is an important remedy in pericarditis and other diseases of the heart, because the provings were conducted with the greatest regard for objective symptoms and the subjective symptoms are by innumerable confirmations proved to be correct. *(C. Hering)*

Has marked elective affinity for the eye, heart, and nervous system. Neuralgia of the fifth nerve is very prominent in its effects. Is especially adapted to anaemic, debilitated, rheumatic and scrofulous subjects. Stabbing pains. Heart affections and neuralgia. Very sensitive to touch, parts feel chilly, send shudder through frame - a remedy for symptoms due to the presence of worms. Child refers to the navel as the most painful part (Granat - Nux mosch).

Head: Pain beneath frontal eminence and temples extending to eyes. Semilateral involving left eye.

Eyes: Pressive pain on turning them - Severe pain in and around eyes, extending deep into socket.

Nose: Discharge through posterior nares. Chronic catarrh.

Mouth: Foul odor from mouth.

Face: Prosopalgia, involving eye, Zygoma, cheek, teeth, temple.

Heart: Pulse weak and irregular, pericarditis. Dyspnoea, must lie on right side with head high.

Rectum: Itching and crawling. Frequent ineffectual urging to stool. Ascarides.

Relation: Spigelia is a chronic Arnica.

Compare: Worm symptom: Sabad, Teucr., Cina.

Dose: 6-30. *(Boericke)*

Spigelia anthelmintica is a common weed in south America; S. Marylandica 'Pink Root' of 'Worm-grass' is a native of southern states of north america. It was known in europe in Hahnemann's time as an anthelmintic - this property of the drug having been learned from the negroes of the Antilles - It is a neuralgia remedy par excellence. 'Spi,' is more left sided than right. Head, eyes, face, teeth and heart are the principal seats of spi. action - The left sidedness of Spi. is shown in its affinity for the heart - I cured with Spi. a case of cardiac neuralgia caused by tobacco - In the eye, neuralgias, inflammation, amaurotic conditions, glaucoma, presenting the symptoms of Spi. - The pains of Spi. are largely out pressing - within outward and below upward - migraine comes from occiput, settles in or over left eye - Masses of Lumbrici have been expelled and also thread worms - Fetid breath and fetid flatus are marked features of Spi. - There is both constipation and diarrhoea - fear of pointed things as pins etc. Sil. has a somewhat similar symptom, but the Sil. patients hunts for pins although afraid of them. Spi. is a Sun remedy, headache beginning at sunrise, at its height at noon, declining to sun set, stammering, repeats first syllable 3-4 times.

Relation: Headache coming and going with sun. Nat. m., Sang., Tab. Headache begins in occiput and goes to left eye (Sang. - to right) - Sil-to both, Worms - Saba, Sin, Teuc., Scirrh., Stn. Tooth ache from tobacco- Plantago. *(JHC)*

Rheumatic diathesis, scrofulous children, afflicted with ascarides and lumbrici sensitive to touch, part touched feels chilly. Afraid of sharp pointed things. Rheumatic affections of heart - Nervous headache, periodical, beginning in morning at base of brain spreading over the head and locating in eye, orbit and temple of left side - headache at sunrise, at its height at noon, declines till sunset - Intolerable pressive pain in eye balls - Prosopalgia- from morning until sun set. Toothache from tobacco smoking. Scirrhus of sigmoid or rectum - dyspnoea - must lie on right side or with head high - palpitation violent, visible and audible. Stammering, repeats first syllable three or four times, with abdominal ailments and Helminthiasis. *(HCA)*

572. *Spiraea Ulmaria*

(Hard hack)

Burning and pressure in oesophagus, feels contracted but not made worse by swallowing. Morbidly conscientious. Relieves irritation of the urinary passages influences the prostate gland, checks fleet and prostatorrhoea, has been used for eclampsia, epilepsy and hydrophobia. Bites of mad animals. Heat in various parts (Salicylic acid is found in spiraea) *(Boericke)*

This agent has been employed in the relief of fleet and prostatic irritation *(Blackwood)*

573. *Spiranthes*

(Lady's Tresses)

Has been used for milk flow in nursing women, lumbago and rheumatism, colic, with drowsiness and spasmodic yawning. Is an anti-phlogistic remedy akin to Acon., its symptoms showing congestion and inflammation. Acidity and burning in oesophagus with eructation.

Female: Pruritus, Vulva red, dryness and burning in vagina. Burning pain in vagina during coition. Leucorrhoea bloody.

Extremities: Sciatic pain, especially right side. Pain in shoulders. Swelling of veins of hands. Pain in all articulations of hands, coldness of feet and toes. Fever: Flushes of heat, sweat on palms hands alternately hot and cold.

Dose: 3rd potency. *(Boericke)*

The genus to which this orchid belongs, received its name from the spiral arrangement of the flowers - The secretions of urine and milk were first diminished, afterwards increased. *(JHC)*

This remedy has been employed in the relief of yawning and paroxysms of sleepiness during the day. It is useful in lumbago and rheumatism, also in dryness and burning pain in vagina, with pruritus of the parts. *(Blackwood)*

574. *Spongia Tosta*

(Roasted sponge)

A remedy especially marked in the symptoms of the respiratory organs, cough, croup, etc. Heart affections and often indicated for the tubercular diathesis. Children with fair complexion, lax fibre, swollen glands, exhaustion and heaviness of the body after slight exertion, with orgasm of blood to chest, face. Anxiety and difficult breathing.

Mind: Anxiety and fear. Every excitement increases the cough.

Throat: Thyroid gland swollen, worse after eating sweet things - Tickling causes cough. Clears throat constantly.

Stomach: Excessive thirst, great hunger.

Male: Swelling of spermatic cord and testicles with pain and tenderness - orchitis - epididymitis.

Female: Palpitation, during menses, wakes with suffocative spells - amenorrhoea with asthma.

Respiratory: Great dryness of all air passages - Hoarseness. Larynx dry, burns, constricted. Cough, dry, barking, croupy, larynx sensitive to touch. Croup, worse during inspiration and before midnight - Respiration, short, panting, difficult, feeling of plug in larynx - cough abates after eating or drinking, especially warm drinks. The dry chronic sympathetic cough or organic heart disease is relieved by Spongia. Irrepressible cough from a spot deep in chest as if raw and sore - chest weak-can scarcely talk - laryngeal phthisis - goitre with suffocative spells. Bronchial catarrh, with wheezing asthmatic cough, worse cold air, worse lying with head low and in hot room. Oppression and heat of chest with sudden weakness.

Heart: Awakened suddenly after mid-night with pain and suffocation - Surging of heart into chest as if it would force out upward-hypertrophy of heart, especially right with asthmatic symptoms.

Skin: Swelling and induration of glands, also exophthalmic - cervical glands swollen.

Sleep: Awakes in fright and feels as if suffocating - Generally worse after sleep or sleeps into an aggravation.

Mod: (Worse) ascending, wind, before midnight, (Better) descending; eating amel: cough.

Relation: Merc Prot iod. (Goitre)

Dose: 2x or Tincture to 3rd potency. *(Boericke)*

According to Hahnemann, roasted spong was first mentioned as a specific for goitre - it was generally given mixed with other substances and had fallen into disuse, when Hahnemann proved it - Virtues of Spongia have been attributed to the iodine contained in it and partially liberated by the presence of roasting-best suited to, blue eyed, fair haired patients. Key note of the spongia is dryness of mucous membrane-cough is caused by dryness. Sounding like a saw, being driven through a pine board - dry asthma. patient rouses up generally after midnight with fear of suffocation and death - The sputa cannot be raised, must be swallowed; swallowing relieves, Agg: after sleep - rouses up in sleep as if in a great fright. Cough is excited by talking, by dry cold winds amel: by eating or drinking, by swallowing especially amel: by warm food sweets agg. The action of Spongia on the respiratory organs s closely connected with its action on the glandular system, the lymphatics, the thyroid and testes are indurated. Perfect picture of exophthalmic goitre is produced - Hypertrophy of the heart is frequently met by Spo. especially indicated when the right heart is affected and when asthmatic symptoms are associ-ated with it - Nash gives this key note of Spong. in valvular diseases - Awakes out of sleep from a sense of suffocation with violent loud cough, great alarm, agitation, anxiety, and difficult respiration - Spo, meets also thickening of joints after rheumatic fever - In orchitis, with heavi-ness and screw like squeezing pain in cord and testicles - Scratching does not amel: biting itching - lying with head low agg, and amel: warm food or drink, Agg: at full moon and Agg: periodically every night - eating and drinking amel: cough; Agg; sweets and after sleep - Spo. is dry; Hep rattling; Spo. before midnight - Hep Agg: after - Iod. is dark; Spo. is fair. *(JHC)*

Synopsis: for the tubercular diathesis, fair complexion, induration of glands, goitre - awakes in a fright and feels as if suffocating - mental excitement Agg: or increases the cough - worse after sleep or sleeps into Agg: (Lach) - sore throat Agg: after eating sweet things - Goitre - Great dryness of mucous membranes of air passages - dry as horn - every thing is perfectly dry, no mucous rale. Cough dry, sibilant, like a saw driven through a pine board Agg: sweets, cold drinks, smoking, lying with head low Amel: eating or drinking warm things - croup anxious, wheezing agg: during inspiration Agg: before midnight (Agg: before morning - Hepar) awakened suddenly after midnight with suffocation - valvular insufficiency, before or during menses - spermatic cord swollen, painful, testicles swollen, bruised, squeezed, orchitis. *(HCA)*

575. *Squilla Maritima*

(Sea-onion)

A slow acting remedy. Corresponds to ailments requiring several days to reach their maximum. Persistent, dull, rheumatic pains permeate the body - A spleen medicine, stitches under left free ribs. Important heart and kidney medicine - Broncho-pneumonia.

Acts especially on mucous membranes of the respiratory and digestive tracts and also upon the kidneys. Valuable in chronic bronchitis of old people with mucous rales, dyspnoea and scanty urine.

Eyes: Feel irritable, child bores into them with fists.

Respiratory: Fluent coryza, margins of nostrils feel sore. Sneezing, throat irritated, short, dry cough, must take a deep breath, dyspnoea and stitches in chest, and painful contraction of abdominal muscles, violent, furious, exhausting cough, with much mucus, profuse, salty, slimy expectoration and with involuntary spurting of urine and sneezing - child rubs face with fist during cough-Cough provoked by taking a deep breath or cold drinks, from exertion, change from warm to cold air, cough of measles, frequent calls to urinate at night, passing large quantities, sneezing with coughing.

Heart: A cardiac stimulant.

Urinary: Much watery urine, involuntary, spurting of urine when coughing.

Mod: (Better) rest; (worse) motion.

Dose: 1-3 potency. (Boericke)

576. *Stannum*

(Tin)

Chief action is centered upon the nervous system and respiratory organs. Debility is very marked when Stannum is the remedy especially the debility of chronic bronchial and pulmonary conditions, characterised by profuse muco-purulent discharges upon tuberculosis basis - Talking causes a very weak feeling in the throat and chest. Pains that come and go gradually, call unmistakably for stannum. Paralytic weakness, spasms, paralysis.

Mind: Discouraged.

Head: Pain Agg: motion gradually increasing and decreasing. Ulceration of ring hole in lobe of ear.

Throat: Much adhesive mucus, difficult to detach.

Stomach: Smell of cooking causes vomiting, bitter taste, sensation of emptiness in stomach.

Abdomen: Colic relieved by hard pressure.

Female: Bearing down sensation, prolapsus with week sinking feeling in stomach, menses early and profuse-leucorrhoea.

Respiratory: Violent dry cough in evening until midnight, cough excited by laughing, singing, copious green, sweetish expectoration, sore chest feels weak, phthisis mucosa, hectic fever.

Sleep: With one leg drawn up, the other stretched out.

Extremities: Paralytic weakness, drops things, limbs suddenly give out when attempting to sit down. Dizziness and weakness when descending, spasmodic twitching of muscles of forearm and hand, fingers jerk when holding pen, neuritis, typewriters' paralysis.

Fever: Exhausting night sweats, especially towards morning.

Modalities: (Worse) using voice (laughing, talking, singing) lying on right side, warm drinks (better) coughing or expectorating, hard pressure.

Comple: Puls.

Dose: 3-30 potency. *(Boericke)*

Stannum is the Jupiter of alchymists - The ancients have recorded wonderful cures of the most serious diseases with Tin says, Hahnemann, but until he proved it its only use was as a vermifuge. A number of worm symptoms appear in the pathogenesis, sinking, empty, all gone feeling, diaphragmatic and abdominal pains, tendency to excessive mucous secretions, pale sunken, sickly countenance with dark rings around eyes, convulsions. Many of these symptoms occur in conditions not due to helminthiasis and Stan. will be the remedy - Colic Amel: by hard pressure as by laying the child, with its abdomen across the knee or on the point of the shoulder - Stannum has weakness, exhaustion of mind and body - the chest is so weak as to make talking impossible - she drops into a chair instead of sitting down, while dressing in the morning has sit down several times to rest. An important remedy for singers and public speakers - weakness felt much more on going downstairs than on going up - The relaxation of tissue is probably responsible for uterine prolapse - Nausea and vomiting from smell of cooking. Deep, hollow, shattering cough, expectoration profuse, like white of egg, sweetish, salty, sour putrid, musty, yellow - green pus, deep, husky, hollow voice amel. for the time by hawking or expectorating mucus. The yellowness of the stannum secretions is worth noting - the tongue is yellow sputa and leucorrhoea are also yellow. The convulsions are opisthotonic, the thumbs are drawn in - they are such as are met with in teething children, or in children who masturbate or who have worms. Scratching arm produces an intolerable sensation of pleasure in genital organs, which extends to uterus and produces orgasm. The uterine and vaginal prolapse of Stan has this distinguishing feature - it is Agg: during stool, especially during pressure- Monday constipation - that is constipation occurring on days following rest days - Stan. Agg: warm drinks Spo. Agg: cold drinks - Prolapsus uteri Agg: during stool.

Causation: Emotions, fright, masturbation, dentition, using voice. *(JHC)*

Sad, despondent, feels like crying all the time - going down stairs Agg. Lumbrici, passes worms - prolapsus, worse during stool, weak, she drops into a chair. While dressing in the morning has to sit down several times to rest. Great weakness in chest Agg: from talking, laughing, reading aloud, singing, so weak, unable to talk. Empty sensation in chest - expectoration, profuse, like the white of an egg, sweetish, salty, sour, putrid, musty - Sweat - mouldy, musty odor after 4 a.m. every morning on neck and forehead - very debilitating. Agg: drinking anything warm. *(HCA)*

577. *Staphisagria*

(Stavesacre)

Nervous affections with marked irritability, diseases of the genito-urinary tract and skin, most frequently give symptoms calling for this drug. Acts on teeth and alveolar periosteum. Ill effects of anger and insults, sexual sins and excesses. Very sensitive lacerated tissues. Pain and nervousness after extraction of teeth. Sphincters lacerated or stretched.

Mind: Violent outbursts of passion, very sensitive as to what others say about her. Dwells on sexual matters, prefers solitude, child cries for many things and refuses them when offered.

Head: Sensation of a ball of lead in fore-head. Itching eruption above and behind ears.

Eyes: Heat in eye balls, dims spectacles - Recurrent styes, chalazae (Platanus) - Margins of lids itch.

Throat: Stitches flying to the ear on swallowing, especially left.

Mouth: Teeth black and crumbling, salivation, spongy gums, bleed easily-after eating feels sleepy, pyorrhoea (Plantago).

Stomach: Desire for stimulants, flabby and weak, craving for tobacco, canine hunger even when stomach is full.

Abdomen: Colic after anger, severe pain following an abdominal operation, constipation, (2 drops tincture night and morning), haemorrhoids with enlarged prostate.

Male: Persistent dwelling on sexual subjects, spermatorrhoea.

Female: Parts very sensitive, irritable bladder in young married women, leucorrhoea, prolapsus with sinking in the abdomen, aching around the hips.

Urinary: Cystocele, ineffectual urging to urinate in newly married women. Sensation as if a drop of urine were rolling continuously along the channel. Burning in urethra during micturition. Prostatic troubles, burning in urethra when not urinating, urging and pain after urinating.

Skin: Eczema of head, ears, face and body, thick scabs dry and itch violently, scratching changes location of itching, Figwarts pedunculated, arthritic nodes. Inflammation of phalanges, night sweats.

Extremities: Muscles, especially of calves, feel bruised, backache worse in morning before rising.

Modalities: Worse, anger, indignation, grief, mortification, loss of fluids, onanism, sexual excesses, tobacco, least touch on affected parts better after breakfast, rest, at night.

Dose: 3-30 potency. *(Boericke)*

As an exterminator of vermin this seed was called by the Greeks-Unguentum pediculosum - this last is the only use of Staph, now known to orthodox medicine - Taste found Staph. (6th dilution), like Coccul, a remedy for sea sickness. To be successful Staph. had to be taken at the moment when dizziness and nausea commenced before vomiting set in - It is noteworthy that Staph and Coccu. are both head remedies and both effective against head lice. Both also affect the genitals, Staph. more especially and both are remedies for crab lice. An application of a dilution of the Tincture of the strength of 1 to 4 with water will destroy the parasites, though the state which favours their presence needs internal treatment (probably) with a dilution of the same remedy at the same time - Taste cured with Staph. effects of tobacco smoking. It produces both physical and moral sexual disturbances, provokes an irregular sexual appetite, a tendency to masturbation and a physical state corresponding to the effects of that habit. Removing the habit of masturbation in children - for removing improper appetites in adults. In women coition is painful because the external parts are excessively sensitive. I have seen staph 30. give unspeakable relief in such cases - Constant urging to urinate in young married women - Burning in urethra, when not urinating, affections of genital organs of both sexes - prostatis in the man - Stitching towards groin and testicles. Staph is not only a remedy for ovarian and other affections, it also meets the conditions following operations on ovaries - Staph. is a remedy for anger and for the effects of anger, especially if the indignation cannot have its natural expression, was insulted, being too dignified to fight, swallowed his wrath, and went home sick, trembling and exhausted - The touchiness may take the form of sudden, violent outbreaks provoked by mere trivial causes. I have known Staph - 30 remedy this state, when the impulse to throw things at persons who had caused a trifling or imaginary irritation and had almost passed into mania. Colic of screaming, ugly, pot bellied children, especially if they suffer much from their teeth which turn black with tender spongy gums Agg: from least food or drink. This applied to vomiting, colic or dysentery. The action of Staph on the teeth is only one of many points in which it touches Merc; and which makes it one of the best antidotes to Merc - Teeth turn black and have dark streaks through them. Cannot be kept clean, crumble, decay on edges. The stomach and abdomen feel as if hanging down, relaxed. There is extreme hunger when the stomach is full - craving for tobacco - inability to perspire is one of the notes of Staph. Exostoses and gouty nodes of fingers and toes - sycotic and syphilitic condylomata. Seed warts. As if a round ball in forehead. As if head would burst. As if brain were compressed. Caust, Coloc., Staph follow well in this order.

Causation: Anger, suppressed or reserved, injury, falls, clean cut wounds, operations, coitus, masturbation, sexual abuse, sexual craving, emissions, dentition, tobacco, mercury. *(JHC)*

For the mental effects of onanism and sexual excesses. Very sensitive to slightest mental impression, least action or harmless word offends. Great indignation about things done by others or by himself, grieves, about consequences. Ailments from pride, envy or chagrin. Ill humoured children cry for things, which after receiving, they petulently push or throw away. Was insulted, being too dignified to fight, subdued his wrath and went home, sick, trembling and exhausted (the rev. of Nux) - Sensation of a round ball in forehead, sitting firmly there even when shaking the head - Mechanical injuries from sharp cutting instruments, post-surgical operations, stinging, smarting pains, like the cutting of a knife - Styes, chalazae on eye lids, or upper eye lids one after another, leaving hard nodosities in their wake (Con, Thuja) - Thuja) - Tooth ache, during menses sound as well as decayed teeth, painful to touch of food or drink agg: drawing cold air into mouth, from cold drinks and after eating. Teeth turn black, show dark streaks through them, cannot be kept clean, crumble, decay on edges, scorbutic cachexia - craving for tobacco - Extreme hunger even when stomach is full of food - Sensation as if stomach and abdomen were hanging down relaxed - urging to urinate, has to sit at urinal for hours, in young married women, after coition, after difficult labor, burning in urethra when not urinating, urging and pain after urinating in prostatic troubles of old men, prolapse of bladder - Painful sensitiveness of sexual organs, vulva so sensitive, can scarcely wear a napkin - persistently dwelling on sexual subjects, constantly thinking of sexual pleasures - Spermatorrhoea, guilty abashed look - cough only in the day time, or only after dinner, worse after eating meat, after vexation or indignation - excited by cleaning the teeth - cough excited by tobacco smoke - Backache Agg: at night in bed and in morning before rising - Arthritic nodosities of joints, especially of the fingers - sleepy all day - awake all night - Eczema - yellow acrid moisture oozes from under crusts - new vesicles form from contact of exudation, by scratching one place after itching ceases, but appears in another - Figwarts, dry, pediculated cauliflower - like - after abuse of mercury. *(HCA)*

578. *Stellaria Media*

(Chick weed)

Induces a condition of stasis, congestion and sluggishness of all functions. Morning aggravation. Sharp, shifting, rheumatic pains in all parts very pronounced. Rheumatism, darting pains in almost every part, stiffness of joints, parts sore to touch, worse, motion. Chronic rheumatism, shifting pains (Puls, Kali sulph.). Psoriasis. Enlarged and inflamed gouty finger joints.

Abdomen: Liver engorged, swollen with stitching pain and sensitive to pressure.

Extremities: Rheumatoid pains in different parts of the body.

Mod: Worse mornings, warmth, tobacco.

Better: Evenings, cold air, motion.

Dose: Tincture externally, internally 2x potency. *(Boericke)*

F.H. Brett gave an experience with the tincture applied externally, in the case of his wife, to enlarged, inflamed gouty finger joints, and in his own case a painful, aching great toes. In each case few applications removed the trouble. Brett was led to this use by having heard a rumour that Chick Weed poultices were good for gouty joints - The most prominent symptom, apart from the rheumatic effects, was the pain, swelling and soreness of the liver. The pains were amel: by motion and were accompanied by soreness - shifting rheumatism, pain now in ankle, now in knee, now in arm, wrist or fingers, Stel. 2x taken 3 times a day completely cured in a month. Bellairs suggested that 'Shirting Pains' may be a key note and Kopp. confirms this - Cooper gave much relief with a single dose of 'Q' in the case of a woman, 55, who had psoriasis dating from 21 years back with irritation in the spots, chiefly on flexures of joints, with much irritation of scalp and soreness of eyeballs. *(JHC)*

This remedy is indicated in rheumatism, when the parts are sore to touch, the joints are stiff, and there are darting, shifting pains in all parts of the body. The liver is enlarged and tender.

Compare - Pulsatilla. *(Blackwood)*

579. *Sterculla*

(Kola nut)

Neurasthenia. Regulates the circulation, is tonic and anti-diarrhoeic, regulates cardiac rhythm and acts diuretically - weak heart. The remedy for the drinking habit. It promotes the appetite and digestion and lessens the craving for liquor. Asthma. Gives power to endure prolonged physical exertion, without taking food, and without feeling fatigued.

Relation: Coca.

Dose: 3-10 drops, even one dram doses - 3 doses a day. *(Boericke)*

Kola nut. Habitat, Africa. Mother tincture of the nuts; and dilutions. Of the tincture, 1 to 30 drops, of the fluid extract-mv.

This agent is employed in the relief of the liquor habit, as it lessens the craving for liquor and stimulates the appetite and digestion.

Compare-Coca. *(Blackwood)*

580. Sticta Pulmonaria

(Lungwort)

Offers a set of symptoms like coryza, bronchial catarrh and influenza, together with nervous and rheumatic disturbances. There is a general feeling of dullness and malaise, as when a cold is coming on, dull heavy pressure in forehead, catarrhal conjunctivitis, etc. Rheumatic stiffness of neck.

Mind: Feels as if floating in air, confusion of ideas, patient must talk.

Head: Heavy pressure in forehead and root of nose - catarrhal headache before discharge appears.

Nose: Feeling of fullness at the root of the nose-dryness of nasal membrane - constant need to blow the nose, but no discharge - Hay fever - incessant sneezing.

Respiratory: Dry, hacking cough during night, worse inspiration, worse towards evening and when tired - Pulsation from right side of sternum down to abdomen.

Extremities: Rheumatic pain in right shoulder joint, deltoid and biceps - Inflammation and redness over affected joint.

Dose: Tincture to 6 potency. *(Boericke)*

There cannot be much doubt, when Sticta received its name of Pulmonaria. the likeness of the plant to lung tissue is self evident - it was a popular remedy of great repute in catarrhs and coughs when Hale introduced it to homoeopathy. It was found to cause severe coryza with violent sneezing, intense headache, and conjunctivitis. These attacks were preceded or followed by rheumatic pains and swelling of the small joints. The catarrh of sticta is for the most part obstructs and if there is discharge, it dries quickly and forms crust or scurf. Constant need to blow the nose, but no discharge comes on account of dryness. In syphilis or any other disease where this condition is present stic. will be the remedy - The cough of Stic. is also dry - dry night cough - cough dry, agg: evening and night can neither sleep or lie down, must sit up - Dr. P.C. Majundar cured two cases of whooping cough with stic. "6x". The cough began just after sun set and went on till vomiting occurred and all the contents of stomach were thrown off - hard dry barking coughs following colds. M.D. Young man related a number of cases of catarrhal and pulmonary affections cured with Stic. ϕ - Whilst taking Stic. the flow became ample and remained, so long as an occasional dose was being taken - the levitation symptom - the legs feel as if floating in the air. As if she cannot keep her tongue still.

Causation: Fall, haemorrhage. *(JHC)*

Natural order, Lichens - This remedy is indicated in catarrhal affections. There is a dull headache and pressure at the root of the nose before the discharge appears. There is dryness of the nasal membranes and a constant desire to blow the nose, but there is no discharge.)

It is useful in catarrhal bronchitis. The throat is rough and there is a dry hacking cough which is worse at night and during inspiration.

It is of service in rheumatism, when there is swelling, heat, redness and shooting pain in the affected joint. The rheumatic pains precede the catarrhal symptoms.

Compare - Stillingia, Rumex crispus.
(Blackwood)

581. *Stigmata Maydis - Zea*
(Corn-Silk)

Has marked urinary symptoms and has been used with success in organic heart disease, with much oedema of lower extremities and scanty urination. Enlarged prostate and retention of urine. Uric and phosphatic. Gonorrhoea. Cystitis.

Urinary: Suppression and retention. Dysuria, renal lithiasis, nephritic colic, blood and red sand in urine. Tenesmus after urinating. Vesical catarrh. Gonorrhoea. Cystitis.

Shucks (as a decoction used for chronic malaria - teaspoonful doses freely - Dr. E.C. Lowe England)

Dose: Tincture 10 to 50 drop dose.
(Boericke)

Two parts of Maize have been used in medicine, the pistils (Stigmata maidis) and the husks (Shucks), but I think it best to take them together - Corn silk has been used in (1) Irritable conditions of the urinary tract, ureters, bladder urethra. (2) As a powerful diuretic in renal disorders unconnected with cardiac involvement. (3) Heart and urinary conditions combined. Dr. Duments observed: (1) It makes the heart action slower and stronger. (2) Regulates its rhythm. (3) Its diuretic action is manifested first. (4) Its action is more powerful and evident in cardiac affections with dropsy. (5) with the disappearance of the dropsy arterial tension increases and venous tension diminishes - Hansen has confirmed the value of Z.st in 20 drop doses of the fluid extract in organic heart disease with dropsy, much oedema of lower limbs and scanty urination - The other use of Zea (Z. Sh) - Dr. Pruitt learned it from people. Shuck Tea is a popular remedy for chronic malaria - he found, it was in the chronic cases only that it was beneficial.

Zea Mays. Maize. Indian Corn. N.O. Graminea (Tribe, Phalarideae). 1. Stigmata Maidis. Corn silk. Green pistils. Tincture: One part, by weight, of the silk to two of alcohol. Fluid extract. (Z. st) 2. Shucks. Decoction or tincture of the husks of Maize after the removal of the grain. (Z. sh.) Of the mother tincture, 1 to 30 drops. *(JHC)*

This remedy is indicated in renal lithursesis, nephritic colic, with a discharge of small red sand and calculi in the urine, also in chronic pyelitis from calculi.

It is useful in chronic vesical catarrh, when the urine contains an excess of mucus and is ammoniacal, also in chronic gonorrhoea, when the prostatic gland is involved and urination is painful.

It is of service in suppression of the urine when the solids are low, and as a result the specific gravity is low, also in organic heart disease with dyspnoea, anasarca, and scanty urination.

Compare: Chimaphila, Barosma.
(Blackwood)

582. Stillingia
(Queen's Root)

Chronic periosteal rheumatism, syphilitic and scrofulous affections. Respiratory symptoms well marked. Torpor of lymphatics, torpid liver with jaundice and constipation.

Mind: Gloomy forebodings.

Extremities: Aching pains in bones of extremities.

Skin: Ulcer, chronic eruptions on hands and fingers. Enlarged cervical glands. Burning, itching of legs, worse exposure to air, exostosis, scrofuloderma, syphilis, secondary eruption and later symptoms.

Mod: Worse in afternoons, damp air, motion, better in morning, dry air. *(Boericke)*

Still. has long been a popular remedy for syphilis in the southern states of U.S., T.V. Symons introduced it into professional medicine and Hale to homoeopathy. The proving shows an action closely parallel with that of syphilis, attacking the genito urinary organs, throat (Pharynx, larynx and-trachea) mouth, head, and bones. Still. attacks the periosteum and produces pain in the bone. It has removed nodes on the forehead, tibia and elsewhere and arrested carries of the nasal bones. It has a popular repute in scrofula, skin affections, liver diseases, and rheumatism - Dryness is a common feature. *(JHC)*

It is of service in chronic tubercular conditions, as enlarged cervical glands, enlarged abdomen, and tubercular eruptions of the skin. The liver is torpid, and there is jaundice and constipation of the bowels.

Compare: Mercurius, Aurum, Staphisagria. (Blackwood)

583. Stramonium
(Thorn apple - Datura)

The entire force of this drug seems to be expended on the brain, though the skin and throat show some disturbance. Suppressed secretions and excretions. Sensation as if limbs were separated from the body. Delirium tremens. Absence of pain and muscular mobility especially of muscles of expression and of locomotion. Gyratory and graceful motion. Parkinsonism.

Mind: Devout, earnest, beseeching and ceaseless talking, loquacious, garrulous, laughing, singing, sweating, praying, rhyming, sees ghosts, hears voices, talks with spirits. Rapid changes from joy to sadness. Violent and lewd. Delusions about his identity, thinks himself tall, double, a part missing, religious mania, cannot bear solitude or darkness, must have light and company. Sight of water or anything glittering brings on spasm. Delirium with desire to escape.

Head: Raises head frequently from the pillow.

Eyes: Pupils dilated, staring wide open, loss of vision, complains that it is dark and calls for light. Small objects look large. Parts of the body seem enormously swollen. All objects look black.

Face: Expression of terror.

Mouth: Dry, dribbling of viscid saliva, aversion to water, stammering, cannot swallow on account of spasm.

Urine: Suppression.

Male: Sexual erethysm with indecent speech and action. Hands constantly kept on genitals.

Female: Metrorrhagia, with loquacity, singing, praying.

Sleep: Awakes terrified, screams with fright. Deep snoring sleep. Sleepy, but cannot sleep.

Extremities: Graceful, rhythmic motions, chorea, violent pain in left hip.

Skin: Effects of suppressed eruption in scarlatina.

Mod: Worse in dark room, when alone, looking at bright or shinging objects after sleep, on swallowing.

Better: From bright light, company, warmth.

Relation: Compare especially, Hyoscy. and Bel. It has less fever than Bel., but more than Hyos. It causes more functional excitement of the brain but never approaches the true inflammatory condition of Bel.

Dose: 30 and lower power. *(Boericke)*

Grows in vicinity of Cultivation, on rank soil where refuse is deposited, in all parts of the world. Tr. of fresh plant in flower and fruit. Hahnemann says Stram. allays some spasmodic movements and restores suppressed excretions, in several cases in which absence of pain is a prominent symptom - extreme muscular mobility - Nymphomania of lying-in-women-Fixed notion that some uppardonable sin has been committed - the delirium visions of animals enter largely into it - Grasping at imaginary objects before the eyes, when expression frequently became anxious as if the patient was trying to ward off imaginary foes - Hallucinations completes the picture of many cases of hydrophobia. Vomiting of green stuff always induced by bright light. On the other hand the Stram. patient is dependent on light and company, cannot walk in the dark - constriction of the chest, asthmatic symptoms and cough of the whooping cough type - The common practice of smoking Stramonium leaves for asthma is roughly homoeopathic - Stram is suited to: Ailment of young, plethoric persons, especially of children (Chorea, mania, fever, delirium).

Relation: Antidoted by - Lemon-Juice, Vinegar, Tobacco injections - Hands constantly on genitals - Zn. *(JHC)*

Acute mania, convulsions at the sight of a light, a mirror or water and when a cup of drink touches the lips. It is useful in neurotic asthma, when smoking the dried leaves will give temporary relief. Compare - Belladonna, Hyoscyamus. *(Blackwood)*

584. *Strontium Carb*

Rheumatic pains, chronic sprains, stenosis of oesophagus - Pains make patient faint or sick all over. Chronic sequelae of haemorrhages, after operations with much oozing of blood and coldness and prostration. Arterio-sclerosis. High blood pressure with flushed face, pulsating arteries, threatened apoplexy. Violent involuntary start. Affections of bones, especially femur. Restlessness at night, smothering feeling. For shock after surgical operations, neuritis, great sensitiveness to cold.

Head: Vertigo with headache and nausea - Aches from nape of neck, spreading upwards, flushes in face, violent, pulsating. Face red, burns, itches, itching redness and burning of nose.

Stomach: Aversion to meat, craves bread and beer.

Abdomen: Diarrhoea worse at night, continuous urging, burning in anus, lasts a long time after stool.

Extremities: Sciatica with oedema of ankle, rheumatic pain in right shoulder, chronic spasms, particularly of ankle joint, oedematous swelling, icy cold feet.

Skin: Moist itching, burning eruption, better in open air, especially warm sunshine, sprains of ankle - joint with oedema, violent perspiration at night.

Mod: Better immersing in hot water, worse change of weather, from being quiet, when beginning to move, great sensitiveness to cold. It is anti-fermentative and neutralizes excessive acidity.

Dose: 6th Trituration and 30 potency. *(Boericke)*

Stro. C. varies in color from white to yellow and pale green; flushing in the face and violent pulsation of the arteries, congestion of heart, lungs and head, Amel: by warmth and wrapping up and Agg: by cold. This also distinguishes the headaches of Str. carb - The diarrhoea is Agg: at night and the stools are yellow. Phlebitis and varicosis - sprains and bone affections - Stro. c. is indicated in chronic sprains of the ankle when oedema exists - Sciatica accompanied by oedema of left ankle - Heat of sun Amel: tension in head - pressure in stomach amel: by eating and Agg: after meals. *(JHC)*

Physiological action - This agent has an anti-putrescent and antiseptic action. The bromide prevents acetic and lactic fermentation; also in epilepsy and hystero epilepsy. Strontia iodide has much the same action as potassium iodide, and has been employed in parenchymatous nephritis, in rheumatic and scrofulous subjects; also in the albuminuria of pregnancy. It should not be employed when the urine is scanty or there are indications of suppression of urine. It is also used in diabetes.

Strontia salicylate is employed in chronic, gouty and rheumatic conditions; also in lithaemia, when there are intestinal disturbances and flatulent dyspepsia.

The carbonate is indicated in threatened apoplexy; when there is violent congestion of the head, with a red face while exercising. There is headache which comes up from the nape of the neck and spreads over the head.

It is useful in diarrhoea, when there is a continuous urging which is worse at night. He is hardly off the vessel before he must return.

It should be remembered in chronic sprains of the ankle joint with oedema.

Compare: Arnica, Silica, Baryta carbonia. *(Blackwood)*

585. Strophanthus Hispidus

(Kombe seed)

Strophanthus is a muscle poison, it increases the contractile power of all striped muscles. Acts on the heart, increasing the systole and diminishes the rapidity. May be used with advantage to tone the heart and run off dropsical accumulations. In small doses for weak heart, it feels enlarged. In mitral regurgitation, where oedema and dropsy have supervened. Strophanthus occasions no gastric distress, has no cumulative effects, is a greater diuretic and is safer for the aged as it does not affect the vaso-motors. In pneumonia and in severe prostration from haemorrhage, after operations and acute diseases. After the long use of stimulants, irritable heart of tobacco smokers. Arterio-sclerosis, rigid arteries of aged. Restores tone to a brittle tissue, especially of the heart muscle and valves. Especially useful in failing compensation dependent upon fatty heart. Hives. Anaemia with palpitation and breathlessness. Exophthalmia goitre. Corpulent persons.

Head: Senile vertigo.

Stomach: Nausea with special disgust for alcohol and so aids in dipsomania 7-drops of Tr.

Urinary: Increased secretion, scanty and albuminous.

Respiratory: Dyspnoea, especially on ascending. Lungs congested. Oedema of lungs. Bronchial and cardiac asthma.

Heart: Pulse quickened, hearts action weak, rapid, irregular, due to muscular debility and insufficiency, cardiac pain.

Skin: Urticaria, especially more chronic forms.

Extremities: Swollen, dropsical, anasarca.

Dose: Tr. and 6x potency. In more acute cases - 5 to 10 drops of the Tincture 3 times a day. *(Boericke)*

Strophanthus is an ornamental, ever-green climbing shrub native of tropical Africa and Asia. It is used as an arrow poison by natives of Africa - gave to a dipsomaniac-63 for weak heart and intermittent pulse in 7-drop dose 3 times a day an infusion of Strop. The first dose caused nausea and a repugnance to alcohol which proved to be permanent - Strop has cured functional disturbance of the heart from alcohol, tobacco and tea (Strop-in 5 drop doses of 1x tincture, in urticaria, which again bears out the gastric relations of strop).

Causation: Alcohol, Tea, Tobacco. (JHC)

Physiological action: This agent is a muscle poison. It increases the contractile power of the striped muscles. The heart muscle receives a greater amount of the drug in a given time than any other muscle and as a result it is more distinctly affected than any other striped muscle. The cardiac systole is increased, and its contractions are slowed by small doses. If large doses are administered the heart is paralysed in a condition of rigid systolic contraction. This condition is produced even when the influence of the cerebro-spinal nervous system is removed.

This remedy is indicated in the active, energetic type of patient whose muscular development is below par. They are always exhausted and overtaxed. Frequently there is a history of some violent exercise or exertion that has left its effect in the form of dyspnoea, praecordial distress, or a painful throbbing in various parts of the body.

It is of service when the heart's action is rapid and feeble, the pulse is irregular and weak, there is severe dyspnoea, and a condition of arterio-sclerosis present. It is useful in nephritis when there is a permanent high arterial tension with senile rigidity of the arteries. The heart's action is weak and irregular.

It is also useful in fatty degeneration of the heart, in hepatic cirrhosis, in the enfeebled heart's action that follows acute fevers, in reflex palpitation in the neurasthenic and hysterical.

It should be remembered in anasarca, when diuresis can be promoted by an increased blood pressure.

It is particularly useful for corpulent persons and for children, those suffering from chlorosis, anaemia, irritability of the heart, and in senile vertigo from cerebral anaemia. If continued for a period it has a favourable influence in many cases of exophthalmic goitre.

It is useful during the climacteric period when there are aching pains through the hips and extensors of the thighs.

It is to be preferred to Digitalis on account of its greater rapidity of action, in having but little if any vaso-motor effects, in having a greater diuretic power, in not disturbing the digestive organs, in not being accumulative, and in being safer for children and for the aged.

Compare: Digitalis, Adonis ver., Crataegus, Sparteine. *(Blackwood)*

586. Strychninum

(Alkaloid of Nux Vomica)

Its primary function is to stimulate the motor centers and the reflex action of the spinal cord. Homoeopathic to spasms of muscles, cramps from an undue reflex excitability of the cord, spasm of the bladder etc. Strychnin stimulates the central nervous system, mental activities, special senses rendered more acute. Respiration increased. All reflexes are made more active. Stiffness in muscles and face and neck. Opisthotonus, Tetanic convulsions with opisthotonus. The muscles relax between paroxysms, worse slightest touch, sound, odor. Influences more directly the spinal cord and is less appropriate invisceral derangements than Nux. Tetanus. Explosive nervousness. The pains and sensations come suddenly and return at intervals.

Head: Over-irritability.

Eyes: Twitching and trembling of lids.

Face: Pale, anxious, livid, jaws stiffened, lower jaw spasmodically closed.

Throat: Deglution impossible, violent itching in roof of mouth.

Female: Desire for coitus, any touch on body excites a voluptuous sensation.

Respiratory: Spasm of muscles about larynx.

Back: Rigidity of cervical muscles, back stiff, icy sensation down spine.

Extremities: Violent jerking, twitching and trembling, tetanic convulsions and opisthotonus, spasms provoked by slightest touch and attempt to move. Shocks in the muscles, cramp like pains.

Skin: Itching of whole body, especially nose - icy sensation down the spine.

Relationship: *Eucalyptus (neutralises ill effects of strychnin).* *(Boericke)*

Poisonings innumerable with strychnine are on record, the symptoms being convulsions of a tetanic nature in the fatal cases ending in asphyxia. The spasms are intermittent and the least touch or movement is sufficient to induce an attack. Lying on the back is the only tolerable position - Opisthotonus, cries, terror, hippocratic countenance and frothing at the mouth are common occurrences - The action of strych. On the rectum and genito - urinary organs was as pronounced as that of Ign. and Nux - Hale mentions the following uses of strych and it salts:

1) In the tetanic spasms of cerebro-spinal meningitis strych-6. (2) Amaurosis from atony of retina. (3). Diplopia and night-blindness, facial neuralgia and neuralgic headache (Strych. sul. or Strych Val). (4) Spasm of oesophagus in hysterical women strych. (5) Brain exhaustion of

women in whom high nervous erethism exists (Strych Val. 2x) (6) Chorea, when the convulsions do not cease during sleep (Strych 12 or 30).

There is much itching of the whole body and violent itching in roof of mouth which should prove a useful symptom - jerkings twitchings and shocks in all parts run throughout the pathogenesis. *(JHC)*

Strychnine is an alkaloid obtained from Nux vomica, Ignatia, and other plants of the order.

All the reflexes are increased. Tetanic convulsions - over irritability and restlessness - spermatorrhoea-atonic dyspepsia, progressive muscular atrophy.

Compare: Cicuta virosa, Arnica montana. (Blackwood)

Strychninum Ars - Lack of nerve force, anaemia, tendency to oedema, prostrate, asthmatic bronchitis.

Strychninum Nit. - Removes the craving for alcohol, 2x or 3x. Use it for 2 weeks.

Strychninum Phos. - Anaemic, weak and debilitated, irritation of the spinal cord - feet and hands cold and clammy - Pregnancy.

Strychninum Val: Exhaustion of brain power, women of high nervous erethism. *(Blackwood)*

587. Succinic acid

Hay fever, paroxysmal sneezing, dropping of watery mucus from nostrils, Asthma, inflammation through respiratory tract, causing asthma, chest pains, etc. Itching of eyelids and canthi and nose. worse drafts.

Use. 6-30 Potency. *(Boericke)*

Dr. Morris Weiner quoted, 'Succin ac.- the fumes of the crude acid, are inflammable and produce asthma, cough, sneezing, weeping, dropping of watery mucus from nostrils, pain in chest and headache'. On this indication he treated thirty persons suffering from hay fever and cured them all and saved them the necessity of making an annual exodus. He gave one or two grains of the 3x trit of succinum itself diluted in twelve teaspoonfuls of water, a teaspoonful every two hours. *(JHC)*

588. Sulphonal

(A coal tar product)

Sulphonal is a synthetic hypnotic. It comes in colourless prismatic crystals. The great use of this remedy has been in 20 grain doses as a hypnotic. It is given in a hot fluid about two hours before the desired result is expected. It should not be repeated that day. It is indicated in ataxia with staggering gait and trembling of the legs. There is extreme restlessness and muscular twitching. The knee reflexes are lost - It is useful in nephritis, the urine contains albumen and casts, is scanty and high coloured.

It is also useful in cerebral diseases when the patient is apathetic, alternately happy and despondent. There is mental confusion and illusions.

Compare: Trional. (Blackwood)

Sulfonal was at first regarded as one of the safest of hypnotics, but many cases of poisoning by medicinal doses have occurred and my Schema is made up of reported effects produced on patients. *(JHC)*

589. *Sulphur*

(Sublimated Sulphur)

This is the great Hahnemannian antipsoric. Its action is centrifugal from within outward having an elective affinity for the skin where it produces heat and burning with itching, made worse by heat of bed. Inertia and relaxation of fibre, hence feebleness of tone characterises the symptoms. Ebullitions of heat, dislike of water, dry and hard hair and skin, red orifices, sinking feeling at stomach about 11 a.m. and cat-nap sleep, always indicates sulphur homoeopathically. Standing is the worse position for sulphur patients, it is always uncomfortable. Dirty filthy people, prone to skin affections. Aversion to being washed. When carefully selected remedies fail to act, especially in acute diseases, it frequently arouses the reactionary powers of the organism. Complaints that relapse, general offensive character of discharges and exhalations. Very red lips and face, flushing easily. Often great use in beginning the treatment of chronic cases and finishing the acute ones.

Mind: Thinks rags as beautiful things - that he is immensely wealthy. Busy all the time - Childish peevishness in grown people - irritable—very selfish - no regard for others - Sulphur subjects are nearly always irritable, depressed, thin and weak, even with good appetite.

Head: Heat on top of head-tinea capitis, dry form, scalp dry falling of hair, worse washing, itching, scratching causes burning.

Eyes: Burning ulceration of margin of lids - Halo around lamp light. Heat and burning in eyes - Black notes before eyes - First stage of ulceration of cornea. Chronic ophthalmia.

Ears: Whizzing in ears. Bad effects from the suppression of an otorrhoea - Oversensitive to odors.

Nose: Stuffed indoors, imaginary foul smells, alae red and scabby, chronic dry catarrh, dry scabs and readily bleeding, polypus and adenoids.

Mouth: Lips dry, bright red, burning, bitter taste in morning - swelling of gums, tongue white, with red tip and borders.

Throat: Pressure as from a lump, as from a splinter, as of a hair, burning, redness and dryness.

Stomach: Complete loss of or excessive appetite, food tastes too salty, drinks much, eats little, milk disagrees, great desire for sweets, great acidity, sour eructation, very weak and faint about 11 a.m., must have something to eat.

Rectum: Itching and burning of anus, piles, frequent unsuccessful desire, hard knotty, insufficient, redness around the anus, with itching, morning diarrhoea, painless, drives out of bed, with prolapsus recti. Haemorrhoids, oozing and bleeding.

Urine: Frequent micturition, especially at night, enuresis especially in scrofulous, untidy children. Parts sore over which it passes, must hurry, great quantities of colourless urine.

Male: Itching of genitals when going to bed. Organs cold, relaxed and powerless.

Female: Pudenda itches. Menses too late, short, scanty and difficult, thick black, acrid, making parts sore. Menses preceded by headache or suddenly stopped, leucorrhoea burning, excoriating, nipples cracked, smart and burn.

Respiratory: Oppression and burning sensation in chest - difficult respiration, wants windows open, loose cough, worse talking, morning, greenish, purulent, sweetish expectoration, much rattling of mucus. Pleuritic exudations - Oppression as of a load on chest, dyspnoea in middle of night, relieved by sitting up - pulse more rapid in morning than in evening.

Back: Drawing pain between shoulders, stiffness of nape, sensation as if vertebrae glided over each other.

Extremities: Trembling of hands. Hot sweaty hands. Rheumatic pain in left shoulder. Burning in soles and hands at night, sweat in arm pits, smelling like garlic-drawing and tearing in arms and hands. Stiffness of knees and ankles. Cannot walk erect - Stoop shouldered - ganglion.

Sleep: Talks, jerks and twitches during sleep, vivid dreams, wakes up singing, wakes frequently and becomes wide awake suddenly, cat naps, slightest noise awakens - Cannot sleep between 2 and 5 a.m.

Fever: Frequent flashes of heat violent ebullitions of heat throughout entire body - dry skin and great thirst. Night sweat on nape and occiput - Perspiration of single parts. Disgusting sweats. Remittent type.

Skin: Dry, scaly, unhealthy, every little injury suppurates; Freckles, itching burning worse scratching and washing. Pimply eruption, pustules, rhagades, hang nails, excoriation, especially in folds. Feeling of a band around bones, skin affections after local medication. Pruritus, especially from warmth, in evening, often recurs in spring time, in damp weather.

Mod: (Worse) at rest, when standing, warmth in bed, washing, bathing, in morning, 11 a.m., night, from alcoholic stimulants, periodically. (Better) dry warm weather, lying on right side, from drawing up affected limbs.

Relation: *Comple: Aloe, Psorin, Acon, Pyrarara* (a fish caught in the Amazon, clinically used for various skin affections).

Compare: Acon, (Sulph often follows in acute diseases) Merc. and calcarea are frequently useful after sulphur, Not before.

Magnetis polus arcticus: Anxious coldness of eyes as if a piece of ice lay in orbit, increased flow of saliva, constipation, sopor, trembling, abdominal flatulence.

Magnetis Polus Australis: Dryness of lids, easy dislocation of ankles, in growing toe, nails, aching in patella, shooting in soles.

Compare: Adenoids - Agraphis.

Dose: Acts in all potencies from the lowest to the highest and not too frequent doses. Excellent results obtained from the higher. The 12th potency is a good one to begin treatment with, going higher or lower according to the suceptibility of the patient. In chronic diseases 200 and upward. In torpid eruptions the lowest potencies.

(Boericke)

A saturated solution of sulphur in absolute alcohol constitutes the tincture. The reputation of sulphur as a remedy is perhaps as old as medicine. As early as 2000 years ago, says Hahnemann, Sul. had been used as the most powerful specific against the itch - especially itching in the joints and in the night. Antipsoric action independent of its power of bringing out rashes. The psoric poison may be present and active in a case of disease and apparently well indicated remedies may fail to act in consequence. In such cases one or two doses of Sul. will frequently antidote, as it were, the Psora, and either clear up the case, or open the way for the action of other remedies. In such cases there will almost certainly be some Sul. indications present - irregular distribution of the circulation, flushes of heat-redness of orifices and parts near orifices, red ears, red nose, red eyelids, and red borders, around eyelids, brilliant red lips, bright red anus in children, red meatus urinarius, red vulva. Feeling of emptiness - faint sinking all gone sensation at 11 a.m. (Sul. 30) - Heat at vertex, dyspepsia, portal congestion - piles; constipation with ineffectual urging, constipation alternating with diarrhoea. Agg: is most noticeable by warmth of bed - when ever a patient says he is all right till he gets warmth of bed, Sul. must be examined, it will generally cover the case - Sul. is related to both the sun and the moon, which makes it one of the most important of periodics - Cooper cured many cases of neuralgia Agg: at noon or at midnight. He regards every twelve hours as the most-characteristic periodicity, but it may be multiples or divisions of twelve. Cooper recalls the fact that workers in Sulphur mines, though in malarial districts, enjoy a complete immunity from intermittent fevers - Sul. is the chronic of Acon - I have frequently cured ganglion of the wrist with Sul. CM and lower, given on general indications - It is the remedy for a large number of periodical headaches, occurring every week, every month, sick headache - Aversion to be washed always Agg: after a bath - Complaints that are always relapsing (menses) leucorrhoea etc. Burning soles, must find a cool place for them at night, hot head with cold feet. Lutze finds that Sul. 1M will make feet that have been cold for years comfortably warm - Diarrhoea after midnight, painless, driving out of bed early in morning as if bowels were too weak to contain their contents - Skin itching, voluptuous, scratching Amel: (feels good to scratch)- Poor breakfast eaters - Sul. Agg: much more in high dilutions than in lower ones, especially where extensive collections of disease tissue exist, a single globule of 200th will often set up violent disturbance - As of water in ears - skin excessively sensitive to atmospheric changes. Children who cannot bear to be washed or bathed - emaciated - big bellied - restless-hot-kick off clothes at night-have worms-people with hot sweaty hands - ragged philosophers - dirty looking persons who are always speculating on religious or philosophical subjects - People who refer all their sufferings to the epigastrium Agg: before a storm Agg after sleep, from milk, sweets and alcohol Amel: eating, Agg: after - Sul, frequently serves to rouse the reactive powers when carefully selected remedies fail to act, especially in acute diseases - in chronic Psorinum. Sul, Calc, Lyc-follow in this order.

Sul, Sars, Sep. - follow in this order.

If a patient is sleepless , Sul. may be given at night - if the patient sleeps well, it is best given in the morning, as it may disturb sleep if given at night - Nux. may be given at night and Sul. in the morning.

Sul. complements Rhus in paralysis.

Complements Ant. T. and Ipeca in lung affections.

Pso. compliments Sul. - Psor. loves heat, Sul. hates it.

Early morning diarrhoea. Bry as soon as he moves. Nat. sul with much flatus. Pod. Stool changeable, go on all day though agg: at noon. Sul., raw, sore anus.

Itch - Merc., Sep, Causticum.

Dyspepsia: Nux, Sep.

Excessive venery, Masturbation - Nux, Calc.

Yellow brown spots - Sep, Lyco., Curare.

Rheumatism, Paralysis - Rhus.

Sour stools, sore anus - Chamo.

Paralysis from cold - Aco., Caust., Rhus.

Bad effects of mental exhaustion - Sel. (Sel is a cognate element of Sul. and close analogue - Sel. Agg: from tea - Sul. Agg: from coffee - Sel. has tingling spots).

Wetting bed in deep sleep - Bel.

In first sleep - Sep.

Rhagades of hands - Nat. C.

Hard horny hands - NM, Graph. (Opp- to above) Calc.

Tall slender people - Phos.

With a stoop - Sul.

Aversion to be washed - Ant. c., Clem., Hep., Rhus., Sep., Spi. Like to be washed - Puls.

I have been frequently asked by patients taking Sul not to give them that medicine again as it made them see faces generally described as horrible. Passes almost pure blood from rectum - Merc, Aco,

Excessively sensitive to atmospheric changes - Hep, Kali carb., Psorinum. *(JHC)*

Synopsis: Standing is the worst position for sulphur patients, they cannot stand dirty filthy people-always agg: after a bath - cannot bear to be washed or bathed. When carefully selected remedies fail to produce a favourable effect - complaints that are continually relapsing - sensation of burning on vertex - constant heat on vertex, with burning soles at night - Bright redness of lips - Weak empty, gone, or faint feeling in the stomach at 11 a.m., (10 or 11 a.m.) amel. by eating (nat. c.) - driving out of bed early morning. Constipation, stools hard, knotty, dry as if burnt, large, painful - child is afraid to have the stool on account of pain-parts around anus red excoriated - all the orifices of the body are red - Menorrhagia - has not been well since her last miscarriage - A single dose at new moon - Lippe - boils coming in crops in various parts of the body -skin itching, voluptuous scratching causes burning Agg: from heat of bed.

Compatible: Calc, Lyc, Pul., Sars, Sepia. Agg: At rest, when standing, warmth, in bed, washing, bathing, changeable weather, amel: Dry warm weather, lying on the right side. *(HCA)*

590. Sulphur Iodatum

(Iodide of Sulphur)

Obstinate skin affections, notably the barbers' itch and acne, weeping eczema.

Throat: Uvula and tonsil enlarged and reddened, swollen, tongue thick, parotid hypertrophied.

Skin: Itching on ears, nose, and in urethra - Papular eruption on face, cold sores on lips, boils on neck, barbers' itch, acne, lichen planus, arms covered with itching rash. Hair feels as if erect.

Dose: 3rd Trituration. *(Boericke)*

Sul. Iod was proved by Kelsall on himself and some others - Hale has used it in obstinate skin diseases, notably barbers itch for which it is almost a specific - Pustular eruption on upper lip and erythema on chin - Hale used the 3x trit internally and applied a cerate - Suppurating acne. Weeping eczema - associated with varicose veins of the leg and pronounced itching - Also a child with eczema of arms - key note in all is dark red, swollen, and weeping eczematous surface which itches terribly. Agg: in morning. Hair feels as if erect - Hypertrophy of parotids after parotitis, lichen planus, chronic and simple - stricture after gonorrhoea, chordee, very painful urination. Twisted stream - yellow discharge. *(JHC)*

This remedy is indicated in skin affections, acne, lichen planus, barbers' itch, and erythema on the chin. The patient complains of apathy. There is a thick, green mucus secreted in the nostrils. The face is dry, hot, and of a yellowish color with yellow pustules and painful sores over it which soon disappear in dry scales. *(Blackwood)*

591. *Sulphuricum Acidum*

(Sulphuric acid)

The debility common to acids shows itself here, especially in the digestive tract giving a very relaxed feeling in the stomach with craving for stimulants, tremor for weakness, every thing must be done in a hurry — Hot flushes followed by perspiration, with trembling. Tendency to gangrene following mechanical injuries. Writers cramp. Lead poisoning. Gastralgia and hypochlorhydria - purpura haemorrhagica.

Mind: Fretful, impatient, unwilling to answer questions hurried. Compressive pain inside of occiput, relieved by holding the hands near the head. Trust in right temple as if plug were pressed in.

Mouth: Aphthae, gums bleed readily, offensive breath. Pyorrhoea.

Stomach: Sour eructations, sets teeth on edge, craving for alcohol, water causes coldness of stomach - relaxed feeling in stomach - averse to smell of coffee - hiccough.

Abdomen: Feeling as if hernia would protrude.

Rectum: Diarrhoea, fetid, black with sour odor of body and empty faint feeling in abdomen.

Female: Menstruation early and profuse, erosion of cervix in the aged, easily bleeding. Acrid, burning leucorrhoea, often of bloody mucus.

Respiratory: Respiration rapid and shooting in cervical muscles and movement of wings of nose. Larynx moves up and down violently. Bronchitis in children.

Extremities: Cramp-like paralytic contraction in arms and hands, jerking of fingers while writing.

Skin: Purpura haemorrhagica, livid, red, itching blotches. Haemorrhage of black blood from all outlets. Cicatrices turn red and blue. Carbuncles, boils and other staphylococcic and streptococcic infections.

Mod: *Worse* from excess of heat or cold in forenoon.

Relationship: Comple: Puls.

Dose: Sulphuric acid mixed with three parts of alcohol 10-15 drops - 3 times daily for several weeks, has been successfully used to subdue the craving for liquor. For homoeopathic purposes - 2 to 30th potency. *(Boericke)*

Hahnemann proved Sul. ac. and says that it has cured affections characterised by tension in the eyelids, in the morning, short sightedness, hardness of hearing, inguinal hernia, chronic looseness of bowels, profuse menses, metrorrhagia, roughness in the throat, asthma, swelling of the feet, coldness of the feet, water is not tolerated, often qualified with alcohol, it chills the stomach. Hurry, hasty, quick, sullen, impatient, angry because things move so slowly - A chemist in a convent garden used to use a lotion of sulphuric acid, well diluted for all the cases of itch that came before him and they were many - The piles of Sul. ac. are external, sensitive to touch and accompanied by itching - Sul. ac. is a great haemorrhagic, there is bleeding from every orifice - with sul. ac. 30 a dose every night, I gave great help to a delicate woman, who had nightmare, waking in a fright, before each menstrual period - The local weakness of Sul. ac. may amount to prolapse of vagina and uterus. It also removes long lasting black and blue spots with soreness and stiffness of the parts - Easy sweating is a note of Sul. ac, and the sweat affects mostly the upper part of the body. The body odour of Sul. ac. is sour and cannot be washed off. As if white of egg had dried on face - Jerking on falling asleep -Carbo veg. is a putrid remedy; Sul. ac. is more sour. Acidity sets teeth on edge - Prolapse of vagina (Staph.). *(JHC)*

Flushes of heat in climacteric years - Feels a great hurry, everything must be done quickly - Child has a sour odor, despite careful washing (mag. c., Rheum) - Gums bleed readily, ulcers painful, offensive breath. Chronic heart burn, sour eructations, sets teeth on edge. (Rob) - Water drunk causes coldness of the stomach - Bad effects from mechanical injuries, with bruises, chaffing and livid skin, prostration - Ecchymosis, cicatrices turn blood red, or blue (turn green ledum) - Blue spots livid, red, itching blotches - Haemorrhage of black blood from all the outlets of body - After led. in ecchymosis. *(HCA)*

There are aphthous conditions of the mouth, gums and buccal cavity. The gums are painful and bleed easily. Hypochlorhydria. Lichen, prurigo, and urticaria when there is a distressing itching, tingling and formication of the skin. *(Blackwood)*

592. Sumbul

(Musk root)

This agent is a nerve tonic, it stimulates the appetite and facilitates digestion.

It is useful in nervous palpitation of the heart, the pulse is irregular and there is neuralgia around the left breast - it is of service in ovarian neuralgia. The abdomen is distended and painful.

This remedy is indicated in hysteria and neurasthenia in anaemic women. There is constrictive choking and a constant swallowing and belching of gas from the stomach.

Dose of the mother Tincture. 1-60 drops. *(Blackwood)*

Has many hysterical and nervous symptoms and is of use in neuralgic affections and anomalous, functional, cardiac disorders. Numbness on becoming cold. Numbness on left side. Insomnia of the delirium tremens (15 drops of Tr), sensation as if water dropped down spine. Asthma. A tissue remedy for sclerosed arteries.

Dose: Tr. to 3rd potency. Dr. W. Mc. George advises the 2x every 3 hours for arteriosclerosis.

Compare: *Asaf, Mosch.* *(Boericke)*

Sumbul, as its name - Musk root, implies it has an odour resembling that of musk. The resemblance is so close that sumbul is used to adulterate Musk. Hysterical mood, easy fainting nervous palpitation are common to both. *(JHC)*

593. *Symphori Carpus Racemosa*

(Snow berry)

This drug is highly recommended for the persistent vomiting of pregnancy. Gastric disturbances, fickle appetite, nausea, water brash, bitter taste. Constipation. Nausea during menstruation. Nausea worse any motion - averse to all food. Better lying on back.

Dose: 2nd and 3rd potency; 200th has proved curative. *(Boericke)*

Dr. S.P. Burdick gave the Tincture to a lady who said its effects were precisely like the morning sickness - she used to have during pregnancy - Qualmishness and indifference to food, deathly nausea, vomiting continuous, violent retching. One patient was Amel: lying on back - no particular morning Agg: observed. The smell or thought of food was repugnant to the extreme - symph. 200 in the middle of a violent paroxysm - In a few minutes she stopped vomiting, In half an hour nausea began again but a few pellets checked promptly - A few more doses completed the cure. *(JHC)*

Mother Tincture. of the fresh ripe berries - This agent appears to act upon the uterus and from this reflexly upon the stomach and has produced a nausea similar to that of pregnancy.

This remedy is of service in the nausea of pregnancy, which is relieved by lying in* bed in the horizontal position and perfectly quiet. There is deathly nausea with vomiting and retching which is so violent that it produces haematemesis. The smell or thought of food is unendurable. She is constipated.

Compare: Ipecac and Piper Nigrum. (Blackwood)

594. *Symphytum*

(Comfrey-knit bone)

The root consists of a crystalline solid, that stimulates the growth of epithelium on ulcerated surfaces. It may be administered internally in the treatment of gastric and duodenal ulcers. Also in gastralgia and externally in pruritus and injuries to sinews and the periosteum. Acts on joints generally, neuralgia of knee.

Of great use in wounds, penetrating to perineum and bones, and in non-union of fractures, irritable stump after amputation. Irritable bone at point of fracture. Psoas abscess, pricking pain and soreness of periosteum.

Eyes: Pain in eye after a blow of an obtuse body. For traumatic injuries of the eyes, no remedy equals this.

Relation: Compare - Arn., Calc. phos.

Dose: Tincture.

Externally as a dressing for sores and ulcers and pruritus ani. *(Boericke)*

Symphytum may be considered the orthopaedic specific of herbal medicine - that it will solder and glue together meat, that is chopped in pieces, seething in pot, and make it in one lump - Gerarde - The black rind of root is scraped off and the mucilaginous root is then scraped carefully into a nice even pulp, this spread of thickness of crown piece upon cambric or old muslin is wrapped round the limb and bandaged over; it shortly stiffens and forms a casing; superior to starch, giving support and strength to the part - never removed the bandage after the first dressing until the limb was well.

1. When the bone or periosteum has been injured and the soft parts have recovered from the bruised soreness under Arn., the remaining pain and soreness of periosteum may be promptly relieved by Symph.

2. In traumatic injuries of bone or periosteum (as from snow ball or any thing else on the face) Symph was the only remedy Lippe has seen efficient - He cured many cases after others had used Arn. and failed.

3. Next to bone injuries in importance are injuries to ball of the eye. (H.C. Allen) - Allen gives to these indications. (Severe pain in globe of eye, after an injury by a blunt instrument or snow ball, cane, point of umbrella, infants fist) - the soft parts remaining intact - injuries of the bones are healed most promptly with Sympt. 30, internally once a day - Sir William Thomson of Dublin relates a case of malignant tumour of the antrum which had extended to the nose - Microscopical examination proved it to be round celled Sarcoma - the man applied poultices of comfrey root and the swelling disappeared. Eases pains in the back from violent motion as wrestling or from excessive sexual indulgence even when spermatorrhoea has been induced thereby.

Arnica - Soft parts injuries, painful swelling with discolouration, sore, bruised, lame.

Symphytum: Hard parts. Without discolouration, prickling, stitching, jagging pains. *(JHC)*

This agent, through the tannic acid, starch and asparagine which are found in it, has an action on affections of the bone and periosteum, the result of traumatism; also irritable stumps after operations, when there is soreness of and pricking pains in the periosteum; also in non-union of fractures.

It is of service in injury to the eyeballs, when there is severe pain and haemorrhage into the vitreous, the result of trauma.

It is indicated both locally and internally in periostitis, when due to injury.

Compare: Arnica, Calcarea phos.
(Blackwood)

595. *Syphilinum*

(The syphilitic Virus - A Nosode)

Utter prostration and debility in the morning - shifting rheumatic pains. Chronic eruptions - Ichthyosis, syphilitic affections. Pain from darkness to day light, decrease and increase gradually. Hereditary tendency to alcoholism - Ulceration of mouth, nose, genitals, skin, succession of abscesses.

Mind: Loss of memory, remembers every thing previous to his illness - feeling as if going insane or being paralysed. Fears the night. Despairs of recovery.

Head: Pains from eyes backward. Falling of the hair. Top of head feels coming off.

Eyes: Chronic recurrent Phlyctenular inflammations of cornea - Pain intense at night.

Mouth: Teeth decay, excessive flow of saliva, it runs out of mouth when sleeping.

Stomach: Craves alcohol.

Rectum: Feels tied up with strictures, enemas very painful, fissure, prolapse.

Extremities: Sciatica, worse at night, better about day break - Rheumatism of shoulder joint at insertion of deltoid. Run-around. Severe pain in long bones - redness and rawness between toes - always washing the hands. Muscles contracted in hard knots.

Female: Ulcers on labia, leucorrhoea profuse thin watery, acrid with sharp knife pain in ovaries.

Respiratory: Aphonia, chronic asthma in summer, wheezing and rattling - cough dry, hard, worse at night. Lancinating pains from base of heart to apex at night.

Skin: Reddish, brown eruption with disagreeable odor.

Mod: (Worse) at night, sundown to sun shine, sea shore, in summer.

Better - Inland and mountains, during day, moving about slowly.

Dose: The highest potencies only and in infrequent doses. *(Boericke)*

It has been mainly, almost exclusively, employed by those who are familiar with the use of high attenuations - I have used no potency lower than 200, and rarely repeat the dose more often than once a week.

(1) First in importance is the night Agg., pain from darkness to day light, begin with twilight and end with day light. All symptoms Agg: at night - terrible dread of night on account of mental and physical exhaustion on awaking. In ophthalmia, the pains are Agg: at night and during the night, the lids glue together, neuralgia and headache, asthma, coughs Agg: from sunset to sunrise, whether syphilitic or not will be benefited by Syph; which vies with Sul. as a sleep restorer.

(2) Next to the night Agg: is ulceration, this may affect mouth, nose, genitals, or skin, and the ulcers have greyish bases, in the nose, they produce the most offensive form of ozaena with discharge of fetid clinkers. Fetid discharges from the ear come in the same category. (3) Abscesses with foul secretions. Succession of abscesses is one of the grand key notes of the materia medica. Teeth decay at the edge of the gums and break off, are cupped, have serrated edges, dwarfed in size and converge at their tips - The typical eruption of Syph. is copper - coloured spots - Leucorrhoea, profuse, soaking through napkins and running to heels. Craving for alcohol in any form - Hereditary tendency to alcoholism - obstinate constipation for years - rectum seems tied up with strictures. When enema was used the agony of passage was like labour. "Thomas Wildes" says, in chancre he gives Syph. 1M (Swan), one dose every night. The chancre increases for the first two weeks and then gradually fades away not being followed by secondaries - where the edges of chancre assume the appearance of proud flesh in the 3rd or fourth week, and become everted, jagged and angry dark red, he gives Lac. can. CM (Swan), every night for 10 to 14 days until the

sore takes on a more natural appearance - when Syph. 1 M is again given to finish the case - For any remaining induration Nit ac. 30 four times a day is given - Swan says he gave crying infants, when they developed this propensity immediately after birth and did not cease, one dose of Symph, CM and it was difficult to make them cry after that.

Mod: Agg: Sea side: Amel: In mountains, averse to consolation (Nat. M.) - Shoulder rheumatism Agg: raising arm laterally (Rhus and Sang. Rt. shoulder). Ferrum (left) Urtica ur. - Dentition trouble Agg: night (Med. Agg: early morning).

(JHC)

Pain from darkness to day light - All symptoms are worse at night - Eruptions, dull, red, copper - coloured spots. Cannot remember names of books, persons or places, arithmetical calculation difficult - Sensation as if going insane - Leucorrhoea, profuse, soaking through the napkins and running down to the heels - headache, neuralgic in character, falling of hair, acute ophthalmia neonatorum Amel: by cold bathing - Ptosis - Diplopia - Teeth decay at edge of gum and break off - dwarfed in size, converge at their tips - craving alcohol in any form, obstinate constipation - rectum seems tied up with strictures - Fissures in anus and rectum, prolapse of rectum - Rheumatism of the shoulder joint Agg: from raising arm laterally - Syphilitics or patients who have had chancre treated by local means and as a result have suffered from throat and skin troubles for years are nearly always benefitted by this remedy. Agg: - at night from twilight to day light.

(HCA)

596. *Syzygium Jambolanum*

(Jambol Seeds.
Enlexing-active principle)

Has an immediate effect of increasing the blood sugar - glycosuria results. A most useful remedy in diabetes mellitus. No other remedy causes in so marked degree the diminution and disappearance of sugar in the urine. Prickly heat in the upper part of the body, small red pimples itch violently. Great thirst, weakness, emaciation. Very large amount of urine, specific gravity high - Old ulcers of skin - Diabetic ulceration. The seeds powdered-10 grains - 3 times a day - also the tincture.

Relation: *Compare:* Insulin. An aqueous solution of an active principle from pancreas which affects sugar metabolism. If administered at suitable intervals in diabetes mellitus, the blood sugar is maintained at a normal level and the urine remains free of sugar. Over dosage is followed by weakness and fatigue and tremulousness and produces sweating.

(Boericke)

Tr. of the seeds (fruit stones) - Syz. J is a native of India. It has an edible fruit, the powdered stones of which have a popular use in India as a remedy for diabetes. The dose in 5 grains of the powdered stones three times a day. Dudgeon used Syz. in the lower homoeopathic attenuations with marked success, which has been repeated by many others. Hansen mentions as having cured with Syz. the ulcers of skin, probably of diabetic foundation. Dudgeon relates this case. A scientific man, 56, complained of prickly heat, all over upper part of body and arms. The skin was covered with small red papules, which itched, so intensely he could get no rest. He felt very weak which was perhaps due to his having abstained from all animal food and confined himself to bread, farinaceous food, vegetables and fruit. There was much thirst and great flow of urine, which he was obliged to pass every two hours, night and day, mouth very dry, Urine 1036, very saccharine. He was ordered chiefly, animal diet, very little bread and no sugar. Syz. ϕ mixed with 3 times the quantity of alcohol was given. Of this 2 drops every 3 hours. The specific gravity of the urine steadily declined, sugar disappeared and all the symptoms passed off - and this in spite of the fact that dietetic rules were relaxed. *(JHC)*

597. Tabacum

(Tobacco)

The symptomatology of Tabacum is exceedingly well marked. The nausea, giddiness, death like pallor, vomiting, icy coldness and sweat, with the intermittent pulse, are all most characteristic. Has marked antiseptic qualities, anti-dotal to cholera germs.

Complete prostration of the entire muscular system. Collapse, gastralgia, enteralgia, seasickness, cholera infantum, cold, but wants abdomen uncovered vigorous peristaltic activity, diarrhoea. Produces high tension and arteriosclerosis of the coronary arteries. Should prove the most homoeopathic drug for angina pectoris; with coronaritis and high tension (Cartier), constriction of throat, chest, bladder, rectum, pallor, breathlessness, hard-cord like pulse.

Mind: Very despondent.

Head: Vertigo on opening eyes.

Eyes: Amaurosis.

Face: Covered with cold sweat. Throat: Hoarseness of public speakers.

Stomach: Incessant nausea, worse, smell of tobacco smoke, vomiting, during pregnancy with much spitting, sea sickness, terrible faint, sinking feeling at pit of stomach.

Abdomen: Wants abdomen uncovered, it lessens the nausea and vomiting, incarcerated hernia.

Rectum: Constipation, rectum paralysed, prolapsed, diarrhoea, sudden, watery, with nausea and vomiting, prostration and cold sweat.

Urinary: Renal colic, violent pain along ureter, left side.

Heart: Palpitation when lying on left side. Pulse intermits, feeble, imperceptible. Angina pectoris, pain in precordial region. Pain radiates from centre of sternum, tachycardia, bradycardia.

Respiratory: Difficult, violent constriction of chest. Praecordial oppression with palpitation and pain between shoulders. Cough followed by hiccough. Cough dry, teasing, must take a swallow of cold water.

Extremities: Legs and hand icy cold.

Sleep: Insomnia with dilated heart with cold clammy skin and anxiety.

Fever: Chills with cold sweat.

Mod: Worse, opening eyes.

Better: Uncovering, open fresh air.

Antidote: Vinegar, Sour apples.

Ars: Chewing tobacco.

Ign.: Smoking.

Sepia: Neuralgia and dyspepsia.

Lycopod: Impotency.

Nux: Bad taste due to tobacco.

Calad. and Plant: Cause aversion to tobacco.

Phos: Sexual weakness, tobacco heart.

Dose: 3-30 and higher potencies. Tab. 200 or 1000 for the craving of tobacco, and when discontinuing its use. *(Boericke)*

Dr. M.E. Douglass mentions that palliative for Bee stings and mosquito bites. A portion of a leaf is moistened with vinegar and applied to the part. This is interesting as Ipe., one of the antidotes of Tab. has a similar reputation. For headache, leaves of tobacco are moistened with vinegar or camphor solution and applied to the force head and nape - The pain is allayed and sleep induced. The local application over the pit of the stomach relieves nausea. Prostatorrhoea and impotence are also among the effects of Tab - Rectal tenesmus and there is also paralysis and prolapse of Ani - The power of Tab. to paralysis, sphincters and also morbid constrictions account for its traditional use in cases of strangulated hernia and obstruction of the bowels, which has been confirmed in homoeopathic practice. Tab. produces a number of skin affections, notably pruritus. *(JHC)*

This agent produces a relaxation and paresis of the involuntary muscular system, there is distress in the cardiac region, with pallor of the surface, icy coldness and sweat, nausea, nervous trembling and debility.

Deathly nausea, vomiting, icy coldness and cold sweats and intermittent pulse, praecordial distress.

Seasickness, nausea from any cause, sinking feeling at the pit of the stomach; during pregnancy, yellow or green and slimy diarrhoea. Amaurosis, atrophy of the optic nerve; violent constriction of the chest, with palpitation of the heart.

Compare: Veratrum alb., Arsenicum alb., Camphora. *(Blackwood)*

598. *Tanacetum Vulgare*

(Tansy)

Abnormal lassitude. Nervous and tired feeling. Half dead, half alive feeling all over. Of use in chorea and reflex spasms (worms) said to be a specific against effects of poison ivy.

Dose: Tr. to 3 potency. *(Boericke)*

Gerarde says that the seeds kill and expel worms of every sort - the root is good in gout, and being drunk with wine. Tan. relieves pain in the bladder and dysuria, when a man is only able to urinate by drops, like Senec - Tan. has an action on the female generative organs and a large proportion of the observations with it have been on women who have taken it to procure abortion - Experiments on animals show that Tan. induces all the cardinal features of rabies, convulsions without loss of consciousness, opisthotonus, spasms of pharynx, larynx and thorax, abundant salivation, sensual excitability, tendency to bite, hoarse cry, diminished sensibility and mobility, momentary paralysis, sub pleural ecchymoses, infraction of the liver - whether the convulsions of Tan. be rabic or epileptic, they are sufficiently similar to render the drug useful in either conditions - Pierson treated with it every case of epilepsy, which came to him with drop doses of the fluid extract of Tan. 4 times a day and with marked success.

This agent is an emenagogue, diuretic and anthelmintic.

This remedy is indicated in chorea, reflex spasms and twitching during sleep and waking, dependent upon intestinal parasites. It is useful in amenorrhoea and dysmenorrhoea, with bearing down pain, tenderness and drawing in the joints.

It is of service in dysentery; there is pain in the bowels which is relieved by stool. The desire for stool is renewed by taking food.

Compare: Cina, Absinthium, Cimicifuga.
(Blackwood)

599. *Taraxacum*
(Dandelion)

The young leaves of the Dandelion are sometimes eaten in salads. They have a bitter chicory like taste as also has the root. Children eat the flowers, although they are supposed to cause bed wetting. This has given rise to one of the popular names of the plant. Its chief traditional uses are as a remedy for jaundice, liver obstruction, in dysentery, involuntary emissions and in difficulties in passing water. Hahnemann's proving brought out these leading symptoms-painless urging to urinate, and frequent urging to urinate with copious discharge of urine. Hahnemann points out that this with the thirst may indicate Trx. in some cases of diabetes. Pain in both splenic and liver regions, jaundice with enlarged indurated liver. Disordered digestion-mapped tongue-the tongue is coated white and clears off in patches-the bright yellow flowers of Trx open in the morning between 5-9 Of' clock and close in the evening between 8-9 Of' clock-hands and nose cold at 8' PM, cold finger tips - Almost all symptoms appear when sitting, lying down, resting, Hahnemann's dosage was a single drop of the Tincture. *(JHC)*

This remedy is indicated in cases, where there is loss of appetite, with weak digestion, gastric headache and bilious attacks. The tongue is coated white. This comes off in spots, leaving sensitive aphthous patches, mapped tongue.

It is of service is hepatic congestion and atonic dyspepsia, when the liver and spleen are enlarged and the liver is indurated. The patient complains of sharp stitching pains in the hepatic region, there is tympanitis and jaundice, a bitter taste and eructations and salivation. It is useful in neuralgia of the knee that is relieved by pressure.
(Blackwood)

600. *Tarentula Hispanica*
(Spanish Spider)

Remarkable nervous phenomena, with chlorosis, chorea, dysmenorrhoea, spinal irritability. Bladder tenesmus, constriction, sensation of formication. Extreme restlessness, must keep in constant motion even though walking aggravates.

Hysterical epilepsy. Intense sexual excitement.

Mind: Sudden alteration of mood, destructive impulses, moral relaxation; Must constantly busy herself or walk. Sensitive to music, averse to company, but wants some one present. Ungrateful discontented, guided by whims.

Head: Intense pain, as if thousands of needles were pricking into brain, vertigo, wants hair brushed or head rubbed.

Male: Sexual excitement, lasciviousness, reaching almost to insanity, seminal emissions.

Heart: Palpitation, sensation as of heart twisted and turned around.

Female : Vulva dry hot, with much itching, profuse menstruation, with frequent erotic spasms, Pruritus vulvae, nymphomania, dysmenorrhoea, with very sensitive ovaries.

Relation : Compare - Agar, Ars, Cupr, Mag. Phos.

Antidotes : Lach.

Dose : 6-30 Potency. *(Boericke)*

The name Tarentula covers a number of poisonous spiders, but in homoeopathy, unless otherwise distinguished, it refers to Tarentula Hispanica, Lycosa Tarentula. Tarentula is a dance, named from the city of Tarentem - Tarentism is a dancing mania, set up in persons bitten by the Tarentula, or in those who imagine themselves bitten. The cure is music and dancing.

(1) Dark red or purplish coloration and swelling of skin and tissue.

(2) Apparent imminent choking.

(3) Choreic movements, restlessness.

(4) Amel : by music; music at first excites and subsequently relieves.

(5) Periodicity, deep action returning annually on the date of the bite. Desire is excited in both sexes to the point of mania. The sexual desire was so excited in one woman, that when playing or dancing with men she hugged them before everybody and was angry when reproved, but did it again. At times she had a desire to take things which did not belong to her-hysteria in connection with sexual disorders, sighing, yawning, laughing and crying, joking and profound melancholy, twitching, jerking, dancing, great excitability of nerve endings, tips of fingers extremely sensitive. Farrington gives among the mental symptoms; when there are no observers, there is no hysteria; when attention is directed to her, she begins to twitch, cunning attempts to feign paroxysms of wild dancing. The chorea of Trn. is most marked on right side. As if thousands of needle were pricking the brain. Amel: by rubbing head against pillow. Amel: by rubbing is a keynote condition of Trn - Terminals of nerves become so irritated that some kind of friction is necessary in order to obtain relief - But Trn. is not a hysteric remedy only - C. M. Boger cured a case of irritative dry cough with tearing pain in chest Amel: from smoking - diphtheria, tonsillitis of an intensity to threaten suffocation. Septic and intermittent fevers have been successfully met in Trn., on its indications. Stools occur immediately when the head is washed - wetting hands in cold water causes symptoms - Trn. is suited to nervous hysterical patients subject to choreic affections, when whole body or right arm and left leg are involved. Agg: by touch, Amel: rubbing, pressure, music; Agg: rest, must walk about but walking aggravates all symptoms, Agg: washing head, wetting hands in cold water. *(JHC)*

Choreic affections, right arm and left leg (left arm and right leg—Agaricus) Restlessness, could not keep quiet in any position, must keep in motion, though walking aggravates all symptoms. Abscess, boils, felons, bluish colour, atrocious, burning pain - the agony of a felon, compelling patient to walk the floor for nights - Head ache, neuralgic

Agg: by noise Amel: by rubbing head against pillow - Sexual excitement, extreme, even to mania, pruritus vulvae intolerable, Agg: touch of affected parts, Amel: in open air, music rubbing affected parts. Terminal nerves so irritated, friction is necessary to obtain relief. *(HCA)*

This remedy is indicated when there is extreme restlessness; must be constantly on the move, although motion aggravates. It is useful in hysteria with chlorosis, chorea, spinal irritation or dysmenorrhoea; she must be busy with something all the time. She feels relieved while in the open air, from music, bright colors, and from massaging the affected parts.

It is of service in nymphomania and pruritus of vulva. The parts are dry and hot, with much itching and frequent erotic paroxysms and sensitiveness of the ovaries.

Compare : Cimicifuga, Magnesia Phos.
(Blackwood)

601. *Tarentula Cubensis*

(Cuban spider)

A toxaemic medicine, septic conditions, diphtheria - Adapted to most severe types of inflammation and pain, early and persistent, prostration - various forms of malignant suppuration. Purplish hue and burning, stinging pains. Bubo. It is the remedy for pain of death, soothes the last struggle. Pruritus, especially about genitals. Restless feet. Intermittent septic chills, Bubonic plague. As a curative and preventive remedy, especially during the period of invasion.

Dose : 6 - 30 Potency.

This remedy is indicated in septic conditions, with great prostrations. The parts are of a purplish colour, and there are burning, stinging pains. It is of service in carbuncles, when the parts are of purplish hue, are gangrenous and there are burning, stinging pains. It is said to soothe the pains in the last struggle of death.

Compare: Ars, Crotalus, Echinacea.

602. *Tartaricum Acidum*

Found in grapes, pineapple, sorrel and other frutis. It is an anti-scorbutic, antiseptic, stimulating the mucus and salivary secretions - Dullness and lassitude - great weakness, with diarrhoea, with dry and brown tongue.

Pain in heels (Phytol).

Dose : 3rd Trit : The pure acid 10-30 grains dissolved in water. *(Boericke)*

One of the most marked symptoms was intense burning in throat and stomach, feeling as if on fire-tongue brown and dry. Almost constant vomiting. Vomitted matter of deep green colour. Faeces coffee colour. Tearing pain on the soles of the feet, near the heel which prevents him putting his foot on the ground, after luncheon. The pasty taste is Amel: after eating.

An artificial lemonade may be made by dissolving this acid in water and adding a few drops of the essence of Lemon.

(Blackwood)

603. *Taxus Baccata*

(Yew)

In pustular diseases of skin and night sweats. Also in gout and chronic rheumatism.

Stomach: Saliva hot acrid. Nausea. Pain in pit of stomach and region of navel. After eating, cough. Feeling of pins and needles at pit of stomach; of emptiness, must eat frequently.

Dose: Tincture to 3rd potency.

(Boericke)

This poisonous properties of the Yew have been recognised and disputed from ancient times. Gerarde says that in his school days he and his companions ate their fill, of the berries of Yew and slept not only under its shade, but on its branches, without any ill effect. But there is plenty of evidence on the other side - Yew leaves are more poisonous, some time after they have been cut than when fresh - Yew cropped green from the tree has no fatal effect and animals do not eat it fresh, they prefer grass - but if Yew has been cut and allowed to wither, cattle will eat it in large quantities and in that state it is deadly poison - Death from Yew poisoning, says Cooper, is remarkably painless - Empty feeling in the stomach was prominent and it was noted that the digestion was very rapid. Must eat frequently is a characteristic.

The siliva is increased and it also is viscid and there is a viscid sweat - An intense action on the skin was developed and 'Tax' is indicated in pustular skin affections, the pustules being large flat and strongly itching. *(JHC)*

Mother tincture of the fresh twigs and leaves; and dilutions.

Dosage: Of the tincture - 1 to 60 drops.

This remedy is indicated in pustular diseases of the skin. The pustules are large and flat and are attended with much itching. *(Blackwood)*

604. Tellurium

(Metal Tellurium)

Marked skin (herpes circinatus), spinal, eye and ear symptoms - very sensitive back - pains all over body. Offensive discharges. Slow development of symptoms (Radium). Sacral and sciatic pains.

Eyes: Lids thickened, inflamed, itching, Pterygium, pustular conjunctivitis, cataract, following occular lesions, aids the absorption of infiltrations in Iris and Choroid.

Ears: Eczema behind ear, catarrh of middle ear, discharge acrid, smells like fish - pickle, swelling, throbbing in meatus, deafness.

Stomach: Craving for apples. Empty and week feeling, heart burn.

Rectum: Pruritus ani et perinei after every stool.

Back: Pain in sacrum, pain from last cervical to fifth dorsal vertebra, sciatica, worse right side, coughing straining, contraction of tendons in bends of knees.

Skin: Itching of hands and feet, herpetic spots, ringworm, (Tub) ring shaped lesions, offensive odour from affected parts, barbers' itch, stinging in skin, fetid exhalations (Sul), offensive foot sweat, eczema, back of ears and occiput. Circular patches of eczema.

Modalities: Worse while at rest at night, cold weather, from friction, coughing laughing, lying on painful side, touch.

Dose: 6th Potency and higher - Takes long time to develop its action, which is very prolonged. *(Boericke)*

Tellurium occurs in the native state and in combination with gold, silver, lead and antimony. It resembles sulphur and selenium in its chemical reactions. The most notable feature of the proving was the irritation of the skin, including skin of eyelids, and ears, of spinal column and some nerves. The most characteristic form of the skin irritation of Tell. is herpes circinatus, and it has probably cured more cases of ring worm, especially of the face and body, than any other remedy. (I cured with Tell. an indian officer home on furlough, whose body was covered all over with a ring worm like eruption. The odour of the body and of the sweat is offensive and garlic like. In parts where the skin forms openings, as the ear, the effect of Tell. is intensified. The characteristic odour of the ear discharge is that of fish brine. The discharge is so acrid, it vesicates any part of the skin it touches. Tell. is one of the most important remedies in otorrhoea. Nash cured, several cases of post scarlatinal otorrhoea, using the 6th; higher attenuations having failed. Eye lids are inflamed and the vesicating property extends to the eye itself, setting up phlytenular, conjunctivitis - other parts of the skin, affected by Tell are the hair - roots, the breasts, the perineum and the anus. There is itching in the rectum after stool. Tell has caused expulsion of thread worms. The offensiveness of Tell appears in the breath and in the flatus and it is a leading remedy in offensive foot sweat. In addition to the inflammation of the eyes caused by Tell it has pains over the eyes. Skin and nerves are closely allied and Tell is a remedy in many neuralgic conditions, notably sciatica. The right side is most affected. Yawning after retching, drowsy after eating. I once gave Tell. to a child for an eruption and cured it incidentally of constant yawning with which it had been troubled - Sensation as if in air on going to sleep.

Compare : Ring worm, Bac., Sep, Nat mur - Ring worm in clusters, Sep, Glac;

Thread worms : Teucr. *(JHC)*

This is a semi metallic element. It is pinkish white, crystalline and very brittle.

This remedy is indicated in eczema, especially behind the ears, and herpes circinatus; barber's itch, when there is stinging pain and foetid exhalation. It is of service in spinal irritation, with sensitiveness from the last cervical to the fifth dorsal vertebra. The patient fears being touched.

Compare : Arsenicum album, Sepia.
(Blackwood)

605. Terebinthina
(Terpentine)

Has a selective affinity for bleeding mucous surfaces. Tympanitis and urinary symptoms, very marked, Inflammations of kidneys with haemorrhages - dark pressive fetid. Bright's disease, preceded by dropsy (Goullon) drowsiness and stranguary, coma - unbroken chilblains.

Mouth: Tongue, dry, red sore, shining burning in tip, with prominent papilae.

Abdomen: Enormous distention - Haemorrhage from bowels, worms, lumbrici, abdominal dropsy, pelvic peritonitis, fainting after every stool, entero - colitis, with haemorrhage and ulceration of bowels.

Urinary: Stranguary with bloody urine, odor or violets, urethritis with painful erections.

Female: Intense burning in uterine region.

Respiratory: Haemoptysis, blood expectoration.

Back: Burning pain in region of kidneys.

Skin: Acne, erythema, itching, pustular, vesicular eruptions, urticaria, purpura, ecchymosis, dropsies, scarlatina, chilblains, with excessive itching and pulsative pains. Aching soreness of muscles.

Antidote: Phos.

Dose: 1st to 6th Potency. *(Boericke)*

Illness caused by sleeping in newly painted rooms is due to a great part to the turpentine - burning is a constant note and gives the key to many cases calling for Ter, - burning in gums, tongue, mouth, throat, stomach, rectum, and anus, kidneys, bladder and urethra, uterus, air passage, chest and sternum. Cooper has found it indicated in children especially teething children, when they fly into passions - There is irritation of the meninges and often ascarides or other intestinal worms - Ter. is a great haemorrhagic and its haematuria is particularly characteristic, smoky, turbid urine depositing a sediment like coffee grounds. Ter. corresponds to many cases of albuminuria and haematuria after scarlatina and also to the consequent dropsy - burning in uterus is very characteristic. The haemorrhages to Terebinth are generally passive, dark and fetid. Purpura, ecchymoses in great numbers from day to day - Additional key notes. (1) Smooth glossy red tongue as if deprived of papillae. (2) Excessive tympanitis. (3) Drowsiness in capillary bronchitis, the child is drowsy, Ter. antidotes and is antidoted by phos - Pains in the bowels, which cause frequent micturition. Ter. is specially suited to children (dentition, nose bleed, worms.).

Relation : Urticaria after eating shell fish. (Apis, Urtica urens); Burning and drawing in kidneys, bladder and urethra, (Berb., Can. S, Canth.)

Causation : Alcohol. Falls, Strains, Tooth extraction, Damp cellars. (JHC)

606. Teucrium Marum

(Cat-thyme) (Marum Verum)

Nasal and rectal symptoms marked. Polypi - Affections of children. Suitable after too much medicine has been taken-over sensitiveness. Desire to stretch. A remedy of first importance to chronic nasal catarrh with atrophy-large offensive crusts and clinkers- ozaena. Loss of sense of smell.

Eyes: Smarting in canthi, lids red and puffy, tarsal tumor.

Ears: Hissing and ringing otalgia.

Nose: Mucous polypus, discharge of large irregular clinker-crawling in nostrils.

Stomach: Unnatural appetite.

Respiratory: Mouldy taste in throat, hawking up mucus.

Extremities: Pain in toe-nails, as if they had grown into flesh.

Rectum: Itching of anus and constant irritation in the evening in bed, ascarides, with nightly restlessness-crawling in rectum, after stool.

Skin: Itching causes, tossing about all night, very dry skin, suppurating grooves in the nails.

Dose: 1st to 6th Potency-Locally for polypi- snuffing of dry powder. *(Boericke)*

Marked symptoms of helminthiasis, irritation of anus and nose- No remedy meets more cases of thread worms than Teucr. - The nasal symptoms have led to the use of Teuc., in nasal polypus- A snuff of Teuc. has been used in some cases in addition to the internal use of the remedy. - It has removed a fibrous tumour of the eye lid, urethral granulations following gonorrhoea and also uterine fibroids. Worms and polypi suggest a tubercular taint and I have used both Teuc. M. and Teuc. `Scorod' in phthisical cases. Teuc. has the craving hunger of the antipsories and worm remedies. It prevents sleep at night- nervous-irritable. Sensitive- Desires exercise in open air which does not fatigue.

Relation: (Worms) Scirrh., Cin., Spig., (Nasal polypi), Phos., Sang., Sil., - (Nails ingrowing), Mgt., Aust., Nit. acid. (JHC)

This remedy is indicated in polypi of the nose and vagina. There is frequent sneezing with a sensation of crawling in the nose without coryza. It is of service in ascarides with a sensation of creeping and crawling in the rectum, which in worse during the evening and from the warmth of the bed. It is also recommended in rheumatism.

Comparè: Sanguinaria, Cina, Staphisagria. *(Blackwood)*

607. Thallium

(The metal Thallium)

Thallium seems to influence the endocrines, especially the thyroid and adrenaline. Most horrible neuralgic, spasmodic, shooting pains. Muscular atrophy - Tremors - relieves the violent pains in locomotor ataxia, paralysis of lower limbs pain in stomach and bowels, like electric shocks. Paraplegia. Alopecia, following acute exhausting diseases. Night sweats. Polyneuritis - dermal trophic lesions.

Extremities: Trembling, paralytic feeling, lancinating pains like electric shocks. Numbness in fingers and toes, with extension up lower extremities, involving lower abdomen and perineum and inner thighs to feet.

Relation: Lathyr., Caust, Arg. nit., Plumbum. *(Boericke)*

A metallic element. It is a soft, heavy, crystalline metal, rapidly tarnishing in air.

This agent is indicated in locomotor ataxia for the relief of the violent pains. There is paralysis of the lower extremities, with trembling, also pains, as electric shocks in the stomach and bowels.

(Blackwood)

608. Thaspium Aureum - Zizia

(Meadow - Parsnip)

Hysteria, epilepsy, chorea, hypochondriasis, come within the sphere of this remedy.

Mind: Laughing and weeping moods.

Extremities: Chorea, especially during sleep, fidgety legs.

Modalities: Worse during sleep.

Dose: Tincture to 3rd. Potency.

(Boericke)

The meadow parsnip is a common plant, indigenous to the United States on the moist banks of streams in open wet woods, where it flowers in June and July. Symptoms of poisoning. Exhilaration with increased physical strength was noted, but a slight amount of exercise caused fatigue. The spasms and convulsions of the umbelliferae were excited. The generative organs in both sexes were excited.

This remedy is indicated in hysteria and hypochondriasis, when there are suicidal tendencies with mental depression, alternating moods of crying and weeping. There is a great lassitude following coitus. It is also of service in epilepsy and chorea. During sleep the legs are constantly on the move.

Compare: Agaricus muscarius, Aurum met, Tarentula. *(Blackwood)*

609. Thea

(Tea)

Nervous sleeplessness, heart troubles, palpitation and dyspepsia of old tea-drinkers-produces most of the sick head-aches - Tabacum - antidotal. *(Allen)*

Stomach: Faint gone feeling.

Dose: 3 - 30th Potency. *(Boericke)*

The use of Tea has spread from the older civilisations of the east to the new ones of the west - Tea contains an alkaloid. Thein which is by some considered, identical with caffein and both tea and coffee are used to stimulate jaded faculties and enable persons to endure fatigue and get more enjoyment out of themselves than they could obtain by mere food. Excessive tea-drinking is a fruitful source of neuralgia and insomnia. A woman who kept a pot of tea boiling on the stove and drank several bowlfuls every day, developed both suicidal and homicidal mania-impulse to jump out of the window, to cut her baby's throat and throw it down stairs.

Relation: *Antidoted by : Thuja, Ferrum,* Beer-Hering says coffee drinkers should drink wine and tea drinkers beer. *(JHC)*

610. Theridion

(Orange-spider)

Nervous hyperaesthesia. Has affinity for tubercular diathesis. Vertigo, sick headache, peculiar pain around heart region, phthisis florida, scrofula, have all been treated successfully with this remedy. Sensitive to noise, it penetrates the body, especially teeth. Noises seem to strike on painful spots over the body. Rachitis, caries, necrosis. Phthisis, stitch high up in left apex - where the indicated remedy does not hold long.

Head: Pain worse anyone walking over floor - vertigo with nausea and vomiting on least motion. Particularly when closing eyes.

Respiratory: Pain in left floating ribs, cardiac anxiety and pain.

Skin: Stinging thrusts every where.

Dose : 30th Potency. *(Boericke)*

Tincture of the living spider. The spider is found in the West Indies, chiefly in the island of Curacoa. It is about the size of a cherry stone, is found on orange trees, velvety black when young with anterio - posterio lines composed of white dots. On posterior of body, there are three orange red spots; and on the belly, a large square yellow spot. It is very poisonous. It produces a highly sensitive nervous condition with weakness, trembling, coldness, anxiety, faintness and easily excited cold sweat - keynotes. Extreme sensitiveness extends to vibrations of any kind, jar of a step, riding in a carriage or in a boat - Agg: closing eyes. This applies to vertigo and symptoms of the head and stomach. This forms the indication in many cases of sea sickness, of pregnancy. The headaches are severe and affect the eyes especially the left. The ears are highly sensitive. A type of intoxication is induced, hilarity, talkativeness. Time passes too slowly is a well marked symptom. Therid. has a peculiar cough. Frequent, convulsive, head spasmodically jerked forward, knees jerked up to abdomen. Agg: from least over work and motion; Amel by keeping quiet in horizontal position. Constipation, stool hard, small, dry.

Vertigo: (Closing eyes) Therid, Lach, Thuja.

Vertigo (Opening eyes): Tab.

Vertigo (Looking up): Puls, Silicea.

(JHC)

This remedy is indicated in periodical headaches. The pain is over the left eye and is throbbing and shooting in character. It is aggravated by the heat of the sun and noises and is attended with vertigo and nausea which is made worse by closing the eyes and from motion. It is useful in acute phthisis, when there are sticking pains in the left chest, extending to the back. There is cardiac anxiety, pain. It is of service in sensitive spines, when the patients avoid any pressure at this point. There are stinging pains in various parts of the body.

Compare: Chininum Sulph, Lach., Phosphorus. *(Blackwood)*

611. *Thiosinaminum - Rhodallin*

(A Chemical derived from oil of mustard - seed)

A resolvent, externally and internally dissolving scar tissue, tumors, enlarged glands, lupus, strictures, adhesions, ectropion, opacities of cornea, cataract, ankylosis, fibroids, scleroderma. Noises in ear. Suggested by Dr. A. S. Hard or retarding old age. A remedy for tabes dorsalis, improving the lightning pains, vesicle and rectal crises. Strictures of rectum.

2 grains twice daily *(Boericke)*

Dose: 2x attenuation.

Thio. belongs to the same chemical group as Urea. The colourless bitter crystals are soluble in water, alcohol and ether. Thios. has been used externally and internally for resolving tumors of the uterine appendages. The internal dose of old school practice is 4 - 8 grains a day, given hypodermically in a 15% solution.

(JHC)

This remedy has been employed both locally and internally in case of lumpus, chronic enlarged glands, strictures and for dissolving scar tissue. It has relieved stricture of the rectum, when two grains were given twice a day. Also tinnitus aurium where the ossicles were bound down by fibrous bands. *(Blackwood)*

612. *Thlaspi - Bursa Pastoris*

(Capsella - Shepherds Purse)

Is an anti - haemorrhagic and anti uric acid remedy. Albuminuria during gestation. Chronic neuralgia. Renal and vesical irritation. Haemorrhage from uterine fibroid with aching in back or general bruised soreness. Aching between scapulae. Uterine haemorrhage with cramps and expulsion of clots. Craves butter milk. Effects of suppressed uterine disease.

Head: Eyes and face puffy - frequent epistaxis - Vertigo - Worse rising - Frontal pain-worse toward evening - scaly eruption behind ears. Tongue white coated. Mouth and lips cracked. Sharp pain over right eye - drawing eye upwards.

Nose: Bleeding in nasal operation, especially passive haemorrhage.

Female: Metrorrhagia, too frequent and copious menses. Haemorrhage with violent uterine colic - every alternate period very profuse. Leucorrhoea before and after menses, bloody dark offensive, stains indelibly. Sore pain in womb on rising. Scarcely recovers from one period before another begins.

Urinary : Frequent desire, urine heavy phosphatic, chronic cystitis, dysuria and spasmodic retention, haematuria, accumulation of gravel, renal colic, brick dust sediment, urethritis, urine runs away in little jets. Often replaces the use of the catheter.

Dose: Tincture to 6th potency.

(Boericke)

'Shepherds', purse says Gerarde 'stayeth bleeding in any part of the body, whether the juice or the decoction, thereof be drunk or whether it be used poultice wise or in both or any way else. In a clyster it cureth the bloody flux, it health green and bleeding wounds, it is marvellous for inflammations new beginning and for all diseases which must be checked back and cooled.' Gerarde adds that the decoction will stop diarrhoea, blood spitting, haematuria and all other fluxes of blood. Thlaspi is the white man's faithful friend. A native of Europe; it has accompanied Europeans in all their migrations and established itself, wherever they have settled to till the soil. It does not refuse to grow in the poorest soils, but it luxuriates in the richest. Burnett noticed that it flourished best in the neighbourhood of dung hills and the odour of the tincture is much suggestive thereof. Some have seen in the seed vessel the signature of the shape of the uterus and Burnett found in it an organ remedy of vast importance. The Q/TR, he said is the best thing to give for menses, that have been checked, for uterine haemorrhages he preferred the attenuations. He has observed, it causes sexual excitement like cantharis. It aided Burnett in the cure of an inveterate case of gall - stones, the origin of which he traced to the uterus. The 6th had immediate good effect. Rademachers showing the action of Thlasp on uric acid excretion - Thlaspi. ϕ-30 drops - 5 times a day was given solely with the idea of stopping the haematuria but the result was more copious discharge of urinary sand than ever before. The urine increased the dropsy disappeared. *(JHC)*

This remedy is indicated in haemorrhages, especially those that are uterine in origin, haemorrhage accompanying uterine fibroid, metrorrhagia, with uterine colic, she scarcely recovers from one period before another begins. It is useful in chronic cystitis, dysuria, and spasmodic retention of the urine, also renal colic, gravel; brick dust sediment and phosphatic deposits in the urine.

Compare: Urtica Urens, Crocus Sativa, Trillium, Ipecac, Millefolium. (Blackwood)

613. *Thuja Occidentalis*

(Arbor Vitae)

Acts on skin, blood, gastro-intestinal tract, kidneys and brain. In relation to the production of pathological vegetations, condylomata, warty excrescences, spongy tumors it is very important. Moist mucous tubercles. Bleeding fungus growths. Naevus - Excess of venosity.

The main action Thuja is on the skin and genito - urinary organs, producing conditions that correspond with Hahnemann's sycotic dyscrasia, whose chief manifestation is the formation of wart like excrescences upon mucous and cutaneous surfaces. Figwarts and condylomata. Has a specific anti - bacterial action as in gonorrhoea and vaccination. Suppressed gonorrhoea. Salpingitis. Ill effects of vaccination. Sycotic pains i.e. tearing in muscles and joints, worse at rest. Better in dry weather, Worse - damp humid atmosphere. Lameness. Hydrogenoid constitutions, whose blood is morbidly hydroscopic, so that damp air and water are inimical. Complaints from moonlight. Rapid exhaustion and emaciation - Left sided and chilly medicine, Variola, aborts the pustule - prevents the suppurating fever - vaccinosis Viz. inveterable skin troubles, neuralgia etc.

Mind: Fixed ideas, music causes weeping and trembling.

Head: Pain as if pressed by a nail - Neuralgia from tea - left sided headache white scaly dandruff, hair dry and falling out. Greasy skin of face.

Eyes: Iritis - eyelids agglutinated at night, dry scaly, styes and tarsal tumors, acute and subacute inflammation of sclera.

Ears: Painful pressure at root.

Nose: Chronic catarrh, thick green mucus - ulceration with in the nostrils.

Mouth: White blisters on side close to root, painful sore - Teeth decay next to gums. Gums retract. Drinks fall audibly into stomach - Ranula - Pyorrhoea alveolaris.

Stomach: Complete loss of appetite - dislike for fresh meat and potatoes. Rancid eructations after fat food, pain in epigastrium - cannot eat onions - Tea drinking dyspepsia.

Abdomen: Chronic diarrhoea, worse after breakfast, discharges forcibly expelled, gurgling sound, brown spots. Flatulence and distention, protruding here and there. Constipation with violent rectal pain causing stool to racede - piles swollen. Anus fissured - painful with warts - movement as of something living.

Urethra: Swollen inflamed - urinary stream split and small. Frequent micturition accompanying pains. Desire sudden and urgent but cannot be controlled.

Male: Inflammation of prepuce and glans, pain in penis - Gonorrhoeal rheumatism - gonorrhoea - chronic induration of testicles - prostatic enlargement (Ferr Pic, Thiosinaminum, Iod, Sabal).

Female: Vagina very sensitive, warty excrescences on vulva and perineun - profuse leucorrhoea - thick greenish - severe pain in left ovary and left inguinal region - menses scanty, retarded, polypi, fleshy excrescences, ovaritis, worse left side at every menstrual period.

Respiratory: Dry hacking cough in afternoon with pain in pit of stomach - stitches in chest, worse cold drinks. Asthma in children (Nat. Sulph) chronic laryngitis.

Extremities : when walking, limbs feel as if made of wood or glass and would break easily - Tips of fingers swollen, red, feel dead. Muscular twitchings, weakness and trembling. Cracking in joints - Pain in heels and tendo-achilles. Nails brittle - in growing toe nail.

Skin: Polypi, tubercles, warts, epithelioma, naevi, carbuncles, ulcers, especially in ano, genital region. Freckles and blotches. Perspiration, sweetish and strong - Dry skin, with brown spots, Zona, herpetic eruptions. Tearing pains in ganglia -

Glandular enlargement. Nail crippled - brittle and soft - eruptions only on covered parts, worse after scratching - very sensitive to touch, coldness of one side, sarcoma, polypi, brown spots on hands and arms.

Sleep: Persistent insomnia.

Fever: Chill beginning in thighs - Sweat only on uncovered parts or all over except head when sleeping, profuse, sore, smelling like honey. Orgasm of blood in the evening, with throbbing in the blood vessels.

Modalities: *Worse* - at night - from heat of bed; at 3 a.m. and 3 p.m.; from cold damp air, after breakfast, fat, coffee, vaccination. *Better:* left side; while drawing up a limb.

Compare: (Bad effects of vaccination, Sil, Maland) - (Suppressed Gonorrhoea Medorrh.)

Complementary: Sabina, Ars, Nat sulph, Silicea.

Dose: Locally, for warts and excrescences Tincture or Cerate - Internally Tincture to 30 the Potency. *(Boericke)*

The American Arbor Vitae is a spiry ever green attaining a height of 20 to 50 feet, though generally not above 40 and a diameter of about 10 to 20 feet through the greatest breadth of foliage. It grows upon the rocky banks of rivers and in low, swampy spots, blossoming from May until June and maturing its fruit in autumn. The Arbor Vitae assumes a conical form with such true line as to appear clipped, thus forming one of our most valued high - hedge trees. The native habitat of Thuja is not with out its importance in relation to therapeutics. It loves swamps. It is Hahnemann's typical antisycotic and Grauvogl's hydrogenoid. Gonorrhoea. Taste remarks that in the period, when the doctrine of signatures prevailed the resinous callosities of the stems and leaves of Thuja occ. might have seemed an indication, that the plant was the specific for sycosis and warts. He indicates Castor in his Thuja group and gives an instance in which it acted on fig warts - Castor is the product of an animal which subsists on the bark of resionous trees. Burnett says Thuja is the remedy for fatty tumours which he regards as sycotic in nature. Thuja not only produces symptoms of the secondary stage of gonorrhoea and vaccinal affection, it also produces urethritis and a variolus eruption - Agg: by extension is a characteristic of Thuja - it causes cracking in joints. The arm symptoms are also Agg: when the limb hangs down (which is also an extension) - cannot sleep after 3 a.m. - dreams much of falling - feet sweat much, offensive, sweats much about groins - Thuja ϕ - in five to seven drops doses at bed time control nocturnal emission better than any other remedy - nocturnal emission is an emphasised symptom in MMP. Epulis (Fibrous tumour of gum). Scalp tumour in youth of seventeen of the size of bean - Thuja. 30. once in 20 days - in 4 months the youth was cured - left side inguinal hernia after labour - Thuja high. On blowing nose a pressing pain in the hollow tooth - A key note of Thuja is frequent micturition accompany pains. The desire of Thuja is sudden and urgent. The skin is mottled and discoloured, brown or red mottled spots - floating stripes before the vision is a symptom of Thuja - Peculiar sensation are - as if a strange person were at her side. As if soul and body were separated. Eyes were swollen and would be pressed out of head. As of fine sand in eyes - As if living animal were in abdomen - As if anus would fly to pieces during stool - Thuja suited to - Hydrogenoid constitution

- (possessing an increased capacity to contain water, hence rain, cold, damp, weather and food that increase the number of molecule of water in the system) - Lymphatic temperament, in very fleshy persons - left sided medicine (left arm is usually vaccinated) - Agg: after breakfast, after eating, after tea, coffee, Beer, Sweets, Tobacco, Fat meat, Onions. Antidoted by: Sulphur, Mercury. *(JHC)*

Adapted to Hydrogenoid constitution of Grauvogl which is related to sycosis - Fig warts, condylomata, wart like excrescences - fleshy persons - dark complexion - black hair - unhealthy skin - bad effects of vaccination - maltreated gonorrhoea. As if strange person were at his side - as if soul and body were separated - as if a living animal were in abdomen - of being under the influence of a superior power - vertigo when closing eyes (Lach, Theri) - Headache as if a nail had been driven into parietal bone. Agg : from sexual excess; from tea. Sycotic - dandruff, hair dry, ophthalmia neonatorum, large granulations like warts or blisters Amel : by warmth and covering - lye lids agglutinated at night - styes - Tarsal tumors - Ears - otitis, discharge purulent, polypi - Teeth decay at the roots (on edges- Staph) crumble, turn yellow (Syph.) - Ranula - bluish or varicose veins on tongue or in mouth - toothache agg : tea drinking - on blowing the nose; pressing pain in the hollow of tooth - burning pain in left ovarian region-constipation - violent pains in rectum - compel cessation of effort, stool recedes, after being partly expelled - Piles swollen, pain most severe when sitting - diarrhoea early morning, expelled forcibly, gurgling as water from bunghole, after breakfast, coffee, fat food, vaccination, onions - Anus fissured, flat warts, skin dirty, brown, brownish white spots here and there - eruption only on covered parts. Flesh feels as if beaten, from the bones. Urine trickling in urethra. Severe cutting at close of urination - Chill beginning in the thighs - sweat only on uncovered parts or all over except head (Rev. Sil), when he sleeps; stops when he wakes (Rev. Samb.) - Profuse, sore smelling, fetid at night - Perspiration, smelling like honey, on the genitals, sensation as if body, especially the limbs were made of glass and would break easily. Suppressed gonorrhoea, causing articular rheumatism, prostatitis, sycosis, impotence, condylomata and many constitutional symptoms. Nails deformed, brittle (Ant. c.).

Complementary: Med., Sab., Sil.

Compare: Cann. s., Canth., Cop, Staph; Cinnab is preferable for warts on the prepuce.

Follows well: After Med., Merc., Nit. ac.
(HCA)

614. *Thymol*

(Thyme Camphor)

A remedy having a wide field in genito - urinary diseases. It is indicated in pathological emission, priapism and prostatorrhoea. The provings show an action limited to the sexual organs, producing a typical sexual neurasthenia - Specific for hook worm disease (Chenopodium).

Relation: Carbon Tetrachloride - as a remedy for hook worms, according to Dr. Lambert, Suva, Fiji, who employed it in 50,000 cases.

1. Carbon Tetra - chloride is a vermifuge and vermicide of great potency and has shown itself to be the best verifuge for the treatment of hookworm in a country where the disease predominates.

2. It gives little discomfort to the patient, is palatable, requires no preparation of the patient and when pura is apparently not toxic - all of which features are of advantage in a popular campaign. W. G. Smillia and S. B. Pessoa of sao Paulo, Brazil, also have found Carbon Tetra Chloride to be extremely efficient to remove 95% of all the hook worms harbored.

Dose: Thymol - 6th attenuation.

(Boericke)

615. Thymus Serpyllum

(Wild Thyme)

Respiratory infection of children, dry nervous asthma, whooping cough, severe spasms, but little sputum - Ringing in ears with feeling of pressure in head, burning pharynx, sore throat, worse empty swallowing - blood vessels distended, dark.

Dose: Tincture. *(Boericke)*

616. Thyroidinum

(Dried Thyroid gland of sheep)

Thyroid produces anemia, emaciation, muscular weakness, sweating, headache, nervous tremor of face and limbs, tingling sensations, paralysis. Heart rate increased, exophthalmus and dilatation of pupils. In myxoedema and cretinism its effects are striking - Rheumaoid arthritis - infantile wasting. Rickets, delayed union of fractures. In half grain doses twice in a day over a considerable period said to be effective in undescended testicle in boys. Thyroid exercises a general regulating influence over the mechanism of the organs of nutrition, growth and development. Thyroid weakness causes decided craving for large amount of sweets.

Of use in psoriasis and tachycardia - arrested development in children. Improves the memory - goitre - excessive obesity - acts better with pale patients, rather than those of high color. Amblyopia. Mammary tumor - uterine fibroid - great weakness and hunger and yet loses flesh. Nocturnal enuresis, agalactea. Begin treatment early in pregnancy.

Dose: 1½ gr; 2 to 3 times daily. Vomiting of pregnancy (give early morning before patient gets up) Fibroid tumors of the breast - 2x trit. Dilates arterioles (Adrenaline contracts them). Sensation of faintness and nausea. Marked sensitiveness to cold. Hypothyroidism after acute diseases i.e. weakness, easy fatigue, weak pulse, tendency to fainting, palpitation, cold hands and feet, low blood pressure, chilliness and sensitive to cold (Thyroid 1x - 3 times daily). Has a powerful diuretic action in myxoedema and various types of oedema.

Head: Persistent frontal headache, eye balls prominent - face flushed - lips burn tongue thickly coated. Fullness and heat-face flushed-bad taste in mouth.

Heart: Weak frequent pulse with inability to lie down - tachycardia, anxiety about chest, - as if constricted - palpitation from least exertion - severe heart pain-ready excitability of heart - heart's action weak with numbness of fingers.

Stomach: Desire for sweets and thirst for cold water - flatulence, much flatus in abdomen.

Urinary: Increased flow - polyuria, some albumen and sugar - enuresis in weakly children who are nervous and irritable (½ gr. night and morning), urine smells of violets, burning along urethra - increase of uric acid.

Extremities: Rheumatic arthritis with tendency to obesity - coldness and cramps of extremities - peeling of skin of lower limbs - cold extremities - Aching pain - oedema of legs, trembling of limbs and entire body.

Skin: Psoriasis associated with adiposity (not in developing stage) - skin dry, impoverished - cold hands and feet - eczema. Uterine fibroids. Browny swelling - swelling of glands of stony hardness - sluggish cases - jaundice with pruritus. Ichthyosis - Lupus - itching without eruption - worse night.

Relation: Spongia, Calc, Fucus, Lycopus, Iodothyrine (the active principle isolated from thyroid gland, a substance rich in iodine and nitrogen, affects metabolism - reducing weight, may produce glycosuria. Use cautiously in obesity, for a fatty heart may not be able to maintain the accelerated rhythm. Milk contains the internal secretion of the thyroid.

Thymus gland extract (arthritis deformans, metabolic osteoarthritis) - 5 gr. tablets 3 times daily - High potencies very efficient in exophthalmic goitre.

Dose: Crude thyroid at times - better 6-30 potency - if crude thyroid is taken (2-3 grains or more daily) the pulse should be watched-must not be given in physiological doses where with feeble heart there is high blood pressure and not in tubercular patients. *(Boericke)*

With Thyr. 1M (FC) Skinner cured a case of dysmenorrhoea in a goitrous subject. The connection between the heart and the thyroid gland is very close as seen in exophthalmic goitre. Many cases of the latter affection have been cured with Thyr - In myxoedema, cachexia strumipriva, cretinism and similar conditions, the thyroid gland is absent or defective and the idea of the thyroid feeding is to supply a physiological want. A state of puffiness and obesity may therefore be regarded as a key note indication for Thyr. In a case of universal and very aggravated psoriasis in a school boy, fair, very chilly, cold, clammy hands and feet, Thyr. 3x and later 30 (which seemed to act better than the lower attenuation) completely cured after a prolonged course. An obese lady aet 60 developed diabetes. I cured her completely of the diabetes with Thyr. 3x and 30. Skin cases in great variety have been cured with Thyr. in substantial doses. Pityriasis rubra, intense redness and scaliness of legs and also with intense itching, ichthyosis, syphilitic eruptions, scleroderma - Thyr. has increased the flow of milk in nursing women, when the flow has been deficient - Thyr. is antagonistic to adrenaline - in that the latter contracts, whilst the former dilates the arterioles. Myxoedema patients lose their hair as a rule, and Thyr. when successful restores the growth - persons suffering from skin diseases were found tolerant of much larger doses than myxoedemics. Thyr. treatment nearly always raises the bodily heat.

Relation: Myxoedema - Psoriasis etc. Ars. (I permanently cured a case of Myxoedema with Ars. high before the thyroid method was introduced). (Arsenic has been found to be a normal contituent of the healthy thyroid gland).

Phthisis, Bac. (I have found Bac. follows Thyr. well-found tuberculosis very common in myxoedemics) - "Young" of Switzerland has cured cretinism with Bac. - (Goitre exophthalmic; Spo., Iod., Spi.) Thyr. for dilated arterioles (Adren. Opp.) *(JHC)*

The function of the Thyroid is the splitting up of the iodine containing molecules on any compound which enters the body and the conversion of this into the thyroid product, Thyroxin - Plummer has found that the maximum physiological effects of the single dose in a myxoedematous patient is not reached before the 10th day and in some cases, it is three weeks, before a single dose has ceased its function. He also found that in a patient of 150 pounds weight, 0.001 gm of Thyroxin would increase the metabolic rate by 2%. The size of the gland is no indication as to its secretory function - Goitres are common in girls about puberty. The most pronounced cases of hypothyroidism and hyperthyroidism occur in women. If the thyroid is hyper-secreting, iodine will aggravagte the case - Hyperthyroidism symptoms are tachycardia, tremor, nervous irritability, insomnia, hot flushes, with perspiration, exophthalmus and digestive disturbances. In some cases there is a hyperchlorhydria and hypertension, the temperature may be increased one or two degrees and the patient is apt to be too hot or too cold. Many of the other glands show disturbance as the thymus. Parathyroids, pancreas, ovaries, pituitary and suprarenals. In some the secretion is increased while in others it is diminished. In some of these cases, there is glycosuria and an increased nitrogen output.

Hyposecretion is indicated by cretinism and myxoedema and many symptoms that are not as easily recongnised. Cretinism is an absence of thyroid or its secretion in infancy. With a subthyroid secretion in young children, there is a slow growth, a general lack of mental and physical development. With these the skin is dry and at times stimulates, ichthyosis or eczema. There may be amenorrhoea, chlorosis, hysteria, nausea and vomiting. Epilepsy may develop in these cases during infancy, puberty or the menopause.

After the 45th year the secretion of the thyroid is lessened. If it has not increased at menopause in women, they are disturbed by hot flushes, rapid heart action and general circulatory disturbances. Should the secretion diminish too rapidly, the women become obese and this is also true in men together with senility - if there is marked hypo-secretion - By the term senility is understood a sluggish mentality, a dry skin, hard arteries, and a reduced metabolism. A normal sexual function in the female is dependent upon a normal thyroid gland. In subthyroid the hands and feet are cold - menstruation is often scanty and delayed, while in others menstruation is absent, they become obese, are more or less apathetic and sleepy, especially during the day and have a morning backache. In hypothyroidism, thyroid in some from is indicated and will improve the condition of the patient and increase the basal metabolism. Thyroxin can be obtained for administration by mouth. It contains 65% of Iodine. The indications for its use are the same as those for the dry thyroid extracts.

Infantile obesity often requires thyroid in combination with small doses of pituitary. These patients may require small doses of thyroid at puberty, if menstruation does not develop at the proper time or chlorosis develops.

Nocturnal enuresis may be annoying when small doses of the thyroid alone or combined with pituitary often benefit.

Myxoedema is a common condition if looked for and small doses of thyroid is the remedy. It must be kept up.

Epileptic attacks are often benefited when there is evidence of a subthyroid condition.

Hypertension is benefitted by thyroid when there is dry skin and evidence of senility, also asthma and constipation in the aged. *(Blackwood)*

617. *Thyroiodinum*

(Iodo - Thyrinum. Trituration)

Thyroiodinum is now more generally, named iodothyrin, but I retain the former as more covenient. It is present in only small quantities in the thyroid of the sheep. It is completely free from albuminous substances, stable and directly assimilated. The iodine exists in organic combination and Thyri. contains 0.003 parts of Iodine to every gramme. The general effects of the drug are increased secretion of urine and corresponding loss of flesh - enlargement and induration of all lobes of thyroid. Thyri. 5 grains tablets - once every evening - at the end of a week twice daily. After using twenty five tablets the gland was smaller and softer, the previously hard and resistant nodules were elastic, after two more weeks only remnants of the goitre remained. *(JHC)*

618. *Titanium*

(The metal)

Is found in the bones and muscles. Has been used in lupus and tuberculosis processes externally, also in skin disease, nasal catarrh etc. Apples contain 0.11% of titan - imperfect vision - the peculiarity being that half an object only could be seen at once. Giddiness with vertical hemiopia, also sexual weakness with too early ejaculation of semen in coitus. Bright's disease. Eczema, Lupus' rhinitis.

Dose : Lower and middle potencies. *(Boericke)*

Titanium stands midway between silicon and Tin in some of its relations and in other respects it is closely related to iron, chromium and aluminium. The crystals proved by "Sharp" were originally believed to be the pure metal, but were proved later to be the cyanonitrid. One symptom of the proving is remarkable - imperfect vision, the peculiarity being that, half an object only could be seen. Sexual weakness. Too early ejaculation of semen in coitus. *(JHC)*

619. *Tribulus Terrestris*

(Ikshugandha)

An east Indian drug - Useful in urinary affections, especially dysuria and in debilitated states of the sexual organs, as expressed in seminal weakness, ready emissions and impoverisheu semen. Prostatitis, calculous affections and sexual neurasthenia. It meets the auto - traumatism of masturbation, correcting the emissions and spermatorrhoea. Partial impotence caused by over indulgence of advancing age or when accompanied by urinary symptoms, incontinence, painful micturition etc.

Dose : 10-20 drops of the Tincture. TDS. *(Boericke)*

620. *Trifolium Pratense*

(Red clover)

Produces most marked ptyalism - Feeling of fullness with congestion of salivary gland, followed by increased copious flow of saliva. Feeling as if mumps were coming on, crusta lactea, dry scaly crusts, stiff neck, cancerous diathesis.

Mouth: Increased flow of Saliva.

Respiratory: Hoarse and choking, Chills with cough at night, whooping cough, paroxysms, worse at night.

Compare: Trifolium repens - white clover - prophylactic against mumps, feeling of congestion in salivary glands, pain and hardening, especially submaxillary, worse lying down, mouth filled with watery saliva, worse lying down, taste of blood in mouth and throat.

Dose: Tincture. *(Boericke)*

Red Clover - In the cancer cases an extract of the blossoms of the first crop is used. This extract, says Cooper, is made from boiling down the flowers till nothing but an inspissated residue is left. In this condition, it seems to be caustic and for this reason is used by herbalist. I doubt its utility.

Tri. P. has a reputation among eclectics in whooping cough and coughs of measles and phthisis - T. C. Duncan and others proved it and elicited some very decided respiratory symptoms, dry, tickling cough, oppressed breathing and fever. One peculiar symptom was cough followed by hiccough. Many symptoms of congestion appeared. Cooper says of Tri. P. that it causes salivation in horses and diarrhoea, if tney eat much of it and that it cures mumps and affections of the pancreas and salivary glands. Hale says it causes heaves in horses. Felter gives it to persons disposed to cancer. He finds it retards the progress of cancerous tumors and improves the general conditions of the patient. It keeps cancer from ulcerating. After ulceration has occured Tri. p. does no good. Another indication of Felters is scaly and ulcerated conditions of the tibial region of the old.

This remedy is indicated, where there is pronounced ptyalism. The salivary glands are congested and this is followed by a profuse flow of saliva. It is useful when there is an irritable condition on the larynx as observed in spasmodic cough, whooping cough and the cough of measles. It is also useful in coryza with hoarse and choking spells, coughing on going into the open air. It has been employed extensively in the cancerous diathesis.

Dose: Tincture 1-60 drops.*(Blackwood)*

621. Trillium Pendulum

(White beth-root)

A general haemorrhagic medicine with great faintness and dizziness. Chronic diarrhoea of bloody mucus, uterine haemorrhage. Threatened abortion - Relaxation of pelvic region, cramp like pains. Phthisis with purulent and copious expectoration and spitting of blood.

Head: Nose bleed (Millef, Melilot).

Mouth: Haematemesis.

Stomach: Haematemesis.

Rectum: Chronic diarrhoea, discharge bloody, dysentery, passage almost pure blood.

Female: Uterine haemorrhage, with sensation as though hips and back were falling to pieces, better tight bandages. Gushing of bright blood on least movement. Haemorrhage from fibroids. Prolapse, with great bearing down, leucorrhoea, copious, yellow, stringly, metrorrhagia and climacteric. Lochia suddenly becomes sanguinous.

Respiratory: Cough, spitting of blood, haemoptysis.

Relationship : Trillium cernum (Eye symptoms-everything looks bluish-greasy feeling in mouth) 'Ficus' - (Haemorrhages, menorrhagia, haematuria, epistaxis, haematemesis, bleeding piles) 'Sanguisuga' - Leech (Haemorrhages, bleeding from anus) Ipc, Sab., Lach., Ham.

Dose : Tincture and lower potencies.
(Boericke)

According to Millspaugh, T. Pendulum is the white variety of T. Erectum. The chief use of Trill, comes to us from the eclectics, who learned some of them from the native Indians. The popular name Birth - root, sufficiently indicates one part of its reputation. In haemorrhage, ante - partum, post partum and climacteric, in fibroid tumour and in haemorrhages of all kinds Trill has been found curative. Both the white and the purple varieties have been used - haemorrhage of Trill. is accompanied with faintness and sinking at the stomach - flooding with fainting is a key note - haemostatic in epistaxis and for bleeding after tooth extraction - the haemorrhages of Trill are copious, either active or passive , usually bright red and profuse. Trill is suited to women, who flood after every labour, flabby subjects.

Relations: Calc Phos (menstrual and haemorrhagic affections) - Haemorrhages Chi, Calc, Ham, Secal, Ust, Sanguis - Bright red blood - Ipc, Milli - Bleeding after tooth extraction - Ham, Kreo. Menses profuse every two weeks and lasting a week or longer—Calc phos - Flow profuse gushing, light red Agg : least movement - Sabi. Flow dark clotted - Thlasp. As if bones of pelvis broken - Aesc. h. *(JHC)*

This agent acts as an astringent, tonic and anti-septic and a said to produce both an active and passive haemorrhage.

Relaxation of tissues, accompanied by mucus discharges active and passive haemorrhages - menorrhagia, when the menses appear every two weeks and lasts from seven to eight days and in the interval there is a profuse yellow creamy or bloody leucorrhoea - uterine prolapsus - haemorrhages from uterine fibroids - haemoptysis - incipient phthisis - chronic diarrhoea - the passages are bloody, also in cases of dysentery when the passage consists of pure blood. *(Blackwood)*

Haemorrhage, copious, both active and passive, usually bright red from nose, lungs, kidneys and uterus (Ipc, Mill); Epsitaxis, profuse, passive, bright red-Bleeding from cavity after extraction of a tooth (Ham, Kreo). Menses profuse, every two weeks, lasting a week or longer (Calc Phos) - Flooding with fainting - Menorrhagia, flow profuse, gushing, bright red, at the least movement (Sab), from displaced uterus, at the climacteric every two weeks, dark, clotted (Thlas - Ust). *(HCA)*

622. Triosteum
(Fever-Root)

Triost. is an energetically acting drug and has been proved by Williamson, Neidhard, Gatchell and other experienced provers. The name fever Wort (Rool) tells its traditional reputation. Hale says it is one of the ingredients of the fever powder of the eclectics. Talmadge, one of the provers, found it of great value in typhoid and gastric fevers. It produced acute rheumatic symptoms and an intense urticaria. Talmadge says of the effect on himself: It acted promptly and emphatically, causing aching pains in nearly every part of the body, especially of lower limbs and head.

The right side of the head was more affected than the left. The stomach was very much disordered. The vomiting and pain in the stomach was very severe. At the anus there was itching and exudation of mucus. A peculair concomitant of the evacuations was, numbness of the lower limbs after stool. Many symptoms came on in the early morning hours. *(JHC)*

This remedy is indicated in sick headache . There is nausea and vomiting of bilious material. The pain is worse in the occiput and upon the right side. It is useful in diarrhoea when the stools are watery and frothy and are attended with colicky pains, nausea and vomiting. It is to be remembered in influenza with aching pain all over, heat in the limbs, also urticaria when it is dependent upon gastric derangement. *(Blackwood)*

Dose : 6th potency. *(Boericke)*

623. Triticum - Agropyron Repens

(Couch - Grass)

An excellent remedy in excessive irritability of the bladder, dysuria, cystitis, gonorrhoea.

Nose: Always blowing nose.

Urinary: Frequent, difficult and painful urination - gravel deposits - Catarrhal and purulent discharges (Pareira) - Strangury, pyelitis, enlarged prostate - chronic cystic irritability - incontinence, constant desire - urine is dense and causes irritation of the mucous surfaces.

Compare: Chimaph, Senecio, Populus trem, Buchu, Uva. *(Boericke)*

Frequently in dysuria, from an inflamed state of the urethra, I found Trit. r. Q-10 drops in a little water, frequently repeated, of prompt effect, often giving complete relief in a few hours, and if the ailment is primarily in the urethra, the relief is an abiding cure; if from a tugging of the heavy womb, it is only relief. *(JHC)*

This agent is a mild and soothing diuretic, increasing the watery portion of the urine.

This remedy is indicated when the urine is of a high specific gravity and causes irritation of the mucous surfaces of the bladder and kidneys. It is of service in cystitis and in frequent and difficult urination, also in pyelitis, strangury and prostatitis, when the specific gravity is high and irritation of the mucous surfaces is resulting. It is useful in lithaemic and rheumatic conditions, when the elimination of solids irritates the kidneys and produces much distress.

Compare: Chimaphila. *(Blackwood)*

624. Trychosanthes Dioica

Patel, West Bengal - Mother Tincture of fresh root.

Dilution - 3x and higher.

This agent is an active cathartic. This remedy is indicated in diarrhoea. The stools are profuse, thin, yellowish, watery, offensive. There are cutting pains in the abdomen before, during, following the stool. The face is pale or of a yellow tinge. There is pain in the liver and dizziness following the stool.

Compare: Veratrum Album. Gambogia. *(Blackwood)*

625. Trombidium

(Red Acarus of the fly)

Has a specific place in the treatment of dysentery, symptoms are worse by food and drink.

Adomen: Much pain before and after stool - stool only after eating - Griping in hypochondrium in morning - congestion of the liver, with urgent, loose stools on rising, brown, thin, bloody stools with tenesmus. During stool, sharp pain in left side, shooting downward, burning in anus.

Dose: 6-30 Potency. *(Boericke)*

Tromb is a parasite found singly or in groups upon the common housefly of a bright red colour, neatly circular in shape. The alcoholic Tincture, a brilliant orange in colour, was prepared from specimens about 115, in number, collected in Frankfort, Philadelphia in Sept. 1864 - the potencies used 3x, 6x, 9, 18 and 30. The grand key note of Tromb is Agg: by eating or drinking. The symptoms may be in the nose, teeth or tonsils, this modality is characteristic. On this indication I have cured some of the worst case of diarrhoea and also intestinal pains coming on when the patient eats or drinks - much pain before and after stool, stool only after eating - Tromb. has cured dysentery with brown, thin bloody stools and tenesmus. Congested liver with urgent loose stools on rising from bed - during stool sharp pain in left side, shooting downward. Skin symptoms were prominent, especially itching of scalp and in whiskers. *(JHC)*

626. Tuberculinum

(A nucleo - protein, a nosode from tubercular abscess)

Tuberculinum is indicated in renal affections, but caution is necessary for where skin and intestines do not perform normally even high potencies are dangerous. In chronic cystitis brilliant and permanent results.

Of undoubted value in the treatment of incipient tuberculosis. Especially adapted to the light complexioned, narrow chested subjects. Lax fiber, low recuperative powers and very susceptible to changes in the weather. Patient always tired - Motion causes intense fatigue, averion to work, wants constant changing - when symptoms are constantly changing and well selected remedies fail to improve and cold is taken from the slightest exposure. Rapid emaciation. Of great value in epilepsy, neurasthenia and in nervous children, diarrhoea in children running for weeks, extreme wasting, bluish pallor, exhaustion, mentally deficient children. Enlarged tonsils - skin affections, acute articular rheumatism. Very sensitive mentally and physically. General exhaustion. Nervous weakness, trembling, epilepsy, arthritis.

Mind: Mania and melancholia, insomnia and sopor, irritable especially when awaking, depressed, melancholy, fear of dogs, animals especially. Desire to use foul language, curse and swear.

Head: Subject to deep brain headaches and intense neuralgia as of an iron band around head. Meningitis - when critical discharges appear, sweat, polyuria, diarrhoea, exanthema, repeating the dose only when crises come on. Nocturnal hallucinations, awakes frightened, crops of small boils, intensely painful, successively appear in the nose, green fetid pus.

Ears: Persistent, offensive otorrhoea, perforation in membrana tympani with ragged edges.

Stomach: Averse to meat, all gone hungry sensation, desire for cold milk.

Abdomen: Early morning sudden diarrhoea.

Female: Benign mammary tumors, menses too early, too profuse - dysmenorrhoea - pain increases with the establishment of flow.

Respiratory: Enlarged tonsils, hard dry cough during sleep - expectoration, thick, easy, profuse, bronchorrhoea, sensation of suffocation even with plenty of fresh air, bronchopneumonia in children.

Skin: Chronic eczema, itching intense, worse at night.

Sleep: Poor, wakes early - overpowering sleepiness in day time - dreams vivid and distressing.

Modalities: (Worse) Motion, music, before a storm, standing, dampness, before draught, early morning, and after sleep. (Better) Open air.

Tuberculine Aviare: From birds - Acts on the apices of the lungs - has proved an excellent remedy in influenzal bronchitis, symptoms similar to tuberculosis. Relieves the debility, diminishes the cough, improves the appetite and braces up with the whole organism, acute broncho-pulmonary diseases of children, itching of palms and ears. Cough acute, inflammatory, irritating, incessant and tickling, loss of strength and appetite.

Hydrastis: To fatten patients after tuberculin.

Thuja: Vaccinosis may block the way of action of tuberculin and until thuja has been given and then acts brilliantly.

(Burnett)

Complementary: Calcarea, China, Bryonia.

Dose: Tuberculin needs more frequent repetition in children's complaints, than nearly every other chronic remedy (H. Fergie woods) - 30 - and much higher in infrequent doses - when Tuberculin fails, syphillinum often follows advantageously producing a reaction. *(Boericke)*

TUBERCULINUM - BACILLINUM

Adapted to persons of light complexion, blue eyes, blonde in preference to brunette, tall slim, flat, narrow chest, active and precocious mentality, weak physically, the tubercular diathesis. Best selected remedy fails to relieve or permanently improve - symptoms everchanging, ailment affecting one organ - then another, beginning suddenly - ceasing suddenly - Takes cold easily, without knowing how or where, seems to take cold every time he takes a breath of fesh air (Hep) - Emaciation rapid and pronounced - losing flesh while eating well. Melancholy, despondent, morose, irritable, fretful, peevish, taciturn, sulky, naturally of a sweet disposition, now on the borderland of insanity.

Everything in the room seemed strange as though in a strange place. Headache, chronic, tubercular, pain intense, sharp, cutting from above right eye to occiput - as if an iron hoop around head.

School girls headache Agg: by study or even slight mental exertion, when using eyes in close work and glasses fail to ameliorate.

Acute cerebral or basilar meningitis, with threatened effusion, nocturnal hallucinations, wakes from sleep frightened, screaming (Apis, Hell, Sulph).

Crops of small boils, intensely painful, successively appear in the nose. Green, fetid, pus.

Plica Polonica, several bad cases permanently cured after Bor. and Psor. failed.

Diarrhoea early morning, sudden, imperative. Emaciating, though eating well. Stool, dark brown, watery, offensive, discharged with great force, great weakness and profuse night sweats.

Menses too early, too profuse, too long lasting, tardy in starting, with frightful dysmenorrhoea in patients with a tuberculous history.

Tubercular deposit begins in apex of lungs, usually the left (Phos, Sulph, Ther).

Eczema, tubercular, over entire body, itching intense, Agg: night, when undressing, from bathing. Immense quantities of white bran like scales, oozing behind the ears, in the hair, in folds of skin with rawness and soreness; fiery red skin, ringworm.

Relation: Comple: Psor, Sulph.

When Psor, Sulph, or the best selected remedy fails to relieve or permanently improve. Follows Psor. as a constitutional remedy in hay fever, asthma.

Belladona, for acute attacks congestive or inflammatory, occuring in tubercular diseases.

Hydrastis to fatten patients cured with Tuber. *(HCA)*

Different Varieties of Tuberculinum.

1) Burriett's Bacillinum: prepared from Tubercular ulcer from Cow's lung.
2) Dr. Kent's Tuberculin: from infected lymp glands of cattle.
3) Koch's Tuberculinum: from cultures of Tubercular Bacilli macerated in glycerine broth.
4) Koch's Lymph: from old Tuberculin of Koch containing T. B. Homnia - Potency above 200.
5) Tuberculin Aviare: from infected liver of chicken.
6) Bacillinum Testicum: from Tubercular Testicles.
7) Deny's Tuberculinum: from Tubercle cultures. Potency: 100, 200, 500.
8) Marmork anti-tuberculous serum: from serum obtained by injecting animals with young cultures of Tubercle germs - Potency - 6, 30, and above. (Systematic Materia Medica - *K. N. Mathur)*

I do not find any appreciable difference between the action of Tub. and that of Bac. My own impression is that they are practically identical and that the one will answer to the indications of the other - Insanity is very frequently a manifestation of the consumptive taint and there is something more than a pyrexial power in Tub. *(JHC)*

SYNOPSIS: Renal affections, incipient tuberculosis, epilepsy, wasting, mentally deficient, enlarged tonsils, skin affection, mania, nocturnal hallucination, otorrhoea, aversion to meat, desire for cold milk, cough acute, inflammatory, best selected remedy fails to relieve, affecting one organ then another, ceasing suddenly, takes cold easily, insanity, headache chronic, school girl headache, wakes from sleep frightened, crops of small boils, plica polonica, diarrhoea early, morning, menses too early, too profuse, night sweats, itching intense, Agg: night, undressing; bran like scales, insanity very frequently a manifestation of consumption.

627. *Turnera*

(Damiana)

Said to be of use in sexual neurasthenia, impotency, sexual debility from nervous prostration - incontinence of old people - chonic prostatic discharge - renal and cystic catarrh - frigidity of females - aid the establishment of normal menstrual flow in young girls.

Dose: Tincture and fluid extract - 10 to 40 drop doses. *(Boericke)*

Hale has collected from old - school sources much experience respecting this drug, showing its power over the genito - uninary system. The herb Damiana (the local name of Turn-a), Turnera Aphrodisiaca has long been a domestic medicine in Mexico where it is used to invigorate the system-Indian hunters discovered that a decoction of it was a great invigorator after wearisome journeys and they also found in it a cure for inability to exercise the reproductive functions in both sexes - Hale gives many cases illustrating the latter. Among the causes of the defect in the cured cases are injury to spine from a fall; sexual excess, syphilis, gonorrhoea, in the men and amenorrhoea, dysmenorrhoea and leucorrhoea, in the women. Douglass reports - incontinence of urine - Turnera 2X in water 4 times a day cured in 2 months.

Relation: Impotence, injuries, over exertion, fatigue - Bellis, Arn. Prostatic affection - Sabal, Solidage. Migraine - Epipheg. *(JHC)*

This remedy is indicated in sexual neurasthenia and frigidity also in renal and cystic catarrh. It has been employed in respiraory disorders when accompanied by profuse secretion. *(Blackwood)*

628. *Tussilago Petasites*

(Butter-burr)

Has some actions on the urinary organs and found useful in gonorrhoea. Affection of pylorus.

Urinary: Crawling in urethra.

Male: Gonorrhoea, yellowish, thick discharge, erections with urethral crawling. Pain in spermatic cord.

Relation: Tussilago fragrans (Pylorus pain, plethora and corpulency)

Tussilago Farfara (Coughs); as an intercurrent remedy in phthisis pulmonalis) see tuberculinum.

Dose: Tincture. *(Boericke)*

Pain about the pylorus, urethritis, with yellow discharge, acute or chronic gonorrhoea, yellow or white thick discharge - crawling in urethra; jerking in spermatic cord and drawing in R. Testicles are additional symptoms of the proving - Rosengberg refers to a writer who says of the plant, that it is macerated in water, the water will not spoil even if kept for years.

Compare: Lumbago, Ant tart, Act. r., Gonorrhoea - Thuja. *(JHC)*

This remedy is indicated in gonorrhoea - There is a sensation of crawling in urethra. The discharge is thick and yellow and there is pain in the spermatic cord. *(Blackwood)*

629. *Upas Tiente*

(Upas tree - Strychnos Tiente)

This remedy is of service in tonic spasm, tetanus and asphyxia. The patient is irritable, there are dull pains in the brain and lancinating pain through the right lung towards the liver. The hands and feet are numb. *(Blackwood)*

Produce tonic spasms, tetanus and asphyxia.

Eyes: Pain in eyes and orbit with conjuctivitis.

Male: Dull backache as after excessive coitus, Antidote - Curare.

Dose: 3-6 Potency. *(Boericke)*

630. *Uranium Nitricum*

(Nitrate of Uranium)

Causes glycosuria and increased urine. Is known to produce nephritis, diabetes degeneration of the liver, high blood pressure and dropsy. Its therapeutic keynote is great emaciation, debility and tendency to ascites and general dropsy. Backache and delayed menses. Dry mucous membrane and skin.

Eyes: Styes,

Stomach: Excessive thirst, nausea, vomiting, ravenous appetite, eating followed by flatulence. Boring pain in pyloric region - gastric and duodenal ulcers, burning pain, abdomen bloated - Gas second only to Lycop.

Urinary: Copious urination - Diuresis - incontinence of urine, diabetes, emaciation and tympanites, burning in urethra and very acid urine - Unable to retain urine without pain - Enuresis (Mullein Oil).

Male: *Compare-* Impotency, with nocturnal emissions - organs cold, relaxed, sweaty.

Relation: Syzygium, Phos ac., Lact ac., Arg nit., Kali bich., Ars., Phloridzin. *(Boericke)*

"Leconte", who found sugar in the urine of dogs, slowly poisoned with Ur. nit. Blake was not very successful in producing sugar, but his proving is not in any way less valuable on that account and clinical use has filled out the picture. Many cases of diabetes have been relieved or cured by Ur. nit; usually in the lower attenuations. In a case of diabetes insipidus, in a young girl Ur. nit 30 gave more relief than any other remedy. Excessive thirst, polyuria and dry tongue are the indications. Glycosuria is by no means an essential part of the indication for Ur. nit. In some of the animals experimented on by Blake the pylorus was found to be affected. With this the symptoms of proving correspond and Ur. nit. has cured both pyloric and gastric ulcer.

Compare: Diabetes - Ph. acid, Syzygium, Thyr, Lac def., Lact ac. Craves tea, Selen. *(JHC)*

This agent produces ulceration of the stomach, glycosuria and dropsical effusions. This remedy is indicated in the ulceration of the stomach, when there is a great burning pain in the stomach with vomiting and flatulence. It is useful in diabetes, when there is great thirst, emaciation, diuresis, incontinence of urine and prostration. *(Blackwood)*

631. *Urea*

The chief solid constituent of the urine of mammals. The failure of kidneys to eliminate urea from blood leads to uraemic intoxication, delirium, convulsions, and coma. On general indications Urea has been used in medicine by both schools. Merck mentions that it is diuretic and is used in cirrhosis of liver, pleurisy, renal calculus. Renal dropsy. Burnett has used both Urea 6. and uric acid 6. in gouty eczema - where the gouty eczema has been the cutaneous out let for the constitution - Burnett gave Urea in gouty cases where the urine was thin and of low specific gravity - it thickens the urine and gives great relief to the patient - Urea, Buch says, is formed in spleen, lymph and secreting gland but principally by the liver - Under the treatment, Lupoid nodules disappeared, tuberculous glands disappeared, tuberculous joints improved. No ill effects of the treatment were noticed - On the countrary the action has evidently been in many cases that of a nervous tonic. *(JHC)*

632. *Uricum Acidum*

(Lithic acid)

Uric ac. has been used on inferential grounds in gouty conditions. Burnett gave it in 5th and 6th attenuations. It is most useful in cases where deposits persist, it stirs them up and helps to eliminate them. It is useful is gouty eczema, where the eczema has been the cutaneous outlet for the constitution - with Uric acid 3x. Mersch cured a case of lipoma, situated on the left side between abdomen and chest, as large as a man's head, only lengthened. Relief was immediate, the tumour disappeared in a month. *(JHC)*

633. *Urinum*

(Urine - dilutions)

Under Urea, Allen gives some symptoms observed on a man, who for a skin affection drank in the morning, the urine he had passed the night before. The symptoms were severe, consisting of general dropsy, scanty urine and excessive weakness. These symptoms I have arranged under Urinum.

Urinotherapy is practically as old as man himself. The Chinese treat wounds by sprinkling urine on them and the custom is widespread in the Far east - Taken internally it is believed to stimulate the circulation and is valued as an active oxytocic. The parturient woman drinks the urine of a male child four to five years old and the part voided in the middle of micturition. The child urinates into three vessels, the woman drinking the contents of the second. In the British Med. Journal of 1900 a number of instances of Western urinotherapy were given (Collected H. W. xxxv, 507). To these Cooper has made some additions. The cases are these (1) A youth for crops of boils which nothing could remedy was recommended to drink every morning, for three morning a cupful of his own Urine. Then after an intermission of 3 days to resume and so on till cured. He was cured on the 9th day. (2) Black head cured in exactly the same way. This patient drank it when fresh. (3) Chronic bronchitis, much relieved. This patient was deaf and misunderstood the doctors direction to bring some of his Urine. He thought drink was the word and acted accordingly (4) Ague in the Lincolnshire Fens. (5) Urticaria. (6) For thrush it was a custom in Yolkshire to wipe the baby's tongue with its own napkin. (7) For pimples and blotches, the negros of Barbados, drink their urine and apply it locally. (8) For ophthalmia in children, it is the custom in Switzerland to bathe the eyes in the children's own Urine. Cooper mentions the case of a man who suffered very much from weak and inflamed eyes until he adopted this plan, which after a time cured him. Cooper also mentions that a celebrated breeder of cattle and horses succeeded in getting his animal's skin into an astonishing condition of fineness by giving them about a tablespoonful of old human urine with every meal - Kraft (AH xxvii-4) mentions that urine has been used as a remedy for croup. S. Mills - Fowler (M. A. xx. 281) mentions the use of urine as a remedy for scurvy in the civil war. These cures are to some extent analogous with nosode cures as the patient drank their own urine, but Urinum, Urea, Uric acid are also medicines on their own account and rank with Sarcodes. The symptoms of Uraemia may be taken as a pathogenesis of Urinum for the use of the attenuations. Urea cured renal dropsy and urinum produced it. The skin action of urinum is remarkable in connection with its use in the dressing of leather, no substitute have been found for it in this.

Relation: Urea (problably Urine owes the chief effect to Urea), *Ur. ac., Urtica urens.*

(JHC)

634. *Urtica Urens*

(Stinging Nettle)

A remedy for agalactia and lithiasis. Profuse discharge from mucous surfaces. Enuresis and urticaria. Spleen affections. Antidotes ill effects of eating shell fish. Symptoms return at the same time every year. Gout and Uric acid diathesis. Favours elimination.

Rheumatism associated with urticaria like eruptions. Neuritis.

Abdomen: Diarrhoea, chronic disease of large intestines, characterised by large secretions of mucus.

Male: Itching of scrotum, keeps him awake, scrotum swollen.

Female: Diminished scretion of milk - Uterine haemorrhage. Acid and excoriating leucorrhoea - Pruritus vulvae with stinging itching - Arrests flow of milk after weaning - Excessive swelling of breasts.

Extremities: Pain in acute gout, deltoid, pain in ankles, wrists.

Skin: Itching blotches. Urticaria, burning heat with formication, violent itching, consequence of suppressed nettle rash - Rheumatism alternates with nettle rash, burn confined to skin. Urticaria nodosa - Burns and scalds - chicken pox - Angioneurotic oedema. Herpes libialis with sensation of heat, itching - itching and stinging of scrotum.

Fever: Fevers of gout - Tropical fever.

Mod: (Worse) from snow air, water, cool, moist air, touch.

Compare: Medusa, Nat. mur, Lac can, Ricin, (diminished mammary secretion) - Bombyx, Rhus, Apis, Chloral, Astac, Puls (Urticaria) Boletus, Luridus and Anacard (Urticaria tuberosa)

Lyco and Hedeoma (Uric acid conditions) - and Formica.

Dose: Tincture and lower pctencies.

(Boericke)

Tincture of the fresh plant in flower - Burnett may be said to have rediscoverd Urtica as a remedy. Its use in gravel and urinary affections is very old. "Being eaten, boiled with periwinkles, it maketh the body soluble, doing it by a kind of cleansing faculty. It also provoketh urine and expelleth stones out of kidneys. Being boiled with barley cream, it is thought to bring up tough humours that stick in the chest." Gerarde quoted: (1) The juice inserted into the nostrils stops nose bleed. It is good against the inflammation of uvula. (2) Pleurisy, Pneumonia, whooping cough. (3) Antidote to Hensbane, Serpents, Scorpions.

The leaves or seeds of any kind of nettle, says Gerarde, do work the like effect, but not with the good speed so assured as the Roman nettle - U. pitulifera - A bundle of nettle, says Cooper, applied to a rheumatic joint or part has long been a favourite country remedy. A leaf of the nettle placed on the tongue and pressed to the roof of the mouth stops bleeding from the nose - Burnetts tincture is made of small nettle - U. Urens - which is the corect one in homoeopathy. Burnett had used Urt. u. a good deal in spleen affections and found patients under its use often passed large quantities of gravel. The middle aged maiden lady who had enlarged spleen and who smelled so strongly of nettles, that it almost nauseated me, whenever it was my duty to examine her. Burnett gave U. Urens - ϕ, whilst taking it, she passed large quantities of gravel. But this did not attract much notice, as the lady was in the habit of passing considerable qunatities of gravel with her motions. Localised abdominal pain, preceeding such an occassion by a number of days. The painful spot just under her spleen, she called her gravel pit - Burnett concluded that Urtica was a remedy for acute gout which should cut short the attack. In a safe manner namely by ridding the economy of the essence of the disease product, its actual suffering producing material. He usually ordered 5 drops of the Tincture in a wine glass full of warm water every two or three hours. Under its action the urine became more plentiful, dark and loaded with uric acid. Burnett remarks of the nettle that it springs up everywhere near human habitation and he has noticed it flourishing more by the side of ditches which carry off fluid sewage. Thus possibly living to some extent on Uric food. A very severe case of Uraemia was cured by him with Urtica. Urt. u. was the sheet - anchor in cases of the fevers of the East - India, Burma and Siam - Urtica causes fevers as well as cures it. Among the rheumatic pains, a pain in the right deltoid muscle is very striking. the action of Urtica in causing flow of milk has been often confirmed. In the case given in Allen it caused swelling of the breasts and profuse flow of milk in a woman years after the birth of her last child. Urt. Urens is one of the best and given internally. Gerarde mentions its antidotal action to snake bites, bee stings. In Sweden nettles are regarded as a remedy for anaemia and fresh nettles are cooked and eaten like spinach for the purpose or a nettle tea is prepared from dry nettles. The juice of nettles with sugar is in vouge for haemorrhages of all kinds. The symptoms are apt to return at the same season every year. Periodicity is a point in the correspondence of Urt. to ague.

Antidoted by - Dock leaves, rubbed on the stung part lessen the pain, also nettles own juice; and juice from the common snail. The relation of Urt. to Nat. m and Urinum is interesting in connection with the fact that nettles do not grow at any distance from human dwellings or away from parts where animals are fed. Is this due to the wetting of the soil with urine? He says, yes and queries further - if the salt in the urine is the efficient agent - recalling from the fact that Barbarossa after destroying Milan, strewed salt over the ruins 'So that nettle might grow there'.

Compare: secretion of Milk - *Ricinus, Puls, Urticaria, Apis, Nat mur, Ast. Fl. Medusa, Homar, Pariet.*

Causation: Burns, Bee stings, Blows, suppressed milk, suppressed nettle rash.
(JHC)

This remedy is indicated in urticaria, dropsical effusions, gout, burns, scalds, and when the milk is diminished. It is useful in urticaria when the skin is elevated. There is a white central spot and a red areola; this is attended with stinging. It is of service in dropsical effusions when the upper portion of the body is greatly swollen, pale, dropsical, and covered with small confluent vesicles that are filled with serum; it is also of service in the anasarca that follows scarlatina when the lower extremities are greatly distended and oedematous. The kidneys are affected and the urine is suppressed.

It should be remembered in erysipelatous inflammation of the extremities when there is burning heat and formication of the skin. The hands and feet are much swollen. It has been employed in menorrhagia, which alternates with an acid leucorrhoea. It has been used in epistaxis and haematemesis. It is a reliable remedy in insufficiency or entire absence of the secretion of milk. It is used in acute gout in ten drop doses.

Compare: Apis mel., Rhus tox., Cantharis, Agnus castus. *(Blackwood)*

635. Usnea Barbata

(Tree - moss) (Bearded Usnea)

Is a remedy in some form of congestive headache; Sunstroke.

Head: As if temples would burst or the eyes burst out of the sockets.

Relation: Glonoine, Bel.

Dose: Tincture and drop. *(Boericke)*

The writer who ate a little of the Moss and had in consequence a severe congestive headache which compelled him to give up his work and go to bed. He got to sleep and woke very well next morning. Two young ladies out picking Cran-Berries had headache from riding in the hot sun and were compelled to lie down. Usnea. b. ϕ one drop in a tumbler of water, a tea spoonful to be taken at once and repeated in fifteen minutes. The second dose stopped the pain. A young married lady subject to headache for 5 years, was almost frantic with the pain. Usn.b. as above, cured in one or two doses. *(JHC)*

This remedy is indicated in congestive headaches, when there is a sensation as though the temples would burst or the eyes would protrude from their sockets. *(Blackwood)*

636. Ustilago Maydis

(Corn Smut)

Burt who proved Ust. on himself and others introduced this remedy to homoeopathy. It has been observed that pregnant animals, feeding on maize affected with smut were very liable to abort - shedding of the hair and some times of teeth, occurred in animals and men - Mules fed on it cast their hoofs and fowls laid eggs without shells. The provings brought out a specific affinity for the generative sphere of both sexes and especially for the left ovary and uterus - Ust. congests the uterus and produces haemorrhages, generally passive or in clots - Uterine haemorrhage, menstrual, post partum and climacteric, Ust. has been used for vicarious menstruation, bleeding from the lungs, bowels, between periods. Loss of hair and nails is a keynote for Ust.

Compare: Bearing down and prolapse of uterus 'Sep' - Pain in right shoulder Urt. ur., Sang. *(JHC)*

Flabby condition of the uterus. Haemorrhage, congestion to various parts, especially at climacteric, crusta lactea (Viola Tric.).

Female: Vicarious menstruation, ovaries burn, pain, swell, profuse menses after miscarriage. Discharge of blood from slightest provocation, bright red, partly clotted, menorrhagia at climaxis, oozing of dark blood, clotted, forming long black strings, uterus hypertrophied, cervix bleeds easily, post partum haemorrhage, profuse lochia.

Skin: Alopecia, small boils, skin dry, eczema, copper coloured spots, pruritus. Sun burn, Psoriasis. (Internally and Externally).

Dose: Tr to 3rd Potency. *(Boericke)*

637. Uva Ursi

(Bear Berry)

Urinary symptoms most important - cystitis with bloody urine - Uterine haemorrhage, chronic vesical irritation, with pain tenesmus and catarrhal discharges. Burning after the discharge of slimy urine. Pyelitis - Calculus, inflammation - dyspnoea - nausea - vomiting, pulse small and irregular, cyanosis, urticaria without itching.

Urinary : Frequent urging with severe spasms of bladder - burning and tearing pain - urine contains blood, pus and much tenacious mucus, with clots in large masses - involuntary, green urine - painful dysuria.

Dose: Tincture 5 - 30 drops - In pyelitis trituration of the leaves. *(Boericke)*

Tincture or trituration of dried leaves and fruit - Tincture of fresh leaves gathered in autumn.

A few experiments have been made with 'Uva' and these have seemed to accentuate its traditional reputation as an astringent used to check excessive secretion of mucus as in urinary and bronchial affections and even in calculus. The keynote indications are - painful micturition with burning sensation. Burning after the discharge of slimy urine - slime passes with blood. In one cured case there were pains shooting through from hip to hip. The bladder symptoms are Amel: lying on the back.

Compare: Arbut, Gaulther. *(JHC)*

This remdy is indicated in cystitis with bloody urine. There is constant urging to urinate, with straining and a discharge of blood, pus and tenacious mucus and large clots of blood. It is serviceable in dysuria and strangury when the urine contains pus or blood.

Compare: Cannabis Sativa.
(Blackwood)

638. Vaccininum

(Nosode - from vaccine matter)

Vaccine poison is capable of setting up a morbid state of extreme chronicity named by Burnett, vaccinosis, symptoms like those of Hahnemann's sycosis. Neuralgias, inveterate skin eruptions, chilliness, indigestion, with great flatulent distention, whooping cough.

Head: Frontal headache.

Relation: Anti vaccinal remedies; Variolin, Malandrinum, Thuja, powerful adjuvants in treatment of malignant disease.

Dose : 6 - 200 Potency. *(Boericke)*

The symptoms of vaccinosis are protean and are for the most part, identical with the symptoms of the sycosis of Hahnemann - vaccinosis is a sycotic disease.

Neuralgias, inveterate skin eruptions, chilliness, indigestion with great flatulent distention are leading features of the Vaccinal dyscrasia and therefore indications for the nosode. There is another disease to which vaccina is related - that is whooping cough. Homoeopathic observers have seen whooping cough follow immediately on vaccination and have cured it with Thuja 30 - where as some years ago an old school observer vaccinated several children while suffering from whooping cough and the whooping cough vanished. *(JHC)*

This is used in the same class of cases as Variolinum *(Blackwood)*

639. *Vaccinium Myrtillus*

(Whortle - Berry, Huckle Berry.)

I have always used it in the Tincture from, generally giving 5 drop doses every 4 hours. It is especially applicable to vaccinal malarial, and dysenteric cases. It is a close relative of Cranberry and the natural order is allied to the Ericaceae. It is a native of healthy and swampy mountainous regions.

Compare: Simaruba, China, Rheum, and Merc. *(JHC)*

Vaccinium Myrtillus - Huckle Berries - dysentery, typhoid, keeps intestine aseptic and prevents absorption and re - infection. *(Boericke)*

640. *Valeriana Officinalis*

(Valerian)

This remedy is indicated in nervous derangements. Hysterical spasm, changeable disposition, irritable, then mild, hallucination as of floating in the air, as if there was a thread hanging down the throat. Gastric disturbances - Sciatica - the pains are worse while standing the foot resting on floor - Rheumatic jerking pain in the heels. *(Blackwood)*

Hysteria, over sensitiveness, nervous affections, when apparently well chosen remedies fail - Hysterical flatulence.

Mind: Changeable disposition, feels light, as if floating in air, oversensitiveness, hallucination at night - irritable - tremulous.

Ears: Earache from exposure to draughts and cold.

Throat: Sensation as if a thread were hanging down throat.

Stomach: Child vomits curdled milk in large lumps after nursing.

Abdomen: Bloated hysterical cramps - thin watery diarrhoea with lumps of coagulated milk with violent screaming in children.

Extremities: Rheumatic pain in limbs - constant jerking, sciatica, pain worse standing and resting on floor - better walking - pain in heels when sitting.

Compare: Asaf, Ign, Croc, Caster.

Dose: Tincture. *(Boericke)*

V. Officinalis is usually found in moist hedge rows or on the banks of ditches and streams. The peculiar fetid odour of Valeriana is probably due to the presence of Valerianic acid. It is especially agreeable to Cats, who become, as it were intoxicated with it. It was the custom among ladies in Germany to take Valerian almost as frequently as coffee and to this practice he attribted no little of the nervous suffering then prevalent. The many inveterated spasms of the stomach and abdomen - the incurable cases of hysteria and hypochondriasis, moral disturbances, passing from one extreme of emotion to another, from the highest joy to the deepest grief, from leniency, kindness and mildness to grumbling, impatience, obstinacy and quarrelsomeness from a sinking of the vital force accompanied by a painful craving for stimulants to the greatest liveliness and extravagance and vice versa. Acceleration of the pulse and congestion of the head. The symptoms of the upper and lower limbs alternate frequently. The principal times of day when Val. produces its symptoms are noon and early afternoon and the hours before midnight - Val. causes several kinds of darting, tearing pains which come and go - Shine before the eyes in the dark, the closed dark room seemed to be filled with shine of twilight, so that he imagined he distinguished the objects in the same - Val. suits to - 1. hysterical women who have taken too much chamomile tea. 2. Nervous irritable hysterical subjects in whom the hysterical faculties predominate and who suffer from hysteria and neuralgia. *(JHC)*

This remedy is indicated in nervous derangements when other remedies have failed, although apparently well indicated. The patient is of a hysterical nervous temperament, and gives to excessive nervous excitability; persons in whom the intellectual faculties predominate. It is useful in hysteria and hysterical spasms, when the patient is of a changeable disposition, irritable, then mild, has hallucinations, feels as if floating in the air, or as if there was a thread hanging down the throat.

It should be remembered in nervous gastric disturbances, in which there is nausea felt in the throat, nausea with hunger, nausea with faintness. Foul eructations, with hysterical cramps and a flat, slimy taste in the mouth early in the morning, insomnia, with muscular spasms, spasmodic asthma, and choking on falling asleep; sciatica, the pains are worse while standing, the foot resting upon the floor. Rheumatic pains in the limbs that are attended with constant jerking pain in the heels.

Compare: Ignatia, Moschus, Pulsatilla, Asafoetida, Castoreum. *(Blackwood)*

641. Vanadium

(The metal)

Its action is that of an oxygen carrier and catalyzer, hence its use in wasting diseases. Increases amount of haemoglobin, also combines its oxygen with toxins and destroys their virulence. Also increases and stimulates phagocytes.

A remedy in degenerative conditions of the liver and arteries - Anorexia and symptoms of gastro - intestinal irritation, albumen casts and blood in urine. Tremors, Vertigo, Hysteria and Melancholia, neuro - retinitis and blindness. Anaemia, emaciation, cough dry, irritating and paroxysmal, sometimes with haemorrhages. Irritation of nose, eyes and throat. Tuberculosis, chronic rheumatism, diabetes. Acts as a tonic to digestive function and in early tuberculosis. Arteriosclerosis, sensation as if heart was compressed, as if blood had no room in the Aorta. Anxious pressure on whole chest. Fatty heart degenerative states, has brain softening. Atheroma of arteries of brain and liver.

Dose: 6 - 12 potency. *(Boericke)*

This remedy is indicated when the hearts action is weak, when there is fatty degeneration of the liver, heart and arterial walls. It is of special benefit in those cases, where anaemia, chronic rheumatism, diabetes, neurasthenia or tuberculosis is the exciting cause. *(Blackwood)*

642. *Vanilla - Panifolia*

(Vanilla)

Marked skin irritation, resembling milk poison-oak, is some times produced by handling the beans, also by local use of Vanilla essence in a hair wash. Vanilla is supposed to stimulate the brain and sexual propensities. Do not use the synthetic Vanilla extract. Various disorders of the nervous system and circulation are produced in workers with Vanilla - Iy is an emmenagogue and Aphrodisiac. Menses prolonged.

Dose: Vanilla 6th and 30th has been found effective in curing the skin affections. *(Boericke)*

643. *Variolinum*

(Lymph from Small pox pustule)

Used for Internal vaccination. Seems to be efficacious in protecting against, modifying and aiding in the cure of small pox.

Head: Morbed fear of small pox - pain in occiput - inflamed eyelids.

Extremities: Excruciating backache. Aching in legs.

Skin: Hot, dry, eruption of pustules, shingles.

Relationship: Vaccin. (Same action) Malandrinum - the morbid product of the grease of horse (a prophylactic of smallpox and a remedy for the ill-effects of vaccination) (Chronic eczema following vaccination).

Dose: Sixth to Thirtieth potency. *(Boericke)*

The cardinal symptoms of smallpox are the keynote symptoms for the use of Variolinum. The backache of smallpox is about the worst backache known and Var. has cured in my practice a number of bad backaches that nothing else seemed to touch - proved an efficient preventive against smallpox contagion and vaccinal infection - (Cardinal symptoms) - Severe cold, chill, chilly creepings as if cold were trickling down the back-violent fever with extremely hot skin with or without high pulse, violent headache, nausea, pain in epigastrium, pain in limbs as if in bones, severe backache, there may be rash or there may not.

Compare: Herpes - Mez., Rhus., Ars.,

Causation: Confusion, enlarged testicles. *(JHC)*

This remedy is employed as a prophylactic against and to modify the course of an attack of small pox - excruciating back ache - great restlessness - aching in legs-fever is intense, profuse, offensive sweat. *(Blackwood)*

644. *Veratrum Album*

(White Hellebore)

A perfect picture of collapse, with extreme coldness, blueness and weakness is offered by this drug. Post operative shock with cold sweat on forehead, pale face, rapid feeble pulse. Cold perspiration on the forehead with nearly all complaints. Vomiting, purging and cramps in extremities. The profuse violent retching and vomiting is most characteristic. Surgical shock - Excessive dryness of all mucous surfaces. Coprophagia -, violent mania, alternates with silence and refusal to talk.

Mind: Sullen indifference, delusions of impending misfortunes - Mania with desire to cut and tear things - cursing howling all night.

Head: Cold sweat on forehead, sensation of a lump of ice on vertex.

Face: Eyes surrounded by dark rings, icy coldness of tip of nose and face, nose grows more pointed, face very pale, blue, collapsed, cold.

Mouth: Tongue - cool sensation as from peppermint, salty saliva.

Stomach: Voracious appetite, thirst for cold water, but is vomited as soon as swallowed, averse to warm food, copious vomiting and nausea, aggravated by drinking and least motion, craves fruit, juicy and cold, things, ice, salt, chronic vomiting of food.

Abdomen: Cold feeling in stomach and abdomen, terrible colic.

Rectum: Stool large, with much straining until exhausted, with cold sweat - Diarrhoea very painful, watery, copious and forcibly evacuated, followed by great prostration, Cholera morbus and true cholera when vomiting accompanied by purging.

Respiratory: Cough on entering warm room from cold air. (Bry).

Heart: Palpitation with anxiety and rapid audible respiration, tobacco heart from chewing - One of the best heart stimulants in homoeopathic doses.

Female: Menses too early, profuse and exhausting - dysmenorrhoea, with coldness, purging, cold sweat. Faints from least exertion, sexual mania precedes menses.

Extremities: Cramps in calves.

Skin: Blue, cold, clammy in-elastic, cold as death, cold sweat, wrinkling of skin of hands and feet.

Fever: Chill with extreme coldness and thirst.

Modalities: Worse at night, wet cold weather.

Relation: Camp, Cupr, Ars, Cuprus ars. (intermittent cold clammy sweat)

Dose: 1 to 30th potency - In diarrhoea not below the sixth. *(Boericke)*

White flowered Veratrum - White Hellebore - The evacuant use of Ver. gives one of the key notes for its homoeopathic use. Its discharges are copious - Copious stools, copious vomiting, copious urine, copious salivation and copious sweat. The discharges drain the tissues like cholera - ranking with Camphor and Cupr. rapid sinking of forces - complete prostration - cold sweat and cold breath - skin blue, purple, cold, wrinkled, remaining in folds, when pinched - nose pointed - hands icy cold - face and legs icy cold. This coldness is another of the keynotes of Ver. Coldness as of a piece of ice on vertex - Cold nose - face cold and collapsed - cold tongue - cold sweat on forehead - blueness of face - it has also heat and redness of face and hands - with the fever delirium and prolonged sleep - fury tears his clothing cursing - stamping - wants to run away - Hahnemann says of Ver. that it has the power to promote a cure of almost 1/3 (one third) of the insane in lunatic asylums - swallows his own excrement - Child had a craze for eating its own faeces or dung lying in the street - Imagines as if she is pregnant - mania for kissing everybody - fainting from emotions. The constipation of Ver. is no less characteristic, no desire, stools large, hard in round black balls, from inactive rectum, frequent desire felt in epigastrium - painful - of infants and children, of women after confinement - Mrs. C. had severe nervous headaches for years

Any over exertion, as riding or working on hot days would excite them. They frequently began in occiput, settling sometimes in one eye sometimes in the other - Spi. and Sil. gave no relief - one day 'Watts' noticed that the brow contracted and eye lids nearly closed with the intensity of the pain - this was cured with Ver - 200 one dose. Heat Aggravates. Cooler the better. The convulsions of Veratrum may be tetanic, with lockjaw or epileptic - leading local symptom is tickling - Electric pains occur in various parts - Lyco. and Nux. in painful constipation of infants - Mania with desire to cut clothes Trn. - (Camph has scanty - Ver copious stools) Delirium, Bell, STram (These have not the cold surface and cold sweat of Ver).

Causation: Fright, shock of injury, disappointed love, injured pride or honour, suppressed exanthema, Opium, tobacco, Alcohol. *(JHC)*

For children and old people, the extremes of life - persons who are habitually cold and deficient in vital reaction, young people of nervous sanguine temperament, rapid sinking of vital forces, complete prostration, collapse - Cold perspiration on the forehead - thinks she is pregnant - mania with desire to cut and tear - Lascivious talk, amorous or religious - sensation of a lump of ice on vertex. Face pale blue, collapsed, features sunken, hippocratic - thirst intense, unquenchable for large quantities of very cold water and acid drinks, wants every thing cold - craving for acids or refreshing things - icy coldness - violent vomiting and profuse diarrhoea - Agg: by drinking - cold sweat on forehead, constipation, no desire, stool large hard - exhausting diarrhoea - bad effects of Opium eating, tobacco chewing - often removes bad effects of excessive use of alcohol and tobacco. *(HCA)*

SYNOPSIS: Collapse, Coldness, Blueness, Cold sweat, Vomiting, Purging, Cramps, Violent mania, Cursing, Howling, Heart stimulant, Cramps, Discharges Copious. As if piece of ice on vertex, Insane, Constipation, Nervous headache, Cooler the better, Tickling, Electric pains, Thirst for very cold water.

645. Veratrum Viride

(White American Hellebore)

Paroxysm of auricular fibrillation - Induces fall of both systolic and diastolic blood pressure. Congestion, especially to lungs, base of brain with nausea and vomiting, twitchings and convulsions. Especially adapted to, full blooded, plethoric persons. Great prostration. Rheumatism, of heart. Bloated, Livid face. Furious delirium. Effects of Sunstroke. Oesophagitis (Farrington). Verat Vir will raise the opsonic index against the diplococcus pneumonia - 70 to 100 percent congestive stage and early manifestations of hepatization in pneumonia. Zigzag temperature. Clinically, it is known that such diseases as Tiegel's Contracture; Thompson's disease, athetosis and pseudo-hypertrophic muscular paralysis present a symptomatology quite like that produced by Veratrum vir. upon muscular Tissues.

Mind: Quarrelsome and delirious.

Head: Congestion, intense, pupils dilated, pain from nape of neck, face flushed, convulsive twitching of facial muscles.

Tongue: Increased saliva.

Stomach: Nausea and vomiting, smallest quantity of food or drink immediately rejected - Hiccough - Spasm of oesophagus.

Respiratory: Congestion of lungs, croup.

Female: Menstrual Colic - strangury.

Heart: Pulse, slow, soft, weak irregular, intermittent, rapid, low tension, beating of pulses throughout body.

Extremities: Aching pain in back of neck and shoulders, acute rheumatism, fever.

Skin: Itching to various parts, heat, sweating.

Fever, hyper-thermy in the evening and hypothermy in the morning.

Dose: 1st to 6th potency.

(Boericke)

Millspaugh, however, says that, though much like Veratrum Alb. in its minor points - Ver. Vir is strikingly different in general appearance having a much more pointed leave, panicles looser and more compound the racemes of Ver. a. being more compact and as a whole cylindrical, those of Ver. v. scattered, compound, and scraggy - Ver. a. flourishes in moutain meadows. Ver. v. grows in swamps and wet meadows and along mountain creeks from Canada to the California. Hale was chiefly instrumental in introducing Ver. v. to homoeopathy using it in fevers and particularly in pneumonia constant aching pains in back of neck and shoulders - the great keynote of Ver. v. is congestion - rapid congestion of the lungs. The localities most congested by Ver. V. are base of brain, chest, spine, stomach - slowing of heart's action is a leading effect - Ver. v. has been used to knock down fever in the same way as Acon. Nash points out that there is some risk in this. In chorea Ver. v. has had many successes - twitching during sleep - constant jerking or nodding of the head - jerking and trembling, threatened with convulsions are other leading symptoms. In muscular and articular rheumatism, it has been used locally as well as internally and in chorea an application to the spine of the tincture diluted with spirit has proved a serviceable adjunct. Head full, throbbing of arteries, sensitive to sound, double or partial vision. A key note symptom is Red streak down the centre of the tongue. Ver. v. has a pronounced action on the oesophagus - it causes a sort of ruminating action or reversed peristalsis. Numbness is prominent among the effects of Ver. V, dim sight - numbness, pain in head as if a tight band were round it - confused feeling in head as if head would burst - Ver. v has marked arterial tension - (Tetanus) Nux, Hyperic. (Nodding of head) Lyc, Stram (Neck muscles weak) Ant. t. Ver. a.

Causation: Sun, suppressed menses, suppressed lochia. *(JHC)*

Geen Hellebore - For full blooded, plethoric persons, congestion, especially to base of brain, chest, spine, and stomach - Acute rheumatism, high fever, full hard rapid pulse, severe pains in joints and muscles (Bry, Sal.ac) - child jerks, threatened with convulsions continual jerking or nodding of the head, congestive apoplexy, hot head, blood shot eyes, slow full pulse, hard as iron - Basilar meningitis - cerebro spinal disease, with spasms, dilated pupils, tetanic convulsions, opisthotonos, cold, clammy perspiration - sun stroke head full, throbbing of arteries, sensitive to sound, double or partial vision - tongue white or yellow with red streak down the middle - pulse suddenly increases and gradually decreases below normal, slow, soft, weak, irregular, intermittent. *(HCA)*

SYNOPSIS: Fall of both systolic and diastolic pressure. Congestion lungs, base of brain - Twitching and convulsions - delirium - sun stroke - twitching of facial muscles - Hiccough - spasm of oesophagus - pulse slow soft - beating of pulse throughout the body - pain back, neck and shoulders - fever, hyper - thermy in the evening and hypo - thermy in the morning - slowing of heart's action - chorea - twitching during sleep - jerking or nodding of the head - red streak down the centre of the tongue - numbness - full hard rapid pulse - apoplexy - basilar meningitis.

646. *Verbascum Thapsus*

(Mullein oil)

Tincture of fesh plant at the commencement of flowering (Mullein oil is prepared by placing the crushed yellow blossoms in a bottle which is corked and allowed to stand in the sun; or by steeping the blossom in oil and keeping in a warm place till the oil has absorbed them - Gerarde)

The thick wooly leaves of V. thapsus the great mullein have a mucilaginous bitterish taste and a decoction of them is employed in domestic practice in catarrhs and diarrhoea. They are also used as emollient applications to hard tumours and in pulmonary complaints in cattle - hence one of its popular names is Bullock's Lungs - Wort. It is also called Adams flannel from its flannel - like leaves. It produced neuralgic pains of great intensity, pressing and lancinating and especially in the facial bones, navel and limbs and a peculiar cough - Cough deep, hollow, hoarse in sound, like a trumpet is Nash's description. He has cured many cases and always used low - more especially in night cough. It occurs in children during their sleep. Some years ago Mullein was brought forward as a popular specific for phthisis, the leaves being boild in milk which was then strained and given warm. Among the traditional uses Gerarde mentions it as a remedy for piles and I do not know a better application for itching haemorrhoids or pruritus ani than an ointment made of the tincture in the proportions of one drachm to one Oz. of Catacean ointment. I generally direct it to be applied at bed time. Gerarde says that the oil of the yellow flowers is also curative in oils. The flowers contain a yellow volatile oil and fatty acid, free Malic and Phosphoric acids and salts of lime, a yellow resinous colouring matter and the general plant consituents including an uncrystallisable Sugar - Cushing prepared from the flowers an oil (1) By putting the blossoms in a bottle and laying the bottle in the sun and later by expression. The mullein oil has found many uses and especially for instilling in the ears in cases of deafness or earache, in cases of enuresis nocturna (Cushing had good success with the 3x) and painful micturition. The provings brought out some very marked symptoms in the ears especially the left ear (Verb is predominently left sided) W. B. Mc Coy gives several illustrations. According to him Verb has a soothing effect on the entire nervous system, in many cases acting as a soporific. In summer diarrhoea he gives 1 to 4 drops in 2 Ounces of warm water, a teaspoonful every hour. In enuresis or dribbling of urine one drop doses in warm water 3 - 4 times a day - salt water collects in mouth is a guiding symptom. *(JHC)*

Mullein oil is a sun distilled extract of the fresh flowers. This remedy is of service in cases of nervous and bronchial irritation with cough, urinary irritation and painful micturition - cases of migraine with a sensation as though the temples were crushed together. Neuralgic pain about the zygoma, ear and temporo - maxillary joint upon the left side. These pains are aggravated by a change of the temperature, talking, sneezing or biting the teeth together.

It is indicated when there is a deep, hollow, hoarse cough that sounds like a trumpet; which is worse towards evening, there is a hoarseness, when reading aloud, also stitching in chest. It is useful in nocturnal enuresis and in constant dribbling of the urine. Mullein oil is used locally for earache. *(Blackwood)*

647. Vesicaria - Communis

This is an old remedy much used in some parts of Germany for all forms of urinary and kidney difficulties, for gravel, for gonorrhoea, both in the male and female. Shafers' - indication for the remedy is a smarting burning sensation along the course of the urethra and bladder, with frequent desire to void urine, often accompanied with strangury - Nephralgia, acute cystis, irritable bladder, following acute cystitis, chronic cystitis - Vesic. ϕ in 15 drop doses every fifteen minutes, gave marked relief in 2 hours, which in six hours was completed. Man, 65, irritable bladder, had to rise 20 to 30 times in the night - Vesic. ϕ in 20 drop doses relieved quickly and cured in 6 weeks. Gonorrhoea with smarting and burning on micturition and thick creamy discharge - Vesic. ϕ a drachm every four hours, soon cured. Mrs. P., general dropsy of years' standing - uraemic spasms when first seen - the kidneys having ceased to secrete urine. Vesic. ϕ was prescribed 15 drops in a teaspoonful of water every 4 hour, till urine was freely secreted, then three times a day. The second day the kidneys were pouring out urine and watery stools were passed. In a week all dropsy had disappeared.

Relation: (In gravel) Oc. c.; Urt. u; Thlaspi. b. pastoris; (Prostatic affections) Hydrang; Solid; Sabal; (Cystitis) Chimaph. u. *(JHC)*

Vesicaria - Urinary and kidney remedy, smarting, burning sensation along urethra and in bladder with frequent desire to void urine often with strangury, cystitis, irritable bladder. Tincture 5 to 10 drops.

Compare - Cantharis. *(Boericke)*

648. Vespa Crabro

(Live Wasp)

Skin and female symptoms marked. Indurated feeling, vasomotor symptoms of skin and mucous membranes.

Dizzy, better lying on back. Fainting, numbness and blindness, nausea and vomiting followed by creeping chills from feet upward. Cramping pain in bowels. Axillary glands swollen with soreness of upper arms. Perspiration on parts laid on with itching.

Face: Chemosis of conjuctiva, swelling of mouth and throat with violent burning pains .

Urinary: Burning with micturition.

Female: Left ovary markedly affected with frequent burning micturition, sacral pains extending up back - Erosion around external os.

Skin: Erythema, intense itching burning, boils, stinging and soreness, relieved by bathing with vinegar, wheals, macules, and swelling with burning, stinging and soreness.

Dose: 3 to 30th Potency.

Vespa Vulgaris - Wasp - Hornet - Yellow - jacket. The symptoms are mostly the result of stings - Oedema of conjunctiva - Chemosis of the right eye - redness of right lower lid - baggy swelling of conjunctiva, partly covering the cornea. E. T. Blake cured with Vespa - 1, the following group of symptoms. Face swollen and puffy, skin transparent and blanched, scalding urine, followed by itching, itching of right arm.

Relations: Antidoted by: Apis, Led, Camph, Salt water, Vinegar.

Incompatible: Arg. Nit. *(JHC)*

This remedy is indicated in erysipelatous inflammation of the eyelids and chemosis of the conjuctiva. The whole face is swollen and painful. It is useful in congestion of the left ovary. Menstruation is preceded by pain and distress.

Compare: Apis. *(Blackwood)*

649. Viburnum Opulus

(High Cranberry)

A general remedy for cramps. Colicky pain in pelvic organs. Superconscious of internal sexual organs. Female symptoms most important. Often prevents miscarriage. False labor - pains - spasmodic and congestive affections, dependent upon ovarian or uterine origin.

Abdomen: Sudden cramps and colic pains. Tender to pressure about umblicus.

Female: Menses too late, scanty, lasting a few hours, offensive in odor, with crampy pains, cramps extend down thighs (Bel). Bearing down pains before. Ovarian region feels heavy and congested. Aching in sacrum and pubes, with pain in anterior muscles of thighs (Xanthox), spasmodic and membranous dysmenorrhoea (Borax). Leucorrhoea excoriating, smarting and itching of genitals, faint on attempting to sit up. Frequent and very early miscarriage, causing seeming sterility - Pains from back to loins and womb, worse early morning.

Urinary: Frequent urging, ciopious, pale, light coloured.

Rectum: Stools large and hard with cutting in rectum.

Extremities: Stiff sore feeling in nape of neck - feels as if back would break - Sacral backache. Lower extremities weak and heavy.

Mod: (worse), lying on affected side, in warm room, evening and night. (Better) in open air and resting.

Compare: Viburnum prunifolium.

Dose: Tincture and lower potencies. *(Boericke)*

Viburnum Opulus, a native of great Britain is widely distributed over the Northern parts of the continent and America. In America, the wild spepcies is called, 'Cramp back' and the knowledge of its curative virtues in painful, spasmodic diseases, especially in dysmenorrhoea is derived from the American aborgines. The tincture has a strong odour of Valerianic acid. Hale derived his knowledge from domestic sources - (1) In spasmodic dysmenorrhoea he gives a few drops of ϕ to 3X TDS (Thrice daily) for a week before the period; every hour when the pains set in, or every fifteen minutes, if the pains are severe. (2) False pains preceding labour. (3) After pains, a dose after each pain. (4) Cramps in abdomen and legs of pregnant women. (5) To prevent miscarriage when the pains are spasmodic or threatening - The left side is much more powerfully affected than the right - Vib. O. is suited to tall, slender, dark or fair haired hysterical subjects.

Compare: Cramp like abdominal pains and menstrual symptoms, 'Caulo' - Pains coming round pelvis to uterus, goneness, bearing down, feeling that organs will escape from vulva and wants support, nervousness. Sep - (with Vib. the bearing down is more violent and culminates in uterus in cramps) - Uterine cramps - (Caul., Sec., Act. r.) *(JHC)*

This remedy is of service in cases where there is irregular spasmodic pain in the region of the uterus and ovaries. It also relieves spasmodic constrictions of the bladder and other abdominal organs which are reflex from uterine irritation.

It should be remembered in uterine irritation that results from hysteria, also neuralgic, membranous and spasmodic dysmenorrhoea with intense cramping pains in the uterus. The menses are often late, they are scanty, spasmodic, lasting but a short time, with a heavy and congested feeling in the ovarian region and pains that extend down the anterior surfaces of thighs. There are hysterical convulsions, general irritation of the nervous system and spasmodic dysuria in hysterical subjects who suffer from uterine or ovarian irritation. It is useful in cramps in the feet after long walks, cramps in the extremities, worse during pregnancy followed by a paretic condition of the part.

Compare: Vib. Prunifolium, Xanthoxylum. *(Blackwood)*

650. Viburnum Prunifolium

(Black Haw)

Hale quotes experiences, showing a close resemblance between Vib. P and Vib.O. E. P. Fowler cured two cases of cancer of the tongue with the decoction of Vib. P. bark, used topically. Phares thinks it perhaps the best remedy in the world of tetanus. Hale used the tincture in the threatened miscarriage, dysmenorrhoea, and spasmodic uterine pains. Phares says of it: It is particularly valuable in preventing abortion and miscarriage, whether habitual or otherwise, whether threatened from accidental causes or criminal drugging and he gives cases in support of each. It entirely antidotes the effects of Gossy. which is much used for procuring abortion in some of the states : one pint of strong decoction of the Cotton root, being sufficient. Vib. P. taken regularly completely neutralises this.

Relation: Antidote to Gossy. *(JHC)*

This remedy should be studied in cases of threatened miscarriage and in cases of habitual abortion, in cases where there is uterine colic and irritability, dysmenorrhoea with scanty menses attended with severe, expulsive, menstrual pain, also in pains of the back, bearing down after pains and the false pains of pregnancy. It is emloyed to prepare women for labor and is said to facilitate labor to control after-pain, prevent post-partum haemorrhage and assist the normal involution of the uterus. It is of service in controlling the morning sickness of pregnancy in relieving sympathetic disturbances of the heart, stomach and nervous system of sensitive females before the menstrual period. It should be given some time before and continued through the period. It is often indicated in the menstrual irregularity of sterile females who are suffering from uterine displacements also. In cases of hysteria and hysterio-epilepsy in those suffering from uterine irritation and menstrual irregularities.

It controls the haemorrhages during the menstrual epoch in those suffering from smallpox.

Compare: Sabina, Viburnum Op., Mitchella. *(Blackwood)*

651. Vinca Minor

(Lesser Periwinkle)

A remedy for skin affections, eczema and especially Plica polonica, also for haemorrhages and diphtheria.

Head: Spots on scalp, oozing moisture, matting hair together. Corrosive itching of scalp, bald spots, Plica polonica, irresistible desire to scratch.

Nose: Tip gets red easily, moist eruption on septum, sores in nose, seborrhoea upper lip and base of nose.

Female: Passive uterine haemorrhage, menorrhagia, continuous flow, particularly at climacteric.

Skin: Corrosive itching, great sensitiveness of skin, with redness and soreness from slight rubbing. Eczema of head and face, pustules itching, burning and offensive odor. Hair matted together.

Relation: Oleand, Staph.

Dose: 1-3 potency. *(Boericke)*

In passive uterine haemorrhages - Vinca has a wide range - Uterine haemorrhage, blood dark red, flow copious, uninterrupted with extreme debility. Chi. and Helon. failed to relieve - Frequent nose bleed is another effect of Vinca., a curious symptom in connection with the nose, which it is well to remember, becomes red from the slightest cause, when least bit angry. There are scabby eruptions about the nose and on the septum, which are part of the general skin effect of the remedy. It causes corrosive itching of the skin, provoking scratching, moist spots and burning in ulcers - crusta lactea, favus and plica polonica - Constipation from induration of faeces - Haemorrhoids constantly sore, smarting after stool - A peculiar symptom was distension of abdomen after-Tooth ache, Amel: in warmth of bed is unusual. Coffea causes nausea. *(JHC)*

This remedy is indicated in eczema of the scalp and face. The spots ooze a moisture which smells offensive. It mats the hair together (Plica Polonica) and crusts from which retain the discharges. It has been employed in the relief of diphtheria and passive uterine haemorrhages, when skin symptoms were present.

Compare: Oleander, Staphisagria.
(Blackwood)

652. Viola Odorata

(Violet)

Has a specific action on the ear. Affects especially dark haired patients, supra-orbital and orbital regions, rheumatism in upper parts of the body, on the right side. Worms affections in children, locally for pain due to uterine fibroids. Also against snake bites, bee stings. Tension extends to upper half of face and ears.

Head: Burning of forehead - scalp tense, must knit the brows, tendency to pain immediately above eye brows. Head ache across the fore-head. Acts upon frontal sinuses.

Eyes: Flames before eyes, fiery serpentine circles.

Ears: Otorrhoea - ear affections with pain in eyeballs.

Respiratory: Dyspnoea during pregnancy.

Extremities: Pressing pain in right carpal and meta - carpal joints.

Urinary: Milky urine.

Compare: Chenopodium.

Dose: 1 - 6 potency. *(Boericke)*

Sweet scented violet-contain emetine and under which Ipec. is some times placed - Tincture of fresh plant in flower.

Aversion to music, especially the violin is one of the peculiar symptoms. Tension of the occiput and forehead -tension of the scalp of occiput, even when not moving, though Agg: bending head forward and backward, painful, compelling him to wrinkle fore-head, lasting several days-oppression in the eyeballs, heat and burning of the eyes-Fiery appearances (Fiery semicircle before the eyes, stinging in the eyes) - (otorrhoea of both ears, Agg: right (from birth) - (Viola odorata ϕ - one dose) - great quantity of ill smelling discharge came from the right ear with immediate improvement - Rheumatism, right sided, affection for the wrist - suited to 'Tall thin nervous girls' 'mild impressive girls of fair complexion'.

Both Viola and Ipec. have been used externally as remedies for stings and snake bites - Teste puts Viola in the Chelidonium group and finds a striking analogy between these two remedies. *(JHC)*

This remedy is indicated in dark complexioned patients with otorrhoea - There is deafness, with sharp stitching pains in the ear, also frontal headache. The scalp is tense, there is burning of the forehead and vertigo. *(Blackwood)*

653. Viola Tricolor

(Pansy)

The principal uses of this remedy are for eczema in childhood and nocturnal emission accompanied by very vivid dreams.

Head: Eczema of sclap - face hot and sweating after eating.

Urinary: Copious, disagreable, cat-like odor.

Male: Swelling of prepuce, burning in glans.

Skin: Impetigo, intolerable itching, eruption particularly over face and head with burning, itching, worse at night, thick scabs, which crack and exude a tenacious yellow pus. Eczema impetigonoides of the face, sycosis.

Mod: Worse winter, 11 a.m. *Compare: Lyco.*

Relation: Compare - Rhus, Calc, Sepia.

Dose: Lower potencies. *(Boericke)*

It had an ancient reputation in Asthma and epilepsy and especially in obstinate skin diseases - Milk crust in children at the breast or recently weaned - Milk crust with violent cough and excessive oppression - Impetigo of hairy scalp and face in children and adult females. Favus and serpiginous crusts in children and adults, with swelling and induration of cervical glands - Large boils all over body in a scrofulous child - Pustules and ichorous exanthema of feet -

squamous spots on skin - Rheumatism and gout - articular rheumatism with itch-like eruption around the joints - Impetigonous exanthema on forehead - ichorous ulcers with viloent itching - Tinea capitis with frequent involuntary urination - Eczema with urinary disturbances, too copious urination or sudden arrest of scretion - urine smelling like cat's urine, is a key note. The male sexual organs were much excited - Swelling, itching and pains in prepuce and glans with erections - Face hot and sweating after eating - Hands twitch and are clenched in sleep. *(JHC)*

This remedy is indicated in crusta lactea with a copious exudation and mats the hair, in eczema, when there is burning and itching which is worse at night. The urine is copious and has the odour of Cat's urine.

Compare: Calc. carb and Rhus tox.
(Blackwood)

654. Vipera
(The German Viper)

Viper poisoning causes a temporary increase in reflexes. Paresis supervenes, a paraplegia of the lower extremities extending upwards. Resembles acute ascending paralysis of Landry (Wells). Has special action on kidneys and induces haematuria. Cardiac dropsy.

Indicated in inflammation of veins with great swelling, bursting sensation. Enlargement of liver.

Face: Excessively swollen, lips and tongue swollen, livid, protruding. Tongue dry brown black, speech difficult.

Extremities: Patient is obliged to keep the extremities elevated - when they are allowed to hang down, it seems as if they would burst and the pain is unbearable (DIAD) - Varicose veins and acute phlebitis - Veins swollen sensitive, bursting pain, severe cramps in lower extremities.

Skin: Peels in large plates - lymphangioma, boils, carbuncles with bursting sensation (relieved by elevating parts).

Compare: Eel Serum heart and kidney disesaes. Failure of compensation and impending asystole.

Dose: 12th potency. *(Boericke)*

Attenuations of the Venom - Vipera affects the blood-vessels, conducing to haemorrhage and inflammation of the vessels themselves - A keynote for Vip. in cases of phlebitis and Varicosis is Agg : on letting the limb affected hang down, as if it would burst with fulness. The region of the vessel affected is inflamed and sensitive - A Goldbeater found the veins of his right arm become exceedingly swollen and painul, so that he could no longer work or let his hand hang down - Vip. cured immediately. A case of varicose vein of the popliteal space with the sensation, as though the leg would burst and a nervous fidgety condition of the feet which kept them in constant motion was cured with Vipera Torva - 30. The bursting feeling appears to be the root of this characteristic. "Swan" said, Vip. was a remedy for all forms of Expistaxis. Vip. has a chronic and periodic action; the symptoms return anually for years. A lady suffering from climateric haemorrhage, flow red with dark clots, excessive to prostration and faintness. She had a small uterine fibroid. A few doses relieved and the excessive haemorrhage did not return. A lady nursing a child prostrated by haemorrhage lasting several weeks, not profuse but continuous, nose bleed nearly every day - Chi. 200 did no good. Vip. CM cured in three doses.

Agg: by touch, pressure, change of weather, letting limb hang down.

Relation : Haemorrhage of fluid blood, Sanguesuga, Agg : hanging down limbs, Calc, Alm, Am. c., Sbi., Thu., (JHC)

This remedy is indicated in phlebitis and varicose veins, when there is a sensation as though the parts would burst. The patient seeks relief by having the extremity elevated. *(Blackwood)*

655. Viscum Alb
(Mistle toe)

Lowered blood pressure. Dilated blood vessels, but does not act on the centres in the medulla. Pulse is slow due to central irritation of the vagus. The symptoms point especially to rheumatic and gouty complaints, neuralgia especially sciatica, epilepsy, chorea, and metrorrhagia - Rheumatic deafness, Asthma, spinal pains due to uterine causes. Rheumatism with tearing pains. Hypertensive albuminuria, valvular disease with disturbances in sexual sphere. Symptoms like epileptic aura and petit mal.

Head: Facial muscle in constant agitation. Persistent vertigo.

Respiratory: Dyspnoea, feeling of suffocation when lying on left side, spasmodic cough. Asthma, if connected with gout or rheumatism.

Female: Climacteric complaints. Pain from sacrum into pelvis, with tearing shooting pains from above downwards. Chronic endometritis, ovaralgia especially left.

Heart: Hypertrophy with valvular insufficiency - Pulse small and weak, unable to rest in a reclining position, low tension, failing compensation, dyspnoea worse lying on left side, weight and oppressin of heart as if hands were squeezing it, tickling sensation about heart.

Extremities: Pains alternate in the knee and ankle with shoulder and elbow. Sciatica, tearing, shooting pains in both thighs and upper extremities. A glow rises from the feet to the head, seems to be on fire. Periodic pains from sacrum into pelvis, worse in bed with pains into thighs and upper extremities. General tremor, as if all muscles were in state of fibrillary contraction, dropsy of extremities.

Relation: Guipsine - active principle - exalts the hypotensive properties of viscum.

Dose: Tincture and lower potencies.

(Boericke)

Mistle toe - Tincture of ripe berries - Tincture of bruised leaves - Tincture of whole plant - developed symptoms resembling epileptic aura and petit mal, which had the additional epileptic feature of recurrence - The bowels being obstinately constipated - The muscles of speech were also paralysed - According to 'Laville' all mistletoes are useful in epilepsy and rabies - Lumbago, from chill, tearing pain, wants something to press aginst it - Lumbago right, extending to right buttock. Agg : by slightest movement - Pain in sacral region, unable to turn either side - applicable to all kinds of Rheumatism, acute and chronic, especially when characterised by tearing pains, in cases occuring in winter, the result of exposure to sharp winds. *(JHC)*

The remedy has been employed in epilepsy, chorea and neuralgia, especially sciatica, also rheumatism when the pains alternate in the knee and ankle, the shoulder and elbow.

Compare: Bry., Pulsatilla. (Blackwood)

656. *Wiesbaden*

(The spring at Wiesbaden in Prussia)

Gout and rheumatism are the chief affections for which wiesbaden is sought.

Hair grows much more rapidly than usual, falls out and grows again rapidly, new growth darker, formerly soft, becómes hard and brittle - Corns and Callosities dropped off. 'Berridge' cured with Wies 200. A 'Miss. B.' 21 of a soft corn between 4th and 5th toes of right foot.

Compare: Nat. m, (Corns) Ferrum pic. (Callosities) Anti crud, (Hair turns darker) Jabor, Pilo, Wild. *(JHC)*

657. *Wyethia*

(Poison - Weed)

Has marked affect on the throat and has proven an excellent remedy in pharyngitis, especially the follicular form. Irritable throats of singers and public speakers. Useful also in haemorrhoids, Hay fever symptoms. Itching in posterior nares.

Mouth: Itching of palate.

Throat: Constant clearing and hemming - dry posterior nares, throat feels swollen, epiglottis dry and burning, difficult swallowing, constant desire to swallow saliva, uvula feels enlongated.

Stool: Itching of anus, constipation with haemorrhoids, no bleeding.

Respiratory: Dry hacking cough, burning sensation in the bronchial tubes.

Dose: 1st to 6th potency. *(Boericke)*

Important place in throat affections - throat feels swollen, epiglottis dry and has a burning sensation, constant desire to swallow saliva to relieve dryness yet affording no comfort, swallows with difficulty - prickling dry sensation in posterior nares - Hale gives these cases from 'Selfridge' (1) Dry asthma in a lady, Wyeth. gave prompt relief in several paroxysms. (2) Chronic follicular pharyngitis with dryness of pharynx and burning in epiglottis. In severe epidemic of influenza

Hale found Wyeth most successful - other noteworthy symptoms are tough, ropy, saliva - peculiar sensations are - mouth as if scalded - uvula as if elongated. Epiglottis feels dry and burning. *(JHC)*

This remedy is indicated in follicular pharyngitis, when there is constant hemming to clear the throat, without relief, there is a desire to swallow. The parts feel dry and as if swollen.

It is of service in the irritated throats of public speakers and singers, also for a dry, hacking cough that is dependent upon a tickling that is referred to the epiglottis. There is a sensation of burning in the bronchial tubes.

It is useful in haemorrhoids that are associated with constipation. There is itching in the anus. *(Blackwood)*

658. *Xanthoxylum Fraxineum*

(Prickly Ash)

This remedy is indicated in chronic rheumatism and catarrhal conditions involving the bile duct and pharynx. It is of service in the ailments of weak delicate women who suffer from profuse menstruation and spasmodic and neuralgic dysmenorrhoea, the pains extending along the course of the anterior crural nerve. It has cured after pains and ovarian neuralgia, when the pain extended down the anterior surface of the thigh. Accompanying these conditions there is mental depression, throbbing headache, a bewildered state of mind, with loss of appetite and a sensation of fulness in the epigastric region.

Compare: Cimicifuga, Gnaphalium. Viburnum. *(Blackwood)*

In dysmenorrhoea Xan. has a wide range - dysmenorrhoea and amenorrhoea - Cullis thinks Xan. especially suited to women of spare habit, nervous temperament and delicate organisations. Leucorrhoea with amenorrhoea, he regards as a strong indication. Uterine fibroid - fetid yellowish white discharge from vagina. Xan - 3x.

Compare: (Uterus) Act. r. (Dysmenorrhoea with reflex neuralgia) Coloc., (Dysmenorrhoea and sciatica, numbness) Gnaphalium; (Dysmenorrhoea), Vib. O., Caulophyllum. *(JHC)*

659. Xerophyllum

(Tamalpais Lily, Basket grass flower)

Should prove curative in eczematous conditions, poison oak, early typhoid states.

Mind: Dull, cannot concentrate mind for study, forgets names, writes last letters of words first, mis-spells common words.

Skin: Erythema, with vesication and intense itching, stinging, and burning blisters, little lumps, skin rough and cracked, feels like leather, dermatitis especially around knees, inflammation resembling poison oak, inguinal glands and behind knee swollen.

Compare: Rhus, Anacard, Grindelia.

Dose: 6th or higher. *(Boericke)*

660. X-ray

(Vial containing alcohol exposed to X-ray)

Repeated exposure to Roentgen (X-ray) has produced skin lesions often followed by cancer. Distressing pain. Sexual glands are particularly affected - Atrophy of ovaries and testicles. Sterility. Changes take place in the blood, lymphatics and bone marrow. Anaemia and leukaemia - Corresponds to stubborness as in burns, they refuse to heel - Psoriasis.

Has the property of stimulating cellular metabolism - Arouses the reactive vitality mentally and physically. Brings to the surface suppressed symptoms, especially sycotic and those due to mixed infections. Its homoeopathic action is thus centrifugal, towards the periphery.

Head: Sticking pains in different parts of head and face. Dull pain in right upper jaw - stiff neck, sudden cricks in neck, pain more severe behind ears. Pain in muscles of neck, when lifting head from pillow. Fullness in ears, ringing in head.

Mouth: Tongue dry, rough, sore throat, painful on swallowing - Nausea.

Male: Lewd dreams - Sexual desire lost, re - establishes suppressed gonorrhoea.

Extremities: Rheumatic pains, general tired and sick feeling, palms rough and scaly.

Skin: Dry itching eczema, Erythema around roots of nails, skin dry, wrinkled, painful cracks, warty growths. Nails thicken, Psoriasis.

Modalities: Worse in bed, afternoon, evening and night, open air.

Dose: 12th potency and higher.

(Boericke)

Hering's reputation in the Homoeopathic world stands out in splendid isolation by his admirable proving of Lachesis. In a similar way we find Beruhardt Fincke having proved X-ray, has left behind him a priceless legacy, in view of the fact that its possibilities in the cure of many of the most obstinate chronic diseases appear limitless.

The administration of this dynamic agent on the constitution of a patient suffering from the chronic deep seated effect of a combination of miasms, leads to the rousing up of the reactive vitality of the system , thereby bringing to the surface the dormant to its reaction on the system, defying the curative effect of indicated remedies, sycotic disorder in particular, would have progressed to culminate in a crisis, especially by producing cancer.

Indications: Desire for sweets, can eat plenty but does not enjoy it - Frequent urination worse after getting to bed - sexual desire lost in a man - Testes relaxed - impotent feeling - Rheumatic pain in right wrist and arm - The antidotes of X-ray are Nux. v and Sulph. and the dynamic potencies of the remedy - Mental processess not clear, writes wrong words in letters would like to kill some body - Sudden cricks attack first one side of the neck, then the other - bloody mucus from the nose - Sulphur vapor sensation in throat and nose - Aversion to meat - Most distress after midday and evening meal - Bitter taste - can't hold things in left hand, powerless or clumsy - Sciatica pain in right hip - Rheumatic pain in limbs - Profuse perspiration of getting into bed, keeping him awake - Symptoms worse when getting into bed, after sun set.*(HCA)*

661. Yohimbinum

(Coryanthe Yohimbe)

Excites sexual organs and acts on central nervous and respiratory centre. An aphrodisiac used in physiological doses, but contra - indicated in all acute and chronic inflammations of abdominal organs. Homoeopathically of service in congestive conditions of the sexual organs. Causes hyperemia of the milk glands and stimulates the function of lactation. Menorrhagia.

Sexual: Strong and lasting erections, neurasthenic impotence, bleeding piles, intestinal haemorrhage, Urethritis.

Sleep: Sleepless, thoughts of events of whole past life, keep him awake.

Dose: As a sexual stimulant - 10 drops of a one percent solution or hypodermic, tabs of 0.005 gms.

Homoeopathic - 3rd potency.

(Boericke)

The natives of West Africa discovered a potent Aphrodisiac in the bark of the Yohimbeha tree and from this an active principle has been isolated and tested in Europe. It is a powerful stimulant of the genital function in males. In animals it causes increased liveliness and cheerfulness, hyperaemia of the conjunctiva, heat and redness of the ears and of the nose in dogs. Eulenburg used Yohimb. in 10 drop doses of a 1% solution and in 5 mg tabs in cases of neurasthenic impotence with excellent results. Yohim. should be a homoeopathic remedy in priapism and congestive state of the sexual organs.

(JHC)

Joshimbin - It greatly increases the sexual desire in men and in animals. Useful for anaemic, thin, nervous and partly impotent men. Neurasthenic impotence. If given in too large doses, it causes, severe feverish conditions. *(Blackwood)*

662. *Yucca Flamentosa*

(Bear Grass)

So called bilious symptoms, with headache, despondent and irritable.

Head: Aches as if top of head would fly off. Arteries of forehead throb, nose red.

Face: Yellow, tongue yellow, coated, taking imprint of teeth (Merc, Podo, Rhus).

Mouth: Taste of rotten eggs (Arnica).

Throat: Sensation as if something hung down from posterior nares, cannot get it up or down.

Abdomen: Deep pain in right side over liver, going through back, stool yellow brown with bile.

Male: Burning and swelling of prepuce with redness of meatus, gonorrhoea.

Skin: Erythematous redness.

Dose: Tincture to 3rd potency. *(Boericke)*

Yocca was proved by Rowell and four others in the 30th. Farrington gives these indications - biliousness with pain going through upper part of liver to back. Bad taste in mouth - Stools diarrhoeic and contain an excess of bile. Much flatus passed by rectum - Frontal or temporal headache with frequent flushing of face. Face sallow. Tongue coated yellow and taking imprint of teeth. Dull ache in centre of liver - Abdomen sensitive. Frequent passage of flatus and of watery, yellowish brown stools. The tongue of Yucca is usually bluish white as with many liver disorders. There is chilliness - cannot bear to be away from the fire. *(JHC)*

This remedy is indicated in hepatic congestion, there is pain through the upper portion of the liver to the back. The face is yellow, the tongue has a yellow coating and takes the imprint of teeth. The stools contain much bile and are diarrhoeic in character. It is also of service in Balanitis and Gonorrhoea, when there is burning and swelling of the prepuce with irritation of the meatus urinarius.

Compare: Podo, Merc., Can sat. *(Blackwood)*

663. *Zincum Aceticum*

Brain feels sore and as if sprinkled with salt - Throat seems too tight and tongue too short - Zinc in Acetic Acid 5 drop doses 3 times a day in water for nurses and others who were compelled to work on an insufficient amount of sleep and also for erysipelas of old people. *(JHC)*

664. *Zincum Brom*

Hale has used it on its double indications for teething children who suffer intensely from pain in nerves of head and face, pains which throw the children into a state of stupor alternating with wakefulness. He used the 3rd and 6th potency. *(JHC)*

665. *Zincum Cyanatum*

The nervous and mental symptoms of Zn. with great intensity - used in convulsions and paralytic conditions in which Zn is indicated. *(JHC)*

This remedy is employed in infantile eclampsia, in meningitis, chorea, paralysis agitans and in hysteria. *(Blackwood)*

666. Zincum Iodatum

Splinter like pain in throat. A cough from tickling in the throat and the more he coughed the worse tickling became. *(JHC)*

667. Zincum Met

(Zinc)

The provings picture cerebral depression. The word fag covers a large part of Zinc action. Tissues are worn out faster, than they are repaired. Poisoning from Suppressed eruptions or discharges. The nervous symptoms are of most importance. Defective vitality, impending brain paralysis. Period of depression in disease. Spinal affections. Twitchings, pain as if between skin and flesh. Great relief from discharges. Chorea from fright or suppressed eruption. Convulsions with pale face and no heat. Marked anemia with profound prostration. It causes a decrease in the number and destruction of red blood corpuscles. Repercussed eruptive diseases. In chronic diseases with brain and spinal symptoms, trembling, convulsive twitching and fidgety feet are guiding symptoms.

Mind: Weak memory, very sensitive to noise - averse to work, to talk, child repeats everything said to it, fears arrest on account of supposed crime, melancholia, lethargic, stupid, paresis.

Head: Headache from the smallest quantity of wine, hydrocephalus, rolls head from side to side, bores head into pillow. Occipital pain with weight on vertex, automatic motion of head and hands, brain fag, headaches of overtaxed school children. Forehead cool, base of brain hot, roaring in head starting in fright.

Eyes: Pterygium, smarting, lachrymation, itching. Itching and soreness of lids and inner angles. Ptosis, rolling of eyes, blurring of one half of vision, squinting, amaurosis, worse inner canthus.

Ears: Discharge of fetid pus.

Face: Pale lips and corners of mouth cracked. Restless and itching eruption on chin.

Mouth: Teeth loose, gums bleed, gnashing of teeth, difficult dentition.

Stomach: Heart burn from sweet things, cannot stand smallest qunatity of wine - Ravenous hunger about 11 a.m. (Sulph), great greediness when eating, cannot eat fast enough, atonic dyspepsia.

Abdomen: Flatulent colic with retraction of abdomen, griping after eating.

Urine: Can only void urine when sitting bent backwards, hysterical retention, involuntary urination when walking.

Rectum: Hard small, constipated stool, cholera infantum, green mucus discharges. Sudden cessation of diarrhoea, followed by cerebral symptoms.

Male: Testicles swell, drawn up, drawing in testicles up to spermatic cord.

Female: Ovarian pain, especially left, can't keep still, nymphomania of lying in women, complaints all better during menstrual flow (Fupion, Lach), all the female symptoms are associated with restlessness, depression, coldness, spinal tenderness and restless feet.

Respiratory: Child grasps genitals during cough, dyspnoea better as soon as expectoration appears.

Back: Dull aching about the last dorsal or first lumbar vertebra, worse sitting, burning along spine, nape of neck weary, from writing or any exertion.

Extremities: Trembling and twitching of various muscles, feet in continued motion, cannot keep still, large varicose veins on legs, soles of feet sensitive.

Sleep: Cries out during sleep, body jerks, wakes frightened, startled, nervous motion of feet, when asleep, loud screaming out at night in sleep without being aware of it. (Somnambulism)

Skin: Varicose veins, especially of lower extremities, formication of feet and legs as from bugs crawling over the skin, preventing sleep, itching of thighs and hollow of knees, retrocession of eruptions.

Fever: Frequent, febrile, shiverings down back, cold extremities, night sweat, profuse sweat on feet.

Mod: (worse) at menstrual period, from touch, between 5 to 7 p.m., after dinner, from wine (Better) while eating, discharges and appearance of eruptions. *Compare:* Amel: by secretions (Lach, Stan, Mosch.)

Dose: 2 - 6 Potency. *(Boericke)*

Zn. poisons the brain and nerve and it corresponds to nerve poisoning of various kinds. The word Fag covers a large part of Zn. action. It may be nerve or brain fag or it may be muscle fag. Fag means that tissues are worn out faster than they can be repaired. This leaves them poisoned by waste products. Zn. meets the effect of brain fag from overstudy, from night watching, fatigue. The common old school use of Zinc ointment to suppress eruptions and Zinc injections to suppress discharges. In homoeopathic attenuations Zn. can reverse this process. Some of the key notes: incessant and violent fidgety feeling in feet or lower limbs, must move them constantly, cannot keep them quiet. These movements may continue even during sleep. Too weak to develop exanthemata or menstrual function, to expectorate, to urinate, to understand, to remember - relief to all suffering as soon as menses begin to flow, or as soon as other excretory functions are restored - Zn. cannot bear any covering during the sweat - Suppression of foot sweat - Zn. has a strong action on the generative sphere - it excites both sexes and causes seminal losses and prostatorrhoea of male associated with varicosis or pruritis of the external genitals - the patient is continually pressing on the pubes or applying the hand to the genitals. Numbness, tingling, formication and fainting spells are other nervous effects of Zn. Hasty eating and hasty drinking - intolerence of wine aggravates all symptoms - Aversions - meat, sweets, cooked or warm food - children cross in the evening - child repeats every thing said to it - Grits teeth as in worm cases - teeth fail to develop. The fidgety feet of Zn are not the only automatic movements of the remedy, though the most characteristic - automatic movements of mouth, arms and hands and general restlessness - Zn. has blueness of surface - the tip of nose easily frost bitten. Hands and feet painful, eruptions, cracks. Lowered state of vitality - As if scalp were drawn together - as if eyes were drawn together by a cord - as if head would burst - as if scalp wrinkled up and kept tightening - Zn. calls - fevers with inflammation of brain meninges.

Compare: Puts hands to genitals - Stramon - Fidgety feet - Trn, Twitching and jerking of single muscles - Agar, Ign., Unconquerable sleepiness - Nux, Op., Causation : Anger, fright, Night watching, suppressions, eruptions, otorrhoea, menses, lochia, millk. *(JHC)*

SYNOPSIS: Persons suffering from cerebral and nervous exhaustion, defective vitality, brain or nerve power wanting, too weak to develop exanthemata, or menstrual function, to urinate to expectorate, to comprehend, to memorise.

Incessant and violent fidgety feeling in feet or lower extremities, must move them constantly.

Always feels better every way as soon as the menses begin to flow, it relieves all her sufferings, but they return again, soon after the flow ceases.

In the cerebral affections, in impending paralysis of brain, where the 'Vis Medicatrix Naturae' is too weak to develop exanthemata (Cup, Sulph, Tub.), symptoms of effusion into ventricles. Child cries out during sleep, whole body jerks during sleep, wakes frightened, starts, rolls the head from side to side, face alternately pale and red.

Convulsions during dentition, with pale face, no heat, except perhaps in occiput, no increase in temperature (Re. Bel) rolling the eyes, gnashing the teeth.

Automatic motions of hands and head or one hand and head.

Chorea from suppressed eruption, from fright.

Hunger, ravenous about 11-12 a.m. (Sul) great greediness when eating, cannot eat fast enough (incipient brain disease of children)

Excessive nervous moving of feet in bed for hours after retiring, even when sleep.

Feet sweaty and sore about toes, foetid, suppressed foot sweat, very nervous. Chilblain painful Agg: From rubbing.

Spinal affections, burning whole length of spine, backache Agg: from sitting, Amel: by walking about (Cobalt, Puls, Rhus).

Spinal irritation, great prostration of strength, cannot bear back touched (Chin. s, Taren, Ther.), can only void urine while sitting bent backwards.

Twitching and jerking of single muscles, weakness and trembling of extremities, of hands while writing, during menses.

During sweat cannot tolerate any coverings. Is followed well by Ign. But not by Nux. which disagrees.

Inimical: Cham and Nux. should not be used before or after. *(HCA)*

Other Keynote Symptoms: Fears of arrest on account of supposed crime - overtaxed school children - Aversions: Wine, Sweets, meat, cooked or warm food - over study, night watching, patient is continually pressing on the pubes or applying the hand to the genitals - as if head would burst - as if scalp wrinkled up and kept tightening.

668. *Zincum Mur*

Things had a putrid smell and taste which were not putrid and faeces had no odour at all. Quinine had no bitter taste and acids and alkalies had no acid or alkaline taste. Insipid things were most relished - no natural appetite, but a morbid craving for something to allay the irritation at the stomach - emaciation *(JHC)*

669. *Zincum Oxy*

Undulating movements in some muscles - Constant impulse to laugh - Farrington says - Zn. is very like Con. in hypochondriasis and melancholy from masturbation. *(JHC)*

670. *Zincum Phos*

Brain fag in buisnessmen - Zn. Ph. 6X has cured irritable kidney with loss of memory in an old man.

Zinc phos. - Herpes Zoster (in 1X).
(Boericke)

671. *Zincum Sulph*

The use of Zn. s. in solution as an eye lotion is founded on a specific relationship and in homoeopathic attenuations, it has cured corneal opacities. Zn. s. has cured many cases of dysentery - burning acute pain in head - immediately sensation as if a strong electric shock passed through head, he expected his brains would have burst through his skull - Irresistable desire to laugh. *(JHC)*

Zinc. sulph not repeated frequently (high potency) will clear up opacities of the cornea. (Mc - Farland) *(Boericke)*

672. *Zincum Valerianum*

(Valerinate of Zinc)

A remedy for neuralgia, hysteria, angina pectoris and other painful affections, notably in ovarian affections. Epilepsy without aura. Hysterical heart pain. Facial neuralgia, violent in left temple and inferior maxillary. Sleeplessness in children, obstinate hiccough.

Head: Intermittent headache, becomes almost insane with pain which is piercing and stabbing. Uncontrollable sleeplessness from pain in head with melancholy.

Female: Ovaralgia, pain shoot down limbs even to foot.

Extremities: Severe pain in neck and spine, cannot sit still, must keep legs in constant motion, sciatic neuralgia.

Dose: 1st and 2nd Trituration - must be continued for some time in treatment of neuralgia. *(Boericke)*

Anti-hysteric medicine - brought out a strong action on the genital sphere, the usual starting point of hysteria. The abdominal symptoms woke him from sleep and he had to rise at 6.30 a.m. to stool which was partly foecal and partly fluid - Patients having piles, who were taking Zn. V. for other troubles had their piles relieved by the remedy - Hale mentions angina pectoris as having been cured by Zn. v. Other conditions are - prosopalgia, spinal neuralgia, sciatica, ovarian neuralgia, cerebro - spinal meningitis and tubercular meningitis - Zn. V. is indicated in hysteria with fidgety feet, groundless fears, epilepsy without aura. *(JHC)*

Neuralgic headache - the pain is so intense, piercing and stabbling that she becomes insane, screams and pulls her hair - insomnia, when there is pain in the head particularly in children. They wake frequently at night - facial neuralgia, sciatic neuralgia, the pains shoot down the limbs to the feet. *(Blackwood)*

673. *Zingiber (Ginger)*

(Mother Tr. of dried root). (Malayalam - Chukku)

States of debility in the digestive tract and sexual system and respiratory troubles, call for this remedy, complete cessation of function in kidneys.

Head: Hemicrania - pain over eyebrows.

Stomach: Taste of food remains long especially of bread and toast. Feels heavy like a stone - Complaints from eating melons and drinking impure water. Acidity (Calc, Robinia).

Abdomen: Colic, diarrhoea, extremely loose bowels - chronic intestinal catarrh - haemorrhoids, hot painful, sore.

Urinary: Frequent desire to urinate, stinging burning in orifice.

Male: Itching of prepuce - sexual desire excited, painful erections, emissions.

Respiratory: Hoarseness, smarting below larynx. Asthma without anxiety worse toward morning, scratching sensation in throat - cough dry hacking, copious morning sputa.

Extremities: Very weak in all joints, back lame, cramps in soles and palm.

Dose: 1st to 6th Potency. *(Boericke)*

The genito urinary and respiratory symptoms are strongly marked - Farrington says, Ginger is not a safe food to give in kidney affections as, it has caused Bright disease. Prolonged retention of urine or complete cessation of the function of the kidneys is an indication of Zing. Farrington gives this indication. Asthma of gastric origin, attacks comes in the night towards morning - patient must sit up to breathe but despite the severity of the paroxysm there is no anxiety - Zing. has a specific action on the digestive organs, causing flatulence and other symptoms of indigestion - Zing. has Agg: from eating melons. It causes diarrhoea. Causation: Melons, Bread. *(JHC)*

* * *

THERAPEUTIC INDEX

Any attempt to select the proper homoeopathic remedy for any case except by the study of the totality of symptoms must prove futile. In order to prescribe homoeopathically, the essentials for so doing must be observed,—i. *e, to let the characteristic symptoms of the individual patient, largely independent of the pathological nature of the case, be paramount in selecting the remedy.*

Such characteristics are found especially

(1) In the location or part affected;

(2) In the sensations;

(3) In the modalities.

The study of the repertory alone will give the indicated remedy. But throughout this work there are numerous suggestions for remedies based on clinical observations or deductions from partial provings, all of which may prove most valuable additions to our Materia Medica if further verified at the bedside. As many of them have no place as yet in our published repertories, I have thought it advisable to give them a place with others in this therapeutic index, in order to bring them to the attention and further study of the physician. At best, a clinical index is but suggestive.

Abortion, threatened.—Caulophyl; Viburnum.

Abscess.—Bellad.; Merc.; *Hepar;* Silica; Ananther.

Acidity.—Calc.; *Robin.;* Sulph. ac.; Nux.v.

Acne.—Kal. br.; Cimicif.; *Berb. a;* Led.; Hydrocot.; Ant. c.; Kali br.

—Rosacca.—Oophor; Kreos.; Sulph.; Carb. an.; Rad. met.

Acromegaly.—Thyr.; Chrysar.

Actinomycosis.—Nit. ac.; Hippoz.; Hecla.

Addison's disease.—Adren; Ars.; Phos.; Calc. ar.

Adenitis.—Bellad.; Merc.; Cist.; Iod.

Adenoids.— Agra; Calc. i.

Adiposity:—Phyt; Fuc.

Adynamia.—Ph. ac.; Chin.

After-pains.—Caulophyl; Mag. p.

Agalactia.—Lact. v; Agn; Urt-u.

Ague.—Nat. m.; Chin; Cedr.

Albuminuria.—Ars.; Kalm; Merc. c.

Alcoholism.—Querc; Aven; Caps; Nux. v.

Alopecia.—Fl. ac.; Pix.

Amenorrhoea.—Puls.; Graph.; Nat. m.

Anasarca.—Oxyd; Elat; Liat.

Anaemia.—Fer. cit.; Chin.; Nat. m.; Calc. p.

— **Pernicious.**—Ars.; TNT.

Aneurysm.—Bar. c.; Lyc.

Angina pectoris.—Lat. m; Cact; Glon.; Bry; Haematox; Ox. ac.; Spig.

Angioma.—Abrot.

Ankylostomiasis.—Card m.

Anorexia.—Nux. v; *Hydr.; China.*

Anthrax.—*Echi.*

Aortitis.—*Aur. ar.*

Antrum.—Hep.; Nit. ac.; Kali. bi.; Euph.; Amyg.

Aphasia.—Bothrops; Stram.; Kali. br.

Aphonia.—Alumn; Arg-m.; Nit. ac.; Caust.; Ox. ac.; Spong; Aur.

Aphthae.—Aeth.; *Borx; Merc.;* Nit. ac.; Kali. m.; Hydr. mur.

Apoplexy.—Op.; Phos.; Arn; Bell.

Appendicitis.—Echi.; Bellad.; Lach.; Iris t.
Arterial tension lowered.—Gels.
Arterial tension raised.—Verat. v.; Visc.
Arteriosclerosis.—Am. i.; Plb. i.; Polyg. a.; Bar. c; Glon 2x; Aur; Card. m; Sumbul.
Arthritis.—Arb.; Sulph.; Bry.; Elat.
Ascarides.—Abrot.; Sabad.; Cina; Spig.
Ascites.—Acet. ac.; Apoc.; Hell.; Apis; Ars.; *Dig.*
Asthenopia.—Nat. m.; Ruta; Croc.; Seneg.
Asthma.—Ip.; Ars.; Eucal; *Adren;* Nat. s.
— **Cardiac**.—Conv.; Iber; Ars. i.
Astigmatism (myopic).—Lil. t.
Atrophy.—Ol. j; Iod; Ars.
Auricular Fibrillation.—Dig.; Quin.
Auto-intoxication.—Skat; Indol.; Sulph.
Azoturia.—Caust.; Senn.
Backache.—Ox. ac.; Aesc.; Rhus t; Puls.; Kali. c.; Cimicif.; Nux. v; Ant. t.; Vario.
Balanitis.—Merc.
Barber's Itch.—Sul- i.; Thuj.
Bed-sores.—Fl. ac.; Arn.; Sul. ac.
Bell's Paralysis.—Am. ph.; *Caust;* Zinc. pic.
Beri Beri.—Elat.; Rhus t.; Ars.
Bilharziasis.—Ant. t.
Biliousness.—Yuc; Euon.; Bry.; Podo.; Merc.; Sulph.; Nux. v; Nyct; Chel.
Bladder (irritable).—*Eup. pur;* Cop.; Ferr.; Nux. v; Apis; Sars.
— **Haemorrhage**.—Amgd. p.; Ham.; *Nit. ac.*
Blepharitis.—Puls.; Graph.; Merc.
Blepharospasm.—Agar.; Phys.
Blood-pressure.—High—Bar. m.; Glon.; Aur; Visc.
Boils.—Bellis. p; Calc. pic.; Ferr. i.; Ol. myr.; *Bellad.;* Sil.; *Hep.;* Ichth.
Bone Affections.—Aur; Calc. p.; Fl. ac.; Ruta; Mez.; Silica; Symph.
Borborygmi.—Haematoxyl.
Bradycardia (slow pulse).—Abies n.; *Dig.;* Kalm.; Apoc.
Brain, Softening.—Salam; Phos.; Bar. c.
Brain-fag.—Anh; Zinc.; Phos.; Anac.; Sil.
Bright's Disease.—Ars.; Ph. ac.; Apis; Merc. c.; Ter.; Kali nit.; Nat. m.
Bromidrosis.—Silica; Calc.; But. ac.
Bronchitis.—Acon.; *Bry.;* Phos.; Ant. t; *Ferr. p.;* Sang.; Pilo.
— **(chronic)**—Amm-c.; Ars.; Seneg.; Sulph.; Ant. i.
Broncho-pneumonia—Kali bi.; Ant. t.; Tub.; Phos.; Squil.
Bronchorrhoea.—Amm-c.; Eucal.; *Bals. p;* Stann.; Bac.
Bulbar paralysis—Gua; Plb.; Botul.
Bubo.—Merc.; Nit. ac.; Carb. an.; Phyt.
Burns—Canth; Urt. u; Pic. ac.
Bursae.—Benz. ac.; Ruta; Sil.
Calculi (biliary).—Chin; Berb; Chel.
— **(renal)**—Berb; Pareir; Sars.
Cancer—(Bladder)—Tarax.
— **(Epithelial)**—Acet ac.
— **(Gastric)** —Ger.
— **(Rectal)**—Ruta; Hydr.; Kali. cy.
— **(Tongue.)**—Fuli.
Cancer.—Semp; *Ars.;* Hydr.; Ant. m.; Gali.
— **Mammae**.—Aster.; Con.; Plb. i.; Carc.
—**Pains**.—Euph.
Cancrum Oris.—Sec.; Kreos.; Ars.; Bapt.
Capillary Stasis.—Caps.; Echi.
Carbuncles.—*Anthraci.;* Led; Tarent. c.; *Ars.;* Lach.; Sil.
Cardiac Dropsy.—Adon; Dig.
Cardiac Dyspnoea.—Acon. f.; Aspidos.
Cardialgia.—Ferr-t.

Cardio-vascular spasm.—Act sp.
Caries.—Aur.; Asaf.; Sil.; Phos.
Car Sickness.—Cocc.
Caruncle, Urethral.—Thuj.
Catalepsy.—Cur.; Hydr. ac.; *Cann. i.*
Cataract.—Cine; *Phos.;* Platan; Quas.; *Naphtin.;* Calc. fl.
Catarrh (chronic).—Anemps; Nat. s.; *Aur.; Eucal.; Kali bi.;* Puls.; Sangin. n.; Nat. c.
Cellulitis.—Apis; Rhus t; Vesp.
Cerebro-spinal Meningitis.—Cic.; Zinc. cy.; Cupr. act.; Hell.
Chancre.—Merc. i. r.; Merc. i. f.; Merc.; Kali i.
Checked Discharges.—Cupr.; Psor.
Cheyne-Stokes Respiration.—Grin.; Morph.; Parth.
Chicken-pox.—Ant. t.; Rhus-t.; Kali m.
Chilblains.—Abrot.; *Agar.;* Tam; Plan.
Chloasma.—Sep.; Paul.
Chlorosis.—Ars.; Ferr.; Helon.; Cupr.; Puls.
Cholelithiasis.—Chion; Hydr.
Cholera.—Camph.; *Verat.;* Ars.; Cupr.
Cholera Infantum.—Aeth.; Cup; Calc. p.
Chordee.—Canth.; Sal. n; Yohim.; Lup.; Agav. a.
Chorea.—Absin.; Agar.; Hipp.; Mygal.; Tanac.; Tarent.; Ign.; Zinc.; Cimic.
Cicatrices.—Thios; Graph.
Ciliary Neuralgia.—Prun; Spig.; Sapo.; Cinnb.
Cirrhosis of Liver.—Nast.; Nat. chor.; *Merc.*
Climacteric Flushings.—Aml n.; *Lach.;* Sang.; Cimicif.; Sep.
Coccygodynia.—Caust.; Sil.
Cold Sores.—Camph; Dulc.
Colic.—Cham.; Mag. p.; Dios.; Plb.
Colic, Renal.—Eryn.; Pareir.
Colitis.—Merc. d.; Aloe; All s.
Collapse.—Camph.; Morph.; Verat.; Ars.
Color-blindness.—Ben.; Carbn. s.
Coma.—Op; Pilo.; Bell.
Comedones.—Abrot.; Aethi. a.; Bar c.
Condylomata.—Cinnb.; Nat. s.; Nit. ac.; *Thuj.*
Conjunctivitis.—Acon.; Puls.; Euphr.; Guar.
Constipation.—Op.; *Hydr.;* Iris; Verat.; Mag. m.; Nux v; Paraf.; Lac d.; Tan. ac.; Mag. p.; Sulph.; Alum; Verat.
— **(in children)**—Aesc.; Coll.; Bry.; Alum; Paraf.; Psor.
Convulsions.—Hydr. ac.; Cyst-l.; *Cupr.;* Cic.; *Bellad.;* Oean.
Corns.—Ant. c.; Graph.; Sil.
Coryza.—All c; Pen.; *Nat. m.; Quill; Gels.;* Euphr.; Acon.; Ars.; Kali ox.
Cough (dry). —Alum.; Bellad.; Hyos.; Laur.; Con.; Menth; Rumx; Spong.; Stict.
— **(laryngeal)**—Nit. ac.; Brom.; Caps.; Caust.; Lach.
— **(hoarse)**—Bry.; Hep.; Phos.; Samb.; Spong.; Verb.
— **(loose)**—Kali. s.; Ant t.; Ip.; Merc.; Puls.; Squil.; Stann.; Coc-c.
— **(phthisical)**—All. s.; Crot. h.; Phell.; Naja.
— **(nervous)**—Ambr.; Ign.; Hyos.; Kali br.
— **(spasmodic)**—Cor. r.; Dros; Meph.; Cupr.; Mag. p.; *Bell;* Ip.; Coc-c.
Cracked Lips.—Graph.; Nat. m.
Croup.—*Acon.; Hep.;* Alum.; Sil; *Spong.;* Brom.; Iod.; Kali bi.; Sang.
Cyanosis.—Ant. t.; Carb-v; Cupr; Lach.; Laur.; Op.
Cystitis.—Epig; Saur.; Pop.; *Canth.;* Chim.; Ter.
Cysts.—Iod.; Apis.
Dandruff.—Kali. s.; Ars.; Lyc.; Bad.

Day-blindness.—Both.

Deafness.—Calen.; Puls.; Hydr.; Graph.

Debility.—Chin.; Ph. ac.; Ars.; Cur; Kali p.; Alf.

—**(after gout)**—Cypr.

Delirium.—Bellad.; Hyos.; Agar.

Dentition.—Bellad.; *Calc. p.; Ter.; Cham.*

— **(drooling)**—Trif-p; Merc.

Diabetes.—Ars. br.; Coca; Cod; Hell.; Syzyg.; Phlor.; Uran. n.; Phos.; Aur.

Diaphragmitis.—Cact; Nux v.

Diarrhoea.—Camph.; *Verat.; Ip.; Chin;* Puls.; *Ph. ac.;* Merc.; Manz; Nat s.; Sulph.; Podo.

— **(chronic)**—Liat; Chap; Coto; Nat. s.; Sulph; Calc.

— **(teething)**—Arund.; *Cham.;* Calc. p.

Diphtheria.—Lach.; *Merc. cy.;* Merc. i. r.; Phyt.; Carb. ac.; Apis; Vinc; Nit. ac.; Echi.

— **(nasal)**—Am. caust.; *Kali. bi.*

Diplopia.—Bellad.; Gels.; Olnd.; Hyos.

Dipsomania.—Caps.

Dissecting Wounds.—Crot-h.; Ars.; Echi.

Dropsy.—Apis; *Apoc.;* Cain; *Samb. c.;* Oxyd.; Hell.; Dig.; Ars.

Dupuytren's Contraction.—Gels.; Thios.

Dysentery.—Ascl. t.; *Aloe;* Ip.; *Merc. c.;* Tromb.; Coloc.; Colch.; Ars.; Canth.

Dysmenorrhoea.—Apiol.; Puls.; Caul.; *Vib*urnum.; Mag. p.; Aquil.

— **(membranous)**—Calc. act.; Borx.

Dyspepsia.—*Nux-v.;* Hydr.; Graph.; Petr.; *Anac.;* Puls.; Lyc.; Hom.; Carb v.

Dyspepsia—(Acid.) —Rob.

— **(Atonic)**—Hydr.

— **(Fermentative)**—Sal. ac.

— **(Nervous)**—Ign; Anac.

Dysphagia.—Bellad.; Lach.; Merc.; Caj.; Cur.; Epil.

Dyspnoea.—Apis, Ars.; Ip.; Queb.; Spong.

Dysuria.—Tritic.; Fab.; *Canth.;* Apis; Sars.; Camph.; Bell.

Ear-ache.—Bellad.; Cham.; Verb.

Ear—(discharges)—Kali-m.

— **(very offensive)**—Elaps.

Ecchymosis.—Aeth; *Arn.;* Rhus t; Sul. ac.

Eczema.—Arb.; Clem.; Dulc.; *Rhus t.;* Sulph.; *Ars.;* Bov.; Nat. ar.; *Anac.;* Olnd.; Petr.; *Psor.*; Aln.; Graph.

Elephantiasis.—Elae; Ars.; Hydrocot.; Lyc.

Emphysema.—Am. c.; Ant. ar.; Lob.

Empyema.—Arn.

Enteritis (acute).—Chin.; Crot-t.; Podo.

— **(chronic)**—Ars.; Sulph.; Arg. n.

Enuresis.—Benz. ac.; Caust.; Sulph.; Rhus a.; Equis.; Lup.; Uran. n.; Physal; Bell.

Epididymitis.—Sabal; Puls.

Epilepsy.—Absin.; Art. v.; Sol. c.; Ferr. cy.; Cupr.; Hydr. ac.; Sil.; Calc. ar.; *Oenan.*

Epistaxis.—Ambro.; Nat. n.; *Arn.;* Ip.; Bry.; Ham.; Ferr. p.; *Nit. ac.;* Phos.

Epithelioma.—Abr.; Ars.; Thuj.; Chr ac.

Erotomania.—Orig.; Phos.; Pic. ac.; Stram.; Plat.

Erysipelas.—Ananther.; Bellad.; *Apis;* Canth.; Graph.; *Rhus t;* Verat. v.

Erythema.—Bellad.; Mez.; Antip.

—**nodosum**—Apis; Rhus t.

Eustachian Deafness.—Kali. s.; Rosa; Hydr.

Exophthalmic Goitre.—Lycps. v; Pilo.

Exostosis.—Hecla; Calc. f.

Exudative Pleurisy.—Abrot.

Eyes—(Inflamed).—Acon.; Euphr.; Ruta.

— **(Detachment of retina)**—Naphthal.

Fever.—*Acon.;* Agrosti. a; Spira; Gels.; Bapt.; Verat. v.; Ferr. p.

Fibroids.—Calc. i.

Fibroma.—Tril. p.; Ergot; Lap. a.

Fissures.—Led.; Graph.; Petr.

Fistula.—Fl. ac.; Nit. ac.; Sil.

Flatulence.—Carb. v.; *Asaf.; Nux m.;* Mosch.; Lyc.; Chin.; Carb. ac.; Caj.; Arg. n.

Framboesia.—Jatr.; Merc. n.

Freckles.—Bad.; Sep.

Galactorrhoea.—Salv.; Calc.

Gall-stones.—Chin.; Calc.; Berb.; Chion.; Cal. ren, (8-10x trit.)

Ganglion.—Ruta; Benz. ac.

Gangrene.—Euph.; Lach.; *Sec.;* Carb-v.

Gastralgia.—Bism.; Carb v.; Cocc.; Nux. v; Cup. ar.; Petr.; Phos.

—(recurring)—Graph.

Gastric Ulcer.—Ger.; Arg. n.; Ars.; *Atrop.;* Kal. bi.; Uran. n.

Gastritis.—Ars.; Nux v; Ox. ac.; Phos.; Hydr.

Gastro-enteritis.—Arg. n.; Ars.

Glanders.—Hippoz.; Merc.

Glands, Swollen.—Bellad.; Merc. i.; Phyt.; Kali ox.; Aln.

Gleet.—Thuj; Sep; Santal.; Puls.; Abies c.

Glossitis.—Laches.; Mur. ac.; Apis.

Globus hystericus.—Ign.; Asaf.

Gonorrhoea.—Cann. s.; Gels.; 0l. sant.; Tus. p; Petros.; Merc.

Gout.—Amm. be.; Lyc.; Urt. u.; Form.; Colch.; Led.; Lith.; Frax.

— **(Retrocedent)**—Caj.

Gravel.—Hydrang.; Solid; Lyc.; Berb.

Growing Pains.—Ph. ac.; Guaj; Calc. p.

Gumboil.—Bellad.; Merc.; Hecla; Phos.

Haematemesis.—Ip.; Ham.; Phos.; Mill.

Haematuria.—Canth.; Ham.; Ter.; Nit. ac.

Haemoglobinuria.—*Pic. ac.; Phos.*

Haemophilia.—Nat. sil.; Phos.

Haemoptysis.—Acal.; Ferr. p.; Ip.; Mill; Sec.; Erig.; Ger.; Hydrin. m.; All. s.

Haemorrhages.—Adren.; Hydrin-s.; Ip.; Chin.; Sabin; Ham; Mill.; Crot. h.; Tril.p.

— **(chronic sequelae)**—Stront. c.

Haemorrhoids.—Neg; Scroph n.; *Aloe; Mur. ac.; Ham.;* Fl. ac.; *Nux-v.;* Aesc., Coll.

Hallucinations.—Antip.; Stram.; Bell.

Halophagia.—Nit. sp. d.; Ars.; Phos.

Hay-fever.—Ambro.; Aral.; Cupr. act.; Naph.; Arund.; Rosa.; *Sabad.;* Lin; Phle.

Headaches.—**(anaemic)**—Chin.; Ferr. p.

— **(bursting)**— *Usn;* Glon.

— **(congestive)**—Acon.; Bellad.; Glon.; Lach.; Meli.; Gels.

— **(nervous)**—Cimicif.; Ign.; Coff.; Guar.; Cann. i.; Zinc.; Nicc. ol.

— **(sick)**—Iris; Sang.; Nux v.; Chion.

Heart Affections.—Acon.; *Cact.; Naja; Dig.; Crat.;* Lyc.; Spig.; Spong.; Adon.; Conv.; Phase.

Heartburn.—Ger.; Carb-v.

Heart Failure.—Stry. s., (1/60-1/30 gr.); Spartin s., (1/4 gr.); Agaricin, (l/10 gr.); hypodermically.

Hectic Fever. —Bapt.; Ars.; Chinin. ar.

Hemicrania.—Ol. an.; Onos.; Sep.; Stann.; Coff.

Hemiplegia.—Olnd.; Cocc.; Both.

Hemopia (vertical).—Titan.

Hepatitis.—Bry.; Merc.; Lach.; Nat. s.

Herpes—(Circinatus).—Sep.; Tell.

Herpes Labialis.—Caps.; Nat. m.; Rhus-t.

— **(preputialis)** —Hep.; Nit. ac.

— **(pudendi)**—Calad.; Nat. m.; Nit. ac.

— **Zoster.**—Carb.o.; Menth; Ran. b.; Rhus t.

Hiccough.—Gins; Rat.; Nux. v; Sul. ac.

Hoarseness.—Acon.; Bry.; Dros.: Carb v.; Phos.; Caust.

Hodgkin's Disease.—Ars. i.; Phos.; Iod.
Homesickness.—Caps.; Ign.
Hookworm.—Chen. a.; Thymol.
Housemaid's Knee.—Stict; Slag.
Hydrocephalus.—Hell.; Iodof; Zinc.
Hydrocele.—Rhod.; Graph.; Puls.
Hydrophobia.—Xanth; Anag; Canth.
Hydrothorax.—Lact. v; Ran. b.; Kali c.; Merc. sul.; Fl. ac.; Adon.
Hyperchlorhydria.—Chinin. ar.; Robin.; Orex; Arg. n.; *Atro.;* Anac.; Iris.
Hysteria.—Aqui.; Castm.; Mosch.; Ictod.; Plat.; Sumb.; Valer.; Ign.; Asaf.
Hysterical Joint.—Cot.
Ichthyosis.—Ars. i.; Syph.
Impetigo.—Ars.; Ant. t.; Mez.
Impotence.—Agn; Calad.; Onos.; *Ph. ac.;* Con.; Lyc.; Sel.; *Yohim.*
Indurations.—Carb. an.; Plb. i.; Alumn.
Inflammations.—Acon.; Bellad.; Ferr. p.; Sulph.
Influenza.—Ery. a.; Bapt.; Eucal.; Lob. c.; *Gels.; Rhus t;* Eup. per.; Bry; Ars.
Insomnia.—*Coff.;* Cypr.; Daph.i.; Ign.; Passi.; *Aqui.*
— **(delirium tremens)**—Sumb.
Intermittent Fever.—Helia.; *Chin.; Ars.;* Ip.; *Nat. m.;* Caps.; Tela.
Iritis.—Bellad.; Merc.; Clem.; Syph.; Dub.; Sarcol. ac.
Jaundice.—Chion.; Chol.; Bry.; Chin.; Myric.; Podo.; Merc.; Chel.; Kali pic.; Nat. p.
— (**infantile**)—Lup; Cham.
— **(toxic)**—Trinit.
Keloid.—Fl. ac.
Kidneys (congestive)—Bellad.; Ter.; Canth.
Lagophthalmus.—Phys.
Laryngitis (**acute**).—Acon.; Hep.; Spong.; Phos.; Caust. Arum. t.
Lectophobia.—Cann. s.
Leprosy.—Elae; Hydrocot.; Crot. h; Pyrar.
Leucocythaemia.—Ars.; Pic. ac.; Thuj.
Leucoderma.—*Ars. s. r.*
— —(**chronic**)—Dros.; Sel.; Mang.; Arg. m.
Leucorrhoea.—Alum.; Calc.; Hydr.; Sulph.; Puls.; Kreos.; Sep.; Hydr.; Eucal.; Thuj.
— **(in little girls)**—Calc.; Cub.; Hydr.; Asper.
Lithiasis.—Aspar.; Lyc.; Sep.
Liver (**congestion**).—Berb.; Bry.; Card. m.; Chel.; Lept.; *Merc.;* Mag. m.; Podo.; Sulph.
Liver-spots.—Nat. hyposulph.
Locomotor Ataxia.—Zinc. p.; Plb.; Arg. n.; Ox ac.; Chr. s.; *Arag.*
Lumbago.—Guaj.; Hyos.; *Rhus t;* Ant t.; Macro.; Phyt.; Kali ox.
Lungs, Congestion.—Acon.; Verat. v.; Ferr. p.
— **Oedema**.—Am. c.; Ant. t.; Ars.
Lupus.—Am. ar.; Ars.; Hydroc.; Thuj.
Lypothemia.—Ign; Nux m.
Malaria.—Alst; Am. pic.; Corn.
Malnutrition.—Alf; Calc. p.
Mania.—Bellad.; Hyos.; Stram.; Lach.
Marasmus.—Abrot.; Iod.; Nat. m.; Ars. i.
Mastitis.—Bellad.; Phyt.; Con.
Mastoid.—Caps.; Onos.; Hydr.
Measles.—Gels.; Puls.; Ferr. p.; Kali. m.
Megrim.—Menis.; Coff.; Sep.; Stann.
Meniere's Disease.—Carbn. s.; Chen. a.; Nat. sal.; Sal. ac.; Silica; Pilo. m.
Meningitis (**tubercular**).—Bac.; Cupr. cy.; Iodof.
Menorrhagia.—Chin.; Sabin; Croc.; Calc.; Plat.; Sed. ac; Tell; Sanguiso.
Menstruation.—(**cessation**)—Lach.; Puls.; Graph.; Sang.
— (**delayed**)—Puls.; Calc. p.; Caul.; Nat. m.

— (**painful**)—Bellad.; Viburnum.; Mag. p.

— (**profuse**)—Cham.; Ip.; Tril. p.; Bellad.; Sabin.

Metritis, Chronic.—Aur. m. n.; Mel. c. s.; Merc.

Milk-leg.—Bufo; Ars.; Puls.; Rhus t; Ham.

Miscarriage.—(**repeated**)—Syph.; Bac.

— (**threatened**)—Sabin; Viburnum.

Morning Sickness.—Amgd. p.; Nux v.; Ip.; Cuc. p.; Cocc.; Apom.; Alet.

Morphine Habit.—Aven.

Morvan's Disease.—Aur. m.; Thuj.

Mountain Sickness.—Coca.

Mumps.—Bellad.; Merc.; Pilo.; Rhus t.

Muscae Volitantes.—Caust.; Cypr.; Chin.

Mushroom Poisoning.—Absin.

Myalgia.—Acon.; Bry.; Macro.; Rhus t.

Myelitis.—Ars.; Plb.; Ox. ac.; Sec; Dulc.

Myocardial Degeneration after Influenza.—Nux v; Gels.

Myocarditis.—Dig.; Ars. i.; Aur. m.

Myositis.—Arn.; Mez.; Rhus t.

Myxoedema.—Thyr.

Naevus.—Fl. ac.; Thuj.

Nephritis.—Methyl.; Tub. k.; Berb.; Kali chl.; Canth.; Merc. c.; Phos.; Ter.; Apis; Eucal.

Nephrolithiasis.—Pareir; Senec.

Neuralgia.—Am. val.; *Acon.;* Bellad.; *Spig.;* Kalm.; *Ars.;* Coloc.; Phos.; Zinc. val.

— (**lumbo-abdominal**)—Aran.

— (**periodic**)—Nicc. s.; Ars.; Cedr.

—(**spermatic cord**)—Ol. an.; Ox. ac.; Clem.

Neurasthenia.—Anac.; *Zinc. pic.;* Stry. p.; Phys.

— (**gastric**)—Gent. l; Anac.

Neuritis.—Stann.; Plb.; Hyper.; Thal; Ars.

Nictalopia.—Bellad.; Hell.

Night-sweats.—Acet. ac.; Nat. tel.; Pop.; Agar; Picro.; Salv; Pilo.

Nipples, Ulcerated.—Cast. eq.; Eup. a.; Rat.

Nodosities of Joints.—Am. p.

Nymphomania.—Robin.; Canth.; Hyos.; Phos.; Murx.

Obesity.—Am. br.; Fuc; Calc.; Phyt.; Thyr.

Oedema.—Apis; Ars.; Dig.

— (**of lungs**)—Ant. t.

— (**pedum**)—Prun.

Oesophagus.—Caj.; Cund.; Bapt.

Onychia.—Silica; Psor.

Orchitis.—Puls.; Bellad.; Rhod.; Spong.; Aur.

Osteitis.—Conch.

Osteomalacia.—Ph. ac.

Otitis Media (chronic).—Chen. a.; Caps.; Bellad.; Merc.; Puls.; Calc.

Otorrhoea.—Kino; Merc.; *Calc.; Puls.;* Sulph.; Hydr.; Tell.

Ovaralgia.—Zinc. val.; Apis; Lach.

Ovarian Cyst.—Ov.; Kali. br.; Apis.

Ovaritis.—Apis; Lach; Plat; Coloc.; Sep; Xan.

Oxaluria.—Senn; Nit. m. ac.

Ozaena.—Alum.; Hippoz.; Aur.; Nit. ac.; Merc.; Hydr.; *Cadm. s;* Sulph.

Panaritium.—Am. c.; Fl. ac.; Sil.

Pancreatic Troubles.—*Iris.*

Paralysis Agitans.—Aur. s.; Hyosin. hbr.; Merc.

Paralysis.—(**post-diphtheritic**)—Gels.; Cocc.; Lach.; Aur. m.; Arg. n.

Paraplegia.—*Mang. o.;* Kali. t.; Lath.; Thal.; Hyper.; Anh.

Paresis.—Aesc. g.; Badiag.

— (**pneumo-gastric**)—Grin.

— (**respiratory**)—Lob. p.

— (**senile**)—Aur. i.; Phos.

— (**spinal**)—Irid

— (**typewriter's**)—Stann.

Pellagra.—Bov.

Pemphigus.—Calth; Manc.; Ran. s.

Pericarditis.—Ant-ar.; Ars.; Bry.; Colch.; Spig.; Dig.

Periostitis.—Asaf.; Aur.; Kali bi.; Merc,: Phos.; Mez.; Sil.; Apis.

Peritonitis.—Apis; Bellad.; Bry.; Coloc.; Merc. c.; Sin. n.; Sangin. n.; Wye.

Pharyngitis, follicular.—Aesc.; Hydr.; Sang.; Wye.

— **(sicca)**—Dub.

Phimosis.—Merc.; Guaiac.

Phlebitis.—Ham.; Puls.

Phthisis.—Acal.; Gall. ac.; Nat. cac.; Polyg. a.; Silph; Calc. ar.; Kreos.

— **(laryngeal)**—Dros.; Stann.; Sel.; Nat. sel.

Plague.—Ign; Oper.

Pleurisy.—Acon.; *Bry.;* Squil.; Asc. t.; Kali. c.

— —**(effusion stage)**—Apis; *Canth.;* Ars.; Sulph.

Pleurodynia.--Bry.; Cimicif.; Ran. b.

Plica Polonica.—Vinc.; Lyc.

Pneumonia.—Bry.; Phos.; Sang.; Iod.; Chel.; Lyc.; Pneu.

Poison-oak.—Anac.; Xero.; Grin.; Cypr.; Rhus-t.; Crot. t.; Graph.; Erech.

Poliomyelitis.—Lath; *Bung;* Kali p.

Polychrome Spectra.—Anh.

Polypi.—Phos.; Calc.; Sang.; Thuj.

— **(nasal)**—Lem. m; *Calc.; Teucr.*

Polyuria.—Arg. m.; *Ph. ac.;* Murx; Squil.; Uran-n; Rhus a.

Portal congestion.—Aesc. g.

Priapism.—Pic. ac.; Canth.

Proctitis.—Ant. c.; Coll.; Aloe; Podo.

Prosopalgia.—Cact; Verb.; Kalm; Puls.

Prostatic Hypertrophy.—Ferr. pic.; Thuj.

Prostatitis.—Merc. d.; Sabal.; Pic. ac.; *Thuj;* Tritic.; Staph.

Prurigo capitis.—Calc. m.

Pruritus.--Antip.; Carb. ac.; Dol.; Fago.; Sulph.; Rhus t; Pulx.; Rad. met.

Psilosis.—Frag.

Psoriasis.—Kali. ar.; Kali. br.; Thyr.; *Ars.;* Graph.; *Borx;* Sulph.; Emet. 1/2 gr.

Pterygium.—Zinc.; Rat.; Sulph.

Ptomaine Poisoning.—Ars.; Kreos.; Pyrog.

Ptyalism.--Merc.; Iris; Iod.; Trif.

Purpura.—Crot. h.; Phos.; Ars.; Ham.; Naja.

Pyaemia.—Ars. i.; Chinin. s.; Lach.; Pyrog.

Pyelitis.—Merc. c.; Hep.; Ter.; Cupr. ar.; Epig; Juni. v.

Pyorrhcea.—Emet.; Staph.; Plan.

Pyrosis.—Gall ac.; Bism.; Caps.

Rachitis.—Calc.; Iris; Phos.; Sil.

Ranula.—Thuj; Calc.; Fl. ac.

Raynaud's Disease.—Ars.; Sec; Cact. tincture.

Rectal pockets.—Poly. h.

Respiration (Cheyne-Stokes).—Antip.

Rheumatism.—Colch.; Prop.; Acon.; *Bry.;* Dulc.; Merc.; *Rhus-t.;* Cimic.

— **(chronic)**—Stel.; Ol. j.; *Sulph.;* Visc.

— **(gonorrhoeal)**—Irisin.; Sars.; Thuj.

Rhinitis (atrophic).—Lem. m.

Riggs' Disease.—Cal. ren.

Ringworm.—Sep; Tell.; Ars.; Bac.

Scarlatina.—Bellad.; Rhus t; Stram.

— **(malignant)**—Am. c.; Mur. ac.; Lach.; Ail.; Crot. h.; Bapt.; Nit. ac.

Sciatica.—Cot.; Visc; *Coloc.;* Rhus t; *Gnaph.*

Sclerosis, multiple.—Aur. m.

Sclerotic Degeneration.—Bar. m.; Plb.; Aur. m.

Scrofula.--Aethi. m; Ferr. i.; Cist; Merc.; Calc.; Sulph.; Ther.

Scurvy.—Acet. ac.; Agav. a; Phos.; Merc.

Seasickness.—Apom.; Petr.; *Cocc.;* Nux v; Tab.

Seborrhoea.—Hera.; Ars.; Graph.; Vinc; Nat m.

Senile Decay.—Ov.; Bar. c.

Sepsis.—Crot-h.; Bapt.; Echi.; Ars.; Lach.

Sleeping Sickness.—Nux m.; Op; Gels.; *Atox.*

Sleeplessness.—Tela.; *Coff.*; Ign.; Cimicif.; Gels; Op (high); Daph; Hyos. hydr.

Snake-poison Antidotes.—Euph. po.; Cedr.; Gymne.; Gua; Salag.

Somnambulism.—Kali p.; Kali br.

Spermatorrhoea.—Sal. n; Chin.; Ph. ac.; Staph.

Spleen Affections.—Cean.; Querc; Helia.; Nat. m.; Polym.

Sterility.—Agn; Nat. m.; Borx.

Stomach Dilatation.—Hydrin. m.

Stomatitis.—Borx; Arg. n.; Kali. m.; *Nit. ac.*

Subinvolution.—Frax.; Aur. m. n.; Epip.

Sycosis.—Aster; Thuj; Nat. s.; Aur. m.

Synovitis.—Apis; Bry.; Calc. f.

Syphilides.—Ars. s. f.; Kali. i.; Nit. ac.

Syphilis.—Calo; Cory.; Plat. m.; Merc.; Kali. ox.; Aur.

—(**latent**)—Ars. met.; Syph.

—(**nodes**)—Cory.; Still.; Kali. i.

Tachycardia.—*Abies n.;* Agn.

Tape-worm.—Fil; Cina; Ioduretted Pot. iod.

Tetanus.—Stry.; Upas; Passi.; Phys.

Thrombosis.—Both.; Lach.

Tinnitus.—Antip.; Cann. i.; Carbn. s.; Sal. ac.

Tobacco-craving.—Daph.

Tonsillitis.—Am. m.; Guaj.; Bar.act.; Bellad.; Merc.; Phyt.

Toothache.—Plan; Mag. c.; Bellad.; Cham.

Torticollis.—Lachn.

Traumatism.—Arn; Bell-p.

Trismus.—Lin.

Tuberculosis.—Ars. i.; Phell.; Tub.; Calc.

Tumors.—Calc. f.; Con; Bar m.; Thuj; Merc. i. r.; Hydr.; Phyt.; Plb. i.

Tympanitis.—Lyc.; Ter.; Asaf.; Erig.

Typhoid.—Bapt.; Mur. ac.; Ars.; Ph. ac.; Bry.

— (**diarrhoea**)—Epil.

Ulcers.—Nit. ac.; Sil.; Ars.; Como.; Kali. i.; Lach.; Paeon.; Calen.

Uraemia.—Am. c.; Cupr. ar.; *Morph.*

Urethral Caruncle.—Cann. s.; *Eucal.*

Urethritis.—Acon.; Apis; *Canth.*

— (**in children**)—Dory.

Uric Acid Diathesis.—Hed.; Oci.

Urticaria.—Ant. c.; Antip.; Apis; Astac.; Bomb.; Cop.; Frag.; Nat. m.

Uterine Displacement.—Abies c.; Eup; Helio.; Sep.; Puls.; Frax.; Ferr. i.

— (**Induration**)—Aur. m.; Kalm.

— (**tumors**)—*Aur. m. n.*

Vaginismus.—Cact.; Plb.; Bell.

Varicose Veins.—Calc. f.; Ham.; Puls.

Variola.—Ant. t.; Sarr.

— (**haemorrhage**)—Crot. h.; Phos.; Ars.

Vascular Tension.—Acon.; Bellad.; Verat. v.

— (**with arterial lesion**)—Adren.; Bar. m.; Tab.; Plb.

— (**rapid reducers**)—Glon.; Aml. ns.; Nat. n.; Trinit.

Vertigo.—Gels.; *Gran.;* Phos.; Cocc.; Con.

Venous Stasis.—*Aesc.*

Warts.—Ant. c.; Caust.; Nit. ac.; *Thuj;* Sal. ac.

Wens.—Thuj; Benz. ac.; Bac.

Whooping-cough.—Castn. v.; *Dros.;* Cupr.; Mag. p.; Pert.

Worms.—Calc.; Cina; Santin.; Spig.; Teucr.; Naph.

Wrist Rheumatism.—Act sp.; Viol. od.

Writers' Cramp.—Arg. m.; Sul. ac.

Weil's Disease.—Chel.; Phos.

Yellow Fever.—Cadm. s; Ars.; Crot. h

(Boericke)

* * *